Assistive technology assessment
handbook

INCLUDES CD

ATE DUE

Assistive Technology Assessment Handbook

REHABILITATION SCIENCE IN PRACTICE SERIES

Series Editors

Marcia J. Scherer, Ph.D.

President
Institute for Matching Person and Technology

Professor
Orthopaedics and Rehabilitation
University of Rochester Medical Center

Dave Muller, Ph.D.

Executive
Suffolk New College

Editor-in-Chief
Disability and Rehabilitation

Founding Editor
Aphasiology

Published Titles

Assistive Technology Assessment Handbook,
edited by Stefano Federici and Marcia J. Scherer

Paediatric Rehabilitation Engineering: From Disability to Possibility,
edited by Tom Chau and Jillian Fairley

Forthcoming Titles

Ambient Assisted Living, *edited by Nuno M. Garcia, Joel Jose P. C. Rodrigues,*
Dirk Christian Elias, Miguel Sales Dias

Assistive Technology for the Visually Impaired/Blind,
Roberto Manduchi and Sri Kurniawan

Computer Systems Experiences of Users with and without Disabilities:
An Evaluation Guide for Professionals,
Simone Borsci, Masaaki Kurosu, Stefano Federici, Maria Laura Mele

Multiple Sclerosis Rehabilitation: From Impairment to Participation,
edited by Marcia Finlayson

Neuroprosthetics: Principles and Applications, *Justin C. Sanchez*

Rehabilitation Goal Setting: Theory, Practice and Evidence,
edited by Richard Siegert and William Levack

Quality of Life Technology, *Richard Schultz*

Assistive Technology Assessment Handbook

Edited by
Stefano Federici and Marcia J. Scherer

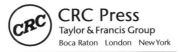

CRC Press
Taylor & Francis Group
Boca Raton London New York

CRC Press is an imprint of the
Taylor & Francis Group, an **informa** business

CRC Press
Taylor & Francis Group
6000 Broken Sound Parkway NW, Suite 300
Boca Raton, FL 33487-2742

Printed in the United States of America on acid-free paper
Version Date: 20120117

International Standard Book Number: 978-1-4398-3865-5 (Hardback)

Library of Congress Cataloging-in-Publication Data

Assistive technology assessment handbook / editor[s], Stefano Federici, Marcia Scherer.
    p. ; cm. -- (Rehabilitation science in practice series)
    Includes bibliographical references and index.
    ISBN 978-1-4398-3865-5 (hardback : alk. paper)
    I. Federici, Stefano. II. Scherer, Marcia J. (Marcia Joslyn), 1948- III. Series: Rehabilitation science in practice series.
    [DNLM: 1. Self-Help Devices. 2. Technology Assessment, Biomedical. 3. Disabled Persons--rehabilitation. WB 320]

617'.033--dc23   2012000644

Visit the Taylor & Francis Web site at
http://www.taylorandfrancis.com

and the CRC Press Web site at
http://www.crcpress.com

This book is dedicated to the psychotechnologists of today and the

future, regardless of the country in which they work.

Contents

Section III   Assistive Technology Devices and Services
S. Federici and M. J. Scherer

Foreword

Global Perspectives and Emerging Themes in Assistive Technology Assessment

I am delighted and privileged to be asked by the eminent editors of this text, Stefano Federici and Marcia J. Scherer, to write a foreword. These colleagues are at the forefront of work within the field of assistive technology and have pioneered much of the current thinking resulting in both the delivery of services to individuals and transformational research. The emergence and importance of this field can be demonstrated through the emergence of *Disability and Rehabilitation: Assistive Technology* as a standalone journal affiliated with *Disability and Rehabilitation*. This journal, which embraces the broad field of assistive technology, is edited by Marcia J. Scherer, ably assisted by Stefano Federici as an editorial board member.

These two journals, like this book, are characterized by their international coverage, multiprofessional publications, and interprofessional research of the highest quality. This edited volume includes contributions from five continents and reinforces the global approach to responding to the needs of individuals and in some cases communities requiring support and intervention.

This is no easy challenge, and the need remains to recognize both the integrity of those contributing disciplines and individuals along with the emerging integrative approach to rehabilitation.

What this text does is set a framework for future practice and research within the field of assistive technology assessment. It is clearly structured into three sections, the first of which sets the context, the second brings together perspectives from those professions working in the field, and the third focuses on assistive technology devices themselves and the positive outcomes that can emerge. Each section of this book has a separate introduction, and these contributions themselves are not only informative but reflect the vision of the editors for this field of work.

Having been asked to write this introduction, it was with pleasure that I was able to read the chapters prior to their publication, and rather than repeating or simply reiterating what can readily be assimilated, I found myself reflecting on some of the emerging cross-cutting themes. Although not comprehensive, the four themes that stood out for me characterize the need to develop innovative approaches within this field while recognizing the individuality of both the user and those professionals engaged.

In many ways the topic all of the authors are addressing and the field of enquiry is relatively straightforward. The advances in technology and the potential benefits that can accrue highlight the need to undertake purposeful and sophisticated forms of assessment of individuals to understand their need and how they can benefit from the wide range of available devices. These individuals themselves in different ways are looking for better outcomes in response to their disabilities and broadly through the rehabilitative process to improve in some way or other their quality of life. Therefore, assessment is the first stage of this process and facilitates an evaluation of the effectiveness of the intervention that must be undertaken on a regular basis. What then emerges from my initial reading of these outstanding chapters from individuals working in this field?

Assistive Technology Is Increasingly Complex and Sophisticated, Which Needs to Be Reflected in the Assessment Process

Although this actually states the obvious, it still provides one of the greatest challenges in undertaking the assessment of individuals to determine how best to deploy technology. Chapters 16, 17, and 18 highlight the sophistication emerging within the fields of technology and the potential benefits to individuals.

Nevertheless, the more complex both the assessment process and the technological aids themselves become, there is a danger that they become less accessible, and a number of authors throughout this text remind us through their work of "abandonment," with one of the greatest problems being that individuals stop using the devices. Furthermore, the more complex the assessment process, the less motivated individuals can become given their need and their understandable desire to have access to available facilities and support. And not only is the complexity difficult for the user and those professionals undertaking the assessments, but there remains the danger that they become more costly and hence have lower impact.

Indeed, the process of assessment itself is costly given the number of professionals who potentially need to be engaged, and there is an "opportunity cost" issue here in terms of direct therapeutic intervention as compared with careful assessment and planning. Therefore, one of our conundrums is that the more complex and greater technological advances we make, there remains a potential threat of the extent to which these can be applied in practice, which in turn affects the vulnerability of those with disabilities.

The Need for Inter- and Multidisciplinary Approaches to Assessment

For me, this is then the second major issue. It is clear from this text that the assessment process is critical to future success, but that it involves a wide range of disciplines and in some cases the emergence of new interdisciplinary approaches. For example, Chapter 9 introduces for the first time to myself the role of the "psychotechnologist." I am sure there are other integrated professional approaches yet to be brought together. As knowledge within the professional fields involved with assistive technology becomes more sophisticated and our knowledge simply grows exponentially, the capacity to introduce shared professional education and training becomes increasingly difficult.

Furthermore, we do need to recognize and indeed value the different perspectives offered by the vast range of individuals working within this field through their initial education, training, and postgraduate study. There are different paradigms ranging from those working primarily in the field from a medical perspective, through to those in focused but relatively multidisciplinary professions, and on to those making such enormous contributions through their technological rather than social skills.

No one person or profession can any longer cover this breadth, and we therefore need to find new ways of working together.

Fortunately, it is not the case that people cannot do this, but it is a time-consuming, resource-intensive process, and the outputs as prioritized and measured need to demonstrate the effectiveness of such an approach.

I know that myself and Marcia J. Scherer are proud to be editing journals that encourage multidisciplinary approaches and perspectives on different aspects of rehabilitation and work hard to include contributions from diverse cultures and backgrounds. In reflecting upon these issues, we should not forget the range of professionals not included in this text, particularly those working in the field of employment, advocacy, insurance, and related business professions. There is nothing negative about recognizing the changing roles of professionals, but the challenge remains to help all of us take different perspectives and to give away some aspects of our own understanding to work better with others.

The Impact of the Environment and the Context

Individuals and indeed communities both embrace and are constrained by the context in which they live. The assessment of an individual has to take this into account, and both place and context are integral to this process. In relatively structured rehabilitation, there are well-worked processes and procedures within which to undertake assessment and to draw upon the services and opportunities presented by the environment within which this is done. However, there are circumstances in which the assessment process is either limited through the resources that are available or by the requirement to respond at a pragmatic level. Community-based programs are often limited by personnel and resources and rely much more upon those living and working within that particular environment. Disasters such as those recently affecting Japan and Haiti require swift and emergency response mechanisms in which the assessment process might be less important when looking to provide assistive technologies to help support the vast numbers of individuals clearly in need. These issues are not confined to the environment or the context but to the interpersonal connections of the individual being assessed.

Chapter 5 highlights the impact on caregivers and the family, but we should add to this the wide range of individual contacts, including friends, peers, and those in the workplace.

This also affects the social context and influences those outputs by which the effectiveness of any intervention is judged, including economic well-being. Underpinning this in many cases is a commitment to enhance the quality of life, often through participation in the world of others with the view to retaining and playing a respected role within wider society.

What the User Wants and How Can It Be Measured?

The importance of participation and enhancing the quality of life as much as alleviating some aspects of disability was referred to in the previous section. In many cases these measures are more important to the individual and more greatly affect the way in which the success of having access to assistive technology is measured. Chapter 15 is an excellent overview of the "user experience framework." Any perceived improvement through the use of assistive technology must be recognized and valued by the individual himself or herself for the impact to be measured effectively.

Many studies are published that do show improvement on a range of variables, and although these are important in demonstrating the efficacy of particular techniques without recourse to simply measuring the impact on the individual from his or her perspective, they do lack an element of validity.

This is not to say that publications of this kind should not be published; it just further reinforces the complexity of working in the field of rehabilitation. The more recent emphasis on goal-setting both jointly with professionals and individually is a positive way forward in terms of measuring impact. There is both a realism to goal-setting and the opportunity to be aspirational and to go beyond that which perhaps others think possible. The goal of employment is not unlikely to remain critical to many for reintegration into the life experienced prior to the disability. This might not always be possible, but without understanding the perspective of the user, the success or otherwise of intervention cannot fully be understood.

At the heart of undertaking an assessment of an individual for the use of assisted technology is where this person is starting from, where they want to go or believe they can get, aspirational thinking to take them further, and the journey itself. I judge that this book in the way it has brought together such a wide range of committed individuals has as its underpinning philosophy a commitment to listening to and responding positively to the voice of the individual participant. Resources are still given to rather than owned by those requiring them, and as in other changing areas such as education and social care there may yet be a further strengthening of the role of the user by providing resources from which they can choose or even purchase.

I found this book stimulating, and I am proud to have had an opportunity to contribute a few thoughts. Thank you to Marcia and Stefano for this opportunity to join you in contributing to this debate.

Dave J. Muller
Editor-in-Chief, Disability and Rehabilitation
Suffolk New College, United Kingdom

The collaboration between Marcia J. Scherer and the Centre for Technological Aid and Research Ausilioteca of the Leonarda Vaccari Institute in Rome was born when Marcia, accompanied with Stefano Federici, visited our institute. On that day, a warm empathy between me and Marcia was born. An interesting brainstorm about the various activities took off: activities that we could carry out together because we realized that we share the same visions. The activities of the Leonarda Vaccari Institute—with its multidisciplinary team—reflected the working methods for the Matching Person and Technology model carried out by Professor Scherer.

Almost a year later, I went to Rochester University to see Marcia again, and it was there that we managed to bring the drafting of the handbook to reality. The Ausilioteca di Roma (Centre for Technological Aid of Rome) put itself at the authors' disposal to verify the assistive technology assessment process model and the new competencies that had to be given to the new specific figure of the psycotechnologist.

The following are just a few words to understand what the Leonarda Vaccari Institute does and, in particular, what the Ausilioteca di Roma stands for. The Leonarda Vaccari Institute, the oldest nonprofit educational institution in Italy, addresses the special needs of children, adolescents, and adults with disabilities. Founded in 1936 by Professor Marchesa Leonarda Vaccari to help children affected with polio, today the institute provides comprehensive service to hundreds of individuals each year. The Leonarda Vaccari Institute is acknowledged as the Moral Entity with Royal Charter No. 2032 and public noncommercial initiative certified by the Region of Lazio; the institute functions under the National Health Service. Established 75 years ago, today the institution is one of the most experienced centers for the rehabilitation of people affected by severe mental and/or physical disabilities between the developmental stages of childhood and adulthood. On December 8, 2007, the President of Italy, Giorgio Napolitano, awarded the Leonarda Vaccari Institute with the Gold Medal of Merit for Public Health Service. In the same year, the center was included in the 2° "Eurispes survey" among the 100 Italian Centres of Excellence. The Vaccari Institute is certified with the ISO 9001-200 IMQ/CSQ 9211.LVA quality.

The intent to provide a comprehensive diagnosis and to help people with disabilities with their special needs have been one of the initiative's main concerns since its foundation. In accordance with the institute's 1936 Constitution, treatment extending to the various aspects of disability can be synthesised in three procedures: medical care, education, and integration into the labor market. Since then, the Leonarda Vaccari Institute has been expanding its activities throughout comprehensive and individualized interventions, bringing a multidisciplinary analysis to every single case. Each day, the Vaccari Institute provides support to more than 300 people who require re-education and rehabilitation care within the framework of full-time hospital care, day care, or outpatient services. The institute provides a large number of therapies such as kinesitherapy and logotherapy, alternative communication, psychosensory stimulation, respiratory exercises, drama, etc., all charged to the National Health Service. The diagnostic team is composed of experienced clinical and school psychologists, psychotechnologists, psychiatrists, neuropsychiatrists, neuropsychologists, pediatricians, orthopedists, rehabilitation therapists, and other professionals working in specific relative fields.

In 1996, the Vaccari Institute founded the Ausilioteca di Roma, a center for technological aid and research. The sector of technological devices is characterized by a fast evolution, by the complexities of solutions that need to be found, and by the necessity to personalize these solutions. This innovative vision leads to different procedures for the various rehabilitation, welfare, and educational processes. To find an international model of assistive technology assessment, the institute has therefore initiated a fruitful collaboration with Stefano Federici of the University of Perugia, Olivetti Belardinelli of the Sapienza University of Rome, and Marcia J. Scherer of the Institute for Matching Person and Technology of Webster, NY. The success of this assistive technology assessment process lies primarily in the selection and implementation of technical aids determined by

- The quality of the assignment's processes,
- The quality of assistive proposals, and
- The taking into account of the specific context of use.

The development of this sector finds its cultural motivations and improvement in the recent declaration of intents issued at the European level (e.g., Madrid 2002; *European Year for People with Disabilities* 2003), at the national level (e.g., *Guidelines for the Rehabilitation* released by the Ministry of Health in 1998), and at the international level [e.g., the International Classification of Functioning, Disability, and Health (ICF), promoted by the World Health Organization].

Digital devices are instruments of an extraordinary importance apt to satisfy the needs of autonomy and quality of life of people with disabilities and their families. They also guarantee a suitable proposal by adding value to the right solutions and giving a permanent help to health service professionals and users. Moreover, a good assistive technology match can also guarantee the efficiency of the public expenses in this sector.

The Ausilioteca is a highly specialized service center that operates together with the National Health Service, various public entities, and schools, sustaining different projects and the use of advanced technologies aimed to the best inclusion of people with disabilities in schools and other life environments.

The handbook, realized in collaboration with academic professionals from different countries (United States, Europe, Australia, Brazil, and Japan), contains a scientific pattern for the assignment of assistive technologies to people with disabilities founded under the ICF model. The fulfillment and achievement of the model described in the handbook—together with the highlighted procedures—are one of the best practices carried out by the highly specialized personnel of the Leonarda Vaccari Institute.

It is with satisfaction and gratitude that I thank the authors of the handbook and in particular the editors, Marcia J. Scherer of the Institute for Matching Person and Technology and Stefano Federici of the University of Perugia, for their useful and splendid work.

Saveria Dandini De Sylva
Executive President
Istituto Leonarda Vaccari

Preface

This book is the result of scientific collaboration and sincere friendship that was born in 2001 and has gradually strengthened over time.

The collaboration begins with the creation, at the Faculty of Psychology, Sapienza University of Rome, of the first course in psychotechnology that was held in Italy. This course aimed to combine multiple topics, bringing together technological and ergonomic arguments and issues concerning the psychology of rehabilitation to train competent psychologists within assistive technology provision.

The course was designed by Stefano Federici and held at the Sapienza University of Rome from 2001 to 2008. The term "psychotechnology," with the meaning adopted and introduced in the psychology of rehabilitation by Federici, initially sounded like a neologism. In fact, the objective of the course was to integrate technology and ergonomic aspects with those more specific of cognitive ergonomics, reread under the lens of the biopsychosocial model of disability, to train psychologists with both psychological and technological expertise and who were able to lead a user to meet their needs. Only in this way would it have been possible for the user to search and find a technological product that not only was satisfactory to his or her own person, but was also able to support him or her in the integration process within its milieu, by preventing, compensating, monitoring, relieving, or neutralizing disability and social barriers. Therefore, the psychotechnologist should possess those skills to be spent in centers for technical aid that, at the end of the last millennium, have begun to be characterized as autonomous centers of technology device assessment and assignment for an individual's disability and independent living.

The main theoretical difficulty in designing the psychotechnology course was to integrate technological-engineering models—not dissimilar in some way by certain models of cognitive functioning that tend to generalize and idealize the individual—with the biopsychosocial model of disability. The ergonomic approach to technology, both of cognitive and engineering types, indeed often tends to neglect the emotional, motivational, and social user experience so that it does not take into account those factors that very often affect it with a higher rate of incidence in the successful outcome in device use.

The discovery by Federici of the Matching Person and Technology model by Marcia J. Scherer was like the key to squaring the circle. It is a model that has combined people with disabilities' needs with assistive technologies in a user-centered context, without neglecting the functional and ergonomic features of the device. The answer to that fateful question was found, namely, that the psychotechnologist usually turned to him- or herself to find an effective integration of knowledge. As Federici was used to repeating in the psychotechnology course at the Sapienza University of Rome: "This course could also be called 'Matching Person and Technology from the psychologist's standpoint'."

The collaboration between the Sapienza University of Rome and the Institute for Matching Person and Technology has produced dozens of theses and several doctoral dissertations concerning the adaptation and validation of the Matching Person and Technology model and tools or related to the professional profile and role of the psychologist in the assistive technology assessment and assignment processes. Some of those researchers and students are now successful professionals in psychotechnology. Furthermore, many authors who took part in writing of the chapters of this book come from that experience of study and research.

However, the collaboration and friendship between Marcia and Stefano has not only led to the sharing of ideas and research projects, but they have also created a scientific network among Italian, American, and other nations' scholars who have formed the scientific community that has allowed such a large participation of authors in the writing of this work.

As the editors, let us now respond to the reasons for this book, which certainly was not intended to be a history of this social network or a biography of its editors. This book is a challenge for us: to develop an international ideal model of the assistive technology assessment process that gathers the most recent scientific developments in the assessment and provision of technical aids for an outcome that, if reached, would be a real success—the well-being of the disabled person. Therefore, this model intends to express in an idealized and essential form an assessment process performed in a center for technical aid because it provides such tools for the assessment and the professional profiles that we might also define as "psychotechnological."

Of course, just because we speak of "challenge," we reveal our awareness about the problems and limitations of an "international" ideal model. For example, one of the unsolved problems is the difficulty, already met several times, in defining the features of a center for technical aid. The modeling process of a center for technical aid is difficult if one takes into account the extraordinary variety of systems of regional and national health and social care, both public and private. This variety influences in different ways the specific characteristics that are required at a center. Furthermore, the different nature of the center for technical aid makes problematic the definition itself of the individual who addresses to it: user, patient, client, or consumer? The user (for convenience we use this definition, a little more generic than the others) of a center for technical aid could be a patient of a physician (physiatrist) who operates in a national system of health care and sends him or her to a specialized facility, the center for technical aid indeed, for a more thorough assessment of a particular device. This assessment can be provided free of charge if the center is part of a national health system or by paying out money if the center is part of a private health system. Furthermore, the product chosen by the user could be sold or assigned directly from the center for technical aid or, alternatively, the device provision may be made later by other providers, external and independent from the center for technical aid.

These are just some of the issues to be discussed by the authors of this book. In fact, other issues will be also addressed that are even more problematic from a scientific viewpoint. We refer to those that are intrinsically linked to the design of an international model. Because of the difficulty in finding an adequate and effective synthesis of the various models proposed by specific national systems of public health and welfare, the scientific community faces a modeling of assistive technology system delivery that will be increasingly individualized with respect to either the social and cultural diversity of users or to the necessary adjustment of the center for technical aid's functioning to the local health system. However, it should be noted that this particularization of the models clashes with some trends that are aimed at instead promoting their globalization (for example, this occurs both in social and health policies of the European Community and in those of the World Health Organization). The internationalization of a model is indeed advantageous because it often emerges as a synthesis of experiences and know-hows of regional models. Moreover, it offers the opportunity, by sharing the theoretical model and evaluation criteria, to share data essential to scientific research, planning, and evaluation of national and international policies and verify the quality of public services.

A goal that we set in the writing of this project was to narrow the topics, trying to legitimate the choice made. In fact, our intention was not only to provide a theoretical text that aims to develop an ideal model of assistive technology assessment processes, but also to provide an operational tool that is able to outline both the specific space of applicability of the model itself and the main characteristics of a center for technical aid's functioning, a tool-kit for a proper assessment, and profiles of professionals acting within the center. Moreover, it even seemed essential for us to compare our model with some of the most advanced researches in technologies for rehabilitation and supports for independent living. However, we were well aware that a detailed description of all matters regarding the functioning of a center for technical aid (i.e. assessment tools, professional profiles, the latest technology devices for rehabilitation and independent living) would have required an encyclopedia and not a manual such as this book. Therefore, and this could be read both as a limit and as well an advantage of this book, we have chosen, for each of the three areas mentioned—the tools of evaluation, the experts of the evaluation in a center for technical aid and new technologies—the aspects of the current state of the art that we judged as the most representative or innovative. So, we not only identified for each topic the leading experts and invited them to write about their topic, but also, where possible, we tried to ensure that each chapter was written by more hands, concerted and promoting cross-cultural viewpoints. For this reason, the reader should certainly not be surprised if he or she will not find mention some professions among those that could be treated in such a manual. We tried to give more prominence to the definition, training, and professional role of the new profession of psychotechnologist, as well as to highlighting the professional profile of the speech language pathologist because of the relevance of dysfunctions in language in today's international health and social policies.

Finally, we would like to stress that this book does not intend to model the assistive technology assessment process as a result of a mere academic mental exercise, but it has even faced an applied research of the model. This is for two main reasons: The theoretical view of the authors' chapters and editors emerge from experimental research applied to rehabilitation and assistive technologies. In addition, the international ideal model of the assistive technology assessment process is already applied in centers for technical aid. Thanks to scientific and clinical collaboration, economic and operational support of the Centre for Technical Aid of Rome, Leonarda Vaccari Institute—which, in turn, is part of the Italian Network of Centres Advice on Computer and Electronic Aids and cooperates with the Institute for Matching Person and Technology and Columbia University, with whom it shares the principles that underlie the assistive technology assessment process—it was possible to define the assessment model proposed in this book because the model is already operative in the Centre for Technical Aid of Rome. This center offers a noncommercial advisory and support on assistive technology and computers for communication, learning, and autonomy. The service is free of charge for users who access it through the Italian National Health Service. Several scientific projects granted by the institute are in progress at the center to verify not only the advantages of a systematic application of the Matching Person and Technology tools in the assessment process, but also the application of the assistive technology assessment process model. Some results will be presented and discussed in the chapters of this book.

Sincere thanks go to the authors of the chapters who have welcomed with enthusiasm our model, enriching in many parts the initial draft of this work and giving it a wide-ranging speech that is updated and credible. Special thanks also go to the publisher, Taylor & Francis, who accepted the project with competence, supporting the long process of drafting and revising the work. Again, special thanks go to many peer-reviewers of the chapters, who have played a generous and valuable role, such as guarantors for the scientific nature and validity of each contribution as well as representatives of the international scientific community in this area.

Contributors

M. Adya
Burton Blatt Institute
Syracuse University
Syracuse, New York

R. Amantis
Leonarda Vaccari Institute for
    Rehabilitation
Integration, and Inclusion of Persons with
    Disabilities
Rome, Italy

G. Basili
Department of Pediatrics
Senigallia General Hospital
Senigallia, Italy

N. Birbaumer
Institute of Medical Psychology and
    Behavioral Neurobiology
Eberhard-Karls University
Tübingen, Germany

and

IRCCS, San Camillo Scientific Hospital
    Institute
Venezia Lido, Italy

S. Borsci
Department of Human Science and
    Education
University of Perugia
Perugia, Italy

and

School of Information Systems, Computing
    and Mathematics
Brunel University
Uxbridge, United Kingdom

and

Mathematics for Match Plus Project Brunel
    University Uxbridge,
United Kingdom

L. W. Braga
Director, Neurosciences and
    Neurorehabilitation Division
SARAH Network of Neurorehabilitation
    Hospitals
Brasilia, Brazil

C. M. Capio
Institute of Human Performance
University of Hong Kong
Hong Kong, China

B. Cordella
Department of Dynamic and Clinical
    Psychology
Sapienza University of Rome
Rome, Italy

F. Corradi
Leonarda Vaccari Institute for
    Rehabilitation Integration,
    and Inclusion of Persons
    with Disabilities
Rome, Italy

V. Corsi
F.A.R.E—Specialist Centre for Dyslexia
    and Learning Difficulties
Perugia, Italy

G. Craddock
Centre for Excellence in Universal Design
Dublin, Ireland

I. L. de Camillis Gil
Neurological Rehabilitation Division
SARAH Network of Neurorehabilitation
    Hospitals
Brasilia, Brazil

D. de Jonge
Division of Occupational Therapy
School of Health and Rehabilitation
    Sciences
University of Queensland
Brisbane St. Lucia, Queensland, Australia

L. Demers
School of Rehabilitation
Université de Montréal
Montréal, Quebec, Canada

E. Di Giacomo
Department of Computer Engineering
University of Perugia
Perugia, Italy

A. Eldridge
Division of Occupational Therapy
School of Health and Rehabilitation
    Sciences
University of Queensland
Brisbane St. Lucia, Queensland, Australia

S. Federici
Department of Human Science and
    Education
University of Perugia
Perugia, Italy

and

CIRID - Interdisciplinary Centre for
    Integrated
Research on Disability
Sapienza University of Rome
Rome, Italy

A. Gossett Zakrajsek
Occupational Therapy Program
School of Health Sciences
Eastern Michigan University
Ypsilanti, Michigan

M. Grasso
Department of Dynamic and Clinical
    Psychology
Sapienza University of Rome
Rome, Italy

F. Greco
Department of Dynamic and Clinical
    Psychology
Sapienza University of Rome
Rome, Italy

K. Hill
Performance and Testing Teaching
    Laboratory
School of Health and Rehabilitation
    Sciences
University of Pittsburgh
Pittsburgh, Pennsylvania

M. Kurosu
Center of ICT and Distance Education
Open University of Japan
Chiba City, Japan

G. E. Lancioni
Department of Psychology
University of Bari
Bari, Italy

G. Liotta
Department of Computer Engineering
University of Perugia
Perugia, Italy

A. Lo Presti
CIRID
Interdisciplinary Centre for Integrated
Research on Disability
Sapienza University of Rome
Rome, Italy

R. Magni
Pragma Engineering Sr1
Perugia, Italy

G. Mascolo
External collaborator at the Department of
    Dynamic and Clinical Psychology
Sapienza University of Rome
Rome, Italy

C. Mazzeschi
Department of Human Science and
    Education
University of Perugia
Perugia, Italy

P. Mecocci
Institute of Gerontology and Geriatrics
University of Perugia
Perugia, Italy

M. L. Mele
ECoNA—Interuniversity Centre for
    Research on Cognitive Processing in
    Natural and Artificial Systems
Sapienza University of Rome
Rome, Italy

F. Meloni
CIRID
Interdisciplinary Centre for Integrated
    Research on Disability, and Department
    of Psychology
Sapienza University of Rome
    Rome, Italy

K. Miesenberger
Institute Integriert Studieren
University of Linz
Linz, Austria

M. Mirza
Institute for Healthcare Studies
Northwestern University
Chicago, Illinois

M. Morris
Burton Blatt Institute
Syracuse University
Syracuse, New York

B. W. Mortenson
School of Rehabilitation
Université de Montréal
Montréal, Quebec, Canada

M. Olivetti Belardinelli
Department of Psychology and CIRID
    Interdisciplinary Centre for Integrated
    Research on Disability
Sapienza University of Rome
Rome, Italy

and

ECoNA Interuniversity Center for
    Research in Cognitive Processing in
    Natural and Artificial Systems, and
    Department of Psychology
Sapienza University of Rome
Rome, Italy

D. Oliva
Lega F. D'Oro Research Center
Osimo, Italy

M. F. O'Reilly
Meadows Center for Preventing
    Educational Risk
University of Texas at Austin
Austin, Texas

M. Orlandi
Vision Research Center of Rome
Rome, Italy

E. Pasqualotto
Institute of Medical Psychology and
    Behavioral Neurobiology
Eberhard-Karls University
Tübingen, Germany

M. Pigliautile
Institute of Gerontology and Geriatrics
University of Perugia
Perugia, Italy

and

Department of Psychology
Sapienza University of Rome
Rome, Italy

K. S. Pinto
Pediatric Rehabilitation Division
SARAH Network of Neurorehabilitation
    Hospitals
Brasilia, Brazil

D. Samant
Burton Blatt Institute
Syracuse University
Syracuse, New York

M. J. Scherer
Institute for Matching Person &
    Technology, Inc.
Webster, New York

and

Burton Blatt Institute
Syracuse University
Syracuse, New York

P. S. Siebra Beraldo
Clinical Research Division
SARAH Network of Neurorehabilitation
    Hospitals
Brasilia, Brazil

J. Sigafoos
School of Psychology and Pedagogy
Victoria University of Wellington
Wellington, New Zealand

N. N. Singh
American Health and Wellness Institute
Verona, Virginia

C. H. P. Sit
Institute of Human Performance
University of Hong Kong
Hong Kong, China

and

Department of Sports Science and Physical
    Education
Chinese University of Hong Kong, China

A. Stella
Department of Comparative Cultures
University for Foreigners
Perugia, Italy

L. Tiberio
Institute for Cognitive Science and
    Technologies
National Research Council of Italy
Rome, Italy

B. Turella
Department of Psychology
Sapienza University of Rome
Rome, Italy

P. M. Wielandt
Department of Occupational Therapy
School of Health & Human Services
Central Queensland University
Rockhampton, Australia

S. Zapf
Children's Journey to Shine, Inc.
Houston, Texas

Section I

The Assistive Technology Assessment Model and Basic Definitions

S. Federici and M. J. Scherer

Introduction

As a part of the human condition, "Disability is complex, dynamic, multidimensional, and contested" (WHO and World Bank 2011, p. 3). The concept of disability conveys a very wide set of different and correlated issues: from disability models to individual functioning and its measurement, from social barriers to the digital divide, from the objective quality of life to subjective experience, to concepts of functioning, activity and participation, human rights and poverty, health and well-being, morbidity, and quality of life (WHO and World Bank 2011). Because of the multidimensionality of disability, the International Classification of Functioning, Disability, and Health (ICF) would like to make clear that disability (and its correlated term "functioning") must be understood as an umbrella term, "encompassing all body functions, activities and participation" (WHO 2001, p. 3).

Disability's multidimensionality and complexity entails a kind of "definitional paradox" (Madans and Altman 2006): On the one hand, any theoretical definition of disability implies aporia, and on the other hand, operational meaning is determined by the purpose of research. In fact, Mont explains:

> [If] each domain represents a different area of measurement and each category or element of classification within each domain represents a different area of operationalization of the broader domain concept, [then] to generate a meaningful general prevalence measure one must determine which component best reflects the information needed to address the purpose of the data collection. (2007, p. 4)

In other words, disability is a multidimensional construct because its measurement is multidimensional and it cannot be held to a "gold standard" valid for any context and for any purpose. The only appropriate measure is the one that best suits the purpose and the context to which it is addressed and not to the concept of disability in the abstract. Moreover, the variety of measurement tools and the flexibility to change the measurement procedures, adapting them to different people, contexts, and purposes, provide the most reliable scientific approach.

Madans and colleagues identify, at the aggregate level, three main classes of reasons for measuring (see Chapter 2). Here, "providing services" (2002, slide 11)—including the development of programs and policies for service provision and their evaluation—is the first among the three classes. More specifically, the assistive technology assessment (ATA) process can be viewed as one aspect of the first-mentioned class.

Assitive technology (AT)* plays a key and fundamental role in facilitating the social integration and participation of people with physical, sensory, communication, and cognitive disabilities. The process of matching AT and person requires a well-designed and well-researched sequential set of assessments administered by professionals with different areas of expertise: The success of the matching is strongly affected by the evaluation protocol/model and by the skills of the multidisciplinary team members. For this reason, the first section opens the present handbook, providing readers with useful guidelines to develop a set of functioning and disability screening tools for assessment in a center for technical aid. The authors of Sections I and II embrace the model proposed as follows.

The Assistive Technology Assessment Model

The introduction of AT into people's lives is a delicate and long-term process, which presupposes teamwork as much as professionalism, time, and experience. The aim of the ATA model is to suggest guidelines to follow to reach valid results during the AT selection and assignment process. The ATA process that has emerged is the result of the integration of

- The AT/aid assignment process, adopted by the aid center of an Italian rehabilitation institute, the "Leonarda Vaccari" Institute in Rome, a model shared through the years with other Italian AT/aid assignment centers, coordinated by the Rete Italiana dei Centri di Consulenza sugli Ausili Informatici ed Elettronici (GLIC; Italian network of advice centers on computer and electronic aids).

- The process, although it has some operating peculiarities, contains the steps common to the centers for technical aid within itself: access to the service stage, evaluative or planning stage, decision or choice stage, providing and customization stage, support and follow-up stage.

---

* We use assistive technology (AT), except where otherwise stated, as an umbrella term (WHO 2004), with the meaning more commonly attributed to the "Assistive Technology device" term, as stated by the *United States of America's Assistive Technology Act* (United States Congress 2004) and acknowledged by the World Health Organization in the recent *World Report on Disability* (WHO & World Bank 2011) as follows: "Any item, piece of equipment, or product system, whether acquired commercially, modified, or customized, that is used to increase, maintain, or improve functional capabilities of individuals with disabilities."

- The AT/aid assignment's processes were implemented by the Italian Public Health Service, in which there are two legal systems, a national and a regional (which decides itself how many local services must be established). The regional system decides the operating guidelines within which each local health service can define its own work processes. Over time, this system has led to a heterogeneity of processes, with similarities mainly deriving from the regional guidelines and from the national legal obligations (e.g., Federici and Borsci 2011): the initial request, the fitting (for some aids and prostheses and for some local services only), the supply, and heck on follow-up of use (for some aids and for some local services only).

- The assessment process, Matching Person and Technology (Scherer 1998; Scherer and Craddock 2002), containing the unique validated Assistive Technology Device Predisposition Assessment mentioned in the literature for matching the AT to the consumer, which allows one to assess the features of a person, environment, and technologies that interact when the AT assignment is considered.

The new model is the result of a decennial collaboration among the Sapienza University of Rome and the University of Perugia (Italy), the Institute for Matching Person and Technology of Webster (NY, United States), and the Leonarda Vaccari Institute in Rome (Italy). In that period various processes have been integrated within the biopsychosocial model of the ICF. The theoretical model created by these processes was shared with all of the authors of the guide (professionals and researchers studying AT/aids from many nationalities) that have been able to verify it and integrate it through the analysis of the processes existing in real life. The proposed model that is presented here is therefore the result of cross-cultural studies, both clinical and experimental, collected during this long-standing cooperation. This model, far from seeking to prefigure a "gold standard," instead sought to create a structure that allows one to build or to change the existing processes so that they can consider more variables, such as the nature of disability, personal motivation and enthusiasm of the person with a disability and family members, and social and political context and availability of human and financial resources within user-driven processes and in the context of the biopsychosocial model of the ICF.

The ATA Process Under the Lens of the ICF Biopsychosocial Model

The ICF (WHO 2001) and ICF-CY (WHO 2007) provide a unified standard framework for an ATA process in centers for technical aid, allowing them to seek the best match of user/client-assistive solution by means of a comprehensive set of clinical measures, functional analysis (see Chapter 3 and 4), and psycho-socio-environmental evaluations (see Chapter 5). The best assistive solution can be achieved only by taking into account the specific context of use, with the AT as a mediator of quality of life: In this way, the ATA process, whether from the perspective of the user/client or from the perspective of the center for technical aid, must be read under the ICF biopsychosocial model (Figure I.1). Both the user's perspective and the actions of the centre for technical aid are illustrated as follows:

A. User
   a. The user (request) seeks a solution for one or more ICF components: body functions and structures (health conditions), activities and participation, both with a context of personal and environmental factors.
   b. The user request triggers the user-driven process.

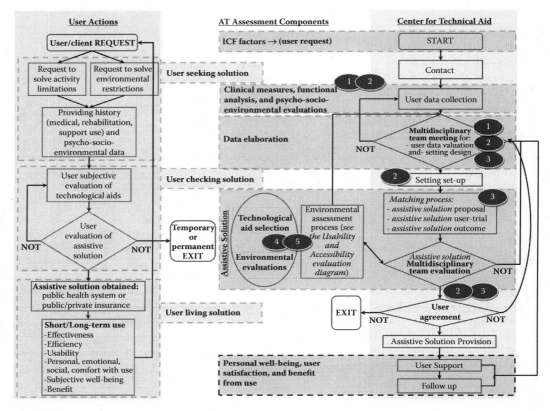

FIGURE I.1
(See color insert.) Flow chart of Assistive Technology Assessment (ATA) process in a Centre for technical aid: The ATA process can be read both from the perspective of the user/client or from the perspective of the Centre for Technical Aid. In the central column are indicated the ATA components. Numbered button signs refer to the chapter in Section I. Their position in the flow chart show an ideal matching with the ATA process.

    c. The user-driven process begins with the ATA for an assistive solution.

    d. The assistive solution is facilitated by the comprehensive utilization of clinical measures, functional analysis, and psycho-socio-environmental evaluations.

    e. The user request is satisfied with the best matching of user/client and assistive solution (including user well-being and realization of benefit from AT use).

    f. The center for technical aid verifies the user's satisfaction and realization of benefit by activating support and follow-up. User well-being continues as long as the solution, with support and follow-up, remains a good match.

  B. Center for Technical Aid

    a. The center for technical aid welcomes a user's request by activating an initial meeting at a time and location that is satisfactory to the user/client population.

    b. The initial interviewer is focused on gathering the user's background information and psycho-socio-environmental data.

    c. When the user provides data to the center for technical aid, data are collected and the case is opened and transmitted to the multidisciplinary team.

    d. The multidisciplinary team evaluates the data and user's request.

        i. If the data provided by the user are not sufficient for a "matching process," the user is requested to convey more information and the process returns to point b.

        ii. If the data provided by the user is sufficient for a "matching process," the multidisciplinary team proceeds by setting and scheduling an appointment for a meeting with the user.

    e. The multidisciplinary team arranges a suitable setting for the matching assessment.

    f. The multidisciplinary team, along with the user, assesses the assistive solution proposed, tries the solution, and gathers outcome data.

    g. The multidisciplinary team evaluates the outcome of the matching assessment.

        i. If successful, the team proposes an assistive solution to the user and schedules a new appointment.

        ii. If not successful, the team restarts at point d.

        iii. When the proposed assistive solution requires an environmental evaluation, the team initiates the environmental assessment process.

    h. The multidisciplinary team proposes the assistive solution to the user (efficacy).

        i. If not a good match (temporary), the user does not agree with the proposed solution and requires a new one. The process restarts at point d.

        ii. If not a good match and an alternative solution does not exist or cannot be found, then the user/client may choose to exit the process. If a good match, the team provides the assistive solution.

    i. Assistive solution provision.

    j. When the technological aid is delivered to the user/client, follow-up and ongoing user support is activated (effectiveness).

AT Abandonment: The Service Delivery System in Different Countries

The most relevant studies on AT abandonment (Philips and Zhao 1993; Scherer 1996; Kittel et al. 2002; Scherer et al. 2004, 2005; Dijcks et al. 2006; Verza et al. 2006; Federici and Borsci 2011) have been effected in different contexts with different national service delivery systems* (Stack et al. 2009; Estreen 2010; Mathiassen 2010). In some cases, such national service delivery systems have been divided according to the model underlying the service delivery itself: medical-oriented model, social-oriented Model, or client-oriented Model (Stack et al. 2009). On the other hand, the service delivery process has been analyzed by others from the public or private health service point of view so that we can distinguish among private insurances, donations, and direct acquisition (Estreen 2010). As an example, Table I.1 quotes the service delivery systems and models of some countries from which the previously mentioned works originate.

---

* "Service delivery" refers to professional advice and treatment activities, as well as the physical delivery of the technical aid to the person with a disability, including training and setup if required. In the AT industry, the term service delivery is used to identify the facilities, procedures, and processes that act as intermediaries between the AT product manufacturers and AT end-users" (Stack et al. 2009, p. 28).

TABLE I.1

Service Delivery System and Model

Country	Service Delivery System[a]	Service Delivery Model[b]
Australia	Private system	Consumer[c]
Austria	Public system and private system for self-employed	Social and medical
Denmark	Public system (health and municipalities)	Social
Finland	Public system (health)	Medical
France	Public system	Medical, social, and consumer
Germany	Private system and partially public system	Medical and social
Greece	Public and private system	Medical and consumer
Italy	Public system (health)	Medical and social
Netherlands	Private and public system	Medical and social
Norway	Public system (municipality)	Medical
Spain	Public system (health and social by regions)	Social, medical, and consumer
Sweden	Public system (health and county councils and municipalities)	Medical
United Kingdom	Private and public system (health and social)	Medical, social, and consumer
United States	Private system	Consumer

In almost all cases, the AT for schools in the private system is managed with a public service delivery system.

[a] Survey performed between 2010 (Estreen 2010) and 2011 by the Leonarda Vaccari Institute in Rome, Italy.

[b] Stack et al. (2009).

[c] Free market model in which there is no intermediary between the patient/consumer and his or her solution (Stack et al. 2009).

In general, we can observe that in European countries, a public health system is more diffused where the person with a disability is considered a patient/user. Inside of these systems, the person who effects the matching does not sell AT but acts as an intermediary between the patient/user and the AT societies by providing an assessment and support service. In Anglo-Saxon countries (such as the United States and Australia), it may occur that the person with a disability is considered a client inside of a private system, to which the assessment center will sell some products. The first model ensures more neutrality in assessing the best AT matching; the second model fosters a user-centered satisfaction with the best matched product. In general, when there is a public system, the financing is bound to a "prescription" effected by a specialist. Moreover, the doctor who prescribes must carry out many duties that, in reality, should be the competence of other experts: engineers, psychotechnologists, psychologists, psychotherapists, etc. On the other hand, in the private service, the client may benefit from well-prepared professionals but without having the necessary services at their disposal. Notwithstanding the diversity of service delivery systems (public/private), recent studies prove that both systems share high AT abandonment percentages—between 12% and 38%, with some exceptions for certain types of devices, such as electric wheelchairs, for which the abandonment rates can be as little as 5% (Wressle and Samuelsson 2004)—a high degree of user dissatisfaction, and a large waste of money. All of this induces the scholars of this sector to pursue a critical elaboration of ATA process models, which, starting from the modeling of the preexisting services, allows us to develop some guidelines to optimize the matching process (Ripat and Booth 2005).

Presentation of the Chapters of Section I

The chapters presented in this section aim to discuss both features and different aspects of the ATA process to set up a standard structure that can be shared among the centers for technical aid that aims to reduce both the abandonment and disuse of their assigned assistive technologies. Specifically, in Chapter 1, "Assessing Individual Functioning and Disability," the authors present an overview of the historical evolution of different models of disability, from the medical to biopsychosocial, to explain the theoretical background underlying the ATA process. The biopsychosocial (or universal) model embraced by the ICF is deepened here: From this new perspective, the concepts of "functioning" and "disability" are redefined in reference to the complex interaction between personal and environmental factors. Under the lenses of this holistic model, the authors aim to explain the function of assistive solutions, which are conceived here as a mediator between the multidimensionality of the specific health conditions of an individual and their effective functioning in the ATA process (see also Section III).

A close examination of the role of individual functioning, and how to measure it, is presented in Chapter 2, "Measuring Individual Functioning." The authors discuss both issues and principles related to the measurement of the individual functioning with special attention to its application to the ATA process. Starting from a discussion of the complexity of the definition of disability, the authors suggest different guiding principles to help professionals work on centers for technical aid in choosing and applying the set of measures that better fit with the aims of the ATA process. Different measures for clinical, functional, and psycho-socio-environmental factors are suggested here for the different evaluation steps of the ATA process. Different tools and techniques are presented to facilitate the multidisciplinary team-building process by means of the characterization of each profession required during the assessment (and measurement) process, with the ultimate aim of ensuring the well-being of the user/client (see also Section II).

In Chapter 3, "Measuring the Assistive Technology Match," the problem of measurement in the matching process between user and AT is discussed. In the first paragraph, the authors focus on the description of two models, the MPT (Figure I.2; Scherer 1998, 2005) and the ICF models, to provide a comprehensive overview of the main standard frameworks of measures and tools currently being used. The aim of this work is to explain how the ATA process is integrated with the MPT model to achieve the best assistive solution because they both share a user-driven approach under the biopsychosocial model of the ICF (see also Section III).

The relation among environment, accessibility, usability, and sustainability between a user and an AT is explained in Chapter 4, "The Assessment of the Environments of Use: Accessibility, Sustainability, and Universal Design." In this chapter, an UX model and the environment evaluation model are discussed as two of the main important steps in the ATA process. Moreover, the environmental assessment in the ATA process is both introduced and exemplified as a step-by-step decision-making process set up by the multidisciplinary team for collecting data about the environment(s) of use, in which the users go to work with the AT (see also Sections II and III).

Chapter 5, "Measuring the Impact of AT on Family Caregivers," concludes this section. It gives an overview of the literature about the impact of AT on informal caregivers of children and adults and describes the relationship among outcomes for assistance users, their informal caregivers, and the related assistive solutions. By means of two hypothetical illustrative vignettes, this chapter aims both to provide recommendations for practice and suggest future developments in this field.

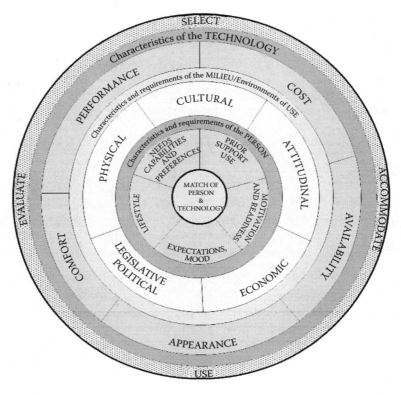

FIGURE I.2
The matching person and technology model (Scherer, 2005). The "Match of Person and AT" (the smallest circle) equals the assistive solution when quality of life and well-being raise from.

Chapters of Section I

Chapter	Topic
1	Assessing Individual Functioning and Disability (Federici, Scherer, Meloni, Corradi, Adya, Samant, and Morris)
2	Measuring Individual Functioning (Federici, Meloni, and Corradi)
3	Measuring the Assistive Technology Match (Corradi, Scherer, and Lo Presti)
4	The Assessment of the Environments of Use: Accessibility, Sustainability, and Universal Design (Mirza, Gossett, and Borsci)
5	Measuring the Impact of AT on Family Caregivers (Demers and Mortenson)

Conclusions

The ATA is a user-driven *process* through which the selection of one or more technological aids for an *assistive solution* is facilitated by the comprehensive utilization of clinical measures, functional analysis, and psycho-socio-environmental evaluations that address, in a specific context of use, the personal *well-being* of the user through the best *matching* of user/client and assistive solution. Because the assistive solution represents the outcome of a user-driven process aimed toward the improvement of individual functioning, it can be considered as a mediator of quality of life and well-being in a specific context of use. For these reasons, it is important to underscore that the assistive solution does not coincide with AT because the first one is a complex system in which psycho-socio-environmental factors and AT interact in a nonlinear way by reducing activity limitations and participation restrictions by means of one or more technologies.

The definition of ATA represents the core definition of this handbook, summarizing the properties of the ATA process. All of the chapters in the section first refer to this definition and follow a guiding reference model (see Figure I.1).

References

Dijcks, B. P. J., De Witte, L. P., Gelderblom, G. J., Wessels, R. D., and Soede, M. (2006). Non-Use of Assistive Technology in the Netherlands: A Non-Issue? *Disability and Rehabilitation: Assistive Technology, 1*(1–2), 97–102. doi:10.1080/09638280500167548

Estreen, M. (2010). *Europe with Free Choice of Assistive Technology. the Provision of Assistive Devices in Specific European Countries.* Retrieved from www.hi.se/bestall

Federici, S., and Borsci, S. (2011). The use and non-use of assistive technology in Italy: A pilot study. In G. J. Gelderblom, M. Soede, L. Adriaens, and K. Miesenberger (Eds.), *Everyday Technology for Independence and Care: AAATE 2011* (Vol. 29, pp. 979–986). Amsterdam, NL: IOS Press. doi:10.3233/978-1-60750-814-4-979

Kittel, A., Di Marco, A., and Stewart, H. (2002). Factors Influencing the Decision to Abandon Manual Wheelchairs for Three Individuals with a Spinal Cord Injury. *Disability and Rehabilitation, 24*(1–3), 106–114. doi:10.1080/0963828011006678 5

Madans, J. H., and Altman, B. M. (2006). *Purposes of Disability Statistics.* Paper presented at the Training Workshop on Disability Statistics for SPECA Countries: UN Special Programme for the Economies of Central Asia, Bishkek, Kyrgyzstan. Retrieved from http://www.unece.org/stats/documents/2006.12.health.htm

Madans, J. H., Altman, B. M., Rasch, E. K., Synneborn, M., Banda, J., Mbogoni, M., et al. (2002). *Washington Group Position Paper: Proposed Purpose of an Internationally Comparable General Disability Measure.* Retrieved from www.cdc.gov/nchs/ppt/citygroup/meeting3/WG3.6a%20Madans_Altman.ppt

Mathiassen, N.-E. (2010). *Assistive Technology: Service Delivery Systems, Presence and Future.* [Aids and Solutions for Quality of Life in a Changing Society: Challenges and Opportunities]. Paper presented at the Ausili e soluzioni per la qualità della vita in una società che cambia: Sfide e opportunità, Bologna, Italy. Oral presentation retrieved from http://www.ausilioteca.org/

Mont, D. (2007). *Measuring Disability Prevalence. Special Protection Discussion Paper No. 0706.* Retrieved from http://siteresources.worldbank.org/DISABILITY/Resources/Data/MontPrevalence.pdf

Philips, B., and Zhao, H. (1993). Predictors of Assistive Technology Abandonment. *Assistive Technology, 5*(1), 36–45. doi:10.1080/10400435.1993.10132205

Ripat, J., and Booth, A. (2005). Characteristics of Assistive Technology Service Delivery Models: Stakeholder Perspectives and Preferences. *Disability and Rehabilitation, 27*(24), 1461–1470. doi:10.1080/09638280500264535

Scherer, M. J. (1996). Outcomes of Assistive Technology Use on Quality of Life. *Disability and Rehabilitation, 18*(9), 439–448. doi:10.3109/09638289609165907

Scherer, M. J. (1998). *Matching Person & Technology. A Series of Assessments for Evaluating Predispositions to and Outcomes of Technology Use in Rehabilitation, Education, the Workplace & Other Settings.* Webster, NY: The Institute for Matching Person & Technology, Inc.

Scherer, M. J. (2005). Cross-walking the ICF to a measure of Assistive Technology Predisposition and Use. Paper presented at the 11th Annual North American Collaborating Center (NACC) Conference on the International Classification of Functioning, Disability and Health (ICF), Rochester, NY, US.

Scherer, M. J., and Craddock, G. (2002). Matching Person & Technology (MPT) Assessment Process. *Technology and Disability, 3*(14), 125–131. Retrieved from http://iospress.metapress.com/content/g0eft4mnlwly8y8g

Scherer, M. J., Cushman, L. A., and Federici, S. (2004, June 1–10). *Measuring Participation and the Disability Experience with the "Assistive Technology Device Predisposition Assessment"*. Paper presented at the North American Collaborating Center 10th Annual Conference on ICF: NACC 2004, Halifax, Canada. Retrieved from http://secure.cihi.ca/cihiweb/en/downloads/10NACC_Conf_Report_FINAL_e.pdf

Scherer, M. J., Sax, C. L., Vanbiervliet, A., Cushman, L. A., and Scherer, J. V. (2005). Predictors of Assistive Technology Use: The Importance of Personal and Psychosocial Factors. *Disability and Rehabilitation, 27*(21), 1321–1331. doi:10.1080/09638280500164800

Stack, J., Zarate, L., Pastor, C., Mathiassen, N.-E., Barberà, R., Knops, H., et al. (2009). *Analysing and Federating the European Assistive Technology ICT industry. Final Report*. Retrieved from European Commission website: http://ec.europa.eu/einclusion

United States Congress. (2004). *Assistive Technology Act (Public Law 108–364)*. Retrieved from http://www.ataporg.org/atap/atact_law.pdf.

Verza, R., Carvalho, M. L. L., Battaglia, M. A., and Uccelli, M. M. (2006). An Interdisciplinary Approach to Evaluating the Need for Assistive Technology Reduces Equipment Abandonment. *Multiple Sclerosis, 12*(1), 88–93. doi:10.1191/1352458506ms1233oa

World Health Organization (WHO). (2001). *ICF: International Classification of Functioning, Disability, and Health*. Geneva, Switzerland: WHO.

World Health Organization (WHO). (2004). *A Glossary of Terms for Community Health Care and Services for Older Persons*. (WHO/WKC/Tech.Ser./04.2). Retrieved from http://whqlibdoc.who.int/wkc/2004/WHO_WKC_Tech.Ser._04.2.pdf

World Health Organization (WHO). (2007). *ICF-CY: International Classification of Functioning, Disability, and Health—Children and Youth Version*. Geneva, Switzerland: WHO.

World Health Organization (WHO), and World Bank. (2011). *World Report on Disability*. Geneva, Switzerland: WHO.

Wressle, E., and Samuelsson, K. (2004). User Satisfaction with Mobility Assistive Devices. *Scandinavian Journal of Occupational Therapy, 11*(3), 143–150. doi:10.1080/11038120410020728

1

Assessing Individual Functioning and Disability

**S. Federici, M. J. Scherer, F. Meloni, F. Corradi,
M. Adya, D. Samant, M. Morris, and A. Stella**

CONTENTS

1.1 The Universal Model of Disability

The origins of the biopsychosocial model date back to the proposal put forward by psychiatrist George Engel in 1977 to integrate within the medical model the dominant social and psychological variables:

> The dominant model of disease today is biomedical, and it leaves no room within its framework for the social, psychological, and behavioural dimensions of illness. A biopsychosocial model is proposed that provides a blueprint for research, a framework for teaching, and a design for action in the real world of health care. (1977, p. 130)

Engel made the leading theoretical contribution to building the biopsychosocial model, identified in von Bertalanffy's general systems theory (von Bertalanffy 1950). According to this approach, the unifying principles in the scientific context are not a reduction of but the organization that explains a scientific phenomenon. It is not sufficient to divide a scientific phenomenon into a simpler unit of analysis and study such units one by one, but it is necessary to study the interrelations among these units. We contrast the old scientific method, which refuses all forms of teleology and is based on linear causality and relations between an independent variable and a dependent variable. On the contrary, we claim an approach that examines the interrelations among many variables, some of them unknown, and takes into consideration the organicistic characters of life and considers concepts such as order, organization, differentiation, and orientation to a purpose. As a result, human beings are also seen as systems ecologically plunged into multiple systems (Gray et al. 1969). In the biopsychosocial model, the definition of the state of health or illness is therefore the outcome of the interaction of processes that operate at the macro level (e.g., the existence of social support for depression) and the processes that operate at the micro level (e.g., biological or biochemical derangements).

Thus, it is impossible from this perspective to isolate disability from the functioning of an individual and vice versa, or rather hypothesize one without the other, not only at the level of social organization but also at the level of a single individual. Disability implies functioning and vice versa. When I. K. Zola in "Toward the Necessary Universalizing of a Disability Policy" (1989) expresses hope for the demystification of the "specialness" of disability and the admission that "people with a disability have long been treated as an oppressed minority" (p. 19), he assumes a conception of disability that is fluid and contextual: "Disability is not a human attribute that demarks one portion of humanity from another (as gender does, and race sometimes does); it is an infinitely various but universal feature of the human condition" (Bickenbach et al. 1999, p. 1182). The issue of disability for individuals "is not whether but when, not so much which one, but how many and in what combination" (Zola 1993, p. 18).

There is not, according to Zola's approach that is close to the biopsychosocial model, a dichotomy between ability and disability, but rather a continuum in which complete ability or complete disability represent nothing but a borderline case possible only in theory. The unique borders to delineate on this continuum should have political and economic purposes and produce functional distinctions to redistribute resources within society. Evidently, we are talking about boundaries that could be criticized and modifiable in the course of time. According to Zola, developing "universal policies" is a matter of urgency that recognizes an indisputable fact: the entire population is "at risk" because of the extraordinary concomitance of chronic illnesses and disability (1989, p. 1). Beyond a universal perspective, we seriously risk creating and perpetuating a model of segregated and separated society, which is also characterized by a progressive accentuation of inequalities:

> Only when we acknowledge the near universality of disability and that all its dimensions (including the biomedical) are part of the social process by which the meanings of disability are negotiated will it be possible fully to appreciate how general public policy can affect this issue. (Zola 1989, p. 20)

The rapid aging of the world population, now more than ever before, confirms what Zola claimed. In most of the World Health Organization's (WHO) recent documents, the spread of disability as a condition correlates with the progressive aging of the population is dramatically shown:

> Life expectancy is increasing in most countries in the Region and the populations are therefore ageing rapidly. In 2050, one third of the population is projected to be 60 years and older. [...] Whereas much of old age is a healthy period, there may be ill health, which leads to disability and dependence, especially in late old age (WHO 2011, p. viii);
>   Global ageing has a major influence on disability trends. The relationship here is straightforward: there is higher risk of disability at older ages, and national populations are ageing at unprecedented rates (WHO and World Bank 2011, p. 35).

Moreover, disability belongs to the human condition not only on a biological level but also on a cultural one because "across the world, people with disabilities have poorer health outcomes, lower education achievements, less economic participation and higher rates of poverty than people without" (WHO and World Bank 2011, p. xi). According to the recent *World Report on Disability*, it estimates that between 110 and 190 million people (from 2.2 to 3.8%) have very significant difficulties in functioning (WHO and World Bank 2011, p. 44).

1.2 Classification, Declaration, and International Definitions of Functioning and Disability

In the International Classification of Functioning, Disability, and Health (ICF; WHO 2001), conceptually founded on the biopsychosocial or universal model, an interactive model (holistic) is proposed. In this model, a person's functioning and disability are considered to be the product of the dynamic interaction between health conditions and contextual factors, which include personal factors as well as environmental ones. In the ICF, concepts such as "functioning" and "disability" are defined in reference to the relation between an individual and his or her context, or rather the complex interaction between personal and environmental factors: "A person's functioning and disability is conceived as a dynamic interaction between health conditions (diseases, disorders, injuries, traumas, etc.) and contextual factors" (WHO 2001, p. 8).

Actually, it is impossible to talk about a person's functioning and disability as if he or she lived in a social, cultural, political, and economic vacuum. This vacuum is filled by the introduction of the contextual factors in the ICF's biopsychosocial inter-relational model of disability. The multidimensionality of the ICF is guaranteed by the fact that contextual factors are a basic and integral component of the human functioning model based on the classification, body functions and structures, and activity and participation. The positive aspects of the relationship between an individual and his or her context are defined by the umbrella term "functioning," by which we mean all nonproblematic or positive aspects of health and health-related individual conditions. On the other hand, all negative aspects that characterize the relationship between an individual and his or her context are defined by the umbrella term "disability." Both terms have in the classification a neutral meaning (or rather are meant as traced back to their original semantic value) beyond any possible social-cultural encrustation that justifies their use as "umbrella" terms.

Overall, the ICF individuates four components related to human functioning and its restrictions: the functioning and disability components, subdivided into i) body functions and structures and ii) activities and participation, and the contextual factor components, which encompass iii) personal and iv) environmental factors. Each component consists of different constructs or qualifiers and is subdivided into domains and categories at different levels. Health and health-related states may be classified using an alphanumeric code system: b = body functions, s = body structures, d = activities and participation, and e = environmental factors. Separated by a dot, on the right of the alphanumeric codes, the ICF requires the use of one or more qualifiers, which denote, for example, the magnitude of the level of health or severity of the problem at issue (WHO 2001, Annex 2).

In accordance with the biopsychosocial model and the ICF, the Convention on the Rights of Persons with Disabilities adopted on December 13, 2006, by the General Assembly of the United Nations resolution (hereafter Convention) recognizes that:

> Disability is an evolving concept and that disability results from the interaction between persons with impairments and attitudinal and environmental barriers that hinders their full and effective participation in society on an equal basis with others ... [and hopes for:] (a) Respect for inherent dignity, individual autonomy including the freedom to make one's own choices, and independence of persons; (b) Non-discrimination; (c) Full and effective participation and inclusion in society; (d) Respect for difference and acceptance of persons with disabilities as part of human diversity and humanity; (e) Equality of opportunity; (f) Accessibility; (g) Equality between men and women; (h) Respect for the evolving capacities of children with disabilities and respect for the right of children with disabilities to preserve their identities. (UN 2006, Preamble)

By founding a concept of disability marked by the international value of human rights, the universal value of the Convention seems to have heeded the wishes of the late Irving Zola regarding the need for a shared approach to policies on disability at the international level. From this perspective: "human rights are applicable to everyone, and to everyone equally, independently of all contingent differences between people—race, religion, language, culture, geographical location, and so on, including disability" (Bickenbach 2009, p. 1112). The unique criterion to be recognized as a beneficiary of a human right is, precisely, that of the human race. Nonetheless, it is undeniable that such a perspective questions several practical issues concerning its application to different human cultures. The concept of disability and functioning are socially constructed, or rather, the meaning of both terms is enriched with different values and denote cross-cultural differences:

> What it means to be disabled, in short, fundamentally includes what it means to be *viewed as disabled* by others, and this is contingent on features of one's society, system of economic exchange, culture, language and many other things besides. (Bickenbach 2009, p. 1112)

Thus, risks of incommunicability or mutual misunderstanding between individuals and institutions from different social, cultural, and political contexts are anything but unrealistic. The possibility of such incommunicability is manifested, at a theoretical level, in the opposition of two different radicalisms: on the one hand, the absolutism of rights and, on the other, cultural relativism. For political reasons the Convention avoided adopting clearly defined terms or excessively binding statements in defining disability. Nonetheless, it seems clear that the Convention is based on the ICF from an epidemiological and an operational viewpoint. Indeed, the ICF and the Convention share

> The core idea [...] that disability is the outcome of, often extremely complex and little understood, interactive relationships between intrinsic features of the person (which, in the ICF are understood as aspects of the person's health state) and features of the overall context in which person lives, works, and interacts with others. Environmental factors, the constituent elements of this context, are not only natural and physical, but also attitudinal, structural, political, social and cultural. (Bickenbach 2009, p. 1121)

Just taking into account the disability concepts of complex interaction, claimed by the ICF (2001) and the Convention (UN 2006) and more recently by the *World Report on Disability*

(WHO and World Bank 2011), it is possible to overcome the aporia of approaches radically opposed:

> As cultural differences are examples of environmental factors that are productive of kinds and levels of disability it is essential to take them into account in practice. A health practitioner cannot understand the nature and severity of the disability of a client without understanding the client's environmental context, including his or her cultural differences. Whether these differences actually make a difference in either the nature or severity of the disability is a practical and empirical question that needs to be answered on a case-by-case basis. (Bickenbach 2009, p. 1121)

In other words, the conflict is not in the contents (i.e., it does not concern the rightness of both engaged positions), but rather in the political and/or ideological radicalism of both:

> I argue that the conflict between universalism of rights and cultural sensitivity exist only if these positions are expressed in extreme form: rights absolutism and cultural relativity. If more sensibly spelled out—in the form of progressive realisation of rights and situational sensitivity of difference—there is no conflict at all. Indeed, these more reasonable positions are mutually supportive. (Bickenbach 2009, p. 1111)

It is now an unquestioned fact that the seriousness of a disability as well as the level of an individual's functioning are largely determined by the context in which the individual lives. The cultural sensitivity, given the universal foundation of human rights, is an operative horizon to which all professionals of rehabilitation should pay attention.

The necessity of better measurements of the effects of environmental factors, to improve the rehabilitation outcome and, therefore, the well-being and satisfaction of a person with a disability and the quality of life achieved, led to the implementation of more and more accurate models of functioning. Concerning this, it is of a great importance that the 2002 American Association on Mental Retardation's (AAMR) *Definition, Classification, and System of Supports*, the 2002 System (Luckasson et al. 2002), aimed to pick out a shared assessment model of assistive technologies. Beyond the specificity of the intellectual disability (preferred term to "mental retardation") the relevance of the 2002 System's model lies in the fact that "support" is considered a basic element of mediation between the multidimensional features of disability (i.e., in this specific case, the intellectual one) and individual functioning. The 2002 System recognizes as a common basis, as does the ICF, the biomedical, functional, and ecological aspects of disability. Both tools, by defining the disability in terms of functional and ecological outlook, represent the raising of a new paradigm that has "its focus on functional skills, personal well-being, the provision of individualized supports, and the concept of personal competence (that is enhanced through skill acquisition, environmental modification, and/or use of prosthetics)" (Schalock and Luckasson 2004, p. 137).

In the 2002 System, the basic meanings are represented by human beings, the environment, and supports. Such meanings explain the condition of disability and individual functioning. In particular, the dimensions by which human functioning is defined are intellectual abilities; adaptive behavior; participation, interaction, and social roles; health; and context. The supports, defined as "resources and strategies that aim to promote the development, education, interests, and personal well-being of a person and that enhance individual functioning" (Schalock and Luckasson 2004, p. 142), are integrated in the 2002 System relating four aspects: first, the individual functioning is the result of the interaction between the disability dimension and supports; second, giving support to people improves their independence, relationships, social participation, and global well-being; third, the assessment and selection of supports are carried out by taking into consideration the aspects and domains of a person's daily life; and fourth, the supports defined as "services" are one type of support provided by professionals and agencies. Also the concept of support, like others, is culturally determined and therefore subject to cultural variability in relation to the importance of rehabilitative practice and use, although Schalock and Luckasson highlight that its "conceptual and practical link to assessment is widely observed" (2004, p. 143). It is, then, in the relationship that entails individualized support to the assessment process that we can reach the goal of a diagnosis (i.e., the intervention) so that the primary purpose of diagnosis is intervention (Schalock and Luckasson 2004, p. 143).

1.3 Where Individual Functioning and Disability Are Assessed: Assistive and Rehabilitation Technology Service Delivery Models

The current literature base demonstrates that the appropriate strategy for the design and distribution of assistive technology (AT) depends on many factors, including the availability of personnel, raw materials, and device parts, and the interaction of all of these factors can complicate AT service delivery models. Health-care workers and policy-makers need a knowledge base in the extant ways that AT may be provided to end-users to improve their well-being and participation. The issue is multivariate and complex and various models have begun to be developed that encourage innovation and service delivery. The extensive variety of models may be captured in six overarching categories, but each of these categories is general and made up of many more subcategories of models. In addition, these categories are not perfectly discrete, but rather they are hybridized or "multimodal" types of models that overlap. Nevertheless, the following six overarching categories are an important way to conceptualize the universe of transferring AT to persons with disabilities (Adya et al., in review):

1. *Charity/donation model*: Mass distribution of free recycled or low-cost AT
2. *Community-based rehabilitation model*: Providing services for independence and integration through the use of local resources in collaboration with community stakeholders
3. *Individual empowerment model*: Matching the person with the appropriate AT and facilitating empowerment through personal construction of AT using available materials, do-it-yourself instructions, and home-based solutions
4. *Entrepreneurship model*: Local entrepreneur or foreign entity designing a solution to match an identified need, developing distribution networks, and commercializing the solution
5. *Globalization and large-scale manufacturing model*: A product already developed or in development locally or in developed regions is transferred to resource-limited environments (RLEs) through multiple methods, such as workshops and factories

6. *Universal design in public use infrastructure*: Building accessibility into mainstream products, such as cell phones, open-source software, and universally designed devices.

1.3.1 Charity-Based Models

Charity-based programs have been used for decades as a means to provide individuals with material products that they could not access because of their socioeconomic and environmental conditions. Past programs have engaged in mass distribution of different types of AT, including mobility devices and hearing aids. Charities engage in different activities such as developing low-cost prototypes available for free, fundraising to finance the delivery of AT, and refurbishing and recycling of old AT devices. Although mass distributions of AT can be helpful at times, such as when a conflict or disaster results in many acquired disabilities, they often involve products designed with the one-size-fits-all approach, which cannot be customized to the needs of the consumers and their environments, or they have low-quality designs that can lead to secondary injuries and wounds.

1.3.2 Community-Based Rehabilitation Models

Community-based rehabilitation (CBR) was conceptualized and promoted by WHO and related United Nations (UN) agencies in the early 1980s as a means of providing services to people with disabilities in developing countries who had no access to quality rehabilitative facilities, physicians, and other qualified personnel. The original rationale behind CBR was to circumvent the need for expensive institutional care and a lack of government support by providing cost-effective rehabilitation services to people with disabilities within their own homes and communities. Although its inception focused on the need for medical rehabilitative care, it has evolved because of a realization that rehabilitation aimed at promoting independent functioning has to respond to the need for securing equal rights and access to services such as education, employment, health services, and public services and facilities. Because CBR works on the principle of finding solutions through locally available resources, most AT delivered through CBR programs are designed to be affordable, made with locally available materials, and appropriate to the environment of the consumer.

1.3.3 Individual Empowerment Models

In individual empowerment models, consumers "partner" with providers in product evaluation and selection as professionals strive to individualize services, help people achieve their self-determined goals, and ensure people are included in all aspects of community life. To achieve a good match of person and technology and improved rates of optimal AT use, it is important that the potential technology user be paired with a well-informed provider.

1.3.4 Entrepreneurial Models

Entrepreneurial models promote the availability of AT through commercialization, and this transfer of technology can occur using either top-down or bottom-up approaches. In the top-down entrepreneurial model, the technology solution is brought into the local market by a foreign or external entity. Top-down distribution of AT can also include local franchising and adaptation to the local culture.

1.3.5 Globalization Model

Globalization models refer to the expansion of multinational and international companies into new markets in resource-limited environments to create new supply chains for the delivery of technology solutions that may or may not be adapted to local needs. Manufacturing in most globalization models is done in-country at a large scale. Solutions can be designed in collaboration with international, national, and local designers. It has to be noted that this model is mainly suited for the one-size-fits-all solutions, even when they are adapted to local context and needs.

1.3.6 Universal Design Models

The universal design approach is based on the understanding that designing products to match a mythical average of human abilities and conditions is in conflict with the fact that all human users are diverse and experience different personal and environmental circumstances. Inaccessible mainstream products and services designed with a focus on a narrow subset of human functioning, such as information and communication technologies (ICT), medical equipment, and physical infrastructure can impose significant barriers on people with disabilities and people who are aging. Universally designed public use products and infrastructure are also necessary to ensure that people with disabilities have equal access to all activities irrespective of the existence of AT because many times individuals cannot use mainstream technologies that do not match their AT devices.

1.4 Assessing Individual Functioning Within a Rehabilitation Process

The international scientific literature presents a wide variety of rehabilitation models from different authors. Some of these models—generally elaborated in the last decade—are conceptually compatible with the universal approach to disability, the biopsychosocial model, and the ICF. The assessment process as a full evaluation of functioning and disability of an individual can be considered as an aspect of any rehabilitation process so that any rehabilitation model encompasses an assessment model also. For this reason, before presenting the assistive technology assessment (ATA) process model of assessment, it might be useful to explore the most relevant models of rehabilitation described in the international scientific literature. Below some of the most important contributions to the conceptualization of a rehabilitation process are briefly described with a special focus on, when possible, the stage of the assessment.

Gracey and colleagues (2009) proposed a "Y-shaped" theoretical model in which to ground a rehabilitation intervention. The starting point of the authors is to identify a biopsychosocial approach to assessment, formulation, and rehabilitation after acquired brain damage. The result is an original theoretical synthesis of existing work drawn from rehabilitation and psychotherapy studies that is also helpful in clinical use. The process of adaptation and reintegration in society is determined by overcoming the social, personal, and interpersonal discrepancies—represented by the two branches of the Y—that often follow a traumatic event. The Y-shaped model is so called because the progressive move toward a new awareness and acceptance of existing health conditions is graphically represented by the conjunction of the two branches of the Y. The process of awareness and resolution of discrepancies made by the client must be supported to consolidate their postinjury sense of self and their psychological growth. The vertical trunk of the Y represents this part of the path. During the process, the client can discover aspects of continuity with the preinjury self and can develop new adaptive and personal meanings arising as a result of the injury and related experiences.

Gracey et al. (2009) suggest that at the very top of the Y, it is possible that many clients will experience a discrepancy by trying to keep a sense of identity through the negation of the difficulties. In the long run, this leads to the loss of relationships and social networks. Customers often deny the presence of difficulty, even with rehabilitation professionals. In the Y-shaped model, social and interpersonal factors can play a role in overcoming personal discrepancies, in reaching a new awareness, and in developing coping resources. Nevertheless, findings from many studies suggest that the focus in rehabilitation may go beyond compensation for deficits and perhaps should more explicitly incorporate a focus on growth and personal meaning.

In the Y-shaped model, the key phases of the process of rehabilitation correspond to (1) the development of safety; (2) the understanding of, engagement with, and reduction of social, interpersonal, and intrapersonal discrepancies; and (3) supporting psychological growth. For each key phase the authors (Gracey et al. 2009) identify the social, interpersonal, cognitive, and emotional variables involved and the corresponding rehabilitation activities and strategies. In conclusion, the authors believe that the meaning of life experiences is key to well-being—psychosocial outcome measures that focus solely on the amount or level of activity might not reflect meaningful personal change for the individual.

Steiner and colleagues (2002) proposed the Rehab-CYCLE, a modified version of the Rehabilitation Cycle developed by Stucki and Sangha (1998). It leads the health-care professional with a logical sequence of activities to successful problem-solving or individual goals achieved. The Rehab-CYCLE identifies the patient's problems and needs and relates the problems to relevant factors of the person and the environment. It is useful to define therapy goals, to plan and implement interventions, and to assess the effects.

To have a conceptual framework for ordering and understanding what disease means to a patient, the authors (Steiner et al. 2002) developed an extension of the Rehab-CYCLE (Stucki and Sangha 1998) that they called the "Rehabilitation Problem-Solving Form" (RPS-Form). The RPS-Form consists of a single datasheet that is based on the ICF. It is divided into three parts: (1) a header for basic information, (2) an upper part to describe the patient's perspective, and (3) a lower part for the analysis of the health-care professionals. The RPS-Form is designed to distinguish between the perspectives held by the patient and those of the health-care professional. The patient's view is recorded in the upper part of the form denoted with "Patient (or Relatives): Problems and Disabilities," and the health-care professional's views are noted in the lower part denoted with "Health Professionals: Mediators Relevant to Target Problems." The rehabilitation team attempted to identify those characteristics of the patients or their environment that caused or contributed to their problems.

The multiple interactions between patient and environment and between all components of the patient's organism require thinking in terms of causal networks rather than in straight lines where A causes B, which leads to C. When it is unclear whether a variable is directly responsible for a disability or whether it is an element that contributes to certain processes involved with the disability, the RPS-Form uses the term "mediator" to describe such variables (Steiner et al. 2002). The main task of the rehabilitation team is to discern the target mediators (i.e., those mediators that are supposed to have the greatest potential to solve the target problems) through the analysis of the RPS-Form as a basis for the team to discuss each case in the framework of the ICF model of functioning and disability.

In 2002, the AAMR released its *Mental Retardation: Definition, Classification, and Systems of Supports* (Luckasson et al. 2002) in which human functioning and intellectual abilities are described as influenced by five factors: (i) intelligence; (ii) adaptive behavior; (iii) participation, interaction, and social roles; (iv) health; and (v) context. Intelligence is defined as "a general mental ability that includes reasoning, planning, solving problems, thinking abstractly, comprehending complex ideas, learning quickly, and learning from experience" (Luckasson et al. 2002, p. 51). Adaptive behavior is defined as "the collection of conceptual, social, and practical skills that have been learned by people in order to function in their everyday lives" (Luckasson et al. 2002, p. 73). The participation and interaction concern the degree of commitment of the person in daily activities and his or her involvement in the surrounding environment. Social roles regard the set of activities that are considered normal for a specific age group. The definition of health, meant as a state of complete physical, mental, and social well-being, is in line with the one determined by WHO. Finally, the context is a concept adapted from Bronfenbrenner's theory (1979) and describes the relationships in which the person is involved, including "the person, family, and/or advocates; the neighborhood, community, or organization providing education or habilitation services or supports; and the overarching patterns of culture, society, larger populations, country, or sociopolitical influences" (Schalock and Luckasson 2004, p. 142). The 2002 System claims for the multidimensionality of the intellectual disability (ID) and assigns a central role to the supports as a mediator between the multidimensional aspects of ID and the individual functioning. In the 2002 System, "supports are defined as resources and strategies that aim to promote the development, education, interests, and personal well-being of a person and that enhance individual functioning" (Schalock and Luckasson 2004, p. 142) so that the individual functioning is determined by the interaction of the supports with the five dimensions listed earlier. The supports are provided with the main purpose of enhancing personal outcomes related to independence, relationships, contributions, school and community participation, and personal well-being of people with ID, and the assessment process is based on everyday life activity areas. An important aspect of the assessment process in the 2002 System is represented by the clinical judgment, defined as

> A special type of judgment rooted in a high level of clinical expertise and experience that emerges directly from extensive data. It is based on the clinician's explicit training, direct experience with person with whom the clinician is working, and familiarity with the person and the person's environment, including his/her family. (Schalock and Luckasson 2004, pp. 143–144)

1.5 Assessing Individual Functioning and Disability in the ATA Process

In the ATA process model, the assessment is defined as

> A user-driven *process* through which the selection of one or more technological aids for an *assistive solution* is facilitated by the comprehensive utilization of clinical measures,

functional analysis, and psycho-socio-environmental evaluations that address, in a specific context of use, the personal *well-being* of the user through the best *matching* of user/client and assistive solution. (See Conclusions, Section I, this volume.)

Consistent with the ICF model of functioning and disability, the 2002 System, and the ATA process, the individual's well-being is the rationale of intervention that is guaranteed by the best match between the user/client and the support or AT. Under the lens of the ICF biopsychosocial model, by the means of which the user/client's request and the assistive solution is provided (Figure 1.1), the assessment process evaluates the individual's functioning through "clinical measures, functional analysis, and psycho-socio-environmental evaluations." In particular (Figure 1.2), in the "User data collecting" step, the diagnosis has a central role in the assessment because it is in relation to the diagnosis that the following setup for matching and assessing tools are designed. However, it is only at the meeting with the user/client (matching process) that it is possible to observe the individual's performance, evaluate their functioning in the most relevant aspects of daily life, and to personalize the support by making reference to the socioenvironmental characteristic qualities or barriers (environmental assessment process) within the user/client's life. Finally, the user support and follow-up procedures allow us to assess the functioning recursively and constantly weigh the outcome of assistive solutions in relation to the user's needs and to the changes faced in the functioning domains of everyday life.

Thus, the role of mediation played by supports and assistive solutions between the multidimensionality of the specific health conditions of an individual and their effective functioning in the ATA process seems quite evident. Nor it is to disregard, as a meta-dimensional process, the dynamic interaction between objective (the center for

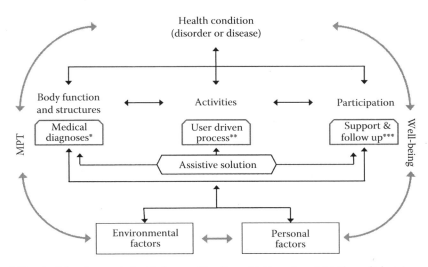

* The physician, the psychologist, the cognitive therapist, the optometrist, the audiologist, the pediatric specialist, the geriatrician

** The psychotechnologist, the occupational therapist, the architect, the engineer

*** The therapist, the special educator, the occupational therapist, the psychologist, the consumer support, speech language pathologist, the physiotherapist

FIGURE 1.1
(See color insert.) Assistive technology assessment under the lens of the ICF biopsychosocial model.

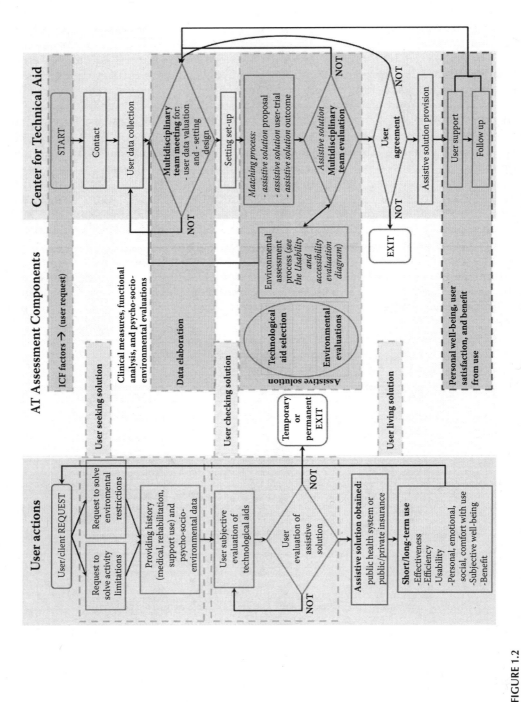

FIGURE 1.2

(See color insert.) The assistive technology assessment process flow chart.

technical aid column, Figure 1.2) and subjective (the user's actions column, Figure 1.2), or rather between the objective and subjective functioning measurements. The features of this dynamic, within the assessment process, tie professionals of rehabilitation to finding solutions that take into consideration the social and cultural context of an individual.

1.6 Conclusions

An ATA model is needed and proposed in this chapter that is consistent with the ICF in that it emphasizes the individual's well-being and the best match between the user/client and the assistive solution. This requires a user-driven process through which the selection of one or more technological aids for an assistive solution is facilitated by the comprehensive use of clinical measures, functional analysis, and psycho-socio-environmental evaluations.

Summary of the Chapter

This chapter discusses the biopsychosocial model as operationalized by the WHO's International Classification of Functioning, Disability, and Health, the Convention on the Rights of Persons with Disabilities, the 2002 AAMR *Definition, Classification, and System of Supports*, and most recently the *World Report on Disability*. A move from the medical to social view of disability requires that assistive technology professionals view disability as existing within a cultural, political, and economic milieu. International models of assistive technology service delivery are reviewed and the need for enhanced assessment of the person with a disability's functioning is highlighted in order to achieve a good match of person and technology.

References

Adya, M., Samant, D., Mofris, M., and Scherer, M. (in review). Assistive/Rehabilitation Technology, Disability, and Service Delivery Models. *Disability and Rehabilitation*.

Bickenbach, J. E. (2009). Disability, culture and the UN convention. *Disability and Rehabilitation, 31*(14), 1111–1124. doi:10.1080/09638280902773729

Bickenbach, J. E., Chatterji, S., Badley, E. M., and Üstün, T. B. (1999). Models of disablement, universalism and the international classification of impairments, disabilities and handicaps. *Social Science and Medicine, 48*(9), 1173–1187. doi:10.1016/S0277-9536(98)00441-9

Bronfenbrenner, U. (1979). *The Ecology of Human Development: Experiments by Nature and Design.* Cambridge, MS: Harvard University Press.

Engel, G. L. (1977). The need for a new medical model: A challenge for biomedicine. *Science, 196*(4286), 129–136. doi:10.1126/science.847460

Gracey, F., Evans, J. J., and Malley, D. (2009). Capturing process and outcome in complex rehabilitation interventions: A "Y-shaped" model. *Neuropsychological Rehabilitation, 19*(6), 867–890. doi:10.1080/09602010903027763

Gray, W., Duhl, F. J., and Rizzo, N. D. (1969). *General Systems Theory and Psychiatry*. Boston: Little Brown.

Luckasson, R., Borthwick-Duffy, S., Buntinx, W. H. E., Coulter, D. L., Craig, E. M., Reeve, A., et al. (2002). *Mental Retardation: Definition, Classification, and System of Supports* (10th ed.). Washington, DC: AAMR.

Schalock, R. L., and Luckasson, R. (2004). American Association on Mental Retardation's *Definition, Classification, and System of Supports* and its relation to international trends and issues in the field of intellectual disabilities. *Journal of Policy and Practice in Intellectual Disabilities, 1*(3–4), 136–146. doi:10.1111/j.1741-1130.2004.04028.x

Steiner, W. A., Ryser, L., Huber, E., Uebelhart, D., Aeschlimann, A., and Stucki, G. (2002). Use of the ICF model as a clinical problem-solving tool in physical therapy and rehabilitation medicine. *Physical Therapy, 82*(11), 1098–1107.

Stucki, G., and Sangha, O. (1998). Principles of rehabilitation. In J. H. Klippel and P. A. Dieppe (Eds.), *Rheumatology* (pp. 11.11–11.14). London: Mosby.

United Nations (UN). (2006). *Convention on the Rights of Persons with Disabilities*. (A/RES/61/106). New York: UN Retrieved from http://www.un-documents.net/a61r106.htm.

von Bertalanffy, L. (1950). An outline of general system theory. *The British Journal for the Philosophy of Science, 1*(2), 134–165. doi:10.1093/bjps/I.2.134

World Health Organization (WHO). (2001). *ICF: International Classification of Functioning, Disability, and Health*. Geneva, Switzerland: WHO.

World Health Organization (WHO). (2011). *European Report on Preventing Elder Maltreatment*. Retrieved from http://www.euro.who.int/__data/assets/pdf_file/0010/144676/e95110.pdf

World Health Organization (WHO), and World Bank. (2011). *World Report on Disability*. Geneva, Switzerland: WHO.

Zola, I. K. (1989). Toward the necessary universalizing of a disability policy. *Milbank Quarterly, 67*(Suppl 2 Pt. 2), 401–428. doi:10.2307/3350151

Zola, I. K. (1993). Disability statistics, what we count and what it tells us: A personal and political analysis. *Journal of Disability Policy Studies, 4*(2), 9–39. doi:10.1177/104420739300400202

2

Measuring Individual Functioning

S. Federici, F. Meloni, and F. Corradi

CONTENTS

2.1 What Individual Functioning Measures

2.1.1 The Best Measure: Is There an Elixir of Measurements for Turning an Assessment into Gold?

In June 2001, the U.N. International Seminar on the Measurement of Disability brought together a large number of experts in disability measurement from developed and developing countries to review the current status of methods used in population-based data collection activities to measure disability in national statistical systems (UN 2001). The seminar developed recommendations and priorities to advance work on the measurement of disability. In particular, the seminar improved principles and standard forms for global indicators of disability for use in censuses and helped to build a network of institutions and experts given the broad consensus on the need for population-based measures of disability for countrywide use and international comparisons. The U.N. international seminar experts selected the International Classification of Functioning, Disability, and

Health (ICF; WHO 2011) as the basic conceptual model. Their work emphasized the fact that the ICF model has established the need for a common language that not only allows a common understanding and use by operators belonging to different professional areas but is also easily applicable to remarkably different environmental contexts, "resolving the apparent tension between respecting cultural and linguistic differences in the meaning of health and providing the scientific basis for an international common language of health" (Üstün et al. 2001a, p. ix; see also Üstün et al. 2001b, 2003b, 2003c).

The real problem encountered by the experts was, paradoxically, the complex definition of disability (Üstün et al. 2003a). In fact, in the ICF disability arises out of activity limitations and restrictions on participation that is determined by the interaction between body function and structure impairments and a disadvantageous context (environmental and personal factors):

> Since only one or two of these dimensions of disability are reflected in measures in any given survey [...], the data will only capture a portion of the population—those who exhibit the specific aspects of disability the questions represent. (Altman and Gulley 2009, p. 544)

In a complex model such as this, each domain represents a different area of measurement and each category or element of classification within each domain represents a different area of operationalization of the broader domain concept. To generate a meaningful general prevalence measure, one must determine which component best reflects the information needed to address the purpose of the data collection (Mont 2007, p. 4).

The "definitional paradox" (Madans and Altman 2006) about the definition of disability is due to the operational nature of the disability concept according to which any theoretical definition implies aporia, whereas any operational meaning is determined by the purpose of the research. Indeed, the outcome of the interaction between a person's state of health and contextual factors, the sum of personal and environmental components, can be described on three levels: (1) body, as impairment of body functions or structures; (2) person, as activity limitations measured as capacity; and (3) society, as participation restrictions measured as performance. For each of these levels it is possible to identify more than one "operational" definition of functioning and disability: In fact, the ICF does not provide a single, unequivocal, operational definition and, consequently, does not point to specific measurement tools. The main consequence is that different operational definitions lead to different and sometimes incoherent assessments:

> Specifically, we are concerned with the similarities and differences in the populations identified as disabled when the conceptualization of disability, the resulting questions, and the methods used to code and analyze the data differ from one set of questions to the next. In addition, we are concerned with disability prevalence estimates when the same sets of questions are asked in two different national populations. (Altman and Gulley 2009, p. 544)

Therefore, there are many different aspects for which the operational measures of disability may vary according to the prevalent notion of disability; the purpose of measurement and application; the characteristic of disability investigated; and "the definitions, question design, reporting sources, data collection methods, and expectations of functioning" (WHO and World Bank 2011, p. 21). Moreover, all of these factors make comparisons of data at national and international levels very difficult. In any case, the need for updated estimates on the worldwide prevalence of disability has led the World Health Organization (WHO) and the World Bank to jointly produce the first ever *World Report on Disability* (2011). This report is based on two large data sources: the WHO *World Health Survey* of 2002–2004 (WHO 2002–2004; Üstün et al. 2003b), from 59 countries, and the WHO *Global Burden of Disease* study, 2004 update (WHO 2008). The first is the largest multinational health and disability survey ever using a single set of questions and consistent methods to collect comparable health data from across countries; the second is an overall assessment of the health of the world's population, providing exhaustive estimates of premature mortality, disability, and loss of health from different diseases, injuries, and risk factors, drawing on available WHO data sources and on information provided by member states.

The *World Health Survey* and *Global Burden of Disease* "based on very different measurement approaches and assumptions, give global prevalence estimates among the adult population of 15.6% and 19.4% respectively" (WHO and World Bank 2011, p. 29). The *World Report on Disability* makes some recommendations to improve the availability and quality of data on disability: (1) adopt the ICF "as a universal framework for disability data collection" (WHO and World Bank 2011, p. 45); (2) improve national disability statistics; (3) improve the comparability of data; and (4) develop appropriate tools and fill research gaps, with particular suggestions for developing "better measures of the environment and its impact on the different aspects of disability" (WHO and World Bank 2011, p. 46) and for coupling the evaluation of disability experience with the measurement of the "well-being and quality of life of people with disabilities" (WHO and World Bank 2011, p. 47).

Moreover, in the field of measurement, the crucial point is not to find the right answer but to answer the right question, and, as Zola conveyed (1993), any attempt to identify standard measures on disability reflects, more than anything else, the effort to consider disability as a fixed and dichotomous entity and not, as the universal model of disability states, a fluid and continuous experience. Indeed, only in a purely theoretical manner might one find in an individual either a full disability or a full ability. In the biopsychosocial model, disability is no longer considered, as medical and social models do, as an identity that defines people or social classes. In the medical model, disability is a negative characteristic belonging to an individual that defines the gap between them and normal standard health. Conversely, the social model identifies disability as a social class of individuals in whom the majority recognizes a stigmatized status of minority (Goffman 1963; Hahn 1985). In the medical model people have a disability because an illness or an impairment is attributed to them and they are called "people with disability" or, much easier, they are wholly identified with the illness (e.g., Down syndrome, deaf, blind); in the social model, people are disabled because they are stigmatized by prejudices of society and one may talk about them as disabled people (not "with disability") or oppressed (not "with oppression") (Oliver and Barnes 1998). The biopsychosocial model moves from the person to his or her functioning, overcoming a causal inference of disability as a result of both the impact of disease or other health conditions (WHO 2001) and a social disadvantage. According to this view, disability is just a way of functioning, expressed by positive wording as the "ability to do" in specific contexts and health conditions.

Individual functioning is also related to the interrelation between a specific environment, personal features, and health conditions: "The issue of disability for individuals [...] is not whether but when, not so much which one but how many and in what combination" (Zola 1993, p. 18). Disability is not a set of immutable characteristics that define a person over another, nor is it predictable by a medical diagnosis because it is not a direct consequence of disease, but it is, instead, a multidimensional process that lasts a lifetime and involves the physical, psychic, and social spheres of the individual:

> Having a disability is not a fixed status, but rather a continually changing, evolving, and interactive process. It is not something that one is or is not, but instead is a set of characteristics everyone shares to varying degrees and in varying forms and combinations. (Zola 1993, p. 30)

The WHODAS 2.0 (World Health Organization Disability Assessment Schedule) (Üstün et al. 2010), as an example of a measure that adopts the ICF's conceptual framework, is a psychometric questionnaire on self-perceived disability that assesses the individual functioning in the "here" of daily life activities and "now" of the last 30 days independently of the background disease or previous health conditions (Üstün et al. 2010, p. 5). Although disability is neither a fixed concept (i.e., aetiologically determined by a diagnosis or immutable in time) nor dichotomous (i.e., ability and disability are not mutually exclusive), it does not mean immeasurable: "Instead, its conception, measurement, and counting differs validly with the purposes for which such numbers are needed. The clearer the outcomes we seek, the clearer it will be what conceptions and measurements are necessary" (Zola 1993, p. 30).

Disability is also a multidimensional construct because its measurement is multidimensional. Therefore, the correct answer to the question posted in the section header is that the elixir of measurement is found when we orient the focus of the research not just on the theoretical definition of disability but also on the clearness of the purpose of our measurements. In other words, you will just measure what you want to find. Indeed, according to the uncertainty principle, the more precisely one property is measured (i.e., capacity), the less precisely the other can be measured (i.e., performance). Thus, with disability being a multiproperty object of measurement, one could not measure all of the properties at the same time with the same tool. As a consequence, the best researcher is one who has clearly defined the property of disability to be measured and the tool required to measure it. For all of these reasons, an elixir of disability measurement is not even desirable. In fact, having a variety of measuring tools and the flexibility to change measurement procedures, adapting them to different people, contexts, and purposes, is the most reliable scientific approach.

2.1.1.1 Fitting Measure for the Purpose of the Assistive Technology Assessment

The purpose of measurement is the guiding principle behind the specification of an operational definition and the choice of a coherent set of measurement tools. Madans and colleagues (2002) identified three major classes of purposes at the aggregate level in their research, asking general census questions on disability in the international context: (1) to provide services, including the development of programs and policies for service provision and the evaluation of these programmes and services, (2) to monitor the level of functioning in the population, and (3) to assess equalization of opportunities. The assistive technology assessment (ATA) process can be viewed as an aspect of the purpose described in point 1. Madans and colleagues stated that "provision of services at the population level includes, but is not limited to, transportation, rehabilitation, providing assistive devices, long term care" (2002, slide 11) and that the fulfilment of this aim "requires detailed information about the person and the environment, as in the case of rehabilitation" (slide 11; please see also Madans and Altman 2006, slide 6). Questions about the need for assistive solutions and problems with accessibility are therefore at the heart of the assessment. Apart from all of this, the ultimate aim of the

ATA process is to "address, in a specific context of use, the personal *well-being* of the user through the best *matching* of user/client and assistive solution" by means of "clinical measures, functional analysis, and psycho-socio-environmental evaluations" (see Conclusions, Section I, this volume.).

2.1.1.2 From the Measures to the Purposes (Well-Being), From the Purposes to the Measurers (Multidisciplinary Team)

This statement indicates two orders of questions that need to be addressed: (1) the nature of the "well-being" concept and measurement, and (2) how to "team up" professionals at the center for technical aid. With regard to 1, it is plain that the nature of the well-being variable is merely subjective; in fact, it "measures 'what people say' rather than 'what people do'. It is true that self-reported well-being has potential shortcomings such as response bias, memory bias and defensiveness" (Uppal 2006, p. 525). Nevertheless, "subjective data have proved to be stable and useful" (Uppal 2006, p. 525) and "there is increasing acceptance of patient-reported outcomes for those constructs where one's subjective reality cannot be objectified (e.g., feelings, pain, energy levels, perceived health and so on)" (Kayes and McPherson 2010, p. 1011). As part of this discussion it is important to point out that, even today, both in the literature and in the different classifications of disability that have succeeded over time, there is no space for the inner world of the individual. In particular, a few authors have focused on the difference between the objective and the subjective dimensions of functioning and disability.

> For example, if people cannot play golf because of impairment (capacity limitation within activity limitation) or because of environmental obstacles (participation restriction), the MEANING of that fact will be quite different from person to person. For a life-long regular golfer it would be disast[e]rous, but for a person, otherwise similar, who has never played it, the fact itself that he is not playing golf would not be essential. It follows that evaluation of meaning or satisfaction (which are both subjective) of the objective activity or participation is indispensable especially for items other than common basic survival needs. (Ueda and Okawa 2003, p. 598)

But what is the subjective experience of functioning and disability? Ueda and Okawa define it as

> a set of cognitive, emotional and motivational states of mind of any person, but particularly of a person with health condition and/or disability. It is a unique combination of, on one hand, a disability experience, i.e. a reflection (influence) of existing health conditions, impairments, activity limitations, participation restrictions and negative environmental factors (obstacles) into the person's mind (negative subjective experience), and on the other hand an experience of a positive nature, which includes, among other things, the psychological coping skills developed, often unconsciously, in order to overcome these negative influences (positive subjective experience). (2003, p. 599)

The assessment of a subjective experience is a focal point in identifying the best assistive solution for a given user/client, and its misunderstanding or underestimation has a major role in abandonment (Elliott et al. 2002). It must also be highlighted that the subjective dimension of functioning and disability does not coincide with the objective dimension, i.e., that one currently coded by ICF. The relationship between the subjective and objective dimensions of functioning and disability is interactive and bidirectional. However, the two dimensions are relatively independent of each other. At present, although it is not possible to introduce a comprehensive codification of subjective experience, this dimension should be carefully considered in the ATA process. However, the attention must be twofold. On the one hand, ignoring the subjective dimension can lead to inaccurate assessments and inappropriate assignments, whereas on the other, as argued by Sen, one must bear in mind that "the internal view of health deserves attention, but relying on it in assessing health care or in evaluating medical strategy can be extremely misleading" (2002, p. 861).

With regard to 2, the choice of a set of measurement tools specifically for the purposes of the ATA process facilitates the multidisciplinary team-building process by means of the characterization of each professional required during the assessment (and measurement) process. In the ATA process the two points are strictly linked. We agree with Kayes and McPherson's statement that "a critical evaluation of one 'objective' measure highlights a number of potential limitations suggesting that the apparent willingness to adopt 'objective' measures with little questioning may be misguided" (2010 p. 1011). In fact, objective measures "are not necessarily invariant across populations" and often produce outcomes that "lack clinical relevance" (Kayes and McPherson 2010, p. 1013); moreover, the administration method can also be affected by the subjectivity of the practitioner.

All things considered, it seems that more than "simplistic dichotomy" among objective versus subjective measures can be useful in determining whether or not a measurement tool is "fit for purpose." In the ATA process, the ultimate aim of ensuring the well-being of the user/client is achieved through the use of many different instruments (clinical measures, functional analysis, and psycho-socio-environmental evaluations). These tools are both subjective and objective, but, in any case, a professional who can interpret the results is always required. For these reasons, many different professionals are involved in the ATA process for each type of user/client and for each step of the process.

In the body function and structure evaluation step—medical diagnosis analysis—the team consists of a physician, a psychologist, a cognitive therapist, and an optometrist, audiologist, pediatric specialist, and geriatrician when the user/client's age or impairment calls for them. In the activity evaluation step, a psychotechnologist, OT, architect, and engineer are primarily needed. Finally, the support and follow-up phases allow us to evaluate the performance of the user/client (participation step) by means of a multidisciplinary contribution from a cognitive therapist, special educator, OT, psychologist, consumer support person, speech language pathologist (if needed), and physiotherapist.

2.1.1.3 What Is Measured Versus Who Measures: Balancing the Power of the Assessment

Apart from all of this, the whole process is "user-driven": Subjective measures are not only considered in the activity or participation evaluation steps but also in medical diagnosis analysis, although making a diagnosis is traditionally characterized by the prevalence and precedence of the objective measurement. Nevertheless, we agree with Mezzich (2002), who cited Lain Entralgo (1982): "Diagnosis is more than identifying a disorder (nosological diagnosis) or distinguishing one disorder from another (differential diagnosis); diagnosis is really understanding what is going on in the mind and body of the person who presents for care" (quoted in Mezzich 2002, p. 162). In other words, we make a claim for a comprehensive diagnosis that "aims to combine the best of objective scientific categorical diagnosis with the unique features, including the strengths and resources as well as difficulties, of individual patients" (Fulford and Stanghellini 2008, p. 10).

There is another big issue in giving such importance to the user/client's subjective perspective in measurement. As Brown and Gordon claimed,

> Measurement and assessment, occurring within both research and clinical service contexts, typically involve an imbalance of power between professionals and persons with disabilities. Power is evidenced in who controls decisions about measurement and whose perspective—the subjective values of the measured person or the objective or normative values of the measurer—is given primacy. (2004, p. S13)

The imbalance of power "can affect the 'something important' that is at stake in measurement because the failure to share power can produce less useful measures" (Brown and Gordon 2004, p. S13). Ordinarily, the imbalance is determined in the selection, use, and interpretation of measures that usually incorporate the preferences and perspectives of the professionals but not of the user/client.

In this context, the person who is measured can have very different positions on many aspects of functioning with regard to the person who measures. For example, the person who is measured "may agree that income is important to his or her QOL but disagree with the societal or normative assumption that a higher income is better" (Brown and Gordon 2004, p. S14).

The point being questioned is the professional-user/client relationship. The ATA process can amplify the relationship's imbalance because the presence of a multidisciplinary team, in which each professional carries out his or her values and preferences, exponentially increases the shadow over the disabled person's point of view. Such a risk can be avoided by adopting a user-driven approach or person-centered planning (Menchetti and Sweeney 1995; Holburn and Vietze 2002; Schalock and Alonso 2002; Steiner et al. 2002; Gzil et al. 2007; Leplege et al. 2007), which places the disabled "at the center of a planning effort, often including a planning group (or circle) comprised of service professionals, family members, and people from the community" (Brown and Gordon 2004, p. S14).

From a professional point of view, namely from this handbook's perspective, a central role in the empowerment of who is measured is played by the psychologist as an expert in human relationships. The psychologist not only administers measures and interprets test results but also plays a key role in both counterbalancing the professional-disabled relationship by paying attention to the powerless at each stage of the assessment process and makes easier connections among the different perspectives of the team of professionals.

2.2 How to Measure Individual Functioning

The purpose of this handbook is not to precisely define a default set of measurement tools that would contradict what we wrote in the previous section. We take responsibility for both pointing out some guiding principles for choosing and applying a set of measures and for suggesting some tools which, together, we believe fit these principles.

2.2.1 Guidelines for Measurement and Assessment

The guiding principles are

- The ultimate purpose of the ATA process is the enhancement of the subjective well-being and the QOL of the user/client through the best match with an assistive solution.

- A comprehensive diagnosis needs both a values-based approach (Fulford and Stanghellini 2008) along with an evidence-based one and an idiographic personalized formulation (Mezzich 2002) together with a standardized assessment.
- When assessing a set of measurements, it would be best "to sacrifice reliability for validity" (Fulford and Stanghellini 2008, p. 12). "Those of us who have worked for several decades to improve the reliability of our diagnostic criteria are now searching for new approaches on understanding of aetiological and pathophysiological mechanisms—an understanding that can improve the validity of our diagnoses and the consequent power of our preventive and treatment interventions" (Kupfer et al. 2002, p. xv). The reliability of diagnostic tools is an essential issue, but it does not guarantee in itself the validity of the treatment, which is the primary purpose of rehabilitation professionals.
- The user/client functioning evaluation should encompass objective and subjective measures for any health or health-related domain.
- Throughout the measurement and assessment process the multidisciplinary team should pay attention to the "power balance" in user/client-professional relationships and in mutual relations between professionals.

The measurement tools that we suggest can be roughly classified into two types: objective and subjective. Although the ICF Checklist (WHO 2003), any ICF Core Set, and the Vineland Adaptive Behavior Scales (VABS; Sparrow et al. 1984) can be considered as objective measures, the WHO-Disability Assessment Schedule II (WHODAS II; WHO 2004), the Matching Person and Technology (MPT) model (Scherer 1998), the Canadian Occupational Performance Measure (COPM; Law et al. 2005), and the Support Intensity Scale (SIS; Thompson et al. 2004) facilitate evaluations of the subjective perspective of the user/client.

2.2.2 Measurement and Assessment in the ATA Process

In Figure 2.1, four orange shapes highlight the steps in the ATA process where a measurement and assessment are required.

From the ATA process perspective, all of these tools can be classified according to the assessment stage in which they are administered. After the ATA process step by step, in the "User Data Collecting" stage (step 1), to reach a comprehensive diagnosis and assessment, both standardized and idiographic, the user/client will provide an ICF Checklist and/or the ICF Core Set related to their specific condition, drawn up by a physician, and the self-administered WHODAS II and SOTU (MPT). At this stage of the ATA process professionals have not yet met the user/client so that the psychologist plays a key role during the "Multidisciplinary Team Meeting" by reading and interpreting all of the data provided (step 2) to both evaluate the individual functioning profile and to set up the "Matching Process." At the time of the Matching Process (step 3), the VABS, the Assistive Technology Device Predisposition Assessment (ATD-PA), and the SIS are administered to the user/client. The Matching Process step is the very first time the user/client meets the professionals of the center to evaluate his or her activity limitations, operationalized as "capacity," and to assess the best match with an assistive solution. Finally, in the "User Support" and "Follow-Up" stages (step 4), the team and the user/client evaluate the participation together, operationalized as performance, and continually check the user/client's need for adjusting the match or for a new match.

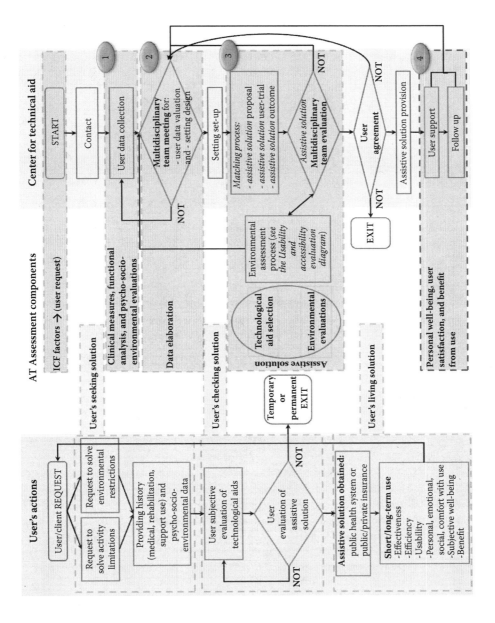

FIGURE 2.1
(See color insert.) The assistive technology assessment (ATA) process and the four steps (orange shapes) of measurement and assessment.

2.2.3 Monitoring Individual Functioning in the Context of an AT Use: The Outcome of the ATA Process

The outcome analysis represents the focal point of the assistive solution matching process and is conducted by the multidisciplinary team of a center for technical aids. It is fundamental to point out some of the factors that can convey important information about the pertinence of an assistive solution to replace, update, and support its adoption by the end-user and prevent its abandonment. The outcome can be analyzed by means of the clinical diagnosis, the functional state, the quality of life, the cost, the satisfaction (DeRuyter 1995), and the comfort (Weiss-Lambrou et al. 1999). In particular, the analysis of two multidimensional constructs enables different degrees of intensity to describe the user's experience of assistive technology (AT): satisfaction (Demers et al. 2000) and comfort (Kolcaba 1992).

Satisfaction is a positive attitude toward psychosocial factors concerning subjective perceptions, evaluations, and comparison processes (Linder-Pelz 1982). The user can describe this kind of positive attitude toward health-care services, products, and providers and toward individual health conditions (Weiss-Lambrou 2002). Comfort can be a physical sensation, a psychological condition, or both things simultaneously (Pearson 2009), and it can generally be reported as a pleasant and positive sensation (Kolcaba and Kolcaba 1991). Another parameter to take into consideration is the environment of use, which involves the user's characteristics and the goals he/she wants to reach with adoption of the AT. An environmental investigation focuses on the person-environment system whereas the user interacts with the given technology (Rust and Smith 2006).

Different studies have highlighted the fact that there are high rates of AT abandonment of up to 75% (Garber and Gregorio 1990; Philips and Zhao 1993; Tewey et al. 1994; Gitlin 1995). However, the causes of abandonment are rarely due to the features of the aid (functioning, manageability, etc.), but they do concern the absence of a user's involvement and/or his/her caregiver in the matching process.

The evaluation process of AT matching must be user-centered and, moreover, it must aim to identify the best correspondence between individual user needs and the features of a particular technology available in a given historical period (Gelderblom et al. 2009). Abandonment can also be due to unnecessary AT; for example, because of the user's recovery, some authors suggested the use of "discontinuity" to describe a possible result of the AT matching process, remarking in this way that the term "abandonment" has a purely negative connotation, whereas the term "discontinuity" generally has a neutral connotation (Lauer et al. 2006).

For all of these reasons, some of the evaluation tools that are able to analyze technical aid matching and that are based on the ICF (Scherer and Craddock 2002) and the client-centered approach have been proposed. The models mentioned highlight the fact that the more we focus on the object (the AT) the more we move away from a good match. In this way, the problem of a good match lies more in the matching process than only in the technology itself; indeed, it is fundamental to involve both users and caregivers in the AT matching process (Long et al. 2003). Starting from this perspective, it is possible to distinguish between AT as a tool and AT as a service. To facilitate both the use of AT and the possibility of examining the chosen technology, it is important to create an assistance network around the user within the evaluation process.

The "Consortium model" describes a matching process centered on the participation of users and caregivers (Long et al. 2003). In this model, the user's family and health workers intervene at the start of the matching process ("Evaluation, identification of outcomes"), taking a fundamental role in the following attainment of a good match between the user and the AT, in which the match is only a component of the outcome.

Verza et al. (2006) also suggested a model focused on the involvement of the user, his or her family, and the rehabilitation team. They highlighted four main reasons for explaining the AT abandonment phenomenon:

1. A change in health conditions,
2. Rejection of the AT,
3. Inadequacy/absence of information and training, and
4. Inappropriateness of the AT.

It follows that a careful outcome analysis of an AT is fundamental for a good match.

2.3 Suggested Measurement Tools for an ATA Process

In this section, we briefly describe some suggested tools. The ICF Checklist (WHO 2003) was developed as a practical tool to elicit clinicians' overall impressions of a patient's condition. It allows the functioning profile of a subject to be described based on 128 codes selected among the thousands forming the whole ICF (WHO 2001).

The ICF Checklist is not a proper instrument for measurement or assessment: It provides the possibility of "opening" the codes on the basis of identifying a person's functional problem and, at the same time, establishes whether or not, and in which measure, the environment acts as a barrier or facilitator for the person's activities. The ICF Checklist is administered to the patient or his or her caregiver. It is structurally divided into four parts: the introductory part, which includes biographical data, the ICD-10 code (WHO 1992), and a specification of the information source; the first part contains a list of codes of body functions (b) and body structures (c); the second part contains a list of codes for activities and participation (d); and finally, the third part contains a list of codes relating to environmental factors (e).

An ICF Core Set (condition-specific) can be defined as

> a selection of ICF domains that includes the least number of domains possible to be practical, but as many as required to be sufficiently comprehensive to cover the pro-totypical spectrum of limitations in functioning and health encountered in a specific condition. (Stucki et al. 2002, p. 281)

In contrast, a generic ICF Core Set allows for a comparison of health across conditions because its domains represent "the most relevant domains to include the least number of domains possible to be practical, but as many as required to be sufficiently comprehensive to cover the general spectrum of limitations in functioning and health" (Stucki et al. 2002, p. 281).

The VABS (Sparrow et al. 2005) are designed to assess the adaptive level of personal and social functioning of any individual, disabled or not. In other words, the VABS measure adaptive behavior, mainly in terms of social competence. The assessment of social competence is made by a developmental perspective and the scales are normalized on samples of males and females aged from 0 to 90. There are currently four versions of the VABS: the Survey Interview Form, the Parent/Caregiver Rating, the Teacher Rating, and the Expanded Interview Form (Sparrow et al. 2005). The Survey Interview Form is administered to a parent or caregiver in a semistructured interview format. The open-ended questions allow more in-depth information to be obtained and facilitate the relationship between the interviewer and the respondent. The Parent/Caregiver Rating Form differs from the Survey Interview Form in that it uses a rating scale format and is the best choice when time or access is limited. The Parent/Caregiver Rating Form is a good tool for progress monitoring when the initial assessment has been made through the Survey Interview Form. The Expanded Interview Form has more items than the Survey Interview Form and is indicated for ages 0 to 5 or to implement specific planning for low-functioning individuals. The Teacher Rating Form assesses adaptive behavior in students. It has a questionnaire format and is completed by the teacher or caregiver. This form differs from Survey Interview Forms in that it also covers content that a teacher would observe more easily in a classroom. The VABS consist of multiple scales organized around four behavioral domains: communication (receptive, expressive, and written), daily living skills (personal, domestic, and community), socialization (interpersonal relationships, play and leisure time, and coping skills), and motor skills (gross and fine, only applicable for children under 6 years of age). There is also a fifth domain, maladaptive behavior, but this is an optional part of the assessment test. The VABS are administered by a psychologist in a semistructured interview format. The VABS have a good concurrent validity with both the Stanford-Binet test and the Wechsler Intelligence Scale for Children. The VABS are a useful tool for assessing adaptive behavior in intellectual and developmental disabilities, autism spectrum disorders (ASDs), attention deficit hyperactivity disorder (ADHD), post-traumatic brain injury, hearing impairment, dementia, and Alzheimer's disease.

The MPT model is a "set of person-centered measures, all of which examine the self-reported perspectives of adult consumers regarding strengths/capabilities, needs/goals, preferences and psychosocial characteristics, and expected technology benefit. There are separate measures for general, assistive, educational, workplace, and healthcare technology use" (Scherer and Craddock 2002, p. 125). The MPT instruments take into account the environments in which the person uses the technology, the individual's characteristics and preferences, and the technology's functions and features. All of these components are analyzed and considered because although a specific technology or a set of technologies may seem the best choice for a particular person, the absence of adequate support or some traits of the personality profile of the customer can cause the failure of the match. The MPT is a user-driven process, and an assessment of the degree of agreement between the user's perspective and that of the provider is planned. Moreover, the quality of life of the customer is a factor that orients the assessment of the influences experienced by the customer when using a specific technology. In the measurement process carried out by the MPT instruments, early recognition of an inappropriate match is crucial. This will limit the phenomenon of abandonment of the aid and reduce the feelings of disappointment and frustration related to this. The MPT set includes a Worksheet, the SOTU (Survey of Technology Use), the ATD-PA (Assistive Technology Device Predisposition Assessment), the ET-PA (Educational Technology Predisposition Assessment), the WT-PA (Workplace Technology Predisposition Assessment), and the HCT-PA (Health Care Technology Predisposition Assessment). The tools included in the MPT are in a duplicate format—one for the technology user and another for the provider of the technology (counsellor, therapist, teacher, employer, or trainer). The ATA process particularly recommends the use of the SOTU and ATD-PA. The SOTU helps to identify technologies that an individual feels comfortable with or has success in using so that a new technology can be built around existing comfort or success. This instrument explores the type of technology that the client already uses, his/her experience, both past and present, and his/her point of view on the technology currently being used. Furthermore, the SOTU values some personal and social characteristics of the user. The client and the provider each independently fill out a version. However, the provider responds by trying to figure out the answers of the client. After administration, the client and the provider discuss the critical discrepancies between the two filled-out forms. The ATD-PA is useful for selecting the most appropriate assistive solution. Each ATD-PA (ATD-PA-Client and ATD-PA-Provider) is divided into two parts: the first part must only be filled out once, whereas the second part must be filled out for each technology. In the client's form version, the client is required to self-evaluate his/her capacity and performance and some personality traits. Furthermore, the client indicates his/her feeling about using a particular AT. For the provider's part, the provider must (1) list what factors and to what extent they can be an incentive or an obstacle to the use of a specific technology, (2) assess whether or not the client's resources are tailored to the characteristics of the specific technology, and finally (3) evaluate what personality traits of the client are particularly implicated in the use of the specific technology.

The WHODAS II (WHO 2004) evaluates disability from a different viewpoint than that of the normal tools of measurement. In fact, whereas the ICF Checklist was developed as a practical tool to elicit clinicians' overall impressions of a patient's condition and to record information on functioning and disability, the WHODAS II directly rates the nature of a disability from the patient's responses. Therefore, the ICF Checklist offers an external (objective) view on disability whereas the WHODAS II offers an internal (subjective) one. The WHODAS II assesses the limitations to activities and the restrictions in participation that are experienced by an individual, independently of a medical diagnosis. Specifically, the instrument is designed to evaluate the functioning of the individual in six activity domains:

1. Understanding and communicating
2. Getting around
3. Self-care
4. Getting along with people
5. Life activities
6. Participation in society

There are several different WHODAS II forms, each of which has been structured in relation to the number of items (6, 12, 24, 12 + 24, and 36), the mode of administration (self-administered or administered by an interviewer), and the user who is to be interviewed (subject, clinician, or caregiver). In any case, WHO recommends the use of the 36-item form, administered by an interviewer, for completeness. The participants who are interviewed are asked to indicate the level of "difficulty" experienced (none, mild, moderate, severe, extreme) by taking into account the way in which they normally perform a given activity, including the use of any support and/or help provided by a person (aids). For every item that receives a positive answer, the next question asks the number of days ("in the last 30 days") in which the interviewee met such a difficulty in terms of a five-point ordinal scale: (1) only 1 day; (2) up to a week (from 2 to 7 days), (3) up to 2 weeks (from 8 to 14 days), (4) more than 2 weeks (from 15 to 29 days), (5) every day (30 days). Then, the person is asked by how much the difficulties interfered with his/her life. The respondents should answer the questions according to the following references:

1. Degree of difficulty (the increase in effort, discomfort or pain, slowness, or any differences in general),
2. Health conditions (disease or illness, injury, mental or emotional problems, those related to alcohol, or problems associated with drug abuse),
3. The last 30 days,
4. The average between good and bad days, and
5. The way in which they normally perform the activity.

Items that refer to activities not experienced within the last 30 days are not included (for further information, please see Federici and Meloni 2010a, 2010b; Federici et al. 2009).

COPM (Law et al. 2005) is an individualized, client-centered measurement tool intended for detecting changes in a client's self-perception of occupational performance over time. COPM allows the user/client to formulate individualized purposes for occupational therapy and to voice their feelings about the appropriateness of their performances, their satisfaction with participation, and the importance of each goal to their lives. The specific focus of the COPM on client-identified problems is intended to facilitate collaborative goal-setting between the therapist and client. COPM is administered through a semistructured interview.

> Once clients have identified their problems, they rate their perceptions of the importance of each activity on a scale from 1 to 10. From this list, clients choose up to five problems they wish to focus on during occupational therapy. For each problem, clients then rate performance and satisfaction with performance, again using a scale from 1 to 10. Higher ratings indicate greater importance, performance, and satisfaction. The performance and satisfaction scores of the selected activities are summed and averaged over the number of problems to produce scores out of 10. (Carswell et al. 2004, p. 211)

COPM is used as an assessment tool in occupational therapy. After an initial assessment of the client and after a period of therapy, the interview is re-administered. If there are changes in scores that exceed a value of 2, the change is considered clinically significant. "Since its initial publication in 1991, the COPM has had two subsequent editions published and has been officially translated into 20 languages. It is in use by occupational therapists in over 35 countries throughout the world" (Carswell et al. 2004, p. 210).

SIS (Thompson et al. 2004) is a standardized assessment tool developed by the American Association of Intellectual and Developmental Disabilities (AAIDD) that measures the pattern and intensity of support that an individual needs. More than a diagnostic test, it is a useful tool for setting up an individualized user-centered plan. The development of SIS is compatible with the official definition of "intellectual disability" drawn up by AAIDD in 2010. This definition no longer contains the term "mental retardation," as was in use until the penultimate definition of 2002 (Schalock et al. 2007). This change reflects the transition from the perception of disability as a "deficit" to another centered on optimizing functioning. The last definition given dates back to 2010: "Intellectual disability is characterized by significant limitations both in intellectual functioning and in adaptive behavior as expressed in conceptual, social, and practical adaptive skills. This disability originates before age 18" (Schalock et al. 2010). SIS completes the 11th edition of the *Definition,*

Classification and Systems of Support for People with Intellectual and Developmental Disabilities, edited by the AAIDD, a tool that allows the theoretical definition of the support-based model to be translated into practice. The support-based model is conceptually compatible with the ICF (Schalock et al. 2010). The ICF domains of body functions (impaired intellectual functioning) and activities (limitations in adaptive behavior) directly relate to the AAIDD definition of intellectual disability. In the two systems, the person is considered as a whole within the context of the person's capacities and the expectations and supportive resources of the environment. The major difference is that the ICF is a general model of disability, whereas the AAIDD system is specific to intellectual disability. SIS consists of three sections that measure the pattern and intensity of support in six life activity domains (home living, community living, lifelong learning, employment, health and safety, and social activities), in protection and advocacy activities, and in 16 exceptional medical conditions and 13 challenging behaviors. In total, 57 various life activities are measured. The tool is administered as a semistructured interview with the user/client and at least other two people who preferably live with the user/client, such as a parent and/or a caregiver. Any other respondents should have observed the person in one or more environments for a substantial period of time. The scale ranks each activity according to frequency, amount, and type of support. Finally, a support intensity level is determined based on the total support needs index, which is a standard score generated from the scores for all items tested by the scale.

2.3.1 Outcome Analysis Tools

The main goal of the multidisciplinary team, after AT provision, is to measure and constantly monitor the effectiveness, efficiency, and safety (appropriateness) of the AT-user/client match to (1) provide support to the user/client, (2) guarantee his or her greatest level of autonomy over time, and (3) justify the resources used. The "efficacy of an assistive technology device is determined by the effect resulting from its use in comparison to the effect claimed beforehand." (Gelderblom and de Witte 2002)

To explain the reasons why an AT is used, disused, or abandoned; to verify the evolution over time of the assistive solution; and, moreover, to create and improve intervention programs for the rehabilitation field, it is necessary to identify and analyze the source of the user's satisfaction/dissatisfaction and comfort/discomfort. In general, the analysis of results obtained by the matching process is fundamental for choosing the best solution if any problem occurs during the evaluation process.

Over the last few years, some tools aimed at measuring the outcome of aids have been designed. However, the corresponding research field is growing slowly and the tools currently being used do not analyze every aspect of the AT matching process because they are only able to investigate some of the dimensions correlated with the quality of life (e.g., satisfaction, comfort, etc.). Among the most frequently used measuring tools we can include the MPT model (Scherer 1998; Scherer and Craddock 2002) and COPM (Law et al. 1990, 2005).

The QUEST questionnaire (Demers et al. 2002) measures the user/client's satisfaction with the use of AT. It can be administered to adolescents, adults, and elderly people with physical or sensory disabilities. The theoretical background of the instrument is the MPT model (Scherer 1998). Several years of implementation and research have confirmed its psychometric reliability and validity as an outcome measure of the user/client's satisfaction about the assigned AT. The QUEST does not evaluate the performance of the user with a device but rather measures his or her satisfaction with the features of the device as well as specific features of the services related to the technology and the match. The tool is not only useful for professionals and researchers but also for AT designers, manufacturers, and retailers. The questionnaire is self-administered and requires approximately 10–15 min to fill out. The minimal writing skills needed are the ability to mark the answer on a points scale and to write a comment. The three main goals of QUEST are (1) to assess the degree of satisfaction that the user attributes to the eight items relating to the aid and to the four items relating to the services, (2) to identify the sources of satisfaction or dissatisfaction of the user, and (3) to determine which aspects of satisfaction are considered most important by the user for evaluating the assistive device. The 12 items about satisfaction are divided in two parts: eight items are related to the device (size, weight control, safety, durability, ease of use, comfort, and effectiveness) and four items are related to the services. Each item is scored by the means of a five-point Likert scale ranging from 1 "not satisfied at all" to 5 "very satisfied." To explore the reasons for user satisfaction/dissatisfaction, there is a space for comments next to each item. After the 12-item list, the user/client chooses the three most important aspects for his satisfaction from within another list of 12 items. The QUEST, depending on the context, can be completed by the evaluator or by the user if the evaluator is sure about the user's understanding of the items. If the user/client does not have the motor, sensory, or cognitive skills required to complete the questionnaire, the professional can interview him/her by asking the client to verbally answer or to indicate the number chosen on the enlarged protocol sheet. If the user/client is aged 0–12 years, a parent or a caregiver may answer in his place. The QUEST provides three scores: one for the aid, one for the services, and a total score. The total score is useful for comparisons with other satisfaction measures and for determining the weight of each subscale score on overall satisfaction. Each score can vary from 1.00 (completely unsatisfied) to 5.00 (completely satisfied). The evaluation fails if the user does not answer more than six items.

The Psychosocial Impact of Assistive Devices Scale (PIADS; Day and Jutai 1996; Jutai and Day 2002) is a self-report questionnaire designed to assess the effects of an assistive device on functional independence, well-being, and quality of life. The PIADS is composed of three subquestionnaires that focus on (1) ability, which measures users' perceptions of their own competence; (2) adaptability, which measures users' willingness to explore new experiences; and (3) self-esteem, which investigates users' emotions, such as happiness, security, and confidence. The subquestionnaire focusing on ability is composed of 12 items that investigate the effectiveness of general skills (feeling of adequacy, efficiency and personal ability, etc.). The subquestionnaire on adaptability consists of six items that aim to investigate the user/client's predisposition toward taking risks and trying new experiences and their perceived feelings of well-being. The subquestionnaire on self-esteem is composed of eight items that are related to general feelings of emotional health, self-esteem, happiness, strength, and control. This questionnaire can be used to assess the impact of AT and rehabilitation processes. It can also be used to evaluate both the impact of aids, regardless of time limits, and as a comparison tool between devices and users. PIADS can be administered to both adults and children over the age of approximately 10 years old. The completion time is approximately 5 min. The participants are asked to read a list of words or phrases describing how the use of an assistive device may affect their life. Each item is rated on a seven-point Likert scale from –3 (strongly untrue) to +3 (strongly true) to indicate the level by which they feel influenced by the AT. Unlike most of the elements, which have positive values, three items—confusion (5), frustration (10), and embarrassment (21)—have a negative rating score. The participants are asked to fill in the questionnaire by ticking the box that best represents the level by which they feel influenced by using the assigned aid. PIADS can also be used to evaluate the user's expectations of the device. The questionnaire is either filled out by the user or a caregiver and can be examined manually or with a specific table to help this process.

The Individual Prioritised Problem Assessment (IPPA; Wessels et al. 2002) is an instrument that assesses both the effectiveness of AT provision and "the extent to which problems identified by an individual assistive technology user in his or her daily activities have been diminished as a result of the provision of assistive technology" (Wessels et al. 2002, p. 141). The instrument is user/customer-centered because it assesses the effectiveness in relation to the operations considered relevant by the user/customer. The IPPA allows variations over time to be checked. After the opening interview, a follow-up telephone conversation is held at least 3 months after the provision of an AT. The initial interview lasts about 10–30 min whereas the follow-up talk takes less than 15 min. During the initial interview, the user/customer has to "identify the problems that he or she experiences in everyday life and that he or she hopes are eliminated or diminished as a result of an AT provision" (Wessels et al. 2002, p. 142). The user/customer is then asked to identify up to seven problems and for each of these to complete an IPPA questionnaire. For each problem, the scores are assigned using a five-point Likert scale in which the scores reflect the importance given by the customer/user to the activities and the difficulty associated with their execution. The total score is calculated by adding the sum of the "importance" scores to the "difficulty" scores for each problem and dividing the result by the total number of issues. The value obtained is "the total average perceived inconvenience experienced by the client with respect to the problems associated with daily activities" (Wessels et al. 2002, p. 142). The higher the score, the more an individual perceives his or her life as being disturbed by these problems. The IPPA score is recalculated during the follow-up interview when the user/customer reassigns a difficulty score for each problem reported in the initial interview. The problem keeps the importance value that was assigned during the first interview. The difference between the total IPPA score before and after the supply of AT indicates the "efficacy" of the match and highlights any changes in the perceived discomfort about the problems reported. The scores also indicate the level of satisfaction the customer/user has regarding their initial expectations.

The Family Impact of Assistive Technology Scale (FIATS; Ryan et al. 2006) measures the multidimensional effects of an assistive device on families who have young children with disabilities through eight related constructs (grouped into subscales) that include child autonomy, caregiver relief, child contentment, performing activities, parent effort, family and social interaction, caregiver supervision, and safety. These constructs analyze the areas of child and family life that ATs can affect, such as the level at which a child can perform activities independently (autonomy), the way he/she interacts with others (family and social interaction), and any requests for attention from family members (supervision). Parents fill out the FIATS, indicating their agreement/disagreement levels with 64 items through a seven-point Likert scale. The FIATS also contains elements of an independent subscale (technology acceptance) to measure the general receptivity of parents to AT devices for their children. The 64 elements are divided into nine subscales. The final FIATS score is calculated by the sum of the averages of the eight subscales. Increasing scores indicate a positive overall impact on the lives of children and families, and decreasing scores suggest a negative effect on the lives of children and families.

The Assistive Technology Outcomes Measurement System (ATOM; Weiss-Lambrou 2002; Lauer et al. 2006) is a device-specific measure that was developed to meet the need for a practical clinical tool to assess AT usability and services. It consists of 19 questions for measuring seven constructs:

1. Use and community (how often an AT device is used within and outside of the home);
2. Comfort in using a device;
3. Hassle (difficulty in setting up, using, and maintaining a device);
4. Self-perceived assessment of function;
5. Assistance and burden of care (assistance required with device set-up and use, and assistance with the functional activities the AT device targets);
6. Service satisfaction (promptness, communication, courtesy, accessibility, and professionalism); and
7. User's knowledge of AT resources.

In addition to the instruments described above, there is a study that helps to assess the quality of the match via guidelines on the process: Empowering USers Through Assistive Technology (EUSTAT; EUSTAT 1999; Andrich and Besio 2002) is a study that was carried out during the period 1997–1999 within the Telematics Application Programme of the European Commission, which addressed the educational needs of end-users of AT. It produced educational material for people with disabilities, members of their family, and personal assistants, as well as guidelines for those who organize or carry out educational initiatives that facilitate the empowerment of end-users, helping them to make informed, appropriate, and responsible AT choices. The EUSTAT had both a technological and social orientation: it stemmed from the idea that people with disabilities must be active participants in the choice of their AT, thus promoting equal opportunities and also introducing direct control by the end-user over the quality of AT services and products.

2.4 Conclusions

In this chapter, we faced a twofold open question regarding the measurement of individual functioning; i.e., what does individual functioning measure, and how should it be measured? The first part is focused on the bigger issue of what variables are used as estimates when measuring functioning and disability, whereas the second part deals with guidelines and tools for measuring individual functioning. These issues arise from the nature of the disability's concept; in other words, it is a complex construct and a "multidimensional experience [that] poses several challenges for measurement" (WHO and World Bank 2011, p. 21).

A comparison of different national and international reports on disability over the course of time shows that each measurement is different and gives rise to dissimilar estimates on the prevalence of the phenomenon not only between different countries but also within the same country and at the same time. Many different aspects can cause the operational measures of disability to vary according to the prevalent notion of disability; the purpose of measurement and application; the investigated characteristics of disability; and "the definitions, question design, reporting sources, data collection methods, and expectations of functioning" (WHO and World Bank 2011, p. 21). For all of these reasons, the *World Report on Disability* (WHO and World Bank 2011) made some recommendations to improve the availability and quality of data on disability, including (1) the adoption of the ICF as a universal framework for disability data collection, (2) the improvement of national disability statistics, (3) the improvement of the comparability of data, and (4) the development of appropriate tools to fill the research gaps. With regard to the latter point, the *World Report on Disability* suggested the development of "better measures of the environment and its impact on the different aspects of disability" (WHO and World Bank 2011, p. 46) and the coupling of the evaluation of the disability experience with the measurement of the "well-being and quality of life of people with disabilities" (WHO and World Bank 2011, p. 47).

Additionally, another crucial point in the field of measurement further complicates the issue. According to Zola (1993), any attempt to identify standard measures for disability reflects the effort to consider disability as a fixed and dichotomous entity more than anything else. Conversely, Zola's universal model of disability indicated that disability is a fluid and continuous experience. Accordingly to Zola's point of view, the *World Report on Disability* repeatedly stressed this point by using the word "experience" in relation to disability and emphasizing a subjective dimension that is not reducible and not due to the level of objective measurement of functioning and disability. Disability is not a set of immutable characteristics that define a person over another or that is predictable by a medical diagnosis because it is not always a direct consequence of disease; instead, it is a multidimensional process that lasts a lifetime and involves the physical, psychological, and social spheres of individuals. Because this is a multidimensional construct, its measurement should also be multidimensional. Therefore, an underlying principle of disability measurement is not even desirable. Instead, a variety of measuring tools and the flexibility to change the procedure of measurement to adapt them to different people, contexts, and purposes provide the most reliable scientific and clinical approach.

In this chapter, we followed the approach stating that the purpose of the measurement is the guiding principle for the specification of an operational definition and for the choice of a coherent set of measurement tools. Indeed, it does not define a default set of tools but points to some guiding principles in choosing and applying a set of measures and in suggesting some tools that fit the ultimate purpose of the ATA process, i.e., "to address, in a specific context of use, the personal *well-being* of the user through the best *matching* of user/ client and assistive solution" via "clinical measures, functional analysis, and psycho-socio-environmental evaluations" (please see *The Best Measure: Is There an Elixir of Measurements for Turning an Assessment into Gold?*). The tools proposed and described in this chapter are from the following two major types: measures of individual functioning and outcome measures. The choice of the tools presented is intended to provide measures that allow the attainment of objective and comparable data in ways that most effectively seize the subjective dimension of the experience of disability.

Summary of the Chapter

This chapter is divided into three main sections. The first focuses on what individual functioning measures should be used with a focus on the principle stating that disability is a multidimensional construct and does not have an underlying principle of measurement valid for every assessment. Additionally, the only guiding principle for a proper measurement is the clarity of the purpose of the measurement. The second section focuses on how to measure individual functioning by both pointing out some guiding principles for choosing and applying a set of measures and by suggesting some tools that fit these principles. The third section suggests some measurement tools for an ATA process used in a center for technical aid.

References

Altman, B. M., and Gulley, S. P. (2009). Convergence and divergence: Differences in disability prevalence estimates in the United States and Canada based on four health survey instruments. *Social Science and Medicine, 69*(4), 543–552. doi:10.1016/j.socscimed.2009.06.017

Andrich, R., and Besio, S. (2002). Being informed, demanding and responsible consumers of assistive technology: An educational issue. *Disability and Rehabilitation, 24*(1–3), 152–159. doi:10.1080/09638280110064778

Brown, M., and Gordon, W. A. (2004). Empowerment in measurement: "muscle," "voice," and subjective quality of life as a gold standard. *Archives of Physical Medicine and Rehabilitation, 85*(2 Suppl.), S13–S20. doi:10.1016/j.apmr.2003.08.110

Carswell, A., McColl, M. A., Baptiste, S., Law, M., Polatajko, H., and Pollock, N. (2004). The Canadian Occupational Performance Measure: A research and clinical literature review. *Canadian Journal of Occupational Therapy, 71*(4), 210–222.

Day, H., and Jutai, J. (1996). Measuring the Psychosocial Impact of Assistive Devices: the PIADS. *Canadian Journal of Rehabilitation, 9*(2), 159–168.

Demers, L., Monette, M., Lapierre, Y., Arnold, D. L., and Wolfson, C. (2002). Reliability, validity, and applicability of the Quebec User Evaluation of Satisfaction with assistive Technology (QUEST 2.0) for adults with multiple sclerosis. *Disability and Rehabilitation, 24*(1–3), 21–30. doi:10.1080/09638280110066352

Demers, L., Weiss-Labrou, R., and Ska, B. (2000). Item analysis of the Quebec User Evaluation of Satisfaction with Assistive Technology (QUEST). *Assistive Technology, 12*(2), 96–105. doi:10.1080/10400435.2000.10132015

DeRuyter, F. (1995). Evaluating outcomes in assistive technology: Do we understand the commitment? *Assistive Technology, 7*(1), 3–8. doi:10.1080/10400435.1995.10132246

Elliott, T. R., Kurylo, M., and Carroll, M. N. (2002). Personality assessment in medical rehabilitation. In M. J. Scherer (Ed.), *Assistive Technology: Matching Device and Consumer for Successful Rehabilitation* (pp. 47–48). Washington, DC: American Psychological Association.

EUSTAT. (1999). *Empowering Users through Assistive Technology: Final Report.* (Project DE3402 EUSTAT). Retrieved from http://www.siva.it/research/eustat/index.html

Federici, S., and Meloni, F. (2010a). A note on the theoretical framework of World Health Organization Disability Assessment Schedule II. *Disability and Rehabilitation, 32*(8), 687–691. doi:10.3109/09638280903290012

Federici, S., and Meloni, F. (2010b). WHODAS II: Disability self-evaluation in the ICF conceptual frame. In J. Stone and M. Blouin (Eds.), *International Encyclopedia of Rehabilitation* (pp. 1–22). Buffalo, NY: Center for International Rehabilitation Research Information and Exchange (CIRRIE). Retrieved from http://cirrie.buffalo.edu/encyclopedia/en/article/299/

Federici, S., Meloni, F., Mancini, A., Lauriola, M., and Belardinelli, M. O. (2009). World Health Organisation Disability Assessment Schedule II: Contribution to the Italian validation. *Disability and Rehabilitation, 31*(7), 553–564. doi:10.1080/09638280802240498

Fulford, K. W. M., and Stanghellini, G. (2008). The third revolution: Philosophy into practice in twenty-first century psychiatry. *Dialogues in Philosophy, Mental and Neuro Sciences, 1*(1), 5–14. Retrieved from http://www.crossingdialogues.com/Ms-A08-03-6.pdf

Garber, S. L., and Gregorio, T. L. (1990). Upper extremity assistive devices: Assessment of use by spinal cord-injured patients with quadriplegia. *American Journal of Occupational Therapy, 44*(2), 126–131.

Gelderblom, G. J., and de Witte, L. P. (2002). The assessment of assistive technology outcomes, effects and costs. *Technology and Disability, 14*(3), 91–94. Retrieved from http://iospress.metapress.com/content/qf91ufxw9nwe003h/

Gelderblom, G. J., Driessen, M., Evers, H., and Claus, E. (2009). Design of a MPT based instrument supporting the quality of procurement of assistive technology. In P. L. Emiliani, L. Burzagli, A. Como, F. Gabbanini, and A.-L. Salminen (Eds.), *Assistive Technology from Adapted Equipment to Inclusive Environments: AAATE 2009* (Vol. 25, pp. 567–561). Amsterdam, The Netherlands: IOS Press. doi:10.3233/978-1-60750-042-1-557

Gitlin, L. N. (1995). Why older people accept or reject assistive technology. *Generations, 19*(1), 41–46.

Goffman, E. (Ed.). (1963). *Stigma: Notes on the Management of Spoiled Identity.* Englewood Cliffs, NJ: Spectrum Book.

Gzil, F., Lefeve, C., Cammelli, M., Pachoud, B., Ravaud, J. F., and Leplege, A. (2007). Why is rehabilitation not yet fully person-centred and should it be more person-centred? *Disability and Rehabilitation, 29*(20–21), 1616–1624. doi:10.1080/09638280701618620

Hahn, H. (1985). Introduction: Disability policy and the problem of discrimination. *American Behavioral Scientist, 28*(3), 293–318. doi:10.1177/000276485028003002

Holburn, S., and Vietze, P. (Eds.). (2002). *Person-Centered Planning: Research, Practice and Future Directions.* Baltimore, MD: PH Brookes.

Jutai, J., and Day, H. (2002). Psychosocial Impact of Assistive Devices Scale (PIADS). *Technology and Disability, 14*(3), 107–111. Retrieved from http://iospress.metapress.com/content/2rc2plwxwbhtcyta/

Kayes, N. M., and McPherson, K. M. (2010). Measuring what matters: Does 'objectivity' mean good science? *Disability and Rehabilitation, 32*(12), 1011–1019. doi:10.3109/09638281003775501

Kolcaba, K. Y. (1992). Holistic comfort: Operationalizing the construct as a nurse-sensitive outcome. *Advances in Nursing Science, 15*(1), 1–10.

Kolcaba, K. Y., and Kolcaba, R. J. (1991). An analysis of the concept of comfort. *Journal of Advanced Nursing, 16*(11), 1301–1310. doi:10.1111/j.1365-2648.1991.tb01558.x

Kupfer, D. J., First, M. B., and Regier, D. E. (2002). Introduction. In D. J. Kupfer, M. B. First, and D. A. Regier (Eds.), *A Research Agenda for DSM-V™* (pp. xv–xxiii). Washington, DC: American Psychiatric Association.

Lain Entralgo, P. (1982). *El Diagnostico Medico.* Barcelona, Spain: Salvat.

Lauer, A., Longenecker Rust, K., and Smith, R. O. (2006, August 18). ATOMS *Project Technical Report—Factors in Assistive Technology Device Abandonment: Replacing "Abandonment" with "Discontinuance."* Retrieved from http://www.r2d2.uwm.edu/atoms/archive/technicalreports/tr-discontinuance.html

Law, M., Baptiste, S., McColl, M. A., Opzoomer, A., Polatajko, H., and Pollock, N. (1990). The Canadian occupational performance measure: An outcome measure for occupational therapy. *Canadian Journal of Occupational Therapy, 57*(2), 82–87.

Law, M., Baptiste, S., McColl, M. A., Polatajko, H., and Pollock, N. (2005). *Canadian Occupational Performance Measure* (4th ed.). Ottawa, Canada: COAT.

Leplege, A., Gzil, F., Cammelli, M., Lefeve, C., Pachoud, B., and Ville, I. (2007). Person-centredness: Conceptual and historical perspectives. *Disability and Rehabilitation, 29*(20–21), 1555–1565. doi:10.1080/09638280701618661

Linder-Pelz, S. (1982). Toward a theory of patient satisfaction. *Social Science and Medicine, 16*(5), 577–582. doi:10.1016/0277-9536(82)90311-2

Long, T., Huang, L., Woodbridge, M., Woolverton, M., and Minkel, J. (2003). Integrating assistive technology into an outcome-driven model of service delivery. *Infants and Young Children, 16*(4), 272–283. doi:10.1097/00001163-200310000-00002

Madans, J. H., and Altman, B. M. (2006). *Purposes of Disability Statistics*. Paper presented at the Training Workshop on Disability statistics for SPECA countries: UN Special Programme for the Economies of Central Asia, Bishkek, Kyrgyzstan. Retrieved from http://www.unece.org/stats/documents/2006.12.health.htm

Madans, J. H., Altman, B. M., Rasch, E. K., Synneborn, M., Banda, J., Mbogoni, M., et al. (2002). Washington Group Position Paper: Proposed Purpose of an Internationally Comparable General Disability Measure, Retrieved from http://www.cdc.gov/nchs/ppt/citygroup/meeting3/WG3.6a%20Madans_Altman.ppt

Menchetti, B. M., and Sweeney, M. A. (1995). *Person-Centered Planning (Technical Assistance Packet 5)*. Gainesville, FL: University of Florida, Department of Special Education, Florida Network.

Mezzich, J. E. (2002). Comprehensive diagnosis: A conceptual basis for future diagnostic systems. *Psychopathology, 35*(2–3), 162–165. doi:10.1159/000065138

Mont, D. (2007). *Measuring Disability Prevalence. Special Protection Discussion Paper No. 0706* Retrieved from The World Bank website: http://siteresources.worldbank.org/DISABILITY/Resources/Data/MontPrevalence.pdf

Oliver, M., and Barnes, C. (1998). *Disabled People and Social Policy: from Exclusion to Inclusion*. London: Longman.

Pearson, E. J. M. (2009). Comfort and its measurement—A literature review. *Disability and Rehabilitation: Assistive Technology, 4*(5), 301–310. doi:10.1080/17483100902980950

Philips, B., and Zhao, H. (1993). Predictors of assistive technology abandonment. *Assistive Technology, 5*(1), 36–45. doi:10.1080/10400435.1993.10132205

Rust, K. L., and Smith, R. O. (2006). Perspectives of outcome data from assistive technology developers. *Assistive Technology Outcomes and Benefits, 3*(1), 34–52.

Ryan, S., Campbell, K. A., Rigby, P., Germon, B., Chan, B., and Hubley, D. (2006). Development of the new Family Impact of Assistive Technology Scale. *International Journal of Rehabilitation Research, 29*(3), 195–200. doi:10.1097/01.mrr.0000210051.94420.1b

Schalock, R. L., and Alonso, M. A. V. (2002). *Handbook on Quality of Life for Human Service Practitioners*. Washington, DC: American Association on Mental Retardation.

Schalock, R. L., Borthwick-Duffy, S., Bradley, V., Buntinx, W. H. E., Coulter, D. L., Craig, E. P. M., et al. (2010). *Intellectual Disability: Definition, Classification, and Systems of Support* (11th ed.). Washington, DC: AAIDD.

Schalock, R. L., Buntinx, W., Borthwick-Duffy, S., Luckasson, R., Snell, M., Tasse, M., et al. (2007). *User's Guide: Mental Retardation: Definition, Classification and Systems of Supports: Applications for Clinicians, Educators, Disability Program Managers, and Policy Makers* (10th ed.). Washington, DC: AAMR.

Scherer, M. J. (1998). *Matching Person & Technology. A Series of Assessments for Evaluating Predispositions to and Outcomes of Technology Use in Rehabilitation, Education, the Workplace & Other Settings*. Webster, NY: The Institute for Matching Person & Technology, Inc.

Scherer, M. J., and Craddock, G. (2002). Matching Person & Technology (MPT) assessment process. *Technology and Disability, 3*(14), 125–131. Retrieved from http://iospress.metapress.com/content/g0eft4mnlwly8y8g

Sen, A. (2002). Health: Perception versus observation. *British Medical Journal (Clinical Research Edition), 324*(7342), 860–861. doi:10.1136/bmj.324.7342.860

Sparrow, S. S., Balla, D. A., and Cicchetti, D. V. (Eds.). (1984). *Vineland Adaptive Behavior Scales*. Circle Pines, MN: American Guidance Service.

Sparrow, S. S., Cicchetti, D. V., and Balla, D. A. (2005). *Vineland Adaptive Behavior Scales* (2nd ed.). Circle Pines, MN: American Guidance Service.

Steiner, W. A., Ryser, L., Huber, E., Uebelhart, D., Aeschlimann, A., and Stucki, G. (2002). Use of the ICF model as a clinical problem-solving tool in physical therapy and rehabilitation medicine. *Physical Therapy, 82*(11), 1098–1107.

Stucki, G., Cieza, A., Ewert, T., Kostanjsek, N., Chatterji, S., and Üstün, T. B. (2002). Application of the International Classification of Functioning, Disability and Health (ICF) in clinical practice. *Disability and Rehabilitation, 24*(5), 281–282. doi:10.1080/10.1080/0963828011010522 2

Tewey, B. P., Barnicle, K., and Perr, A. (1994). The wrong stuff. *Mainstream, 19*(2), 19–23.

Thompson, J. R., Bryant, B., Campbell, E. M., Craig, E. P. M., Hughes, C., Rotholz, D. A., et al. (2004). *Supports Intensity Scale Users Manual.* Washington, DC: American Association on Mental Retardation.

Ueda, S., and Okawa, Y. (2003). The subjective dimension of functioning and disability: What is it and what is it for? *Disability and Rehabilitation, 25*(11–12), 596–601. doi:10.1080/0963828031000137108

United Nations (UN). (2001, June 4–6). *Document Index of the International Seminar on the Measurement of Disability.* Paper presented at the 1st International Seminar on the Measurement of Disability, New York. Retrieved from http://unstats.un.org/unsd/disability/Seminar%202001.html

Uppal, S. (2006). Impact of the timing, type and severity of disability on the subjective well-being of individuals with disabilities. *Social Science and Medicine, 63*(2), 525–539. doi:10.1016/j.socscimed.2006.01.016

Üstün, T. B., Chatterji, S., Bickenbach, J. E., Kostanjsek, N., and Schneider, M. (2003a). The International Classification of Functioning, Disability and Health: A new tool for understanding disability and health. *Disability and Rehabilitation, 25*(11–12), 565–571. doi:10.1080/0963828031000137063

Üstün, T. B., Chatterji, S., Bickenbach, J. E., Trotter II, R. T., and Saxena, S. (2001a). *Disability and Culture: Universalism and Diversity.* Seattle, WA: Hogrefe and Huber.

Üstün, T. B., Chatterji, S., Mechbal, A., Murray, C. J. L., and WHS Collaborating Groups. (2003b). The World Health Surveys. In C. J. L. Murray and D. B. Evans (Eds.), *Health Systems Performance Assessment: Debates, Methods and Empiricism* (pp. 797–808). Geneva, Switzerland: WHO.

Üstün, T. B., Chatterji, S., Villanueva, M., Bendib, L., Celik, C., Sadana, R., et al. (2001b). *WHO Multi-Country Survey Study on Health and Responsiveness.* (Paper Series: No. 37). Retrieved from http://www.who.int/healthinfo/survey/whspaper37.pdf

Üstün, T. B., Chatterji, S., Villanueva, M., Bendib, L., Celik, C., Sadana, R., et al. (2003c). WHO multi-country survey study on health and responsiveness 2000–2001. In C. J. L. Murray and D. B. Evans (Eds.), *Health Systems Performance Assessment: Debates, Methods and Empiricism* (pp. 761–796). Geneva, Switzerland: WHO.

Üstün, T. B., Kostanjsek, N., Chatterji, S., and Rehm, J. (Eds.) (2010). *Measuring Health and Disability: Manual for WHO Disability Assessment Schedule (WHODAS 2.0).* Geneva, Switzerland: WHO.

Verza, R., Carvalho, M. L. L., Battaglia, M. A., and Uccelli, M. M. (2006). An interdisciplinary approach to evaluating the need for assistive technology reduces equipment abandonment. *Multiple Sclerosis, 12*(1), 88–93. doi:10.1191/1352458506ms1233oa

Weiss-Lambrou, R. (2002). Satisfaction and comfort. In M. J. Scherer (Ed.), *Assistive Technology: Matching Device and Consumer for Successful Rehabilitation* (pp. 77–94). Washington, DC: American Psychological Association.

Weiss-Lambrou, R., Tremblay, C., LeBlanc, R., Lacoste, M., and Dansereau, J. (1999). Wheelchair seating aids: How satisfied are consumers? *Assistive Technology, 11*(1), 43–53. doi:10.1080/10400435.1999.10131984

Wessels, R., Persson, J., Lorentsen, Ø., Andrich, R., Ferrario, M., Oortwijn, W., et al. (2002). IPPA: Individually Prioritised Problem Assessment. *Technology and Disability, 14*(3), 141–145. Retrieved from: http://iospress.metapress.com/content/2bm793b7pbdah9bw/

World Health Organization (WHO). (1992). *ICD-10: International Statistical Classification of Diseases and Related Health Problems, 10th Revision* (Vol. 1–3). Geneva, Switzerland: WHO.

World Health Organization (WHO). (2001). *ICF: International Classification of Functioning, Disability, and Health.* Geneva, Switzerland: WHO.

World Health Organization (WHO). (2002–2004). *World Health Survey.* Retrieved from: http://www.who.int/healthinfo/survey/en/

World Health Organization (WHO). (2003). *ICF Checklist Version 2.1a, Clinician Form.* Geneva, Switzerland: WHO.

World Health Organization (WHO). (2004). *WHODAS-II—Disability Assessment Schedule Training Manual: A Guide to Administration*. Retrieved from http://www.who.int/icidh/whodas/training_man.pdf

World Health Organization (WHO). (2008). *The Global Burden of Disease: 2004 Update*. Geneva, Switzerland: WHO.

World Health Organization (WHO), and World Bank. (2011). *World Report on Disability*. Geneva, Switzerland: WHO.

Zola, I. K. (1993). Disability statistics, what we count and what it tells us: A personal and political analysis. *Journal of Disability Policy Studies, 4*(2), 9–39. doi:10.1177/104420739300400202

3

Measuring the Assistive Technology Match

F. Corradi, M. J. Scherer, and A. Lo Presti

CONTENTS

3.1 Introduction

The World Health Organization (WHO) Disability and Rehabilitation Action Plan 2006–2011 (2006) reports that approximately 10% of the world's population experiences some form of temporary or permanent disability. This document highlights that assistive technology (AT) may be a helpful aid for people with disabilities "to increase their level of independence in their daily living and to exercise their rights" (WHO 2006, p. 5). To achieve this goal, it is necessary to further the development, production, distribution, and support to use AT. In particular, the aims of the WHO are to

- Support member states to develop national policies on AT;
- Support member states to train personnel at various levels in the field of AT, especially in prosthetics and orthotics; and
- Promote research on assistive technology and facilitate transfer of technology.

WHO's *World Report on Disability* (2011) affirms this commitment.

Different studies show an average rate of approximately 30% of abandonment of AT within the first year of use, realizing that rates vary depending on the type of AT (Philips and Zhao 1993; Scherer 1998; Kittel et al. 2002; Scherer et al. 2004, 2005; Dijcks et al. 2006). A recent study (Federici and Borsci 2011) found approximately 25% AT abandonment in a local public health system and 12% abandonment in a rehabilitation project. As the authors explain, such a high rate of abandonment/discontinued use can be traced back to not focusing on the user and/or the service delivery process did not foresee a needed support before the device was delivered (Philips and Zhao 1993; Judge 2002; Scherer and Craddock 2002; Lauer et al. 2006).

However, it must be realized that only 5–15% of the population who could benefit from ATs uses them (WHO 2006). WHO hopes for a wider range of people that would benefit from such aids to achieve both functional benefits and participation in desired life situations (WHO 2002). People not receiving the AT that could benefit combined with evidence of AT abandonment highlights the fact that matching is not occurring. Thus, there is a need to perform a matching process that carefully follows an assignation model that encourage centers for technical aid to perform a systematic assessment at each step of the matching process, including post-delivery support and assistance. The need of an assignation model is connected with at least two main objectives:

1. Minimization of financial losses, which would allow more people to take advantage of appropriate technologies
2. The provision of assistive solutions that best fit a user's needs, achieving participation goals

Although a wide number of AT tools and frameworks have been developed, they tend to focus on AT outcome by, for example, the measurement of user satisfaction and/or performance of the assigned assistive technology [e.g. PIADS (Jutai and Day 2002); COPM (Law et al. 2005); QUEST (Demers et al. 1996); IPPA (Wessels et al. 2002); FIATS (Ryan et al. 2006); and ATOM (Lauer et al. 2006)]. Thus, standardized procedures and measures for the match and the assignation of AT at the time of AT selection are still needed. Although some individuals refer to the ICF as a tool that can assist the professional during the matching process (Karlsson 2010), Bernd et al. (2009) consider that even the ICF Checklist is a generic measure not developed for the purpose of assessing and addressing AT needs. A recent analysis of this issue (Bernd et al. 2009) reports a lack of reliable models and tools that can be applicable to the process of selecting AT. In fact, most of the studies in this field are literature reviews or an attempt to develop a valid model of evaluation and do not follow any experimental design criteria. The only validated instrument that is currently mentioned in the literature is the Matching Person and Technology (MPT) model (Scherer 1998). Starting from these considerations, the assistive technology assessment (ATA) process has been developed with the aim of identifying the optimal process to increase both the quality of the match of provided/supplied/purchased AT and users' realization of benefit from its use. Under this perspective, the ATA model is able to identify the steps needed to achieve the optimal match by involving different professional skills and tools for the following activities: clinical analysis, the AT matching process, environmental analysis, the assessment of outcome, and evaluation of the match of the user and selected AT over time (Scherer et al., Early Online). However, the two perspectives adopted by the MPT and the ATA model are different: The MPT process describes what needs to be measured, whereas the ATA process shows how a center for technical aid must be structured to allow for the appropriate match between user/client and AT. Nevertheless, both models share the objective of promoting the personal well-being of the users/clients by ensuring that the AT fits with their needs.

3.2 Measuring the Assistive Technology Match

The Matching Person and Technology (MPT) model is the most published model that is specific to ATA. The MPT model (Scherer 1998) argues that the characteristics of the person, environment, and technology should be considered as interacting when selecting the most appropriate AT for a particular person's use.

3.2.1 The ICF and Other Outcome Measures

The WHO International Classification of Functioning, Disability, and Health (ICF) offers a model to guide and integrate the complex aspects of assessment for AT: the biopsychosocial model, to which the MPT model refers. The ICF conceives of "disability" as the product of the interaction between the individual's characteristics and those of the physical and social environment. The disability is now defined as a "variation" of human functioning along three dimensions: impairments (the organic or psychological deficit), limitations in activity, and restrictions in participation. In particular, the ICF does not classify people, but it describes situations of each person in terms of "health domains and domains associated with it (such as education and work)." For the first time, the WHO model of disability takes into account environmental factors, classifying them systematically, allowing the correlation between health and environment and coming to the definition of disability as a health condition in an adverse environment. Information obtainable by ICF is useful not only to study disability, but also to identify appropriate interventions. For example, if the problem is an impairment, assistance will focus on the individual; if the problem is related to a restriction of participation because of discrimination, then the intervention will be directed to the elimination of social and/or environmental barriers, changing barriers in the environment and also providing facilitators, so as to improve performance in everyday life.

Although the ICF was not specifically developed to guide ATA, the literature shows that it lends itself as a descriptive model for the ATA process. ICF captures the complex aspects of the impact of AT and it can assist the professional in decision making (Bernd et al. 2009). Assessment processes based on the ICF will assist professionals in understanding the intended individual's need, facilitate collaboration across agencies, and prioritize goals for intervention. WHO defines AT as any device or system that enables a person to perform a task that would otherwise be too difficult to execute and that facilitates a task being performed (WHO 2004). AT includes both devices and services. AT services are defined as a service that supports ATA, acquisition, and device use (Bausch and Ault 2008).

Furthermore, the ICF components are well integrated in combination with some assessment instruments, such as the ICF Checklist mentioned earlier. It is compatible with the Canadian Occupational Performance Measure (COPM), the Individually Prioritised Problem Assessment (IPPA), and the Goal Attainment Scale (GAS) (Karlsson 2010). The ICF Checklist is a practical tool to elicit and record information on the functioning and disability of an individual: It elicits what capabilities and limitations the user's experience in activities and participation-related domains. It has a list of mental functions, including sensory function and pain, voice and speech functions, respiratory system, etc. The checklist assists the service provider in knowing if more specific functional assessment will be required. The COPM was developed to capture the client's individual occupational performance; it is not specific to AT, but it looks at the needs of the AT user from a client-centered perspective. Applied with other instruments, it has been found to be a useful tool for ATAs (Bernd et al. 2009). The GAS was introduced to evaluate mental health services; today it is used in pediatrics, rehabilitation, and mental health. It measures the change in response to individual goal-setting. The IPPA is a generic instrument to measure the effectiveness of any AT provision. In sum, the COPM, GAS, and IPPA are sensitive to measure change; a combination of these instruments, along with the ICF Checklist, offers service providers additional evidence-based solutions for outcome measure in AT as an alternative or complement to the MPT (Karlsson 2010).

The only AT model that is based on specific evidence and was developed to match the ICF and its checklist as found in literature is the MPT model (Scherer and Craddock 2002; Bernd et al. 2009), specifically the measure, Assistive Technology Device Predisposition Assessment (ATD PA), in which each item has been mapped to the ICF. The MPT fills a gap that considers the interactions among device characteristics, its user, and the environment. In addition to the COPM, GAS, and IPPA, the literature suggests the use of the Quebec User Evaluation of Satisfaction with Assistive Technology 2.0 (QUEST) and the Psychosocial Impact of Assistive Devices Scale (PIADS) when evaluating contextual factors such as device features and the enhancement of user's well-being, but none of these have each of their items mapped to the ICF.

3.2.2 The Matching Person and Technology Model

The MPT model is a "user-driven" and collaborative model because it is based on technology selection achieved by a partnership of the person with a disability and a professional or team of professionals to create a dialogue and make manifest different perspectives of the person's needs and appropriate supports. For the first time the person with a disability is explicitly involved in AT selection. The traditional one-way process from provider to consumer (medical model) is replaced with an approach acknowledging that the provider is a key element of the environmental influences on AT selection and realization of benefit (social model). Key influences on the selection of the most appropriate AT for any given person is distributed among the following interdependent and interactive elements to achieve a match that is as appropriate as possible (see Figure 3.1):

- Milieu/environment, or the characteristics of the architectural, built, physical, social, cultural, and attitudinal contexts in which the AT is used;
- Characteristics relating to temperament, personality, and preferences of the user; and salient features of the AT itself.

Furthermore, the MPT model contributes to the promotion of GOOD professional practice by emphasizing:

- Get the relevant information;
- Organize that information;
- Operationalize and implement the steps in the matching process of the person and the desired AT; and
- Document, review, and update the impact of the AT.

The MPT process and measures assess the individual predisposition to the use of AT (or other forms of technology) and attempts to assess the extent to which the AT

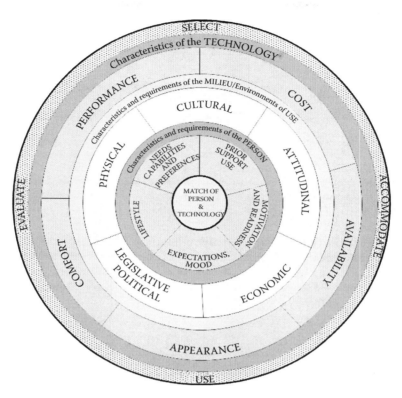

FIGURE 3.1
(See color insert.) The matching person and technology model (Scherer 2005). The "Match of Person and AT" (the smallest circle) equals the assistive solution when quality of life and well-being raise from.

is likely to be accepted and used. It is through a series of worksheets completed by the user and professional (which identify relevant factors related to the environment, technology, and person) that the professional gains information to ascertain the critical factors that influence the acceptance and use of the AT being considered. The goal is to prevent AT nonuse (abandonment) and inappropriate use by gathering information, integrating it, and using it to choose the most appropriate AT and mediate between the needs expressed by the user and those related to the environment of use. For example, use can be forecast to be partial or reluctant because of environmental factors, but good in respect to technology features and characteristics of the person; thus, the environment in which the AT will be used may need modification so that the person can get the most satisfaction and functional gain with the AT. Environmental features extend beyond physical access, often including economic resources and social support, so in the AT selection process it is essential to involve from the beginning all of the people who will be affected by the use of AT (user, caregivers, family members, employers, classmates, etc.).

The MPT perspective emerged from concern about AT abandonment. In the 1980s, scholars began to address the rehabilitation problems related to AT abandonment. The rehabilitation professionals have therefore begun to seriously study the problems of those who use AT and why they use them and those who do not and why they abandon or discard them.

Most of the research on AT use and abandonment took into consideration several factors such as cost of equipment, physical abilities needed for use, demography, product safety, and reliability. Specifically, there are three areas of study: (1) the personal characteristics of users and acceptance of technology, (2) the product features preferred by consumers, and (3) the inquiries about the AT use. Zola (1982) found that consumers prefer devices that promote independence associated with psychological and social freedoms, not only physical functioning. In addition, a number of personal factors have been identified that may affect the AT use and its acceptance, such as motivation, awareness of disability, goals of life, and effort-reward ratio. Devices that allow users to complete important tasks are more likely to be used. In most studies, acquisition cost, durability, reliability, ease of use, security features, aesthetics, ease of repair, handling/portability, and good instructions were the most important features for a good AT.

Usually the factors associated with the person are combined with the technology and environmental features. Philips and Zhao (1993) reported an abandonment of 29.3% for AT, identifying four factors that are significantly related to AT nonuse and abandonment by users regardless of type of disability:

1. Change in user needs,
2. AT was easy to obtain,
3. Low performance of the AT, and
4. Lack of consideration of the user's opinion when selecting the AT.

The highest abandonment rate occurred with mobility aids and mainly in the first year of operation, or after five years, implying an impact both at the individual level in terms of frustration and depression and at the entire health system level in terms of loss of funds and funding (Verza et al. 2006).

Zimmer and Chappell (1999) examined the receptivity of 1400 elderly people in the Canadian province of Manitoba to specific technologies to develop an appropriate model of understanding. The authors found that receptivity is influenced by the following factors: predisposition, need, social support, and the individual's level of concern for problems that could be mitigated through the use of technology. However, on closer analysis the results showed that the primary concern is home security. Older people often have to cope with chronic functional problems that limit their activities and their independence. Therefore, the technology acting on the practical difficulties of the elderly can be an opportunity to improve their quality of life and a means of coping with disability.

Few studies have investigated the use of AT by children (the pediatric population). However, in most children with disabilities, use and abandonment of assistive devices are often influenced by other people close to them, such as parents, teachers, and therapists (Caudrey and Seeger 1983).

Although there are many models in the AT literature, none of these has been proved capable of predicting AT use. Lenker and Paquet (2004) have proposed a holistic conceptual model that is user-centered, predicts AT use in terms of its perceived benefits, and considers it a decision-making process that occurs and is shaped over time and not in a moment. The use of AT has an impact on the user, the environment, and use of the technology, but at the same time, the AT impact predicts its future use.

Similar results were obtained from Verza et al. (2006), who demonstrated how a multidisciplinary approach to the evaluation of patients with multiple sclerosis who require AT can reduce AT abandonment. These authors identified four factors of abandonment: deterioration of physical state, non-acceptance of aid, failure/lack of information and training, and AT inadequacy. Most of the equipment that was abandoned was done so immediately or within the first year of use.

The predisposition to the use of technology is multifaceted and includes the needs, abilities, preferences, previous experiences with technology, personality factors, expectations, and many other variables. A cross-cultural analysis (Federici et al. 2003) confirmed the hypothesis of a relationship between self-representation of disability (assessed with the WHODAS II), coping strategies [measured by the Coping Inventory for Stressful Situation—CISS (Endler and Parker 1999)], and the individual predisposition to the use of AT [assessed with the Survey of Technology Use (SOTU)].

In all studies, we highlight the central role of the user during the whole process of AT selection (aid assignment), by informed choice, trial use, then the use of technology to produce a noticeable advantage in terms of efficiency, satisfaction, acquisition of greater autonomy, and improving the quality and way of life (Lenker and Paquet 2004). The complexity of matching user and technology requires a person-centered approach and, thus, a more complete assessment of the user before the AT selection/assignment. In addition, a better training of professionals and service providers and an appropriate training of users on the ATs will facilitate decisions regarding the AT assignment, thus reducing the likelihood of AT abandonment.

Indeed, the need to assign an AT that enhances the individual skills and quality of life often clashes with the nonuse or abandonment of AT or with the non-optimal use of it.

The MPT is the first theoretical model that has focused on the involvement of the person with a disability in the process of assigning the aid. Because the lived experience of disability is subjective and unique, there is need for a comprehensive user-centered evaluation that gives the user the opportunity to express preferences and individual and psychosocial characteristics (Scherer 2005).

According to Scherer (2002), only through a thorough evaluation can the following be identified:

- The need to change the environment or support from others to enable use of the AT,
- The impact of related limitations,
- The balance between the functional capabilities and limitations,
- The need for training and the identification of contexts for trial use (home, school, and work),
- The most cost-efficient AT for the user in terms of usability and aesthetics, and
- The extent to which the AT meets the needs of the consumer at follow-up and the existence of any unforeseen and undesirable side effects.

The ultimate goal of the selection/assignment process is to improve the performance and quality of life of the individual, in which a quality lifestyle and wellness means "the entire universe of human life domains, including physical, mental and social features that constitute what may be called a good life" (ICF 2001). If the aid does not perform this function, it will not, or rather should not be, used.

3.2.3 The MPT Process and Measures

Table 3.1 lists the MPT process and measures with their intended purpose. It endeavors to follow the GOOD principles.

TABLE 3.1

MPT Assessment Process and Forms

- **Step One:** *Initial Worksheet for the MPT Process* is organized by areas in which persons may experience loss of function (e.g., speech/communication, mobility, hearing, and eyesight) or have important strengths. It identifies initial goals and areas to strengthen through the use of a technology (or other support/strategy) or environmental accommodation. Potential interventions supportive of the goals are written in the space provided on the form. When a new technology is being introduced to a person, it is better to work from an area of strength. Each item should be addressed, regardless if a professional believes it is relevant for this individual or not. You never know what connection will be triggered or what observations will be recollected that will affect later decision-making.

- **Step Two:** *History of Support Use* is used to identify supports used is the past, satisfaction with those supports, and why a new type of support may be better than alternatives. It is organized according to the same areas of functioning as the initial worksheet in step one.

  Although steps one and two do focus on the "separate parts" of the individual, it is believed that unless each area is addressed, key barriers to optimal technology use may be missed. For example, when you focus on communication and are about to recommend a device that requires very good vision, and that has not been assessed, there may be problems if the person does have significant vision loss. The goal is to emphasize the whole person and do a comprehensive assessment considering the whole person, environments of support use, and so on, but to achieve this by considering in turn the many parts that comprise the whole and their relationship to one another.

- **Step Three:** *Specific Technology Matching.* The individual completes his or her version of the appropriate form depending on the type of technology under consideration. The modular nature of the assessments allows for the use of one, two, or more forms as well as sections of forms. The individual versions of the *Assistive Technology Device Predisposition Assessment* and *Cognitive Support Technology Device Predisposition Assessment* have the option for computerized scoring with interpretive guidelines.

  - General:
    Survey of Technology Use-Individual
    Survey of Technology Use-Professional
    A 29-item checklist that inquires into the respondent's present experiences and feelings toward technologies. The questions ask individuals to list all of the different technologies they use and feel comfortable using, the idea being that the introduction of a new technology should build upon and capitalize on existing comfort and skill. Individuals are also asked to provide information about areas regarding their general mood and preferences and social involvement that have been found in research to impact a favorable predisposition toward technology use. The professional version is identical to the students' version.

  - Assistive:
    Assistive Technology Device Predisposition Assessment-Individual
    Assistive Technology Device Predisposition Assessment-Professional
    The ATD PA inquires into individuals' subjective satisfaction with key body functions (9 items), asks individuals to prioritize aspects of their lives in which they desire the most positive change (12 items), profiles individuals' personal factors and psychosocial characteristics (33 items), and asks for individuals' opinions regarding their expectations regarding the use of a particular type of assistive device (12 items). The scales are labeled view of capabilities, subjective quality of life, family support, support from friends, mood and temperament, autonomy and self-determination, self-esteem, and readiness for technology use. The final section allows for the comparison of competing devices and rates the device and person match. The ATD PA (professional form) allows the professional to determine and evaluate incentives and disincentives to the use of the device by a particular person.

  - Cognitive Support:
    Cognitive Support Technology Device Predisposition Assessment-Individual
    Cognitive Support Technology Device Predisposition Assessment-Professional
    The CST PA is structured like the ATD PA above, but it has an additional six items in body functions focused on Specific Mental Functions:
    - Paying attention, not getting distracted
    - Remembering information about people or events

TABLE 3.1 (CONTINUED)

MPT Assessment Process and Forms

- Educational:

  Educational Technology Device Predisposition Assessment-Student

  Educational Technology Device Predisposition Assessment-Teacher

  The ET PA is a 43-item form designed to assess student and educator perspectives in four key areas: (1) educational goal and need, (2) particular educational technology under consideration, (3) psychosocial environments in which the technology will be used, and (4) student learning style and preferences.

- Workplace:

  Workplace Technology Device Predisposition Assessment-Individual

  Workplace Technology Device Predisposition Assessment-Employer

  The 28 items in the WT PA address key characteristics of the technology being proposed, the person or employee, and the workplace.

- Health care:

  Healthcare Technology Device Predisposition Assessment-Professional

  The 42-item HCT PA is a checklist addressing characteristics of the particular health problem, health-care technology, likely consequence of HCT use, personal issues, and attitudes of significant others toward the course of treatment.

  Each of the individual forms may serve as a guide for an oral interview if that seems more appropriate for the situation. The professional completes the professional version of the same form and identifies any discrepancies in perspective between the professional's and the individual's responses. These discrepancies then become a topic for discussion and counseling.

- **Step Four:** The professional discusses with the individual those factors that may indicate problems with his or her acceptance or appropriate use of the technology.

- **Step Five:** After problem areas (barriers, limitations) have been noted, the professional and individual work to identify specific intervention strategies and devise an action plan to address the problems.

- **Step Six:** The strategies and action plans are committed to writing, for experience has shown that plans that are merely verbalized are not implemented as frequently as written plans. Written plans also serve as documentation and can provide the justification for any subsequent actions such as requests for funding or release time for training.

- **Step Seven:** A follow-up assessment is conducted to determine any adjustments or accommodations needed to the technology and to inquire into realization of benefit, goal achievement, and whether the individual consumer has changed priorities. The measures in *Step Three: Specific Technology Matching* are used at baseline/initial assessment and then again at follow-up to determine change over time for a particular person.

The measures in Table 3.1, especially the ATD PA, are consistently reliable and valid (Scherer and Cushman 1995; Vincent and Morin 1999; Goodman et al. 2002; Gatti et al. 2004; Scherer and Sax 2010). Significant correlations are with the following factors: quality of life, mood, support from others, motivation for AT use, program/therapist reliance, self-determination/self-esteem (Scherer et al. 2005), environmental factors of the ICF (Scherer and Glueckauf 2005), Satisfaction with Life Scale (SWLS), Brief Symptom Inventory (BSI) (Scherer and Cushman 1995), and psychosocial aspects (Brown and Merbitz 1995; Brown, 1997).

Furthermore, a recent study aimed at analyzing the use of brain computer interfaces (BCIs) compared with the use of eye-tracking systems in subjects with amyotrophic lateral sclerosis (ALS) found significant correlations between several factors assessed with the ATD PA (AT, environment, disability, character) and other measures such as usability, mood, motivation, and cognitive load. The study highlights the crucial role of the living environment on the use of the assigned AT to promote a satisfactory experience with it.

This study confirms the previously mentioned studies and supports the use of the ATD PA as an appropriate tool for the assessment of the predisposition to AT.

3.2.4 The MPT Model and the ICF

The different measures in the MPT process are compatible with the ICF and allow the assessment of relevant domains affected by the use of technology. Table 3.2 lists the major domains of the ICF, some examples of AT and other forms of support, and the most appropriate MPT measure for the evaluation of each ICF domain (based on Scherer and Glueckauf 2005).

3.2.5 Different Versions of Matching Person and Technology

To provide relevant measures for the various interests and needs of people with disabilities across age groups, there are separate versions of MPT. The evaluation process for Matching Assistive Technology and Child (MATCH) was designed by Scherer (1997) within the MPT model to provide a person-centered approach for the assessment of individual predisposition to the use of AT by infants and children between 0 and 5 years of age with a separate version for those children of school age.

The MATCH process consists of a series of tools designed for those who aim to obtain a better match between the child and support in the form of technologies, i.e., producers and evaluators of AT, social and family care centers, coordinators of centers for technical aid, psychotechnologists, therapists, and parents. Other adaptations of the MPT are designed to address specific disabilities or specific areas of evaluation, e.g., the Cognitive Support Technology Predisposition Assessment (Scherer et al., Early Online).

3.3 The Assistive Technology Assessment Process

AT plays a crucial role in supporting the social integration of people with disabilities. The AT matching process involves a sequential and articulated series of assessments conducted by experts with different professional skills: A successful matching process is determined by both the assessment protocol model and the skills of the multidisciplinary team. The matching process takes place in centers specializing in AT in which a team of experts plays a mediating role between AT and person with a disability. In Western countries, this process is characterized by two seemingly opposing models: In one, more prevalent in some European countries (e.g., Italy), the person who needs an AT is considered as a user/patient; in the other model, more common in Anglo-Saxon countries, the person is rather a consumer or customer. This difference is related to differences in policies toward assistance services. In fact, in the first case, the center does not sell products, but it only provides assistance and evaluation services; in the second case, the center for technical aids may also manufacture and sell the AT that it provides. Compared with the second model, which emphasizes the centrality of customer satisfaction, the first model grants a more neutral approach in the evaluation and the assignation of the technology. The ATA process describes both the skills and functions of the multidisciplinary team involved during the matching process and their mutual interaction. The ATA process can be read both from the user/customer's point of view and from the point of view of the center for technical aid (see Section 3.1).

TABLE 3.2

List of the Major Domains of the ICF, of Some Examples of AT and Other Forms of Support, and of the Most Appropriate MPT Measure for the Evaluation of Each ICF Domain

ICF Activities and Participation	Examples of AT and Other Supports	MPT Measure
LEARNING AND APPLYING KNOWLEDGE: Learning, applying the knowledge that is learned, thinking, solving problems, and making decisions.	Note-taking, real-time captioning services, personal digital assistant (PDA) and laptop computers, audio recording devices, computer software, electronic calculators	SOTU, ET PA, CST PA, MST
GENERAL TASKS AND DEMANDS: Carrying out single or multiple tasks, organizing routines, and handling stress.	Personal assistance, service animals, timers, memory aids	ATD PA Sections B and C
COMMUNICATION: Communicating by language, signs, and symbols, including receiving and producing messages, carrying on conversations, and using communication devices and techniques.	Sign language interpreters, electronic and manual communication devices, computer input and output devices, modified telephones and text messaging devices, radio and television adaptations, signaling and alerting devices	Initial Worksheet, History of Support Use, ATD PA Section B, HT PA
MOBILITY: Changing body position or location or transferring from one place to another by carrying, moving, or manipulating objects; by walking, running, or climbing; and by using various forms of transportation.	Manual and power wheelchairs, canes and walkers, transfer boards, vehicle modifications, lifts, relief maps, global positioning system (GPS)	ATD PA Sections A and B
SELF-CARE: Caring for oneself, washing and drying oneself, caring for one's body and body parts, dressing, eating and drinking, and looking after one's health.	Modified eating utensils, nonslip mats, robotic devices, buttonhooks, liquid soap dispensers, electric toothbrushes	ATD PA Sections A and B
DOMESTIC LIFE: Acquiring a place to live, food, clothing, and other necessities; household cleaning and repairing; caring for personal and other household objects; and assisting others.	Bottle and can openers, tilt tables, modified lighting, support bars and rails, remote- or voice-activated environmental controls	ATD PA Sections A and B
INTERPERSONAL INTERACTIONS AND RELATIONSHIPS: Basic and complex interactions with people (strangers, friends, relatives, family members, and lovers) in a contextually and socially appropriate manner.	Manual and electronic communication devices, life skills coach, sexual aids	ATD PA Sections B and C
MAJOR LIFE AREAS: Tasks and actions required to engage in education, work, and employment and to conduct economic transactions.	Remote control devices, customized workstations, structural modifications, alternative computer access	ATD PA Sections A and B, other MPT measures
COMMUNITY, SOCIAL, AND CIVIC LIFE: Actions and tasks required to engage in organized social life outside of the family in community, social, and civic areas of life.	Signaling and alerting devices, noise reduction devices, adapted recreational and leisure devices, transportation accommodations	ATD PA Sections A and B, other MPT measures

Source: Based on Scherer, M. J. and Glueckauf, R., *Rehabilitation Psychology*, *50*(2), 132–141, 2005. doi:10.1037/0090-5550.50.2.132

The ATA is a user-driven process through which the selection of one or more AT devices for an assistive solution is facilitated by the comprehensive utilization of clinical measures, functional analysis, and psycho-socio-environmental evaluations that address, in a specific context of use, the personal well-being of the user through the best matching of user/client and assistive solution (Scherer et al., Early Online).

ATA under the lens of the ICF biopsychosocial model (see Section 3.1):

- The ICF biopsychosocial model is our lens for viewing the ATA process.
- The user (request) seeks a solution for one or more ICF components: body functions and structures (health conditions), activities, and participation, all within the context consisting of personal and environmental factors.
- The user request triggers the user-driven process.
- The user-driven process begins with the ATA for an assistive solution.
- The assistive solution is facilitated by the comprehensive utilization of clinical measures, functional analysis, and psycho-socio-environmental evaluations.
- The user request is satisfied with the best matching of user/client and assistive solution (including user well-being and realization of benefit from AT use).

The centre for technical aid verifies the user's satisfaction and realization of benefit by activating support and follow-up. User well-being continues as long as the solution, with support and follow-up, remains a good match (Scherer et al., Early Online).

3.3.1 The ATA Process in the Center for Technical Aid and in the Rehabilitation Project

The ATA is the ideal process recommended for a public or private center for technical aid. However, some studies highlight significant data concerning the AT matching in the rehabilitation arena (Verza et al. 2006; Federici and Borsci 2011). Federici and Borsci (2011) have conducted a survey on a large scale on satisfaction with and use of AT within specific public paths (center for technical aid) and within the rehabilitation project. Such a survey highlights a very definite difference between the two processes, showing significantly different abandonment rates: in case of specific paths the abandonment rate is approximately 25% (i.e., below international averages, which show rates of approximately 30%, although it is in line with them if we consider that the ATs studied are only hearing aids and stair lifts). On the other hand, in the case of rehabilitation projects, the abandonment rate goes down to 12%. Moreover, within specific paths without a dedicated rehabilitation service, there is great variability as far as the assignment processes are concerned, which highlights the existence of many possible processes in the assignment of AT. The ATA process allows a general standardization of processes that indicates essential elements in a successful matching path. Actually, according to the analysis of Federici and Borsci (2011), it is clear that they lack some indispensable steps in attaining a good match between user and AT. In particular, all processes registered in the area do not consider as part of the assignment process a follow-up assessment service that is able to manage user-related problems and users' frustrations. The lack of follow-up services is one of the main factors that may cause the abandonment of aids/AT in the research centers.

According to another study conducted in the area of rehabilitation, another relevant factor emerges concerning a low abandonment rate (Verza et al. 2006). A reduction of 28% (9.5% up to 37.3%) was credited to the intervention of a multidisciplinary team (physical therapist, occupational therapist, physician in physical medicine and rehabilitation, and psychologist) and the direct involvement of user and his/her home environment in the AT matching process.

In the same study, the possibility is considered of a further reduction in abandonment by using measurement tools of predisposition to AT such as the MPT. The importance of the main role of the home and personal environment in the use of the matched technology (aid/AT) and an outcome of a satisfactory experience with the AT has also been pointed out by Pasqualotto et al. (2011).

The ATA process sets out the guidelines of the process assignation of an AT and calculates both the intervention of a multidisciplinary team by the involvement of the user and his/her environment and the assistance services as well as recurrent follow-ups, strictly related to the possibility of the need to reassess the used AT.

3.4 The MPT and the Assistive Technology Assessment Process

The MPT process allows the measurement and evaluation of the matching between user and AT through the different measurement tools in the MPT package (SOTU, ATD PA, CSTPA, ETPA, WTPA, and HCTPA). On the other hand, the ATA process is a system of organizing the AT assignment within a center for technical aids and allows professionals to view and manage step by step the articulation of the path that the user follows to achieve the optimal match. In part, the MPT process coincides, or rather is to operate within, the ATA process because both have as their objective the optimal matching of user and AT, except that the MPT process is an assessment method and includes matching measures, whereas the ATA process is a functioning process that guides an AT assignment. The ATA process may thus accompany the successful development of a matching process through the MPT process. The model underlying the MPT and the ATA process is the same, namely a "user-centered" model that is based on a biopsychosocial model of disability (i.e., the ICF). However, the outlook is different: The MPT process describes what should be measured, whereas the ATA process indicates how a center for technical aid is set up in the management of matching user and AT. Specifically, the ATA process provides information and guidelines regarding the setting, the professionals to which the user must contact, the collection of information, the center of technical aid management, the multidisciplinary team involved in the matching process, etc. Within this structured and multidimensional setting, the MPT fits as a model, an assessment tool, and an "outcome measure" of the match achieved. The MPT model underlying the ATA process allows the use of a series of measures that provide a person-centered approach able to identify the best AT that fits the user's needs. This goal can be reached through a collaborative approach in which the user/client and the professional of the multidisciplinary team cooperate during the evaluation processes. Within the ATA process, the different items provided by the MPT can be effectively used by the multidisciplinary team to determine the expectations of user/customer and define the aims (Initial Worksheet and History of Support Use), carry out surveys on the technologies used, and analyze in this way the related users' satisfaction (Survey of Technology Use—SOTU) and carry out assessments of the AT user/customer's predisposition to use and aid/AT (Assistive Technology Device Predisposition Assessment—ATD PA).

In this way, the ATA process is able to guide the work within a center for technical aid and allow professionals to regularly monitor all of the factors that would promote the user/customer's personal well-being through the best combination of their needs and the assistive solution. At the same time, the ATA process would allow obstacles to be identified and overcome that could have a negative impact on the assignation process, such as

- Lack of financial resources for the purchase, evaluation, testing, and training of AT;
- A multidisciplinary team composed of professionals that have not been previously trained to cooperate to the matching process and assist the AT user/client; and
- Processes built that do not consider user/customer's needs, priorities, preferences, and participation in the choice of the AT.

The MPT model aims to help professionals to obtain the best match by using different measures that have been validated within the biopsychosocial context (Scherer and Sax 2010). Both process and measures would contribute to the promotion of user/client personal well-being by identifying the best AT within a well-defined process, with trained professionals and in a completely user-driven model.

3.5 Conclusions

According to Scherer (2002), only through a thorough evaluation can the following be identified:

- The need to modify the environment or support for aid/AT use,
- The impact of limitations on the performance of activities and participation in desired life roles and settings,
- The balance between functional capabilities and limitations,
- The need for training and the identification of contexts for trial use (home, school, work),
- The most cost-efficient AT/aid for the user in terms of usability and aesthetics, and
- The extent to which the AT/aid meets the needs of the consumer and the existence of any undesirable side effects through a follow-up evaluation.

The ultimate goal of the assignment process of an aid/AT is to improve the functioning and quality of life of a person with a disability, and many such individuals, where quality of life and wellness means, in a general sense, "the universe of domains of life, including physical, mental and social features which constitute what may be called a *good life*" (ICF 2001). If the aid/AT does not perform this function, it will not, or rather should not, be used. Using the MPT process within the ATA process could help professionals achieve a better matching between user and AT and, thus, a reduction in AT abandonment.

Summary of the Chapter

In this chapter, the assistive technology assessment (ATA) model has been presented. The ATA model outlines an ideal process that provides reference guidelines for both public and private centers for technical aid provision, allowing them to compare, evaluate, and improve their own matching model. The actions required by the ATA model to centers for technical aid can be divided into four fundamental steps: access to the structure and activation of the process, evaluation and activation of the aid/AT selection, delivery, and follow-up. The ATA is a user-driven process through which the selection of one or more aids/ AT is facilitated by the utilization of comprehensive clinical measures, functional analysis, and psycho-socio-environmental evaluations that address, in a specific context of use, the personal well-being of the user through the best matching of user/client and assistive solution (Scherer et al., Early Online). Because the ATA process and the MPT model and accompanying measures share a user-driven working methodology and embrace the ICF biopsychosocial model, they can be integrated within a path aiming for the best combination of AT to promote user/customer's personal well-being.

References

Bausch, M., and Ault, M. (2008). Assistive technology implementation plan: A tool for improving outcomes. *Teaching Exceptional Children, 41*(1), 6–14. Retrieved from http://cec.metapress.com/content/K57165H1X52W5731

Bernd, T., Van Der Pijl, D., and De Witte, L. P. (2009). Existing models and instruments for the selection of assistive technology in rehabilitation practice. *Scandinavian Journal of Occupational Therapy, 16*(3), 146–158. doi:10.1080/11038120802449362

Brown, D. L. (1997). Personal implications of functional electrical stimulation standing for older adolescents with spinal cord injuries. *Technology and Disability, 6*(3), 199–216. doi:10.1016/s1055-4181(96)00038-6

Brown, D. L., and Merbitz, C. (1995). *Comparison of Technology Match between Two Types of Functional Electrical Stimulation Hand Grasp Systems*. Paper presented at the RESNA '95 Annual Conference: RECREAbility. Recreation and Ability: Explore the Possibilities!, Arlington, VA. Retrieved from http://books.google.com/books?id = d1BRAAAAMAAJ

Caudrey, D. J., and Seeger, B. R. (1983). Rehabilitation engineering service evaluation: A follow-up study of device effectiveness and patient acceptance. *Rehabilitation Literature, 44*(3–4), 80–85.

Demers, L., Weiss-Lambrou, R., and Ska, B. (1996). Development of the Quebec User Evaluation of Satisfaction with assistive Technology (QUEST). *Assistive Technology, 8*(1), 3–13. doi:10.1080/10400435.1996.10132268

Dijcks, B. P. J., De Witte, L. P., Gelderblom, G. J., Wessels, R. D., and Soede, M. (2006). Non-use of assistive technology in The Netherlands: A non-issue? *Disability and Rehabilitation: Assistive Technology, 1*(1–2), 97–102. doi:10.1080/09638280500167548

Endler, N. S., and Parker, J. D. A. (1999). *Coping Inventory for Stressful Situations (CISS): Manual* (2nd ed.). North Tonawanda, NY: Multi-Health Systems.

Federici, S., and Borsci, S. (2011). *The use and non-use of assistive technology in Italy: A pilot study*. In G. J. Gelderblom, M. Soede, L. Adriaens, and K. Miesenberger (Eds.), Everyday Technology for Independence and Care: AAATE 2011 (Vol. 29, pp. 979–986). Amsterdam, NL: IOS Press. doi:10.3233/978-1-60750-814-4-979

Federici, S., Corradi, F., Mele, M. L., and Miesenberger, K. (2011). *From cognitive ergonomist to psychotechnologist: A new professional profile in a multidisciplinary team in a centre for technical aids*. In G. J. Gelderblom, M. Soede, L. Adriaens, and K. Miesenberger (Eds.), Everyday Technology for Independence and Care: AAATE 2011 (Vol. 29, pp. 1178–1184). Amsterdam, NL: IOS Press. doi:10.3233/978-1-60750-814-4-1178

Federici, S., Corradi, F., Lo Presti, A., & Scherer, M. J. (2009). The Adaptation and Use of the Italian Version of the *Matching Assistive Technology and CHild* (MATCH) Measure. In P. L. Emiliani, L. Burzagli, A. Como, F. Gabbanini, and A.-L. Salminen (Eds.), *Assistive Technology from Adapted Equipment to Inclusive Environments: AAATE* 2009 (Vol. 25, pp. 562–566). Amsterdam, NL: IOS Press. doi:10.3233/978-1-60750-042-1-562

Federici, S., Scherer, M. J., Micangeli, A., Lombardo, C., and Olivetti Belardinelli, M. (2003). A cross-cultural analysis of relationships between disability self-evaluation and individual predisposition to use assistive technology. In G. M. Craddock, L. P. McCormack, R. B. Reilly, and H. T. P. Knops (Eds.), *Assistive Technology—Shaping the Future* (pp. 941–946). Amsterdam, The Netherlands: IOS Press.

Gatti, N., Matteucci, M., and Sbattella, L. (2004). An adaptive and predictive environment to support augmentative and alternative communication. In K. Miesenberger, J. Klaus, W. Zagler, and D. Burger (Eds.), *Computers Helping People with Special Needs* (Vol. 3118, pp. 624–631). Heidelberg, Germany: Springer. doi:10.1007/978-3-540-27817-7_144

Goodman, G., Tiene, D., and Luft, P. (2002). Adoption of assistive technology for computer access among college students with disabilities. *Disability and Rehabilitation*, 24(1–3), 80–92. doi:10.1080/09638280110066307

Judge, S. (2002). Family-centered assistive technology assessment and intervention practices for early intervention. *Infants and Young Children*, 15(1), 60–68. doi:10.1097/00001163-200207000-00009

Jutai, J., and Day, H. (2002). Psychosocial Impact of Assistive Devices Scale (PIADS). *Technology and Disability*, 14(3), 107–111. Retrieved from http://iospress.metapress.com/content/2rc2plwxwbhtcyta/

Karlsson, P. (2010). *ICF: A Guide to Assistive Technology Decision-Making*. Paper presented at the ARATA 2010 National Conference, Hobart, Tasmania. Retrieved from http://www.arata.org.au/arataconf10/index.html

Kittel, A., Di Marco, A., and Stewart, H. (2002). Factors influencing the decision to abandon manual wheelchairs for three individuals with a spinal cord injury. *Disability and Rehabilitation*, 24(1–3), 106–114. doi:10.1080/0963828011006678 5

Lauer, A., Longenecker Rust, K., and Smith, R. O. (2006, August 18). ATOMS Project technical report—Factors in assistive technology device abandonment: Replacing "abandonment" with "discontinuance." Retrieved from http://www.r2d2.uwm.edu/atoms/archive/technicalreports/tr-discontinuance.html

Law, M., Baptiste, S., McColl, M. A., Polatajko, H., and Pollock, N. (2005). *Canadian Occupational Performance Measure* (4th ed.). Ottawa, Canada: COAT.

Lenker, J. A., and Paquet, V. L. (2004). A new conceptual model for assistive technology outcomes research and practice. *Assistive Technology*, 16(1), 1–10. doi:10.1080/10400435.2004.10132069

Pasqualotto, E., Federici, S., Simonetta, A., and Olivetti Belardinelli, M. (2011, August 31-September 2). *Usability of Brain Computer Interfaces*. Paper presented at the 11th European Conference for the Advancement of Assistive Technology: AAATE 2011, Maastricht, The Netherlands. Retrieved from http://www.aaate2011.eu/

Philips, B., and Zhao, H. (1993). Predictors of assistive technology abandonment. *Assistive Technology*, 5(1), 36–45. doi:10.1080/10400435.1993.10132205

Ryan, S., Campbell, K. A., Rigby, P., Germon, B., Chan, B., and Hubley, D. (2006). Development of the new Family Impact of Assistive Technology Scale. *International Journal of Rehabilitation Research*, 29(3), 195–200. doi:10.1097/01.mrr.0000210051.94420.1b

Scherer, M. J. (1997). *Matching Assistive Technology and Child: A Process and Series of Assessments for Selecting and Evaluating Technologies Used by Infants & Young Children*. Webster, NY: The Institute for Matching Person & Technology, Inc.

Scherer, M. J. (1998). *Matching Person & Technology. A Series of Assessments for Evaluating Predispositions to and Outcomes of Technology Use in Rehabilitation, Education, the Workplace & Other Settings*. Webster, NY: The Institute for Matching Person & Technology, Inc.

Scherer, M. J. (2005). *Living in the State of Stuck: How Technologies Affect the Lives of People with Disabilities* (4th ed.). Cambridge, MA: Brookline Books.

Scherer, M. J. (Ed.). (2002). *Assistive Technology: Matching Device and Consumer for Successful Rehabilitation*. Washington, DC: American Psychological Association.

Scherer, M. J., and Craddock, G. (2002). Matching Person & Technology (MPT) assessment process. *Technology & Disability, 3*(14), 125–131. Retrieved from http://iospress.metapress.com/content/g0eft4mnlwly8y8g

Scherer, M. J., and Cushman, L. A. (1995). Differing therapist-patient views of assistive technology use and implications for patient education and training. *Archives of Physical Medicine and Rehabilitation, 76*(6), 595. Retrieved from http://download.journals.elsevierhealth.com/pdfs/journals/0003-9993/PIIS0003999395805214.pdf

Scherer, M. J., Cushman, L. A., and Federici, S. (2004, June 1–10). *Measuring Participation and the Disability Experience with the "Assistive Technology Device Predisposition Assessment."* Paper presented at the North American Collaborating Center 10th Annual Conference on ICF: NACC 2004, Halifax, Canada. Retrieved from http://secure.cihi.ca/cihiweb/en/downloads/10NACC_Conf_Report_FINAL_e.pdf

Scherer, M. J., Federici, S., Tiberio, L., Pigliautile, M., Corradi, F., and Meloni, F. (Early Online). ICF core set for Matching Older Adults with Dementia and Technology. *Ageing International*. doi:10.1007/s12126-010-9093-9

Scherer, M. J., and Glueckauf, R. (2005). Assessing the benefits of assistive technologies for activities and participation. *Rehabilitation Psychology, 50*(2), 132–141. doi:10.1037/0090-5550.50.2.132

Scherer, M. J., and Sax, C. L. (2010). Measures of assistive technology predisposition and use. In E. Mpofu and T. Oakland (Eds.), *Rehabilitation and Health Assessment. Applying ICF Guidelines* (pp. 229–254). New York: Springer.

Scherer, M. J., Sax, C. L., Vanbiervliet, A., Cushman, L. A., and Scherer, J. V. (2005). Predictors of assistive technology use: The importance of personal and psychosocial factors. *Disability and Rehabilitation, 27*(21), 1321–1331. doi:10.1080/09638280500164800

Verza, R., Carvalho, M. L., Battaglia, M. A., and Uccelli, M. M. (2006). An interdisciplinary approach to evaluating the need for assistive technology reduces equipment abandonment. *Multiple Sclerosis, 12*(1), 88-93. doi:10.1191/1352458506ms1233oa

Vincent, C., and Morin, G. (1999). L'utilisation ou non des aides techniques: Comparaison d'un modèle américain aux besoins de la réalité Québécoise. *Canadian Journal of Occupational Therapy, 66*(2), 92–101.

Wessels, R. D., Persson, J., Lorentsen, Ø., Andrich, R., Ferrario, M., Oortwijn, W., et al. (2002). IPPA: Individually Prioritised Problem Assessment. *Technology and Disability, 14*(3), 141–145. Retrieved from http://iospress.metapress.com/content/2bm793b7pbdah9bw/

World Health Organization (WHO). (2001). *ICF: International Classification of Functioning, Disability, and Health*. Geneva, Switzerland: WHO.

World Health Organization (WHO). (2002). *Towards a Common Language for Functioning, Disability and Health: ICF The International Classification of Functioning, Disability and Health*. Retrieved from http://www.who.int/classifications/icf/training/icfbeginnersguide.pdf

World Health Organization (WHO). (2004). *A Glossary of Terms for Community Health Care and Services for Older Persons*. (WHO/WKC/Tech.Ser./04.2). Retrieved from http://whqlibdoc.who.int/wkc/2004/WHO_WKC_Tech.Ser._04.2.pdf

World Health Organization (WHO). (2006). *Disability and Rehabilitation WHO Action Plan 2006-2011*. Retrieved from http://www.who.int/disabilities/publications/dar_action_plan_2006to2011.pdf

World Health Organization (WHO), and World Bank. (2011). *World Report on Disability*. Geneva, Switzerland: WHO.

Zimmer, Z., and Chappell, N. L. (1999). Receptivity to new technology among older adults. *Disability and Rehabilitation, 21*(5–6), 222–230. doi:10.1080/096382899297648

Zola, I. K. (1982). *Disincentives to Independent Living*. Kansas City, KS: University of Kansas.

4

The Assessment of the Environments of AT Use: Accessibility, Sustainability, and Universal Design

M. Mirza, A. Gossett Zakrajsek, and S. Borsci

CONTENTS

4.1 Introduction

The role of the environment in inhibiting or supporting full societal participation of people with disabilities is increasingly being acknowledged. Theoretical frameworks of disability such as the social model (Oliver 1990) and the International Classification of Functioning, Disability, and Health (ICF; WHO 2001) recognize the role of the environment in "producing" disability, albeit to varying extents. Even the preamble of the United Nations (UN) Convention on the Rights of Persons with Disabilities affirms that disability results from the interaction between individuals with impairments and environmental barriers (UN 2006).

Furthermore, research studies have repeatedly underscored the dynamic relationship between environmental factors and the community participation of people with disabilities (Egilson and Traustadottir 2009; Verdonschot et al. 2009). In addition, there is a robust body of literature demonstrating that conflict between assistive technology (AT) and its context of use is an important contributor to AT nonuse and abandonment (Philips and Zhao 1993; Day et al. 2001; Kittel et al. 2002; Scherer 2002; Scherer et al. 2004, 2005; Dijcks et al. 2006; Laueret al. 2006; Söderström and Ytterhus 2010). In light of this evidence, any assistive technology assessment (ATA) process would be significantly incomplete without a systematic consideration of how the user's environment influences the acceptance of AT, its utilization, and the user's participation in various life activities.

This chapter provides a rationale and framework for incorporating the environment within the ATA process. In the past, some AT manuals and guides have addressed this area with a primary focus on microenvironments such as the home, school, and workplace (Mann and Lane 1991; Church and Glennen 1992). In this chapter, we take a broader view of the environment and understand the environment to comprise physical, social, cultural, legislative, and economic components. However, our goal is not to prescribe specific measures and tools for evaluating each of these components. Instead, we offer an innovative model for considering the environment within the ATA process more broadly and holistically and along the three dimensions of accessibility, sustainability, and universal design (UD).

This chapter is divided into three sections. In Section 4.2, we introduce the concepts of accessibility, sustainability, and UD and describe two models depicting the interaction between these concepts. In Section 4.3, we discuss how an environmental assessment framework incorporating these three dimensions can inform the ATA process and illustrate a step-by-step evaluation of the environment to support decision-making within the ATA process. Finally, in Section 4.4, we provide an example illustrating how the concepts and processes described in Sections 4.2 and 4.3 can be applied within an actual case.

4.2 Accessibility, Sustainability, and Universal Design: An Overview

Examining the environment in terms of accessibility, sustainability, and UD offers ways of making the ATA process more comprehensive, relevant, and in line with contemporary and future conceptual and geopolitical trends.

4.2.1 What Do We Mean by Accessibility, Sustainability, and Universal Design?

Traditionally, assessments and interventions targeting the environment have tended to draw upon the concept of accessibility. In the United States, the first structured guidelines codifying accessibility of the built environment, known by the acronym ADAAG (Americans with Disabilities Act Accessibility Guidelines), were created in 1990 (U.S. Access Board 2004). Likewise, other countries around the globe have developed accessibility standards, some of which are informed by legislation (Dion et al. 2006). In Europe, through work of the European Institute for Design and Disability (EIDD Design for All Europe) network, the *Build for All Reference Manual* was created in 2006 to organize and promote accessibility within the built environment (Build-for All Project 2006). Build-for-All aims to "enable all people to have equal opportunities to participate in every aspect of society. To achieve this, the built environment, everyday objects, services, culture and information—in short, everything that is designed and made by people to be used by people—must be accessible, convenient for everyone in society to use and responsive to evolving human diversity" (EIDD Design for All Europe 2004; Build-for All Project 2006).

Although these standards and policies were primarily geared toward promoting accessibility for people with disabilities, the current international trend has progressed toward a broader definition of the population that could benefit from "accessible" environments. This broadening definition of the user population is expressed in the philosophy of UD. Universal design is a term used to describe the designing of all products and the built environment in an inconspicuous manner to be both aesthetic and usable to the greatest extent possible by everyone, regardless of their age, ability, or status in life (Mace et al. 1991). Elsewhere, it has been defined as a movement that approaches the design of the environment, products, and communications with the widest range of users in mind (Knecht 2004) and as a process of embedding choice for all people in design (Salmen 2008).

Whereas accessibility is seen as removal of barriers and addition of special features specifically for use by people with disabilities, UD is seen as providing environments that can be fully experienced by all people. Accessibility is based on assumptions of particular barriers for a specific group of people. Conversely, UD is seen as a framework for developing solutions to anticipated needs of all end-users (Knecht 2004).

In addition to accessibility and UD, sustainability is the third dimension that we propose as essential for evaluating the environment. Sustainable design refers to the design and production of objects or buildings in ways that are economical and that minimize harmful effects for the natural environment (Birkeland 2002). For the purpose of this chapter, we have broadened the definition of sustainable design to also encompass the notion of adaptable usage such as the use of products or environments over time and across changing functional abilities and demands.

Although AT professionals and consumers are familiar with the concepts of accessibility and UD, the notion of sustainable design remains unchartered territory, yet one that is becoming increasingly significant within the context of global climate change and resource scarcity. Sustainability is an important concept to consider when designing products and environments for people with disabilities, especially because of recent speculation that this population is likely to be disenfranchised from the global movement addressing the central problem of climate change facing our society (Lovelock 2010).

By incorporating all three concepts within a single framework, this chapter offers an environmental assessment framework that is comprehensive, innovative, and relevant to contemporary trends and demands.

4.2.2 Interaction between Accessibility, Universal Design, and Sustainability

When assessing the environment along the dimensions of accessibility, sustainability, and UD, it is important to understand that these three dimensions do not operate in isolation but instead overlap and intersect (Gossett et al. 2009). The point of intersection between all three dimensions represents the "ideal" design solution for the product or environment being considered—a solution that achieves the highest degree of accessibility, sustainability, and UD. A visual illustration of this point is presented in Figure 4.1.

The intersection model allows one to simultaneously place each decision or design element of the product/environment under consideration in relationship to the three dimensions and to judge it against its approximation to the ideal center. Although the "ideal center" represents the main goal of any design process, previous research (Gossett et al. 2009) has shown that the ideal solution is difficult to achieve. Instead, in most situations there exists a tenuous relationship between these three desired features pulling the design solution in divergent directions. At these times the solution eventually adopted reflects a tradeoff among the three features of accessibility, sustainability, and UD. A visual illustration of this point is presented in Figure 4.2.

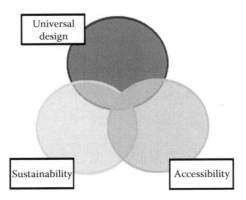

FIGURE 4.1
(See color insert.) The intersection model of conceptual dimensions of accessibility, sustainability, and universal design.

Maximal access	**Accessibility**	No access

No impact/ high efficiency	**Sustainability**	High impact/ low efficiency

Intuitive/ flexible/integrated	**Universal design**	Specialized/ technical/segregated

FIGURE 4.2
(See color insert.) The continuum model of conceptual dimensions of accessibility, sustainability, and universal design.

In Figure 4.2, the dimensions of accessibility, sustainability, and UD each exist along their own continuum. Each design decision can be evaluated in terms of UD, accessibility, and sustainability, falling into various places on the three continua. Evaluation on these continua can help to focus a decision on a critical deciding factor. Both the intersection and continuum models can play an important role in guiding environmental assessments and informing decisions during the ATA process. An environment that falls in the ideal center of the intersection model will have the following characteristics:

- It will facilitate the optimal functioning of a particular AT prescribed to a particular user with a disability (accessibility), thereby promoting the utilization of the prescribed AT by that user. For example, the optimal functioning of a wheelchair and consequently the user's ability to enter and use a building is contingent on the presence of a ramp (accessible) or stairs (inaccessible) at the building's entrance.
- It will seamlessly accommodate the AT as part of its layout or architecture (Center for Universal Design 1997). For example, a building entrance that is level with the sidewalk and textured to allow cane detection eliminates the need for a separate entrance for users of walkers, canes, and wheelchairs, thereby seamlessly

incorporating individuals with a wide spectrum of functional abilities. Most people strive to conform to normative standards of functioning and appearance because we are socialized to minimize or hide our differences (Scherer 2002). This means that aesthetic considerations play an important role in AT acceptance. Therefore, a universally designed environment that aesthetically and inconspicuously supports AT use can minimize potential stigma and promote the uptake and acceptance of the prescribed AT by the user.

- It will support AT use across changing needs, the changing functional status of the user, and across changing weather conditions. It will be easy and economical to maintain and will minimize any negative impact on the natural environment (sustainability). Device adjustability, affordability, and ease of maintenance and repair constitute important features that contribute to long-term AT use (Scherer 2002). However, the extent to which an AT can be adjusted and maintained with ease will be determined to a great extent by its context of use. For example, a height-adjustable worktable that can accommodate pediatric and adult-sized wheelchairs can support the user across the growth curve. Similarly, a carpet that is safe for use with walkers and wheelchairs can support an aging user with declining functional mobility. In addition, if both the worktable and the carpet in the above example can be cleaned with nonchemical agents, they will be easier and economical to maintain without degrading the natural environment.

Thus far, we have introduced the three dimensions of accessibility, sustainability, and UD and described the dynamic interaction between them. The next section describes an environmental assessment framework that is based on these three dimensions and illustrates its incorporation within the ATA process.

4.3 Environment Assessment in the ATA Process Based on the Concepts of Accessibility, Sustainability, and Universal Design

Incorporating the three conceptual dimensions of the environment as discussed above, one has the potential to maximize user participation and satisfaction, thereby affording assistive solutions to users. It is important to note that an assistive solution is the outcome of a user-driven process that aims to improve the user's functioning, quality of life, and well-being in his/her contexts of use. Rather than focusing on AT alone, the assistive solution represents a holistic solution, taking into consideration user needs, the environment(s) of use, and the AT.

The environment represents an important component of the assistive solution and can be evaluated along the dimensions of accessibility, sustainability, and UD described in Section 4.2. An evaluation of the environment along these dimensions must include the following criteria:

- An evaluation of the environment against applicable national/regional accessibility guidelines and design standards;
- An evaluation of social, cultural, political, and economic components of the environment and their potential impact on AT use;

- A user-driven evaluation of how different environments support/hinder the user's participation in various life activities with and without the recommended AT; and
- A determination of possible UD and sustainable strategies for adapting the environment for optimal and flexible AT usage over the long term.

Under the auspices of these four criteria, we present and discuss an environmental assessment (EA) (Üstün et al. 1997) process that provides a way of systematically choosing AT that matches the user's needs while considering the three dimensions of the environment: accessibility, UD, and sustainability. As an ongoing component of the ATA process, the overall aim of this EA process is to help practitioners obtain the best possible match among the user, AT, and environment to arrive at an assistive solution that will optimize user participation and satisfaction in the context of use.

4.4 The Environmental Assessment Process: An Overview

As depicted in Figure 4.3, the EA process should ideally be carried out collaboratively between the AT user and a multidisciplinary evaluation team within a center for technical aid. Acknowledging that the environment is antecedent to the AT and crucial for determining the limits of AT use and functionality, the EA occurs at the beginning of the ATA process, specifically during the user data collection phase. When a user arrives at a center for technical aid seeking an assistive solution, the multidisciplinary team must initiate a systematic process in which they, together with the user, reflect on the environment(s) where the proposed AT will be used and evaluate each environment along the dimensions of accessibility, sustainability, and UD.

When evaluating the environment for accessibility, the multidisciplinary team may ask questions around what accessibility guidelines and mandates are operant at the national and local levels that inform design and modification of buildings, facilities, and programs for people with disabilities. Examples of such guidelines and mandates include the AADAG in the United States and Build-for-All in Europe, as described previously in this chapter. The team may then discuss implications of these accessibility guidelines with the user during the EA process. For example, a multidisciplinary team may use knowledge of physical access laws when evaluating a workplace and seeking an assistive solution with a user who has physical access needs. On the basis of the results of their evaluation, they might need to collectively decide whether the workplace environment needs to be modified to support AT functioning, and consequently the user's productivity, and the extent and costs of modifications required. A knowledge of local policies governing accessibility will also help to determine whether the AT and environmental modifications will be publicly or privately funded, a key factor in determining the feasibility of the proposed assistive solution.

UD is the second dimension to consider when collecting data for the EA process to arrive at an assistive solution. UD represents an aim for the built environment to be both aesthetically pleasing and usable to all (Mace et al. 1991). In evaluating the environment along this dimension, it may be helpful to consider the seven principles of UD as identified by the Center for Universal Design (1997):

1. Equitable use
2. Flexibility in use

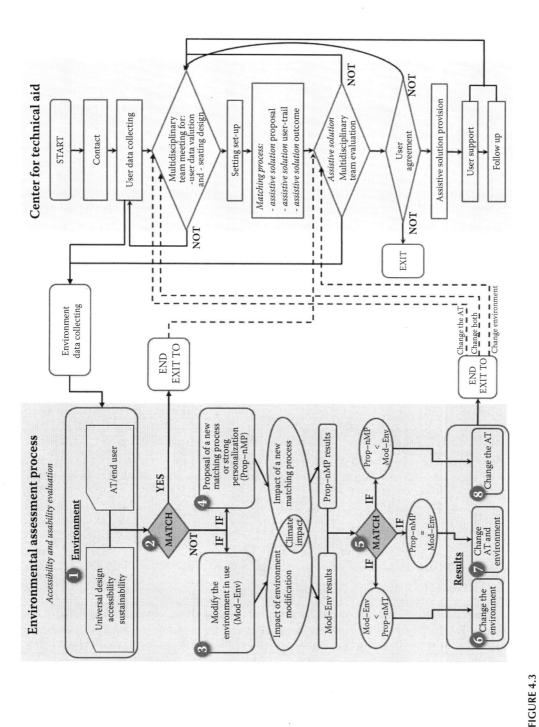

FIGURE 4.3
(See color insert.) Environmental assessment process and interaction with the center for technical aid model.

3. Simple and intuitive use
4. Perceptible information
5. Tolerance for error
6. Low physical effort
7. Size and space for approach and use

These seven principles can guide environmental evaluations by considering the needs of multiple users who may require assistive solutions to participate fully in a given space. This is especially important when considering assistive solutions for communal settings such as schools, which involve multiple users in various capacities, such as students, parents, and administrators. In this example, multiple users of the school could collaborate with a multidisciplinary team of professionals to explore an assistive solution that would be usable to all patrons and visitors of the school. This assistive solution would be reflective of decisions made regarding AT, the environment, and the users while embedding choice for all people in the design (Knecht 2004). For instance, classrooms would be designed so that multiple users with a broad spectrum of functional abilities would benefit from assistive solutions that support full participation for all: AT would support various learning styles; desks and tables would be adaptable to meet the physical and sensory needs of all students, teachers, and parents; and auditory systems would support communication for all participants in the classroom. Incorporating UD philosophy into the EA process offers more inclusive assistive solutions. The UD philosophy also offers a pragmatic way to evaluate environments that most people use in their daily lives but ones that are seldom considered when making AT decisions, such as train stations, airports, schools, museums, and places of worship.

In addition to considering accessibility and UD to support assistive solutions, it is important for the user and multidisciplinary team to evaluate sustainability within the physical, social, economical, ecological, and temporal contexts during the EA process. In evaluating the environment for sustainability specific to environmental impact, some cities, townships, and private authorities have created their own standards. For example, in the United States, the Green Building Council (2011) has developed a green building certification system, entitled Leadership Energy and Environmental Design (LEED). This system offers a useful framework for evaluating and rating new and retrofitted construction in terms of energy efficiency and use of resources and materials that are locally available and easy to maintain. The LEED rating criteria allow projects to achieve a certified, silver, gold, or platinum rating that is based on incorporation of sustainability components into design (U.S. Green Building Council 2011). Although LEED's recognition extends internationally, other sustainability standards offer similar methods of rating "green" design, such as the Building Research Establishment Environmental Assessment Method (BREEAM) in the United Kingdom, Greenstar in Australia, and the Comprehensive Assessment System for Built Environment Efficiency (CASBEE) in Japan (Parker 2009).

We propose that standards of sustainability and green design be applied to both the environment and AT when considering an assistive solution. For example, information may be collected from a user who experiences mobility impairment while at home. During this data collection process, the user and multidisciplinary team can discuss both current and future needs to arrive at an assistive solution incorporating both the AT and the environment into a single "sustainable" solution. In this case, the user may be prescribed a wheeled mobility device made of recycled materials and a ramp constructed of locally grown resources. Additional recommendations may be made to install nonskid flooring that is easy to clean and maintain with nonchemical-based solutions to further minimize any negative environmental impact of the assistive solution.

Considerations of sustainability during the EA process must focus not only on solutions that are ecologically sound and environmental friendly but also on choosing solutions that will meet the user's changing needs over a period of time, ideally a life span. For example, consider the evolving needs of a student with gradually deteriorating vision who is transitioning to college. In thinking about changing needs of this student over the life span, a multidisciplinary team seeking an assistive solution would need to evaluate what would be a better AT for this student: a computer with built-in screen magnification or a computer installed with screen reading software. The final solution would depend on the rate of vision decline and the extent to which alternative learning formats are supported in the college environment.

A potential framework for guiding this "life-span" understanding of sustainability is the evaluation guide for livable communities developed by the American Association of Retired Persons (AARP) Public Policy Institute in the United States (2005). This framework can be used to broadly evaluate the environment and its dynamic interaction with life-span functional changes. Although it was created for aging populations living in urban and suburban United States and would need to be adapted for other age groups and cultures, it may be a useful resource for determining common environments of use and evaluating these environments to meet the needs of users throughout the life span.

Although each of the three dimensions discussed earlier is individually useful in evaluating the environment in the EA process, it is the intersection of accessibility, sustainability, and UD that supports an ideal design solution to enhance the assistive solution for a user. It is in this intersection that AT supports the individual user to fully participate in life (accessibility), is seamlessly incorporated into the environment and useful to all users (universal design), and has a low environmental impact (sustainability).

4.4.1 The EA Process: Step-by-Step Decision Making

The EA process offers a guide for the user and multidisciplinary team to effectively evaluate and determine a best assistive solution for the user's needs. The evaluation of the environmental dimensions of accessibility, UD, and sustainability, along with an assessment of the user's needs and features of the proposed AT, occurs in step 1 of the EA process, as indicated in Figure 4.3. It is at this step that an ATA occurs, the user's needs and desires are assessed, and the environment is evaluated for its impact to support or obstruct full participation for the user. In the assessment of the environment, the three dimensions of accessibility, UD, and sustainability are explored for impediments and opportunities within the environment.

Upon completing the environmental evaluation in step 1, if there is a match among the environment, user, and AT (step 2), the assistive solution is achieved, the EA process ends, and the evaluation is discussed by the multidisciplinary team and user in the ATA process. If a match does not occur at this point in the EA process, possible modifications may be made to the environment (step 3) or the user and multidisciplinary team may reassess the interactions among the environment, user, and AT in a new matching process, thereby determining the impact of this process on the user (step 4). At this point, options to achieve the match are evaluated for the most effective and efficient assistive solution (step 5). This solution may involve modifying the environment to achieve maximal accessibility, sustainability, and/or UD (step 6); changing the AT to match the user's needs (step 8); or making changes to both the environmental dimensions and AT (step 7). This stepwise decision-making process might need to be repeated for each environment or context where the intended use of the AT would occur. The next section describes a case study in which an EA process informed by the dimensions of accessibility, sustainability, and UD was applied in a real-life context to achieve the best assistive solution for multiple users.

4.4.2 Case Evaluation: Considering Accessibility, Universal Design, and Sustainability Within the EA Process

To more fully understand the EA process and the role of accessibility, UD, and sustainability, we share the following case study that resulted from a research project exploring the intersection of these three dimensions of the environment (Gossett et al. 2009). This project began in an effort to document and analyze the decisions that a cross-disability organization named Access Living of Metropolitan Chicago (Access Living) was making during the design a new-construction building. Disabled advocates established Access Living in 1980 to advocate for disability rights, pride, and dignity for people with disabilities. An overall goal of Access Living in designing the new-construction building was to develop a space that was universally designed while maximizing accessibility and sustainability within the design. The dimensions of accessibility and UD were imperative in the project because most users of the future building included staff and consumers with a wide range of disabilities. Sustainability was also important in the project in order to pursue the goal of using "green design" to create environmentally responsible construction in accordance with architectural trends and standards in the city (Kibert 2008). Specific details related to the research project are published elsewhere (Gossett et al. 2009). However, a case example of the decision-making processes involved in designing a conference room within the new building is described here. This case example offers a discussion of the interrelated aspects of the environment, AT, and users of the space within the EA process.

At the beginning of the design process, a multidisciplinary team of architects, disability advocates, and rehabilitation professionals collaboratively assessed the following: (1) users' needs for an assistive solution, with users being defined as all staff and consumers of Access Living services; (2) aspects of access, UD, and sustainability that may/may not be afforded by the environment; and (3) AT options that may contribute to specific needs of individuals using the environment.

Through this initial evaluation process, it was determined that the access needs of the users of the conference room included:

- A room large enough to accommodate large numbers of people using various forms of AT, such as electronic communication devices, wheelchairs, and other mobility devices;
- Ease of communication for people who are deaf/hard of hearing and options for recording and captioning meetings;
- Lighting to meet multiple needs such as focused lighting for sign language interpreters, task lighting for people with low-vision impairments, and nonglare lighting for people with light-sensitivity impairments;
- Electrical outlet options for powering various AT equipment such as real-time interpretation devices, power wheelchairs, and computers; and
- Objects within the environment (tables, chairs, etc.) that offered flexible use and ease of movement throughout the space.

In addition, needs related to sustainability included goals to

- Limit environmental impact of materials and construction procedures;
- Identify energy-saving elements that need to be built into the design during construction, as opposed to incorporating these after construction; and
- Consider long-term needs of the user, including the changing needs of individual users of the space as well as changing needs of the organization, Access Living, (this would offer sufficient flexibility to accommodate changes in staff members, processes, and systems over time).

The seven principles of UD (Center for Universal Design 1997) were also used to guide the environmental evaluation in terms of possibilities for UD, as follows:

- *Equitable use:* The design should meet the needs of all people who would use the space and all conference purposes, such as small and large group meetings, teleconferences, and presentations.
- *Flexibility in use:* Features of the room should be usable for various purposes.
- *Simple, intuitive use:* AT and objects should be easy to use and accommodate a wide range of literacy and language needs.
- *Perceptible information:* Users should be able to effectively and efficiently understand information shared, and activities carried out in the room and features of the room should support alternative forms of communication.
- *Tolerance for error:* Hazards should be limited and use of objects/technology in the room should be intuitive.
- *Low physical effort:* People and objects should be able to freely move around the space with minimal physical effort.
- *Size and space for approach and use:* Design of the room should include adequate space for all to easily enter, exit, and navigate the room.

This evaluation process allowed the multidisciplinary team to develop plans incorporating both environmental decisions and AT into the design to work toward the accessible solution for all users. Decisions made during the decision process were based upon the intersection of the three dimensions of the environment: accessibility, UD, and sustainability. AT was incorporated into the conference room design in ways that decreased costs, targeted long-term needs of the users, maximized accessibility for individual users, and was usable to the greatest extent possible for everyone. The conference room was designed to support and accommodate various types of AT, including video conferencing capability, electronic communication systems, variance of lighting options achieved through overhead lighting and task lighting, manual and power wheelchairs, other types of mobility aids, and augmentative and alternative communication devices. Multiple outlets were installed at wall and floor levels to allow for powering of these various devices.

Furniture included in the designed conference room consisted of chairs and tables made of recyclable materials with powder-coated paints and water-based adhesive. This furniture was also made using volatile organic compound (VOC)-free manufacturing processes. Use of VOC-free manufacturing processes reduces the vapor pressures that negatively affect the environment and human health. In addition, the chairs offered flexibility in use such as removable armrests and seats which can be folded out of the way.

Chairs and tables also offered wheeled capability and could therefore be moved around the room simply and intuitively with low physical effort.

The conference room was also designed in terms of equitable use so that it was large enough to accommodate groups of people with various mobility devices and communication needs who may meet for various reasons. Communication was an important consideration in designing the conference room. The room was designed to abide by the acoustical standards prescribed by ADAAG, making use of microphone options to support communication needs and accommodation of large groups (U.S. Access Board 2004). Light-harvesting options were also used to maximize natural light in coordination with artificial light to minimize the energy costs and maximize applicability to various users.

The case example of the conference room described earlier demonstrates how considerations of accessibility, sustainability, and UD within the environment can be combined with evaluation of users' needs and knowledge of AT features to arrive at an appropriate assistive solution. This case example can be appraised by reflecting back on the intersection model (Figure 4.1) and the continuum model (Figure 4.2) introduced at the beginning of this chapter. All three dimensions (accessibility, UD, and sustainability) were taken into consideration during the EA process when designing the conference room. Each design decision informed by the EA process can be evaluated in terms of whether it fell within the ideal center depicted in Figure 4.1. If it did, then it could be said that an ideal assistive solution was achieved. If not, then we need to determine where the decision fell along the three bars of the continuum model depicted in Figure 4.2. To illustrate this point further, we describe two instances: one in which the design decision achieved the ideal center and one in which the decision initially fell outside of the ideal center, suggesting tradeoffs among the dimensions of accessibility, sustainability, and UD. While appraising the case example in this manner, it is important to bear in mind that within this example, the term "user" refers to the collective of staff and consumers of Access Living.

Let us first consider the conference room seating furniture. When this furniture is rated separately on each bar of the continuum model, it consistently falls on the higher (left) end of each bar. As a UD element, it rates well because of its ergonomic design, that demands low physical effort, flexibility in terms of use as a result of adjustable height, and flexibility in terms of storage as a result of stackability. In terms of sustainability, it rates well because of its recyclabilty and low emission qualities and because it is locally manufactured using VOC-free manufacturing processes. In terms of accessibility, it rates well because of the additional feature of adjustable armrests that allow for easy transfers from other surfaces such as wheelchairs. Therefore, considering all three elements together, this furniture falls in the ideal center on the intersection model and represents an appropriate assistive solution for the various people expected to use the conference room.

A contrasting example is the communication system designed for the conference room. The original design of the communication system made use of microphone capability and an audio frequency induction loop. In terms of accessibility, this design decision rated well because it conformed to standards of communication access recommended for people who are deaf/hard of hearing under the ADAAG and adequately supported technologies needed by this group such as hearing aids. In terms of UD, the communication system did not rate as well because it would be distractive and would pose challenges to people with cognitive disabilities, people attempting to negotiate parallel conversations, and people with hearing sensitivities. In terms of sustainability, the communication system required additional materials but was included in the original design, necessitating few postconstruction modifications. Thus, the original design of the communication system entailed gains in the accessibility continuum (specifically for deaf/hard of hearing users) through a tradeoff with gains in the

UD and sustainability continua. As a result, the communication system in the conference room would fall outside of the ideal center on the intersection model. In other words, the communication system, as originally designed, would offer an assistive solution for deaf and hard of hearing users but not for people with cognitive disabilities and hearing sensitivities.

In the end, Access Living decided against installing the audio frequency induction loop for multiple reasons. The system did not meet local fire safety regulations. Second, the organization's internal research revealed that deaf and hard of hearing users could use portable devices such as personal amplifiers and wireless sound transmitters and receivers as alternatives. Thus, the final design decision for the conference room's communication system was more favorable along the UD continuum.

A final point to bear in mind about this case example is that it describes the EA process for an environment that was in its development stage. This situation offered a perfect opportunity to modify the environment in a way as to approximate the ideal center at the intersections of accessibility, sustainability, and UD to support the participation of multiple users and their varied AT needs. However, such situations are rare, and in most cases AT users have to contend with preexisting and predesigned environments. Nonetheless, the EA process described in this chapter would be just as valuable when applied to such situations because it would guide decisions about modifying the environment(s) or the AT or both to optimize the assistive solution for the user.

4.5 Conclusions

By proposing the assessment of environmental content in the ATA process along the three conceptual dimensions of accessibility, UD, and sustainability, we have presented a model that can be useful in supporting the assistive solution for users. This assistive solution is one in which the ideal center can be achieved by modifying the environment, changing the AT to match the user's needs, or making changes to both the environment and AT. However, this process never occurs without consideration of the interaction between AT, the user, and the environment. Often the goal of achieving the ideal center is elusive, and decisions are made that may incorporate one of the three concepts of the environment over the others. However, the final decision ultimately depends on the contingencies of the situation and the needs of the user.

Summary of the Chapter

This chapter discusses the role of the environment in inhibiting or supporting full societal participation of people with disabilities and provides a rationale and framework for incorporating the environment within the assistive technology assessment (ATA) process. In this chapter, the environment of AT use is viewed broadly as encompassing physical, social, cultural, legislative, and economic elements. Based on this broad definition, the first part of this chapter proposes a model for assessing the environment within the ATA process along the three intersecting dimensions of accessibility, sustainability, and universal design. By evaluating the environment along these three dimensions, one can strive to achieve the "ideal" design solution which will enhance the match between the AT, the user, and his/her environment. The second part of this chapter offers a step-by-step decision-making process to guide the multidisciplinary team to effectively evaluate the environment as an on-going component of the ATA process. The overall aim of this environmental assessment process is to help practitioners arrive at an assistive solution that will optimize user participation and satisfaction in the context of use. The chapter concludes with a case study exemplifying the environmental assessment process in practice.

Acknowledgments

We acknowledge the role of Ann Kathleen Barnds and Daisy Feidt in developing some of the key concepts presented in this chapter. We also thank Joy Hammel and Barbara Knecht for their valuable input and guidance in relation to the UD project that this chapter draws upon. Finally, special thanks to Hsiang-Yi Tseng for her work during the UD project.

References

AARP Public Policy Institute. (2005). *Livable Communities: An Evaluation Guide*. Retrieved from http://assets.aarp.org/rgcenter/il/d18311_communities.pdf

Birkeland, J. (2002). *Design for Sustainability: A Sourcebook of Integrated, Eco-Logical Solutions*. London: Earthscan Publications.

Build-for All Project. (2006). *The Build-for-All Reference Manual*. Retrieved from http://www.build-for-all.net

Center for Universal Design. (1997). *The Principles of Universal Design. Version 2.0*. Retrieved from http://www.ncsu.edu/www/ncsu/design/sod5/cud/about_ud/udprinciplestext.htm

Center for Universal Design. (2008). *The Principles of Universal Design*. Retrieved from http://www.design.ncsu.edu/cud/about_ud/udprinciples.htm

Church, G., and Glennen, S. (1992). *The Handbook of Assistive Technology*. San Diego: Singular Publishing Group Inc.

Day, H., Jutai, J., Woolrich, W., and Strong, G. (2001). The stability of impact of assistive devices. *Disability and Rehabilitation, 23*(9), 400–404. doi:10.1080/09638280010008906

Dijcks, B. P. J., De Witte, L. P., Gelderblom, G. J., Wessels, R. D., and Soede, M. (2006). Non-use of assistive technology in The Netherlands: A non-issue? *Disability and Rehabilitation: Assistive Technology, 1*(1–2), 97–102. doi:10.1080/09638280500167548

Dion, B., Balcazar de laCruz, A., Rapson, D., Svensson, E., Peters, M., and Dion, P. (2006). *International Best Practices in Universal Design: A Global Review*. Ottawa, Ontario, Canada: Canadian Human Rights Commission.

Egilson, S. T., and Traustadottir, R. (2009). Participation of students with physical disabilities in the school environment. *American Journal of Occupational Therapy, 63*(3), 264–272. doi:10.5014/ajot.63.3.264

EIDD Design for All Europe. (2004). Stockholm Declaration. Adopted on 9 May 2004, at the Annual General Meeting of the European Institute for Design and Disability in Stockholm. Retrieved from http://www.designforalleurope.org/Design-for-All/EIDD-Documents/Stockholm-Declaration/

Gossett, A., Mirza, M., Barnds, A. K., and Feidt, D. (2009). Beyond access: A case study on the intersection between accessibility, sustainability, and universal design. *Disability and Rehabilitation: Assistive Technology, 4*(6), 439–450. doi:10.3109/17483100903100301

Kibert, C. J. (2008). *Sustainable Construction: Green Building Design and Delivery* (2nd ed.). Hoboken, NJ: John Wiley & Sons.

Kittel, A., Di Marco, A., and Stewart, H. (2002). Factors influencing the decision to abandon manual wheelchairs for three individuals with a spinal cord injury. *Disability and Rehabilitation, 24*(1–3), 106–114. doi:10.1080/0963828011006678 5

Knecht, B. (2004). Accessibility regulations and a universal design philosophy inspire the design process. *Architectural Record, 192*, 145–150. Retrieved from http://archrecord.construction.com/resources/conteduc/archives/0401edit-1.asp

Lauer, A., Longenecker Rust, K., and Smith, R. O. (2006, August 18). ATOMS Project technical report—Factors in assistive technology device abandonment: Replacing "abandonment" with "discontinuance." Retrieved from http://www.r2d2.uwm.edu/atoms/archive/technicalreports/tr-discontinuance.html

Lovelock, B. (2010). Disability and going green: A comparison of the environmental values and behaviors of persons with and without disability. *Disability and Society, 25*(4), 467–484. doi:10.1080/09687591003755856

Mace, R. L., Hardie, G. J., and Place, J. P. (1991). Accessible environments: Toward universal design. In W. F. E. Preiser, J. Vischer, and E. T. White (Eds.), *Design Intervention: Toward a More Humane Architecture* (pp. 1–44). New York: Van Nostrand Reinhold.

Mann, W. C., and Lane, J. P. (1991). *Assistive Technology for Persons with Disabilities: The Role of Occupational Therapy*. Bethesda, MD: American Occupational Therapy Association.

Oliver, M. (1990). *The Politics of Disablement*. London: Palgrave Macmillan.

Parker, J. (2009). BREEAM or LEED—Strengths and weaknesses of the two main environmental assessment methods. Retrieved from http://www.bsria.co.uk/news/breeam-or-leed/

Philips, B., and Zhao, H. (1993). Predictors of assistive technology abandonment. *Assistive Technology, 5*(1), 36–45. doi:10.1080/10400435.1993.10132205

Salmen, J. (2008). Is universal design really universal? Retrieved from http://www.uigarden.net/english/is-universal-design-really-universal

Scherer, M. J. (2002). The study of assistive technology outcomes in the United States. In K. Miesenberger, J. Klaus, and W. Zagler (Eds.), *Computers Helping People with Special Needs* (Vol. 2398, pp. 131–142). Berlin: Springer. doi:10.1007/3-540-45491-8_152

Scherer, M. J., Cushman, L. A., and Federici, S. (2004, June 1–10). *Measuring Participation and the Disability Experience with the "Assistive Technology Device Predisposition Assessment."* Paper presented at the North American Collaborating Center 10th Annual Conference on ICF: NACC 2004, Halifax, Canada. http://secure.cihi.ca/cihiweb/en/downloads/10NACC_Conf_Report_FINAL_e.pdf

Scherer, M. J., Sax, C. L., Vanbiervliet, A., Cushman, L. A., and Scherer, J. V. (2005). Predictors of assistive technology use: The importance of personal and psychosocial factors. *Disability and Rehabilitation, 27*(21), 1321–1331. doi:10.1080/09638280500164800

Söderström, S., and Ytterhus, B. (2010). The use and non-use of assistive technologies from the world of information and communication technology by visually impaired young people: a walk on the tightrope of peer inclusion. *Disability and Society, 25*(3), 303–315. doi:10.1080/09687591003701215

U.S. Access Board. (2004). *Revised ADA and ABA Accessibility Guidelines*. Retrieved from http://www.access-board.gov/ada-aba/final.pdf

U.S. Green Building Council. (2011). Introduction—What LEED is. Retrieved from http://www.usgbc.org/DisplayPage.aspx?CMSPageID = 1988

United Nations (UN). (2006). *Convention on the Rights of Persons with Disabilities*. (A/RES/61/106). New York: UN Retrieved from http://www.un-documents.net/a61r106.htm

Üstün, T. B., Compton, W., Mager, D., Babor, T., Baiyewu, O., Chatterji, S., et al. (1997). WHO study on the reliability and validity of the alcohol and drug use disorder instruments: Overview of methods and results. *Drug and Alcohol Dependence, 47*(3), 161–169.

Verdonschot, M. M. L., de Witte, L. P., Reichrath, E., Buntinx, W. H. E., and Curfs, L. M. G. (2009). Community participation of people with an intellectual disability: A review of empirical findings. *Journal of Intellectual Disability Research, 53*(4), 303–318. doi:10.1111/j.1365-2788.2008.01144.x

World Health Organization (WHO). (2001). *ICF: International Classification of Functioning, Disability, and Health*. Geneva, Switzerland: WHO.

5

Measuring the Impact of AT on Family Caregivers

L. Demers and B.W. Mortenson

CONTENTS

5.1 Introduction

It is generally understood that assistive technology (AT) has the potential to enhance users' functioning, and, in the process, allow them to be less dependent on the assistance of others. However, for the vast preponderance of ATs, this secondary assumption is not buttressed by systematic evidence (McWilliam et al. 2000; Henderson et al. 2008). To create an enhanced understanding of the impact of AT on caregivers, we need (1) better empirical evidence, (2) an improved conceptual understanding of the inter-relationship of outcomes between assistance users and caregivers, and (3) more developed and refined measurement tools. To address these needs this chapter has the following goals:

- To provide an overview of current literature that explores the impact of AT on informal caregivers of children and adults,
- To offer theoretical contributions that explicate the relationship between AT interventions and outcomes for assistance users and their informal caregivers and

describe an AT provision process that is inclusive of the assistance users and their informal caregivers, and

- To describe two measures in this area and discuss plans for their future development.

By addressing these goals, this chapter will provide clinicians and researchers with an up-to-date understanding of progress in this area and suggestions about how to implement these developments into practice. We have provided two hypothetical vignettes to illustrate more vividly the content of this chapter.

The first vignette is about Charlie, an 8-year-old boy with Duchene muscular dystrophy. He lives in a two-story bungalow with his mother, Susan, his father, Harold, and his 5-year-old sister, Lisa. He has difficulty going up stairs, walking outside of the home, and has problems with fatigue, so his parents carry him when going places outside of the home because when he walks he becomes too tired to do activities. The parents have restricted Charlie's and their own activities to reduce the need to carry him places, but they both report intermittent back pain and ongoing muscle soreness. At school, he can participate in classroom activities, but he has difficulties going to and participating in activities outside of the classroom.

The second vignette is about Bob, a 75-year-old man with osteoarthritis in both knees. He lives with his wife, Jean, who is a 70-year-old woman who is relatively healthy. They live in a one-floor apartment with level entry. Bob is having increasing problems moving around because of knee pain and has had several falls when his left knee "gives out." He is currently waiting for joint replacement surgery and uses a cane. Jean helps Bob get up from low surfaces, helps Bob donning and doffing his socks, and does most instrumental activities of daily living (IADL) tasks around the house, but she does not drive. Bob will drive Jean to go shopping, but he usually waits for her in the car or sits and has coffee while she shops. He is currently following an exercise program recommended by a physical therapist to try to reduce potential deconditioning. Jean has stopped social visits with her friends so she can be available to help Bob and keep him safe around the home, and she reports that she feels tired all of the time.

This chapter begins with an overview of current research in this area, with a specific focus on the impact of AT on informal caregivers. The next section introduces three conceptual models to help explicate the relationship between AT interventions and outcomes for informal caregivers. The first model describes how the personal assistance strategy of individuals with disabilities, which may include AT, simultaneously affects themselves and their informal caregivers. The second model illustrates how AT can moderate caregiver's primary and secondary stressors in a way that influences their participation, health, and quality of life. The third model portrays an AT intervention process that is inclusive of assistance users and their informal caregivers. The penultimate section introduces two tools that measure the impact of AT interventions on informal caregivers of children and adults. In the final section, we illustrate the steps of our AT intervention process and use of the two measurement tools based on the vignettes of Charlie, Susan, Harold, Bob, and Jean.

5.2 Overview of Current Literature

5.2.1 AT and Human Assistance

Assistive device use is common among children and adults with disabilities. According to the Participation and Activity Limitation Study (PALS), a population-based health survey, half of Canadians with disabilities under 15 years and nearly two-thirds of those 15 years or older and used assistive devices (Statistics Canada 2008). A survey of adult consumers of California independent living centers found that devise use increases with age (Kaye et al. 2008). Despite the use of these devices, unmet need appears to be a problem. According to PALS, one-quarter of Canadians with disabilities under the age of 15 had none of the AT they required, and 30% needed additional equipment. Of those 15 years and older, 10% had none of the AT they required and 29% needed additional equipment (Statistics Canada 2008). Agree et al. (2005) found that 72% of older people with activities of daily living (ADL) limitations who used AT also relied on informal care, whereas 54% of non-AT users did. Similarly, 26% of AT users and 12% percent of nonusers relied on formal care. Further analysis indicated that AT use substituted for personal care only for individuals who were unmarried and those with more high school education. In contrast, individuals with cognitive impairments were less likely to substitute AT for informal or formal personal assistance.

Informal caregiving is extremely common and may have detrimental consequences for the care provider. In the United States, more than 50 million informal caregivers, like Jean, Susan, and Harold, assist individuals who are ill or disabled (Houser and Gibson 2008). Informal caregivers of older adults are frequently either spouses or adult children (Department of Health and Human Services 1998), whereas caregivers for children are usually their parents. Because the number of older adults, aged 65 and older, will double in Canada in the next 20 years (Statistics Canada 2005), informal caregivers will likely experience increased demands. To maintain the quality of life of those they help, caregivers may experience a great deal of stress that can lead to their physical or emotional burnout (Egbert et al. 2008). The potential for burnout poses a challenge to our healthcare system because informal caregivers provide their unfunded assistance 4 times more frequently than formal caregivers (Agree et al. 2004). The replacement value of informal caregiver's unpaid contributions has been estimated at $350 billion annually in the United States and $25 billion annually in Canada (Houser and Gibson 2008; Hollander et al. 2009). This value excludes loss of economic productivity associated with time spent providing care and emotional and physical burden. The cost of informal caregiving to employers has been estimated at $33.6 billion annually in the United States (Metlife Mature Market Institute, National Alliance for Caregiving 2006). A meta-analysis found that caregivers have significantly higher stress and depression and significantly lower subjective well-being, self-efficacy, and physical health than noncaregivers (Pinquart and Sörensen 2003).

A principal reason for providing AT is that it reduces dependency on human assistance and decreases caregiver burden. However, despite the use of AT, activities and social participation are likely to remain restricted to some extent, especially for persons with moderate and severe levels of impairments (Fuhrer et al. 2006). There are three main patterns of assistance: (1) the use of AT alone, (2) AT combined with human assistance, and (3) human assistance alone. Harold and Lisa use the third pattern of assistance with Charlie because they carry him places rather than using AT. Bob uses the first pattern of assistance when ambulating with his cane. Bob and Jean use the second pattern of assistance for shopping because Bob uses his cane to get to the car so he can drive his wife to the store, but he does not buy things himself. Indeed, considerable data exist indicating that both AT and human assistance are used by users to enhance their participation (Allen et al. 2001; Taylor and Hoenig 2004; Agree et al. 2005; Østensjø et al. 2005).

5.2.2 Caregivers of Assistance Users

To appreciate the impact of AT on participation, one must understand how provision of AT may affect the human help that is provided. Recognition of the essential role of caregivers in preserving or enabling participation of assistance users began with the emergence of family-centered care in pediatrics (Dunst et al. 1988) and continued with broadening of the term "client" to include family members in definitions of client-centered practice (Townsend et al. 1997). Some scholars have recommended a shift from a patient-focused approach to a patient-and-caregiver approach in the field of AT (Demers et al. 2004; Pettersson et al. 2005; Gooberman-Hill and Ebrahim 2006). Unfortunately, in current clinical practice, the inclusion of caregivers in the AT provision process is rather hit or miss, and scant attention has been paid to the effect of AT on assistance users' human helpers, especially informal caregivers (McWilliam et al. 2000; Henderson et al. 2008).

Some qualitative research has explored the impact of assistive device use on caregivers. Among caregivers of individuals that have had a stroke (Pettersson et al. 2005; Rudman et al. 2006), studies have indicated that caregivers had ambivalent feelings about assistive devices. Although most participants were grateful for the benefits that these devices provided, their use was sometimes accompanied by anxiety about the possibility of injury, accessibility issues, and the social stigma experienced by some individuals who use AT in the community. In contrast, qualitative studies with children and parents have found manual (Glumac et al. 2009) and power wheelchairs (Wiart et al. 2004) to be generally beneficial.

Cross-sectional studies based on national survey data have examined the relationship between AT use and informal caregiving. Data from some of these studies suggest that AT use helps caregivers by substituting for some of the physical and emotional effort entailed in supporting an individual with disabilities (Agree and Freedman 2000; Allen et al. 2001, 2006; Agree et al. 2004, 2005). Although these studies suggest that AT has a positive impact on informal caregivers, there are two principal limitations. The studies rely on cross-sectional data, which limits the development of causal explanations. Furthermore, the impact of AT use on caregivers is inferred from responses to very few queries, principally dealing with the number of hours of assistance provided. This excludes measurement of other important outcomes, such as reduced physical demands on helpers, diminished psychological stress, and satisfaction in providing help. The neglect of such potential outcomes results in an incomplete portrayal of the benefits of AT for caregivers.

Other cross-sectional studies have explored AT use and informal caregiver assistance. Chen and colleagues (1999) examined how physically impaired assistance users ($n = 20$) involved caregivers in accessing or using their assistive devices and how assistance users and caregivers perceived the value of AT. Their results indicated that AT might reduce assistance users' dependence on human assistance and some of the perceived burden of family members and friends. In a descriptive study, Messecar et al. (2002) identified 47 home modification strategies including the use of assistive devices, providing assistance, and making changes to the home environment that were used by caregivers of community-dwelling elders with a variety of impairments. Kane et al. (2001) interviewed 30 caregivers about their perceptions of device use. The caregivers indicated that devices were generally beneficial for assistance users but were not always covered by insurance. Among a subsample of individuals with spinal cord injury that had a decline in physical function over the last five years, half required additional assistance with ADL (Thompson 1999). Among these individuals, family members were the primary form of assistance; however, the use of AT increased over time (Thompson 1999). The internal validity of the above studies is constrained by their use of descriptive rather than experimental designs and by their small sample sizes. Furthermore, in several of these studies, the relationship among the assistance user, assistive device usage, and the caregiver was not explicitly examined.

Two uncontrolled intervention studies have suggested that AT interventions can be beneficial to caregivers. Using a single subject research design, Rigby et al. (2001) found that provision of a rigid pelvic stabilizing bar for children with cerebral palsy reduced caregiver assistance with some bimanual and reaching tasks and reduced their need to perform repositioning during the day. Ryan and colleagues (2009) found that provision of two special-purpose seating devices was associated with a significant improvement in Family Impact of Assistive Technology Scale scores for children and their parents, whereas removal of the devices was associated with a return to baseline scores.

Generally, there are three main limitations with research in this area. First, cross-sectional research designs do not enable causation to be established. Second, the impact of AT is often measured in terms of hours of care, which is a very crude metric. For example, if a caregiver reallocates time saved through the use of AT to other, perhaps more enjoyable caregiving tasks, this change would go unmeasured. Third, outcomes reported in the current literature often provide insufficient detail to capture all of the benefits of providing AT interventions. More studies like those by Ryan et al. (2009) are required to develop a complete understanding of the impact of AT interventions on informal caregivers.

5.3 Conceptual Frameworks on the Impact of AT on Caregivers and Users

In this section, we introduce three conceptual models to help understand the relationship between AT interventions and outcomes for informal caregivers. In the first model, we describe how an assistance user's personal assistance strategy, which frequently includes the use of AT, affects themselves and their informal caregivers. In the second model, we demonstrate how AT can alter caregivers' stressors so that their participation, health, and quality of life can be facilitated. In the third model, we describe an informal caregiver inclusive AT intervention process.

5.3.1 Conceptual Framework 1

On the basis of research and clinical work in this area, we developed conceptual framework 1 to examine the impact of an AT intervention on the assistance user/caregiver dyad (Demers et al. 2007) (see Figure 5.1). The framework starts with a mobility-related AT intervention, which alters the personal adaptive strategy (assistance solution in the Matching Person to Technology model). An assistance user's adaptive strategy consists of two possible components: (1) AT, which includes assistive devices, special equipment, and the services rendered to provide them, and/or (2) the assistance of others, composed of informal support from caregivers and/or formal support. This framework parallels the Matching Person to Technology model in that it acknowledges that selection of assistive devices is facilitated by use of context-specific clinical measures, functional analysis, and psycho-socio-environmental evaluations. This framework extends the Matching Person to Technology model by indicating how the presence of a caregiver creates the potential for a variety of assistive strategies to reduce activity limitations and participation restrictions, which may include caregiver assistance, use of assistive devices, or a combination of the two. The conceptual framework highlights the concomitant effects of an AT intervention on the person with a disability and on his or her caregiver. Caregivers like Jean, Susan, and Harold may have few, if any, opportunities to modify their role unless a new AT or a new way of using available AT is actually adopted by the assistance user. The framework indicates how an inclusive assistance strategy can also be beneficial for the user's informal caregivers. Accordingly, AT use is a vital determinant of benefits such as enhanced activity, participation, psychological functioning, device satisfaction, and well-being of the user and his or her caregiver.

With conceptual framework 1, AT intervention alters the personal adaptive strategy, especially the manner and extent of concerted human help with activity, and, in some instances, wholly eliminates the need for that assistance. The altered helper-related activities encompass (1) the physical and psychological components that are identified in the literature on caregivers (Hoenig et al. 2003; Demers et al. 2009), and (2) the interaction between AT and personal assistance (Chen et al. 1999; Allen et al. 2001; Verbrugge and

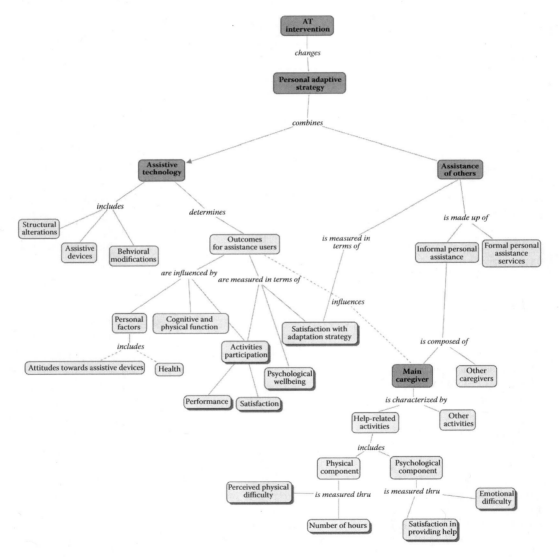

FIGURE 5.1

Model for assistive technology outcomes on an assistive technology user/caregiver dyad.

Sevak 2002; Hoenig et al. 2003; Agree et al. 2005). The physical component includes perceived physical difficulty (Blake and Lincoln 2000; Gallego et al. 2001; Visser-Meily et al. 2004, 2005), frequency of help, and number of hours of help (op Reimer et al. 1998; Chen et al. 1999; Allen et al. 2001; Hoenig et al. 2003; Verbrugge and Sevak 2002; Taylor and Hoenig 2004; Agree et al. 2005). The psychological component of the altered helper-related activities includes participative necessity, satisfaction in providing help (Stuckey et al. 1996; Chappell and Reid 2002), and emotional difficulty (Blake and Lincoln 2000; Gallego et al. 2001; Visser-Meily et al. 2004).

This framework resonates with the assistive technology assessment (ATA) process model in that it identifies the caregiver as a critical component of the environmental milieu, but also emphasizes how an assistance solution that carefully considers the user's environmental context can also influence that context, especially in terms of its impact on user's informal caregivers.

5.3.2 Conceptual Framework 2

Demers et al. (2009) developed conceptual framework 2 to better understand the impact of AT on the AT user's caregiver. According to this framework (see Figure 5.2), model caregivers' primary and secondary stressors have a direct influence on caregivers' outcomes, which include quality of life, physical and psychological health, and social participation. Primary stressors are directly related to the caregiving provided (e.g., types of assistance, number of tasks, time required, safety, and physical effort). Secondary stressors are related to the long-term impact of primary stressors on the caregiver and include role overload, decreased free time, and home modifications required to accommodate an assistance user. Several factors help mediate the relationship between stressors and caregiver outcomes. These include personal resources, coping strategies, and self-efficacy. Other factors can moderate the relationship between stressors and caregiver outcomes by altering the way in which care is provided. AT is one moderating factor that, depending on the device type and amount and manner of use, can decrease the areas of assistance provided, decrease time required, reduce caregiver physical effort, and improve safety. Background and contextual factors also moderate caregiving outcomes. Improvements in social support, environmental accessibility, living arrangement, and quality of relationship can decrease primary stressors by reducing caregiving or perceived stressors that can facilitate positive caregiver outcomes.

In applying conceptual framework 2 to the first vignette, it is evident that carrying Charlie is a primary stressor for Susan and Harold that involves intense physical effort and associated safety issues. The need to carry Charlie results in secondary stressors because this decreases the amount of time they have for other activities. In terms of outcomes, despite their existing personal resources, coping strategies, and a supportive social environment, the stress of caregiving has reduced Harold and Susan's social participation, physical health, and quality of life. Because Charlie will continue to grow larger and less physically able, these outcomes are unlikely to improve unless moderating or mediating factors can be altered.

In the second vignette, Jean experiences multiple primary stressors given all of her caregiving tasks. These likely contribute to secondary outcomes that include role overload and decreased free time. Despite the moderating influences of background and contextual factors and Bob's use of a cane, Jean experiences decreased social participation and reduced physical and psychological health. Until Bob recovers from his surgery, which will not be for several months, it is probable that Jean's outcomes will continue to decline unless moderating or mediating factors are changed in some way.

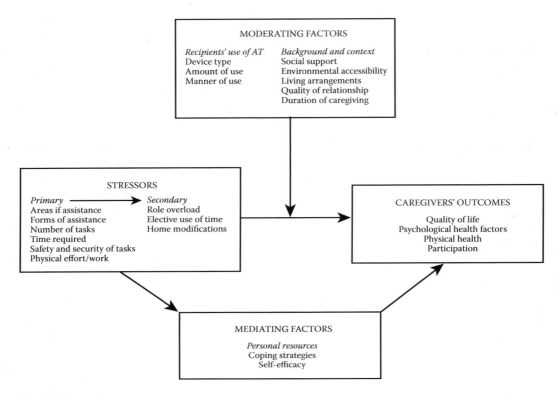

FIGURE 5.2

A conceptual framework for understanding outcomes experienced by caregivers who assist assistive technology users. (Reprinted with permission Demers, L. et al., *American Journal of Physical Medicine & Rehabilitation*, *88*(8), 645–655, 2009.)

5.3.3 Conceptual Framework 3

Given the inter-related outcomes of assistance users and their informal caregivers, it seems logical that informal caregivers should be included as key players in the AT prescription process. Rather than involve informal caregivers in an ad hoc manner, on the basis of our work in the area, we recommend working with assistance users and their informal caregivers using a five-step process (described in Table 5.1). Conceptual framework 3 was developed as part of an experimental study to ensure the intervention was safe, feasible, and relevant to the targeted individuals. To develop this model we used an iterative process that involved delineating the intervention in consultation with clinicians, assistance users, and caregivers and preliminary testing of the intervention with two dyads. This approach is congruent with the ATA process, but it explicitly acknowledged the role of the informal caregiver in this process and is not necessarily based in a center for technical aid. According to this model, the process begins with identification and assessment of problematic activities that have been selected cooperatively by the assistance user and his or her informal caregiver(s). After the identification of potential strategies, the best potential strategy is identified for trial implementation by the user/caregiver dyad. After AT provision and training, desired outcomes are reassessed. The process will continue until an appropriate solution is found or all options have been exhausted.

TABLE 5.1

Process for Identifying Appropriate Assistance Strategies and Assistive Technology Provision Updating and Training for Assistance Users and Their Informal Caregivers

Step	Objectives
1. Identification and assessment of the problematic activities with involvement of the caregiver.	Care givers and clients should agree on the choice of problematic activities and the aspects those activities that make them problematic. Perform baseline measurements and assessments.
2. Identification and exploration of possible strategies.	The caregiver and user should decide together on an AT strategy to addressed the targeted problem. For caregivers and users to make a joint decision to adopt a strategy linked to the ATs, they need to be sensitive to the advantages and disadvantages and take into account: • Their beliefs and values toward technology • Possible impacts on the physical and social environment • Skills required and their actual skills
3. Choice of most appropriate ATs solution.	Decide on strategies related to ATs.
4. Training.	For caregivers and users to become competent in using the strategies related to ATs with targeted activity.
5. Evaluation of the AT solution.	To helpCaregiver's and user's motivation to continue using the strategies related to ATs.

Although the steps in this model are linear, the advent of new problematic activities or environmental changes may require alteration of the process midstream. Furthermore, on the basis of evaluation of the AT solution earlier steps may be revisited. Sometimes new devices may be trialled, but other times, new strategies may be examined or alternative problem activities may be identified. Moreover, with the existence of multiple problematic activities, each step may occur at different times. The steps of this process will be illustrated with the vignettes after the introduction of relevant measurement tools in the next section of the chapter.

5.4　Measurement Tools Adressing AT Impacts on Family Caregivers

Currently there are two tools that measure the impact of an AT intervention on informal caregivers: (1) the Caregiver Assistive Technology Outcome Measure for caregivers of adults, and (2) the Family Impact of Assistive Technology Scale for children and their parents.

5.4.1　Caregiver Assistive Technology Outcome Measure

The Caregiver Assistive Technology Outcome Measure (CATOM) is an 18-item outcome measure with a structured interview format. It was constructed based on a conceptual framework of outcomes for caregivers of assistance users (Demers et al. 2009). The CATOM measures the caregiver's perception of the impacts of AT in his or her life. It may also be used to assess change between assessment and reassessment after an AT-related intervention. The measure is used to record the activities that caregivers provide assistance with and to identify the most demanding one. The measure has three parts. The first part identifies and enumerates all of the care recipient's activities for which the caregiver provides assistance and the forms of assistance given, the second part (13 items) measures the caregiver's frequency (5 = never to 1 = almost always) of elements of burden associated with a dyad-identified activity, and the third part (4 items) captures the caregiver's perceived burden of all of the assistance they provide and overall quality of life. The second part can be administered for each activity that is selected for intervention. The psychometric properties of this instrument are being assessed as part of the feasibility study. Initial results ($N = 29$) indicate that its second part has a Cronbach's alpha of 0.80 and the test-retest interclass correlational coefficient (ICC) for four subjects was 0.80. The 13 domains that are measured with the CATOM are presented in Table 5.2.

5.4.2 Family Impact of Assistive Technology Scale

The Family Impact of Assistive Technology Scale is a 55-item tool that measures parent's perceptions of the impact of assistive device use on children and on themselves (Ryan et al. 2006). The Family Impact of Assistive Technology covers eight domains (n = items per domain): child autonomy (5), caregiver relief (9), child contentment (9), doing activities (child has control over own actions) (5), parent effort (8), family and social interaction (child interacts with others) (4), caregiver supervision (7), and parent's concerns about and safety (8). Parents indicate their degree of agreement or disagreement with each item using a seven-point rating scale in which lower scores indicate better outcomes. The scale was developed with the researchers in consultation with five clinical content experts, and seven parents reviewed preliminary items to establish content and face

TABLE 5.2

Domains for the Caregiver Assistive Technology Outcome Measure

Part 1	Areas of assistance	Assistance provided to the care recipient in relation to mobility, self-care, and communication.
	Forms of assistance	Assistance provided to the care recipient in terms of hands-on help, supervision via verbal cueing, and monitoring at a distance.
	Number of tasks	Number of assistive tasks provided by the caregiver.
Part 2	Time required	Time required for assistance that exceeds the self-perceived capacity of the caregiver
	Safety and security of tasks	Degree of risk associated with the provision of assistance.
	Physical effort/work	Degree of physical energy required to assist the care recipient.
	Physical health	Pain or strain from providing assistance.
	Home modifications	Degree to which assistive technology limits the use of the space within the home.
	Psychological health	Degree to which the caregiver is anxious about the care recipient and degree to which he/she is frustrated by providing assistance.
	Role overload	Degree to which the caregiver feels overwhelmed.
	Elective use of time	Degree to which free time is reduced by caregiving tasks.
Part 3	Participation	Degree to which the social roles of leisure, work, and social life are influenced by the caregiving tasks.
	Quality of life	Caregiver's global evaluation of satisfaction with physical, psychological, and social dimensions of life.

validity. (Ryan et al. 2006, pp. 195–200). The internal consistency of each domain ranges from 0.64 to 0.92 with an overall Cronbach's alpha of 0.94 (Ryan et al. 2007). The ICCs for each domain range from 0.77 to 0.92 and the overall ICC is 0.92 [95% confidence interval (CI) 0.86–0.95] (Ryan et al. 2007). Examples of three supervision questions include "I have little time to get chores done around the house," "I'd like my child to be as independent as possible," and "It is easier to play with my child when someone is holding him/her." An example of a family/social interaction question is as follows, "My child socializes with others at mealtime."

5.4.3 Examples of Outcome Measurement With Vignettes Based on the Assistance Users/Caregiver Dyad Assistive Technology Process Model

5.4.3.1 Vignette 1

Step 1. In concert with the clinician, Charlie and his family decide they would like to improve Charlie's independent mobility.

Table 5.3 provides baseline assessment data using the Family Impact of Assistive Technology Scale regarding their current strategy. For the sake of brevity, description of specific assessments of his physical and cognitive, perceptual status, and postural control are omitted here. As can be noted at baseline in Table 5.3 and Figure 5.3, Susan and Harold are quite concerned about Charlie's autonomy and his performance of activities and about their effort (involved in carrying him places) and limited caregiver relief. Family/social interactions and supervision are less of a concern.

Step 2. Their current strategy of moving Charlie is becoming untenable for Susan and Harold because as Charlie grows, his parents are finding it increasingly difficult to carry him for long distances. Although Charlie can still walk, if he walks far he becomes very fatigued, so this option is no longer realistic. The parents have resisted using AT because of the stigma associated with its use, perceived accessibility issues, and some denial about his diagnosis, but at this point they feel that the benefits would outweigh the disadvantages.

Step 3. There are a variety of options to choose from, including use of a walker, a manual wheelchair, or power mobility. Given the progressive nature of Charlie's condition and

TABLE 5.3

Assessment Data for Charlie's Family with the Family Impact of Assistive Technology Scale

FIATS Domain	Time Domain					
	Baseline		Two Weeks		Six Weeks	
	Score	Mean	Score	Mean	Score	Mean
Autonomy	28	5.6	21	4.2	14	2.8
Caregiver relief	48	5.3	48	5.3	32	3.6
Contentment	40	4.4	38	4.2	26	2.9
Doing activities	26	5.2	27	5.4	14	2.8
Effort	46	5.8	42	5.3	20	2.5
Family/social interaction	12	3.0	13	3.3	10	2.5
Safety	30	3.8	40	5.0	24	22
Supervision	22	3.1	30	4.3	22	3.1
Total (total range 55–385) mean range = 8–56	252	36.2	259	36.9	162	23.2

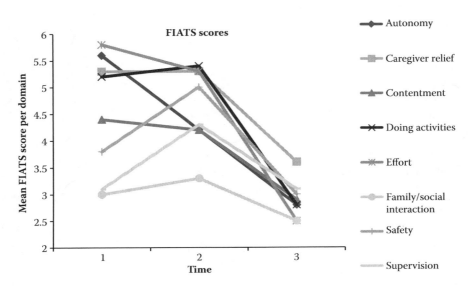

FIGURE 5.3
Family impact of assistive technology scores over time.

growing concerns about his lack of independence, Charlie and his parents decide they would like to trial power mobility for community mobility.

Steps 4 and 5. After a 2-week trial of an appropriately fitted power wheelchair, the parents are somewhat ambivalent about the impact of the device. They are storing the power chair in the garage, and Charlie is able to access it independently, but with difficulty given the stairs he needs to use. They like how the chair gives Charlie more autonomy, but they are more worried about his safety because he has had several minor accidents in the chair and they feel they need to supervise him when driving the chair. Before they used to drive Charlie to school, but because they do not have a lift for their car, they have been accompanying him to school in the power wheelchair, but this takes additional time from their day because it takes over 15 min and the are not sure how they will deal with inclement weather. Charlie can get into the school and into his classroom, but not the washroom. He has hit the walls and doorframes several times with the footrests of his chair. The school staff is worried about the potential for property damage, injury to other students, and issues of what could happen with the wheelchair when Charlie enters the bathroom and leaves it in the hallway.

Steps 4 and 5 repeated. Difficulties identified in step 5 at two weeks suggest additional training is required, so steps 4 and 5 are repeated. With two additional weeks of training and reprogramming of the chair with special modes to facilitate indoor and outdoor mobility, Charlie has become much safer driving the wheelchair and the family has purchased a wheelchair lift so that they can take the chair to school using the car. Charlie has been driving around his home independently and taking part in more activities as a result. Charlie is driving better at school, and teachers have educated other students about the need to leave Charlie's chair alone when it is in the hallway. These changes increase the parent's perceptions of Charlie's autonomy, decrease their safety concerns, reduce their effort, and facilitate caregiver relief as noted below.

Revisiting Step 1 in the future. Given the progressive nature of Charlie's diagnosis, over time other changes will be required to facilitate his ongoing mobility. This will likely include a lift in the home or moving to a level-entry home. The school will need to modify the bathroom to allow Charlie to access it with his power chair. Alternative power wheel-chair control switches and environmental control systems might be necessary.

5.4.3.2 Vignette 2

Step 1. On the basis of the process outlined above in conjunction with their clinician, Bob and Jean have decided they would like to make it safer and less painful for him to (1) get around and (2) perform bathroom transfers. They would also like to see if (3) he could become more independent dressing putting on his shoes and socks. As described in previous chapters, various assessments of the user can be used to help determine the most appropriate AT interventions and evaluate outcomes for Bob, but they will not be described in this chapter.

In looking at the impact on Jean, baseline assessment using the Caregiver Outcome Measure of Assistive Technology provides the following results regarding the current assistance strategy for their three main issues (presented in Table 5.4 and Figure 5.4). At baseline, Jean generally has more frequent concerns with the caregiving she provides. The caregiving burden for dressing is less than the burden associated with mobility and bathroom transfers.

Step 2. After baseline assessment, various strategies for his issues are considered for his mobility and bathroom transfers. Although Bob is independent ambulating with his cane, his falls are a grave concern for Jean and helping him from the floor is a taxing physical

TABLE 5.4

Assessment Data for Jean with the Caregiver Assistive Technology Outcome Measure

CATOM Part 2 and Part 3 Scores	Baseline		Two Weeks		Four Months		Six Months	
	Score	Mean	Score	Mean	Score	Mean	Score	Mean
Mobility-related burden	37	2.8	47	3.6	43	3.3	52	4.0
Bathroom transfers-related burden	34	2.6	55	4.2	47	3.6	59	4.5
Dressing-related burden	50	3.8	53	4.1	51	3.9	53	4.1
Overall caregiving burden	15	3.8	14	3.5	12	3.0	17	4.3

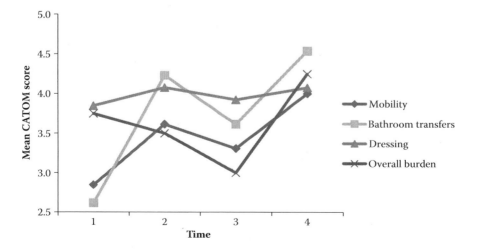

FIGURE 5.4
Caregiver assistive technology outcome measure scores over time.

burden, especially because he is taller and heavier than she is. So providing physical assistance to Bob, especially when he falls, is not sustainable long term. They would like to find a strategy that prevents him from falling. For his dressing of his lower extremities, Jean is their current strategy of choice, but they would like to explore ways to see if he can become independent with this activity again.

Step 3. To facilitate mobility, several AT strategies are considered, but balance problems and instability of his right knee necessitate the use a standard walker for ambulation. To facilitate bathroom transfers, they decide they would like to have a higher toilet seat so that it is easier for Bob to sit down. To make this transfer easier, they would also like to try some toilet armrests so that Bob can use his arms to help him raise and lower himself. For the bathtub, a variety of options are considered. Although it would be possible to have a bath chair in the tub, they are worried he might fall getting over the side of the tub. Instead, they would like to use a tub transfer bench that extends outside of the tub with a tub grab to facilitate bathroom transfers. In terms of dressing options, they decide they would like to trial a flexible sock aide to facilitate donning socks, and a long-handled shoehorn and reacher are trialled to facilitate donning and doffing shoes and socks.

Step 4. The clinicians bring the devices in for trial and over the next two weeks practice using them with Bob and Jean.

Step 5. Although Bob is able to put his socks and shoes on with difficulty with assistive devices, he and Jean decide it is easier for Jean to put on his socks and shoes because, as Jean indicates, "it is much faster and not that much of bother." He decides to keep the reacher because it does enable to him to take his shoes off by himself and pick things up off the floor. At this point scores on the Caregiver Outcome Measure of Assistive Technology indicate that Jean experiences less burden related to mobility and transfers because she is less worried about Bob's safety and has not needed to help him get up from the floor, although she does still worry about the possibility he may fall while ambulating with his walker. One additional activity she needs to do is fold the walker and store it in the car when they drive places, but she does not find this difficult. Because their strategy for dressing is largely unchanged, scores for this activity have remained static.

Four months later (three days after discharge from the hospital), the Assistance Users/ Caregiver Dyad Assistive Technology Process Model was applied again.

Step 1. Mobility and bathroom transfers remained important issues for him after discharge from the hospital.

Step 2. The same potential strategies existed.

Step 3. No new additional equipment needed to be considered, and he used all of his equipment after being discharged.

Step 4. Additional training was required to make sure he could use all of the equipment after his surgery.

Step 5. Jean's re-evaluation with the Caregiver Outcome Measure of Assistive Technology indicates that her burden for the selected issues has increased compared with her 2-week scores and have not returned to baseline levels. Her overall burden is worse than baseline because Bob has felt pretty sick after his surgery and she has needed to perform many additional caregiving duties.

Step 5 repeated two months after surgery. Bob is walking much better, so he has now returned to using only a cane. Because he cannot flex his knee more than 90°, he continues to use the bath bench and the raised toilet seat, especially because he is now waiting for his right knee to replaced. Jean is still a little worried about his safety given his problems with his other knee. She provides physical assistance less, although she still helps with his shoes and socks. Her overall caregiving burden has decreased substantially. In this regard, the surgery and assistive devices have reduced her caregiving burden.

5.5 Future Directions

Much works needs to be done to better understand the impact of AT on informal caregivers. Conceptual models need to be proposed to help understand how AT use impacts the lives of informal caregivers and controlled experimental research, like a study currently underway by the authors, is required to provide causal evidence of their effectiveness (Mortenson et al. 2009). Tools such as the Family Impact of Assistive Technology and Caregiver Assistive Technology Outcome Measure are promising, but additional research is needed to further validate and refine them. Research is currently underway to evaluate the responsiveness of the Family Impact of Assistive Technology Scale and develop tools that are specific to measuring the impact of creative writing technologies and augmentative and alternative communication strategies (Ryan 2010). Work to determine the reliability and validity of the Caregiver Assistive Technology Outcome Measure is currently being undertaken. Mixed methods designs may be required to simultaneously evaluate the effectiveness of AT interventions quantitatively and to understand what are the active ingredients, social processes, and contextual factors that qualitatively influence the outcomes of these interventions on informal caregivers. Additional work is required to conceptualize and evaluate how AT simultaneously influences informal and formal caregiver outcomes, and economic studies are necessary to examine the cost-effectiveness of AT interventions.

5.6 Conclusions

Research to understand the impact of AT on informal caregivers is still in its infancy. It is commonly assumed that AT will provide a trickle-down effect that will reduce the burden associated with informal caregiving. Currently most research that has explored the relationship between AT use and informal caregiver outcomes has used cross-sectional survey or qualitative data, which do not permit such a causal claim to be made. Some studies have indicated that some devices may reduce the hours of care provided, but devices that are more complex may have a less clear-cut influence on caregiver outcomes.

On the basis of the conceptual model we have developed and our clinical experiences, we suggest that for AT interventions to be successful in the long term they need to carefully consider the influence and perspectives of informal caregivers because outcomes for assistance users and their caregivers are inter-related. Assistive solutions that may be beneficial for the assistance user in the short term but negative for the informal caregiver are not self-sustaining. Likewise, an assistance solution that has only a direct benefit on the caregiver by decreasing physical burden (e.g., using an electric rather than a mechanical lift) may create an indirect benefit for the assistance user because it makes the informal caregiver less difficult and more available.

The Family Impact of Assistive Technology Scale and Caregiver Assistive Technology Outcome Measure are two promising measures for capturing the impact of AT interventions on informal caregivers; however, additional research is required to refine them and further test their psychometric properties. Given the stage of development of research in this area, mixed methods research studies may provide invaluable data about the impact of AT on informal caregivers from a variety of perspectives. By developing a thorough understanding of the impact of AT on assistance users and their informal caregivers, interventions that are more suitable can be offered and funding that is more appropriate can be sought.

Summary of the Chapter

In this chapter, we have provided an overview of research that has explored the impact of AT on informal caregivers. We have offered informal caregiver-specific models that help explicate how AT may impact informal caregivers, and we described two measures that are intended to capture this effect. We have proposed that the process of AT provision needs to explicitly acknowledge the role of the informal caregiver. With two vignettes, this chapter provides examples of how these measures could be used to capture the impact of AT on informal caregivers. We have provided suggestions for future work in this area.

Acknowledgments

Dr. Demers is supported by the Fonds de la Recherche en Sante du Quebec as a senior research scholar. Dr. Mortenson is supported via a postdoctoral fellowship for the Canadian Institutes of Health–Institute of Aging. Funding for the development of the CATOM was provided by the National Institute on Disability and Rehabilitation Research through the Consortium on Assistive Technology Outcomes Research (CATOR, http://www.outcomes. org/). (Grant # H133A060062).

References

Agree, E. M., and Freedman V.A. (2000). Incorporating assistive devices into community-based long-term care: An analysis of the potential for substitution and supplementation. *Journal of Aging and Health, 12*(3), 426–450.

Agree, E. M., Freedman, V. A., Cornman, J. C., Wolf, D. A., and Marcotte J. E. (2005). Reconsidering substitution in long-term care: When does assistive technology take the place of personal care? *Journals of Gerontology Series B: Psychological Sciences and Social Sciences, 60*(5), S272.

Agree, E. M., Freedman, V. A., and Sengupta, M. (2004). Factors influencing the use of mobility technology in community-based long-term care. *Journal of Aging and Health, 16*(2), 267–307.

Allen, S., Resnik, L., and Roy, J. (2006). Promoting independence for wheelchair users: The role of home accommodations. *The Gerontologist, 46*(1), 115–123.

Allen, S. M., Foster, A., and Berg, K. (2001). Receiving help at home: The interplay of human and technological assistance. *Journals of Gerontology Series B: Psychological Sciences and Social Sciences, 56*(6), S374–S382.

Blake, H., and Lincoln, N.B. (2000). Factors associated with strain in co-resident spouses of patients following stroke. *Clinical Rehabilitation, 14*(3), 307–314.

Chappell, N. L., and Reid, R.C. (2002). Burden and well-being among caregivers: Examining the distinction. *The Gerontologist, 42*(6), 772–780.

Chen, T., Mann, W. C., Tomita, M., and Nochajski, S. (1999). Caregiver involvement in the use of assistive devices by frail older persons. *Occupational Therapy Journal of Research, 20*(3), 179–199.

Demers, L., Fuhrer, M.J. Jutai, J., Lenker, J., Depa, M., and De Ruyter, F. (2009). A conceptual framework of outcomes for caregivers of assistive technology users. *American Journal of Physical Medicine & Rehabilitation, 88*(8), 645–655.

Demers, L., Fuhrer, M., Jutai, J., Lenker, J.A., and Deruyter, F. (2007). *A Framework for Evaluating Assistive Technology Outcomes on the User-Care Giver Dyad.* Abstract number T0076, Paper presented at the Festival International Conferences on Caregiving, Disability, Aging and Technology (FICCDAT).

Demers, L., Ska, B., Desrosiers, J., Alix, C., and Wolfson, C. (2004). Development of a conceptual framework for the assessment of geriatric rehabilitation outcomes. *Archives of Gerontology and Geriatrics, 38*(3), 221–237.

Department of Health and Human Services. (1998). *Informal Caregiving: Compassion in Action,* Washington, DC: U.S. Department of Health and Human Services.

Dunst, C. J., Trivette, C. M., Davis, M., and Cornwell, J. (1988). Enabling and empowering families of children with health impairments. *Children's Health Care 17*(2), 71–81.

Egbert, N., Dellmann-Jenkins, M., Smith, G. C., Coeling, H., and Johnson, R.J. (2008). The emotional needs of care recipients and the psychological well-being of informal caregivers: Implications for home care clinicians. *Home Healthcare Nurse, 26*(1), 50.

Fuhrer, M., Jutai, J., Demers, L., Scherer, M., Bloch, E., and DeRuyter, F. (2006). Effects of type of locomotive device and disabling condition on device use and disuse among elderly individuals following hospitalization. Abstract. In *Proceedings of the International Conference of Aging, Disability and Independence.*

Gallego, C. F., Roger, M. R., Bonet, I. B., Vinets, L. G., Ribas, A. P., Pisa, R. L., and Oriol, R. P. (2001). Validation of a questionnaire to evaluate the quality of life of nonprofessional caregivers of dependent persons. *Journal of Advanced Nursing, 33*(4), 548–554.

Glumac, L. K., Pennington, S. L., Sweeney, J. K., and Leavitt, R. L. (2009). Guatemalan caregivers' perceptions of receiving and using wheelchairs donated for their children. *Pediatric Physical Therapy, 21*(2), 158–166.

Gooberman-Hill, R., and Ebrahim, S. (2006). Informal care at times of change in health and mobility: A qualitative study. *Age and Ageing, 35*(3), 261.

Henderson, S., Skelton, H., and Rosenbaum, P. (2008). Assistive devices for children with functional impairments: Impact on child and caregiver function. *Developmental Medicine & Child Neurology, 50*(2), 89–98.

Hoenig, H., Taylor Jr., D. H., and Sloan, F. A. (2003). Does assistive technology substitute for personal assistance among the disabled elderly? *American Journal of Public Health: American Journal of Public Health, 93*(2), 330–337.

Hollander, M. J., Liu, G., and Chappell, N. L. (2009). Who cares and how much? *Healthcare Quarterly, 12*(2), 42–49.

Houser, A., and Gibson, M. J. (2008). *Valuing the Invaluable: The Economic Value of Family Caregiving, 2008 Update.* Washington, DC: American Association of Retired Persons, Insight on the Issues 13.

Kane, C. M., Mann, W. C., Tomita, M., and Nochajski, S. (2001). Reasons for device use among caregivers of the frail elderly. *Physical & Occupational Therapy in Geriatrics, 20*(1), 29–47.

Kaye, H. S., Yeager, P., and Reed, M. (2008). Disparities in usage of assistive technology among people with disabilities. *Assistive Technology, 20*, 194–203.

McWilliam, C. L., Diehl-Jones, W. L., Jutai, J., and Tadrissi, S. (2000). Care delivery approaches and seniors' independence. *Canadian Journal on Aging, 19*, 101–124.

Messecar, D. C., Archbold, P. G., Stewart, B. J., and Kirschling, J. (2002). Home environmental modification strategies used by caregivers of elders. *Research in Nursing and Health, 25*(5), 357–370.

Metlife Mature Market Institute, National Alliance for Caregiving. (2006). *The Metlife Caregiving Cost Study: Productivity Losses to U.S Business.* Westport, CT: Metlife Mature Market Institute.

Mortenson, B., Gélinas-Bronsard, D., Roy, L., Plante, M.*, McCabe, D., & Demers, L. (2009). Impacts des aides techniques auprès des usagers et de leurs proches aidants. Résumés des communications de la 7e Journée scientifique annuelle du Réseau québécois de recherche en vieillissement – La recherche sur le vieillissement : Des défis à relever, Québec, p. 33.

op Reimer, S., de Haan, R. J., Rijnders, P. T., Limburg, M., and van den Bos, G. A. M. (1998). The burden of caregiving in partners of long-term stroke survivors. *Stroke, 29*(8), 1605–1611.

Østensjø, S., Carlberg, E. B., and Vøllestad, N. K. (2005). The use and impact of assistive devices and other environmental modifications on everyday activities and care in young children with cerebral palsy. *Disability & Rehabilitation, 27*(14), 849–861.

Pettersson, I., Berndtsson, I., Appelros, P., and Ahlström, G. (2005). Lifeworld perspectives on assistive devices: Lived experiences of spouses of persons with stroke. *Scandinavian Journal of Occupational Therapy, 12*(4), 159–169.

Pinquart, M., and Sörensen, S. (2003). Differences between caregivers and noncaregivers in psychological health and physical health: A meta-analysis. *Psychology and Aging, 18*(2), 250–267.

Rigby, P., Denise, R., Schoger, S., and Ryan, S. (2001). Effects of a wheelchair-mounted rigid pelvic stabilizer on caregiver assistance for children with cerebral palsy. *Assistive Technology, 13*, 2–11.

Rudman, D. L., Hebert, D., and Reid, D. (2006). Living in a restricted occupational world: The occupational experiences of stroke survivors who are wheelchair users and their caregivers. *Canadian Journal of Occupational Therapy, 73*(3), 141–152.

Ryan, S. (2010). Development of an indicator of the impact of assistive devices in children and their families in Canadian Child and Youth Coalition [database online]. Retrieved from http://www.ccyhc.org/hsr_indicators_workshop/presentations/ryan.pdf

Ryan, S., Campbell, K. A., Rigby, P., Germon, B., Chan, B., and Hubley, D. (2006). Development of the new family impact of assistive technology scale. *International Journal of Rehabilitation Research, 29*(3), 195–200.

Ryan, S. E., Campbell, K. A., and Rigby, P. J. (2007). Reliability of the Family Impact of Assistive Technology Scale for families of young children with cerebral palsy. *Archives of Physical Medicine and Rehabilitation, 88*, 1436–1440.

Ryan, S. E., Campbell, K. A., Rigby, P. J., Fishbein-Germon, B., Hubley, D., and Chan, B. (2009). The impact of adaptive seating devices on the lives of young children with cerebral palsy and their families. *Archives of Physical Medicine and Rehabilitation, 90*(1), 27–33.

Statistics Canada. (2005). *Population Projections for Canada, Provinces and Territories, 2005 to 2031.* Ottawa, Ontario, Canada: Statistics Canada, Catalogue no. 91-520-XIE.

Statistics Canada. (2008). *Participation and Activity Limitation Survey 2006: A Profile of Assistive Technology for People with Disabilities.* Ottawa, Ontario, Canada: Statistic Canada, 89-628-X-no.005.

Stuckey, J. C., Neundorfer, M. M., and Smyth, K. A. (1996). Burden and well-being: The same coin or related currency? *The Gerontologist, 36*(5), 686–693.

Taylor, D. H., and Hoenig, H. (2004). The effect of equipment usage and residual task difficulty on use of personal assistance, days in bed, and nursing home placement. *Journal of the American Geriatrics Society, 52*(1), 72–79.

Thompson, L. (1999). Functional changes in persons aging with spinal cord injury. *Assistive Technology 11*(2), 123–129.

Townsend, E., Stanton, S., Law, M., Polatajko, H., Baptiste, S., Thompson-Franson, T. et al. (1997). *Enabling Occupation: An Occupational Therapy Perspective.* Ottawa, Ontario, Canada: Canadian Association of Occupational Therapists.

Verbrugge, L. M., and Sevak, P. (2002). Use, type, and efficacy of assistance for disability. *The Journals of Gerontology. Series B, Psychological Sciences and Social Sciences, 57*(6), S366–S379.

Visser-Meily, A., van Heugten, C., Post, M., Schepers, V., and Lindeman, E. (2005). Intervention studies for caregivers of stroke survivors: A critical review. *Patient Education and Counselling, 56*(3), 257–267.

Visser-Meily, J. M., Post, M. W. M., Riphagen, I. I., and Lindeman, E. (2004). Measures used to assess burden among caregivers of stroke patients: A review. *Clinical Rehabilitation, 18*(6), 601–623.

Wiart, L., Darrah, J., Hollis, V., Cook, A., and May, L. (2004). Mothers' perceptions of their children's use of powered mobility. *Physical & Occupational Therapy in Pediatrics 24*(4), 3–21.

Section II

Assessment Professionals: Working on the Multidisciplinary Team

M. J. Scherer and S. Federici

Introduction

How disability is diagnosed and treated differs according to age at onset and the type of disability. Developmental disabilities, which occur in infancy and childhood, are typically diagnosed after behavioral and maturational anomalies are observed and are then confirmed medically. Acquired disability can occur at any time in the life span and treatment is often initiated in a hospital emergency room. Disability associated with a degenerative condition, typically associated with advanced age, is generally managed by primary care physicians, neurologists, gerontologists, and family members.

Treating Developmental Disabilities

Developmental disabilities such as Down syndrome or cerebral palsy cannot be "cured." However, interventions applied as early as possible can make a great deal of difference in current and future functioning. Orthopedic and neurological impairments can be surgically corrected or medically managed. Often children with developmental disabilities undergo many treatments during their initial development with the goal of strengthening or extending the use of existing capabilities (Scherer 2005). Sensory disabilities can be greatly helped with advances in technology and the means to communicate can be made possible through alternative and augmented communication devices.

The goal today is to help children with developmental disabilities participate in life by playing with other children, attending school and being a valued member of the family and community. This requires that the right blend of technologies, supports, and accommodations are provided in light of the student's needs and strengths (Scherer 2005). In-school interventions may include physical and occupational therapy, speech therapy, and the administration of medications that control seizures, relax muscle spasms, and alleviate pain. This may also include braces and other orthotic devices, communication aids such as computers with voice output, and a wide variety of additional products designed to minimize functional limitations and allow the achievement of academic goals and participation in the full academic curriculum.

Although students with developmental disabilities have educational and physical challenges, their potential is unlimited. The key is to identify abilities and strengths and strengthen them while managing limitations and match students with the opportunities and supports necessary to achieve lives of productivity and quality.

Treating Degenerative Disabilities

The situation is somewhat different at the other end of the life span for those individuals who have a degenerative cause of disability. Until recently, when an aging person was observed putting things in the wrong places and then forgetting where they put them, not performing personal care activities, and saying and doing inappropriate things, then that individual likely moved in with adult children or other relatives to be cared for and monitored. That still occurs today, but just as frequently the individual's primary care physician may recommend the family consider assisted living or a nursing home.

In some ways we have situations, the reverse of what they were traditionally. The families of infants and children with developmental disabilities now assume a major portion of caregiving because placing their child in an institution would be seen by today's society as an irresponsible act. At the same time options for caregivers of aging persons with dementia increasingly include placement in specialized facilities, which, in spite of efforts to lower the staff–patient ratio and create an attractive and homey atmosphere, are institutions for all practical purposes.

Treating an Acquired Disability

Once the person is stabilized medically, he or she may receive medical rehabilitation designed to strengthen remaining capabilities and compensate for those that have been lost. Psychosocial issues (financial, family, housing, or school/work) are viewed with the objective of returning the individual to prior roles and community participation (Scherer 2012).

Rehabilitation centers can be embedded within a larger medical centre or in a free-standing rehabilitation facility. Rehabilitation encompasses not only the therapy provided but also everything else that occurs on the unit, including nursing care, monitoring of behavior, nutritional assessment and planning, and nonpharmacological strategies and techniques employed to foster the optimal environment for recovery. As a result, therapy for the patient occurs 24 hours per day on the unit and provides the opportunity to carry over treatment, strategies, and training all day long and observe the recovery process more closely to adjust to a patient's needs more effectively. Even the physical structure and environment of the unit itself is often used to facilitate management of the patients.

For instance, limiting the points of access onto and off the unit often deters patients from wandering into unsafe areas. In addition, low stimulation settings help decrease agitation and irritability. All of these aspects of management facilitate recovery and help minimize the use of medications and their side effects.

Clinical information, the results of laboratory testing as well as imaging, all aid in the determination of disability. The evaluations done by occupational and physical therapists, speech–language pathologists, psychologists, and so on are equally important. Information from a variety of standardized assessments and tests are used to help determine and guide treatment planning from acute care to community (re)integration.

Outcome measures used to determine the effectiveness of medical interventions and rehabilitation continue to focus primarily on changes over time in body functions and structures and when quality of life is addressed, it is apt to be limited to health-related quality of life (e.g., Maas et al. 2010). A recent study reported, however, that health-related quality-of-life measures are predominantly measures of function that results "in a bias against people with long-standing functional limitations not related to current health" (Hall et al. 2011, p. 98).

As stated by Wilson (2006), improved ways of evaluating rehabilitation are needed that relinquish the dependence on traditional outcome measures that frequently fail to apprehend the real needs of patients and families. It remains the case, however, that too little attention is given to:

- The preferences and goals of individuals with disability and their family members,
- A person's predisposition to benefit from some interventions over others,
- The match of expectations of benefit with realization of benefit from the chosen interventions, and
- Social and environmental factors impacting benefit.

True to a *biopsychosocial approach*, rehabilitation needs to begin with an understanding of the current physical, cognitive, emotional/behavioral, and psychosocial functioning of the individual. This requires a rehabilitation team composed of individuals from the diverse areas of specialty, including neuropsychology, rehabilitation psychology, psychiatry, occupational therapy, speech–language pathology, social work, and vocational rehabilitation counseling. Specialists in sensory loss, such as audiologists and optometrists, may also be included. A key member of the team to include at the outset is the assistive technology specialist. Personal assistance and support from technologies, as well as environmental restructuring and the use of cognitive and behavioral strategies, are important resources. Case managers and disability advocacy organizations can help obtain further appropriate services for those in the community such as transportation, financial management, and housing assistance.

Presentation of the Chapters of Section II

The structure, level of intensity, and services available for rehabilitation vary widely from one area to another, whether comparing facilities, cities, states, and countries. As one illustration, a review of traumatic brain injury rehabilitation, listed the following as comprising the multidisciplinary rehabilitation team (Chua, et al. 2007):

- Person with a disability
- Family or caregivers of the person with a disability
- Rehabilitation physician or physiatrist
- Rehabilitation nurse, rehabilitation technicians
- Allied health professionals: physiotherapist, occupational therapist, speech and language pathologist, clinical psychologist, neuropsychologist, social worker, and counselor
- Paramedical health professionals: dietician, orthotist, and rehabilitation engineer
- Other medical specialists for example: ophthalmologist, gastroenterologist, neurologist
- Vocational rehabilitation services and counselors
- Volunteers from support or spiritual groups

The Joint Committee on Interprofessional Relations Between the American Speech–Language-Hearing Association and Division 40 (Clinical Neuropsychology) of the American Psychological Association (2007) also provided a list of professionals comprising the brain injury "interdisciplinary team:"

- Person with a disability
- Family or caregivers of the person with a disability
- Speech–language pathologist
- Clinical neuropsychologist
- Audiologist
- Rehabilitation psychologist
- Behavioral specialist
- Dietician
- Educator
- Occupational therapist
- Physical therapist (physiotherapist)
- Primary care physician
- Psychiatrist
- Physiatrist
- Rehabilitation nurse
- Social worker
- Case manager
- Therapeutic recreation specialist
- Vocational rehabilitation counselor
- Paraprofessionals

TABLE II.1

Chapters of Section II

Chapter	Topic
6	The Cognitive Therapist (Olivetti Belardinelli, Turella, and Scherer)
7	The Special Educator (Zapf and Craddock)
8	The Psychologist (Meloni, Federici, Stella, Mazzeschi, Cordella, Greco, and Grasso)
9	The Psychotechnologist (Miesenberger, Corradi, and Mele)
10	The Optometrist (Orlandi and Amantis)
11	The Occupational Therapist (de Jonge, Wielandt, Zapf, and Eldridge)
12	The Pediatric Specialist (Braga, de Camillis Gil, Pinto, and Siebra Beraldo)
13	The Geriatrician (Pigliautile, Tiberio, Mecocci, and Federici)
14	The Speech–Language Pathologist (Hill and Corsi)

The Joint Committee states that

> When cognitive, communication, emotional, and psychosocial domains are affected, the team should include at least a clinical neuropsychologist or rehabilitation psychologist, and speech–language pathologist. Team membership will vary with the age of the persons served, the type of impairment, the stage of recovery, and the special training of team members (2007, p. 4).

Thus, there is considerable consistency in these two views of the rehabilitation team, the first from Singapore and the second from the United States.

The nine chapters presented in this section (Table II.1) focus on and describe the role of many professions in the rehabilitation of persons with disabilities and their match with appropriate assistive technologies.

Each chapters was written by an international expert in his or her area of specialty. What unites these authors is not only their commitment to optimal rehabilitation outcomes, but their perspective of the biopsychosocial approach to the assistive technology evaluation, selection, and provision.

Conclusion

The best rehabilitation outcomes are achieved when individuals with shared perspectives, but representing different areas of knowledge and skill, pool their expertise to derive interventions that meet the personal, psychosocial as well as physical needs and preferences of the individual with a disability. This teamwork also needs to be brought to bear on the selection and provision of assistive solutions. Each of the contributors to this section describes how this can be achieved from the viewpoint of their training and practice.

References

Chua, K. S. G., Ng, Y.-S., Yap, S. G. M., and Bok, C.-W. (2007). A Brief Review of Traumatic Brain Injury Rehabilitation. *Annals of the Academy of Medicine, Singapore, 36*(1), 31–42. Retrieved from Annals.edu.sg website: http://www.ncbi.nlm.nih.gov/pubmed/17285184

Hall, T., Krahn, G. L., Horner-Johnson, W., and Lamb, G. (2011). Examining functional content in widely used Health-Related Quality of Life scales. *Rehabilitation Psychology, 56*(2), 94–99. doi:10.1037/a0023054

Joint Committee on Interprofessional Relations Between the American Speech–Language-Hearing Association and Division 40 (Clinical Neuropsychology) of the American Psychological Association. (2007). *Structure and Function of an Interdisciplinary Team for Persons with Acquired Brain Injury [Guidelines].* Retrieved from http://www.asha.org/policy doi:10.1044/policy. GL2007-00288

Maas, A. I., Harrison-Felix, C. L., Menon, D., Adelson, P. D., Balkin, T., Bullock, R., et al. (2010). Common data elements for traumatic brain injury: recommendations from the interagency working group on demographics and clinical assessment. *Archives of Physical Medicine and Rehabilitation, 91*(11), 1641-1649. doi:10.1016/j.apmr.2010.07.232

Scherer, M. J. (2005). *Living in the State of Stuck: How Technologies Affect the Lives of People with Disabilities* (4th ed.). Cambridge, MA: Brookline Books.

Scherer, M. J. (2012). *Assistive Technologies and Other Supports for People with Brain Impairment.* New York, NY: Springer Publishing.

Wilson, B. A. (2006). Recent Developments in Neuropsychological Rehabilitation. *Higher Brain Function Research, 26*(2), 121–127. doi:10.2496/hbfr.26.121

6

The Cognitive Therapist

M. Olivetti Belardinelli, B. Turella, and M. J. Scherer

CONTENTS

6.1 Cognitive Therapy

The origins of cognitive therapy are generally grounded in behavioral therapies. This is true when we consider the original modalities of the behavioral therapies. However, in the frame of the cognitive therapy panorama, we find that it is important now for therapists to consider behavior within a psychodynamic frame.

Behavioral therapy started in the 1940s and 1950s using the conditioning techniques envisaged by Pavlov for human behavior. On this basis, some authors explained human behavior by means of mediators, defined as intervening variables of a biological basis or cognitive type able to interact with antecedents through conditioning to particular consequences. The paradigm of instrumental conditioning afforded the possibility of modifying human behavior. In the first years behavioral modifications were obtained in situations in which it was easy to manipulate the environmental variables, or with subjects characterized with "cognitive simplicity," such as children, psychotics, and "generically disabled people." Afterward, neuroses, emotional problems, and behaviors connected with anxiety and depression were faced.

The name behavioral therapy was given by Lazarus to contrast it with the contemporary psychodynamic therapies. Lazarus based his approach on learning experience and conditioning principles.

Starting in the 1960s, behavioral therapy evolved into cognitive-behavioral therapy, putting greater attention on events internal to the person and to their influence on his or her behavior in relation to the environment. Bandura was the main contributor to this approach, and he put forward the theory of a "reciprocal determinism" between the environment, cognitive processes, and behavior. The restoration of the subject's active role led to the formulation of the concept of "self-efficacy," or the way in which the individual views his or her capabilities and capacity to act with influence. This consideration determines the subject's degree of vulnerability against the adversities of life.

At the beginning of the 1960s in this frame, characterized by a strong behavioristic theme, two new psychotherapeutic theories appeared that set the direction for clinical cognitivism. The first model is Ellis's (1962) and proposes a linear sequence of cognitive, emotional, and behavioral processes. According to the rational emotional behavioral therapy (REBT) beliefs, thoughts and ideas are the causes of the cognitive, emotional, and behavioral consequences that each subject experiences in relation to environmental events. Therefore all individuals are guided by their more or less rational, or distorted, beliefs when selecting their emotional attitudes and reactions. The absolute rule system deriving from beliefs is not always confirmed by everyday experiences; nevertheless, people do not succeed in correcting dysfunctional beliefs because of systematic procedural errors such as arbitrary deduction, selective abstraction, excessive generalization, tendency to magnify or minimize, personalization, or use of absolutist or dichotomous thought (Beck et al. 1979).

The second model is Beck's cognitive psychotherapy. This model culturally unifies many previous contributions with Beck's treatment for depression developed on the premise that the psychological disease and dysfunctional behavior derive from the way the subject is living and interpreting reality. According to Beck, the quality of thoughts and beliefs (schemes and core beliefs) conditions psychological status, which may be emotional dysfunction. The guiding principles of standard cognitive therapy are the following:

- Psychological difficulties are due to cognitive maladjusted processes that rule information processing in a pathological way. Different diagnostic clusters present recognizable patterns of abnormal conditions.
- The different patterns are expressed by automatic thoughts and conscious processing.
- The constructed beliefs and meanings are expressed in thoughts that can undergo logical analysis and empirical verification connected to used or ignored reality data.

The standard intervention is aimed at letting the patient became aware of his or her automatic thoughts, because they occur to the subject spontaneously and without control, appearing obvious and coherent within his or her structure.

Both for Ellis (1962) and Beck (1976), the therapeutic intervention entails the systematic analysis of representations, schemes, thoughts, and conscious and preconscious beliefs that precede, accompany, and follow a certain emotional state that the person experiences as problematic and ego-dystonic (Semerani 2002). However, this approach is flexible and rather diversified among different theorists and practitioners (Durlak et al. 1991; Gonzalez et al. 2004). When considered in continuity with more traditional theories and therapies, the focus is on the present and internal control with the aim of modifying thoughts and behaviors by means of theory teaching (Rait et al. 2010).

The principal differences between Beck's and Ellis's position are tied either to the reference theories, a scientific and evolutionary one for Beck and a philosophical theory for

Ellis, and to their therapeutic theory and technique, with a different consideration of the therapist's role. However, it is generally agreed that Beck and Ellis provided the most systematic and significant contributions to early cognitive psychotherapy and cognitive behavioral therapies.

The main difference between behavioral and cognitive approaches to therapy resides in the object to be changed: the behavior in the first case, and thoughts and emotions in the second.

On the clinical side, cognitive therapy entails many different approaches (Mahoney 1991) that share an emphasis on the ways of processing information, which determines the construction of meaning. In addition to this single commonality, these approaches are very different in many theoretical and epistemological topics determining prominent differences in intervention strategies and techniques. In any case, we underscore that the above-mentioned cognitive theories and therapies are all related to a rationalist matrix stressing the supremacy of cognitive processes.

The rationalist stance was followed by constructivist cognitivism, which stresses personal development processes and the construction of one's own meanings on the basis of emotional experiences. This underlines the interdependence and circular influence among thought, emotion, and action.

In the constructivist perspective, the principle of direct perception of reality and of incomplete correspondence between reality and reality knowledge, defined also as critical realism, is formulated as a principle of match between the two, and in more radical terms as a principle of knowledge fit to reality (von Glasersfeld 1984).

A further step was proposed by the biologists Maturana and Varela (1980, 1987) and by the computer scientist von Foerster (1984). According to them, knowledge is not the product of objectively valid cognitive processing. Rather, it is the result of a subjective interpretation that is valid only in a determinate space and time because it is linguistically generated and socially negotiated.

Such an important revolution of the knowledge paradigm started in the last decades of the past century with the crisis of the empiricist and rationalist epistemologies, not as much for the scientific and clinical results obtained by means of the classic cognitive approach. The results immediately appeared important and relevant because of discontent at a general theoretical level with the hypothesis of the functioning of mind (Olivetti Belardinelli 1973, 1976) and of the meaning of the psychic discomfort (Semerani 2002).

The behavioral approach and the cognitive-rationalist one are based on the assumption that knowledge is the representation of an objective and univocal order that exists independently from our "being in the world." This assumption passed through a crisis and then changed after the publication of work such as that of Mahoney (1980). In his "Psychotherapy and the Structure of Personal Revolutions" he criticizes in six points the behavioral-cognitive therapy giving origin to a new trend in the cognitive psychotherapy. In this study, the author underlines some critical points of the cognitive behavioral model. In particular, he criticized the consideration of rationality and explicit convictions as factors dominating and determining all human experience, both "normal" and pathological, to the detriment of emotional aspects, which are subjective, implicit, and autoreferential. The author maintains that the emphasis on rationality is excessive and unilateral. Moreover, in the therapeutic relation the stress falls on pedagogical and normative aspects, minimizing the complexity of relational events and their role in the therapeutic process. Meanwhile, he proposes a change model in psychotherapy so substantial and significant like those described by Kuhn as occurring during scientific revolutions.

In Italy, Guidano and Liotti (1983) proposed a new model defined as cognitivistic-postrationalist (Guidano 1987, 1991; Liotti 1991, 2001, 2005) to indicate "the relevant modification in the conceptualization of change and in the therapeutic methodology respect to the rationalist perspective" (Guidano 1991, p. 91). According to Guidano's cognitivistic-postrationalist perspective, knowledge is not intended as the result of the cognitive activity of the mind; rather, it is constructed by the mind on the basis of emotional intelligence. Logical and rational processing would be activated starting from a matrix of sensations and actions and would structure beliefs and thoughts, meanings, and explications functionally coherent to the emotional intelligence.

Guidano and Liotti derive their arguments not only from cognitive psychology but also from attachment theory, from developmental epistemology and ethology, and from other clinical theories and approaches. Afterward, thanks to the contribution offered by the theories of complexity and by the second cybernetics as well as that offered by "the theory of knowledge," systemized and developed principally by Maturana and Varela (1980, 1987), Guidano (1987, 1991) states an important epistemological principle: There is no reality or universe valid for everybody, but only a multiverse reality actively constructed by the observer according to rules that ensure identity, uniqueness, and continuity to the individual in his or her own experiences during the lifespan (von Glasersfeld 1984).

Further developments in the theory are tied to the importance attributed to knowledge construction, the concept of the self-organizing system and the principles that regulate its equilibrium (von Bertalanffy 1968; Maturana and Varela 1980, 1987; von Foerster 1984; Bocchi and Ceruti 1985), the use of language and narration (Bruner 1990), and the individual history, particularly of childhood attachment (Bowlby 1979, 1988) and emotional experiences.

The different cognitive formulations we just presented provide unavoidable spinoffs for therapeutic practice with very different ways of considering problems, illness, treatment, and the role of the therapist, as we will see in Section 6.2.

6.2 The Cognitive Therapist

Traditional cognitive psychology, although stating that an individual's own activity is always dependent on him or her and his or her experiences, interprets symptoms and disease as the result of an irrational and distorted belief that the therapist can modify because the presumption is that an external rational order that is univocal and identical for all does exist. For these reasons the traditional cognitive therapies are substantially persuasive because they apply a "method of systematic rational restructuration" aimed at changing "irrational beliefs" that are considered as the cause of the disease. According to the classical cognitive approach, psychological diseases stem from a set of maladjusted schemes or models that pathologically rule information processing. These models are expressed by automatic thoughts and conscious imagery.

In constructivist models, instead, psychopathology has two different possibilities of generation. It may stem from an alteration of functioning of a definite organization of the knowledge of oneself with the other one, centered on a well identifiable semantic nucleus as in the case of meaning organizations. Otherwise it can be generated by a disconnection between episodic and semantic knowledge of one's own self or by obstacles to the processes transforming implicit and emotional knowledge in an explicit one of constructed meanings about oneself and the world. These obstacles may be deficits of knowledge and recognition of emotions, meta-cognitive shortages, or conceptual and language deficiencies (Liotti 2001). Moreover there is a particular psychopathological modality specifically tied to the interactions mediated by the motivational system of attachment. This modality in particular is referred to the disorganized attachment with a representation of oneself with the other one that is dissociated, changing, and emotionally strong (Liotti 1999).

According to Beck (1976), the therapeutic intervention is relieving the psychological disease by means of the correction of wrong beliefs. The standard cognitive therapy (CT) intervention looks for the automatic thoughts and the underlying schemes to perform a critical analysis also by means of alternative thoughts. Patients' tasks are tied to the systematic self-observation technique with an introspective attitude aimed at reaching insight. The patient is taught to register in sequence the principal emotions in a problematic situation; the situation characteristics; and the thoughts and images that preceded, accompanied, and followed the implied emotion. The therapist cooperates with his or her patient at correcting the information processing style. To reach this aim, it is often necessary to help the patient to recognize his or her principal emotions by explaining, for example, which are the somatic correlates of some basic emotions or the tendency to act tied to some emotions (Beck et al. 1985).

Ellis (1962) also maintains that the therapeutic intervention has to detect the cognitive errors (irrational ideas) that cause the emotional disturbance. The correction, substitution, or elimination of such dysfunctional beliefs allow the therapists to "heal" the patient. The patient is invited to register events, beliefs, and consequences by analyzing irrational beliefs by means of the ABC (Activating event, Belief, and Consequences) technique. Therapy is a research in progress that is focused on thought patterns in which the therapist plays the role of an active and directive supervisor.

In the approaches of cognitive-behavioral therapy (CBT), the stress on the possibility of "guiding," "instructing," and "educating" the patient is particularly pronounced. For this reason Ellis also (2003) stated that the future of REBT and more generally of CBTs is tied to formal education. According to these approaches, the therapist knows which are the thoughts and convictions functional to the patient and therefore he affords from outside of the solution to his or her problem. The treatment is aimed at reducing the symptomatology and augmenting the strategies by means of which the patient can become more able to face the problem situations.

In contrast, the cognitive-constructivist approaches maintain that each person-system evolves according to its own rules that guarantee continuity, coherence, and uniqueness toward progressively more complex levels of organization and functioning. Therefore, the equilibrium of the system is not considered to be stable, univocal, and determined all at once; rather, it is considered to be dynamic, changing, and variable according to the numerous variables influencing the system at each particular time (Maturana and Varela 1980, 1987; Guidano 1987). A decompensation occurs in the following cases:

- These perturbing variables determine an alteration of the existing equilibrium that exceeds the system's capacity to return to normality by means of reorganization.
- Experiences and events generate turbulences and emotional fluctuations that go beyond the endurance threshold of the system.
- Reorganization cannot be held within a tolerance threshold and exceeding it renders the experience of being in that reality no more comprehensible and checkable.

The cognitive systems that present more decompensation risk are those characterized by relaxation or rigidity, whereas the more flexible systems, presenting a wider range of variability, are subjected to a minor risk because they are more able to activate effective decompensation strategies in crisis situations of the system (Reda 1986; Guidano 1987, 1991; Cionini 1991, 1998). Because each organization constrains the generative directionality of the personal life span while fixing the range of the tolerable variability, it includes in itself the causes of its own crisis. This is in agreement with the theory of the functioning of complex and autopoietic systems.

A system's functionality depends on its own capability of experiencing reality while constructing the reality. These meanings are dependent on the processing quality with respect to analysis and anticipatory conceptualization. They determine or guide the behavior, defined as the set of actions (including the speculative and emotional ones) aimed at reaching the goals that at each time and in every place the individual maintains must be reached.

The equilibrium, the efficiency, and the health of the system depend on the capacity to process meanings and models of the self that are realistic. These models should allow forecasts about the ways to reach goals, or rather they should indicate the necessity of changing goals, each time allowing that the constructed knowledge again enters the "circle" to feed the incessant process of living in the experience (Reda 1986; Cionini 1998).

In all cognitive approaches referring to Beck's and Ellis' theories, and in general in all cognitive-behavioral approaches, the relationship between the therapist and the patient is not considered the main tool for change; rather, it is appraised according to the treatment outcomes.

In different epistemological approaches the therapeutic relationship is considered as having different functions: support of ego functions, cognitive revealing of unconscious processes aimed at reaching insight and learning, increasing of meta-cognitive functions, and so on. Although all approaches have in common the necessity of creating a therapeutic alliance, an empathetic collaboration between therapist and patient, each of them constructs its experiments in the relationship in a way that is metaphorically similar to what happens in a laboratory (Semerani 2002).

Instead, in Guidano's postrationalist perspective (1987, 1991), the change coincides with a reorganization of the personal meaning and with the construction of a new equilibrium, not predictable in nature and quality but able to assimilate the imbalance through the increase of complexity and self-knowledge. During the therapeutic relationship the therapist avoids being surprised or criticizing the negative emotions tied to the imbalance so as not to confirm the noninvolvement sense experienced by the patient toward these discrepancies. In this sense the systemic approach is aimed at increasing the patient's knowledge of his or her own background and functioning rules using the disturbing emotions as information sources, in the meantime maintaining the internal coherence necessary to the conservation of the personal identity.

However, the change of these cognitive processes, activated by thought processes acting on thinking, develops according to different and speedier rhythms than motivations and emotional backgrounds that form the immediate experience. The systems language-thought and emotiveness-affectivity seem to be processed in distinct ways because the cognitive nucleus entails the application of operative rules of the formal logic whereas the affective aspects seem to combine in a much more stable way, following rules concerning the specific functioning of the person's system that is his or her auto-organization. Therefore, the implicit emotional nucleus can be modified only introducing new emotional tonalities that, while entering structured patterns formed during the life-span experience, are able to change their configuration. In other words, because thinking is able to change only the thoughts and only the emotional feeling is able to change emotions, psychotherapeutic change processes necessarily imply new emotional experiences that will be added to the affective nuclear themes. No change in knowledge and no change in process, in the therapeutic process too can occur without the involvement of emotionality. The person is considered as a complex structure of knowledge that is autonomous and shut from the organization point of view. The person autonomously constructs his or her own meaning on the basis of his or her own experience and these constructed meanings guide the person's future experiences. Therefore, these two levels in which it is possible to operate a change are strictly interconnected. In the patient's narrative it is difficult to discriminate the immediate experience from its explanation. Because this one is a partial and self-referred explanation, it inclines to exclude what is not decodable (Reda 1986; Cionini 1991). The first task of the therapist is to distinguish the immediate experience, the fact, from its explanation, the theory (Guidano 1987). In this way the therapist acts in space, in the interface between these two dimensions (the fact and the theory), and offers to the patient a new element, a new perspective able to upset the patient's structure. As we said, this is easy for thoughts, but to start a true therapeutic change it is necessary that the patient gets emotionally involved with the therapist. This implies that it is the significance of the relationship, its affective valence that guarantees the self-referential function according to which the perceived discrepancy may be referred by the patient to himself or herself rather than to the exterior. The emotional involvement is therefore the condition sine qua non to determine a change. Meanwhile, a change also occurs in the therapist when he or she prepares himself or herself to assume the "responsibility" to be there for the patient. According to Liotti (2001, 2005), the human being is motivated to recover by his or her own sufferings. The patient will recover and therefore activates his or her motivational system of attachment to which the activation of the attending system of the therapist has to match. Once the therapeutic alliance is established, the internal motivational system of joint cooperation is activated thanks to the explicit definition of the common goal. In this joint system there is a meaning sharing and a reciprocal help request because the therapist can also and has to ask for the patient's help; for example, he or she has to check that he or she has understood the patient. The therapist therefore works to detect the organization of the personal meaning in the personal plan and its functioning rules. Although this plan is often outside of the patient's consciousness, it unconsciously guides the patient himself or herself. The new discoveries set up, by means of self-reference, a process of restructuration and personal reorganization, able to "assimilate" the pathological beliefs and the discrepancies appeared with the unbalance and to reveal the innate motivations that are at the basis of the plan as a rule system regulating the personal organization functioning. Each time that during the therapy a pathological belief is rebutted, the process takes a step forward along the planned direction. At the time in which the therapeutic relationship is internalized, the therapeutic experience will sustain the continuity of consciousness outside of the therapist office (Liotti 2005).

During the therapeutic course, the therapist has to abandon the role of external observer, which holds absolute, objective, and right truths. He or she does not have the aim of indiscriminately increasing awareness, because to awareness are connected the loss of spontaneity and immediacy and the emergence of unpleasant and disturbing emotions that stem out from the difficulty of acknowledging oneself. Rather, the therapist aims to obtain an adaptive reorganization, a new homeostatic, wider, and more flexible equilibrium, by means of the minimal modification of the patient's self-knowledge and of the minimal oscillation of his or her identity sense. The goal is to let the patient experience and feel that his or her functioning, personal meaning, and plan determine both his or her world and his or her freedom while being in that world. Therefore according to Guidano, the therapeutic relationship

> evolves in a supervision relationship, as if the patient were a naïf therapist which periodically submit to a more expert colleague the trend of the cases he is healing, with the unique difference that the case he is treating is himself. (1991, p. 184)

6.3 Cognitive Therapy With Individuals Having Cognitive Disability

The efficacy of different types of intervention in the cognitivistic frame may be compared in the treatment of cognitive diseases. The definition of cognitive trouble in the frame of the wider category of disability has to be articulated and precise considering the further distinction between cognitive and intellectual diseases (Schalock and Luckasson 2004).

It is also to underscore that the diagnostic assessment and the intervention also substantially feel the effect of this definition, influencing the attitude of all participants. In fact, in addition to the categorical diagnosis, in the assessment phase the damage of the person system is evaluated (functional and dimensional analysis) to determine the presence/absence of resources necessary for treatment.

The cognitive diseases are generally defined as an alteration of the so-called superior cognitive functions: intelligence, attention, memory, language, reading and writing capacities, visiospatial abilities, praxis abilities, and executive functions (judgment ability, planning, cognitive flexibility, etc.). These diseases are normally the consequences of congenital or acquired brain damage. The most frequent causes of acquired cognitive disability in adults are cranial trauma, degenerative illnesses of the central nervous system (as in dementia and Alzheimer's disease), illnesses of the central nervous system (such as epilepsy and cerebral infections of viral origin), cerebral infarcts (ischemia), brain tumors, metabolic disorders, and other neurological illnesses.

Cognitive disabilities often result in difficulties in social and work adjustment, and they are often accompanied by relational and emotional problems (anxiety, insecurity, depression, etc.). The evaluation is based on anamnesis, on medical and neuropsychological assessments that investigate the damage in cognitive areas by means of behavioral observation, and on the use of sets of standardized tests.

The suitable intervention, in addition to the medical one, is cognitive rehabilitation combined with cognitive-behavioral therapy. Although in the past therapeutic interventions with subjects presenting cognitive disability were considered useless, there is a notable growing interest in structuring interventions focused and adapted to the presented cognitive deficit (Willner and Hatton 2006). It must be emphasized that psychological correlates of cognitive impairment are inevitable and cannot be omitted in a bio-psycho-social integrated approach (Arthur 2003).

Whatever is the adopted approach, it is necessary to adapt the therapy to patients with varying cognitive disabilities by simplifying techniques, language, and tasks while adopting a flexible method characterized by more directivity and at the same time more attachment behavior (Hurley et al. 1998). Only with these adaptations the therapeutic approaches used with the "normal" population, both the psychodynamical and the cognitivistic ones, can be effective with persons with cognitive disabilities. The reference theory determines which adaptations are more often realized in practice. In the CBT approach, the adaptations are mostly related to the technical aspects whereas in the psychodynamic approach they are more often tied to the therapist's attitude and to the countertransference (Whitehouse et al. 2006).

As previously said, the CBT approach is characterized by directivity and teaching to foster improvement of the damaged capacities and to teach the patient specific strategies of deficit compensation by means of the remaining abilities (Taylor 2005; Taylor et al. 2008). Many studies comparing the effectiveness of therapeutic interventions show many limits due to the difficulty of isolating the variables that have produced the change in the treated patients (Heyvaert et al. 2010). The theories, techniques, and strategies used by the therapist that determining the nature of his or her approach cannot be disentangled from his or her own personality variables and from the patient's personality variables, from the quality and significance of their relationship, from their communication and empathy capacity, and the quality/quantity of the problems. Moreover, the efficacy of the intervention is dependent upon external factors because familiar and social resources determine the extratherapeutic environment of the patient. Particular programs for the training of different cognitive abilities (memory, language, attention, etc.) have been developed and are uninterruptedly re-adapted following the demands and characteristics of each patient.

The techniques used in CBT are aimed at producing effects in three spheres: cognition, behavior, and physiology. In the cognitive sphere, the patients learn to activate cognitive reorganizations and to modify negative emotions to render the beliefs more logical and adaptive and the emotions more endurable (McGinn and Sanderson 2006).

The use of cognitive and behavioral principles and techniques that foster learning during the rehabilitation process simultaneously address relational and emotional problems that are obstacles to the success of rehabilitation therapy and the person's adjustment.

6.4 Cognitive Rehabilitation

True to the biopsychosocial approach mentioned earlier, cognitive rehabilitation begins with an understanding of the current cognitive, emotional/behavioral, and psychosocial functioning of the individual. The biopsychosocial approach or model was first articulated by George L. Engel, a psychiatrist at the University of Rochester Medical Center in Rochester, NY (1977). He stated that a pathophysiological view of illness and disability is insufficient for understanding illness and he put forth a systems perspective of treatment that considers the parts, the whole, and the dynamic interaction of biological, psychological (emotional/behavioral), and social factors impacting the individual. Today, the biopsychosocial approach is used to guide all patient treatment and medical education at the University of Rochester Medical Center, as well as many other programs around the world, and is the foundation for the World Health Organization's International Classification of Functioning, Disability, and Health (ICF) (WHO 2001).

With the biopsychosocial approach and the ICF framework as a foundation, the totality of cognitive, emotional/behavioral, and psychosocial functioning of the individual is considered when planning interventions. As mentioned earlier, neuropsychological testing and measurement are imperative to obtaining this understanding. The need to address the individual's unique and individualized pattern of functioning is well recognized.

- People with the same impairments experience different kinds and degrees of incapacity and vastly different restrictions on what actually happens in their lives. Impairments are not proxies for disability; they give only one particular perspective on disability. Disability is the complete lived experience of nonfatal health outcomes, not merely body-level decrements in functioning.

- The converse is also true: People can experience the same restrictions in what they can do in their day-to-day lives although they have different impairments. At the level of actual performance, the contrast is even greater. Impairments as diverse as missing limbs and anxiety can both attract stigma and discrimination that may limit a person's participation in work. (United Nations Economic and Social Commission for Asia and the Pacific 2010).

With the biopsychosocial approach and the ICF framework as a foundation, the totality of cognitive, emotional/behavioral, and psychosocial functioning of the individual is considered when planning interventions. Testing and measurement are imperative to obtaining this understanding. Once an individual with a new cognitive disability is medically stabilized, rehabilitation can begin. True to the biopsychosocial model, rehabilitation encompasses not only the cognitive therapy provided but the consideration of supports for the person's functioning, community living, and social participation.

It has been shown that comprehensive rehabilitation that integrates interventions for cognitive, interpersonal, and functional skills yields greater improvements in self-regulation of cognitive and emotional processes, community integration, employment, and quality of life compared with standard discipline-specific neurorehabilitation treatment (High et al. 2005; Hart 2010) and it has been shown to be effective (Cicerone et al. 2000, 2004, 2005, 2011; Tsaousides and Gordon 2009; Altman et al. 2010). The goal of cognitive rehabilitation is to increase the individual's functioning, adaptation, and quality of life by reinforcing, strengthening, or re-establishing previous learned patterns of behavior and establishing new patterns through compensatory mechanisms.

Problems with memory, conceptualizing, planning, and sequencing thoughts and actions; a lack of concentration, increased anxiety, and irritability; and difficulty interpreting subtle social cues and understanding numbers and symbols are common, as are visual, auditory, and/or vestibular deficits, balance problems, and loss of coordination. Thus, cognitive rehabilitation addresses memory retraining and problem-solving as well as enhanced self-awareness; compensation and coping; social skills; emotional self-regulation; participation in social, work, and leisure activities; health maintenance; and personal care. Personal assistance and support from technologies as well as environmental restructuring and the use of cognitive and behavioral strategies are all important resources.

6.5 Assistive and Cognitive Support Technologies

The ICF is in line with the UN Convention on the Rights of Persons with Disabilities (2006) in recognizing the importance of assistive technology (AT) devices and products for an individual's functioning, performance of activities, and successful participation in desired life roles and situations (Bickenbach 2009).

The World Health Organization recognizes that the ICF does not contain the depth and detail needed by those who specialize in the design, manufacture, distribution, and provision of AT devices. Therefore, in 2003, the ISO 9999 (Assistive Products for Persons with Disability—Classification and Terminology) was accepted as a related member of the WHO Family of International Classifications (WHO-FIC). ISO 9999 is a product of the International Organization for Standardization (ISO 2007) and is an international classification of assistive products in which all products that can be used by persons with disabilities are included. As presented by Heerkens et al. (2010), the definition of an assistive product in the fifth edition of ISO 9999 is

> Any product (including devices, equipment, instruments and software), especially produced or generally available, used by or for persons with disability

- For participation;
- To protect, support, train, measure, or substitute for body functions/structures and activities; or
- To prevent impairments, activity limitations, or participation restrictions (ISO 9999).

The ISO 9999 contains five different types of assistive products:

1. Products that support a function, but are not used as such in the performance of an activity (e.g., nebulizers, oxygen units)
2. Products that are used in the performance of an activity and that support a function or an activity (e.g., walking aids or assistive products for activities of daily living)
3. Products that are a substitute for a function/structure or protect a function/structure, may support a function, are not used in the performance of an activity but can be seen as a prerequisite for participation (e.g., a wig or a cap)
4. Products that are primarily used for training
5. Assistive products that are used to measure/monitor a function/structure, the performance of an activity, or an environmental or personal factor.

Products that are primarily used for training are the ones most pertinent to cognitive functioning, particularly those specific to assistive products for training in cognitive skill defined as assistive products designed to enhance the abilities that underlie reasoning and logical activities (e.g., memory, attention, concentration, and conceptual and applied thinking).

Although some may question the suitability of classifying cognitive support technologies as "products for training," nonetheless this is where they are included. ISO 9999 is used in several national databases of assistive products, including AbleData, which is discussed in Section 6.4.

Cognitive support technology (CST) is a special class of AT products designed to increase, maintain, or improve functional capabilities for individuals whose cognitive changes limit their effective performance of daily activities. CSTs have become more commonplace and diverse (Braddock et al. 2004; Gillette and De Pompei 2004; De Pompei et al. 2008; Bharucha et al. 2009; Sablier et al. 2009).

Broadly defined, CST could refer to very familiar, basic products used by people with and without disabilities to support memory, organization, or other cognitive functions, such as planner books, calendars, labels, post-it notes placed strategically, wristwatches, and shopping lists. Simple and low-cost devices such as magnifying lenses, index cards, and timers/alarm clocks can promote independence and improve the individual's quality of life. Technologies supporting interaction with people or information (telecommunication technologies) are also important resources for individuals with cognitive disabilities and they include telephones, pagers, and the Internet.

There are also specialized devices designed expressly for use by individuals with cognitive disabilities and their caregivers. These specialty products have features that can

- Maintain, organize, and facilitate access to information;
- Present suggestions, instructions, or corrections to the user either on demand or at prescribed times;

- Assume responsibility for task components that have proven too complex for an individual to complete independently so that activities in which those components are embedded can be successfully completed;
- Provide more comprehensive interactive guidance for tasks that are too difficult for the user to initiate or perform, even with other types of modifications and compensatory strategies; and
- Monitor the quality of the user's task performance so errors can be tracked and the CST intervention subsequently modified in an attempt to reduce those errors (Scherer et al. 2005).

Regardless of the sophistication of a device, the primary goal of CST interventions is to improve the performance of functional activities that are critical components of life role fulfillment and participation in community activities, that contribute substantially to subjective well-being and quality of life, and that significantly reduce caregiver burden.

Important aspects of technology selection are knowing the settings in which they will be used and addressing environmental factors and accommodations. Another key is AT service delivery and how to best match a particular individual with the most appropriate technology for his or her use. The following case study illustrates how this can be achieved.

A support selection model has been proposed that takes these factors into account (Scherer 2012; Scherer et al. 2007). It is aligned with the Matching Person and Technology (MPT) model, which is depicted in Figure 6.1.

The goal of the service delivery process is to achieve an optimal match of person and technology. This requires considerations in three domains: characteristics of the person, environments of use, and aspects of the technology product. Getting to know any given person requires a commitment to establishing rapport and exploring strengths, needs, and goals. This is ideally done in partnership with a cognitive therapist. Five examples of key areas to address are shown in the chart, but there are many others that could be added. Some key considerations regarding the characteristics and resources of the individual person include

- *Functional needs:* Does the person have the essential requisite skills to use the technology to maximal advantage? For example, do they have keyboard skills or the requisite ability to read?
- *Lifestyle:* How much will use of the support affect typical routines? How much does that matter to the person?
- *Personal factors:* What is the person's history of prior exposure to and experiences with technologies (and other supports)?
- *Expectations/mood:* What are the person's dreams and goals? When faced with change, does the person generally approach it with a positive attitude, confidence, and self-determination, or with confusion, helplessness, and/or dependence on others?
- *Motivation and readiness:* Does the person view technology (or other support) use as a desirable means of achieving dreams and goals? Does the person perceive a discrepancy between the current and desired situation?

Characteristics of the environments of use as well as of the selected technology itself are the next key areas to address, followed by the cycle of support selection, use, evaluation, and accommodation. Cognitive rehabilitation depends on consistency and the ability to generalize across settings, which sometimes actually means retraining the same skills

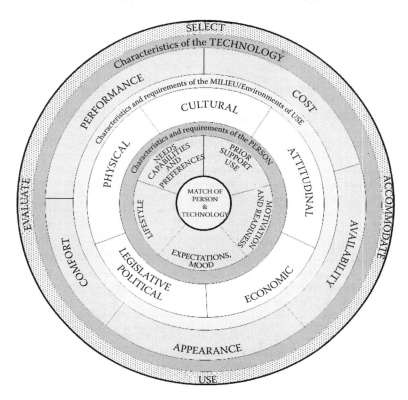

FIGURE 6.1
MPT model: Influences to consider when trying to achieve a good match of person and cognitive support technology. See color Figure 3.1.

when the setting changes. Thus, when there is a change in AT (e.g., different Smartphone or augmentive and alternative communication device), the individual's progress can be affected. This is why this is a cycle and not a one-time assessment. One means of assessing a consumer's perspective of technology use is to have individuals rate their difficulties as well as prioritize their own desired outcomes and progress over time in achieving them. This is the system used in the MPT process (Scherer 1998, 2005), Although individual needs may vary, it is possible to develop standard guidelines to ensure that individual needs and preferences are identified. The MPT assessment process offers one such standard approach. It emerged from a grounded theory research study (Scherer 1986) and has been operationalized by an assessment process consisting of several measures. The items differentiate characteristics of the actual experiences of users and nonusers and they have held up well in additional research studies (Scherer and Sax 2010).

The MPT assessment measures are idiographic and person-focused. They can be used as an interview guide or the consumer can complete the forms independently on paper or on a computer. Assessments range from a quick screen to specialized evaluations (completed in approximately 15 min) to a comprehensive evaluation (completed in approximately 45 min) by someone trained and experienced in their use. The specific steps, with accompanying measures, are shown in Table 6.1. Samples of the actual user forms can be found at http://matchingpersonandtechnology.com.

TABLE 6.1

Matching Person and Technology (MPT) Assessment Process and Forms

- **Step One:** *Initial Worksheet for the Matching Person and Technology Process* is organized by areas in which persons may experience loss of function (e.g., speech/communication, mobility, hearing, and eyesight) or have important strengths. It identifies initial goals and areas to strengthen through the use of a technology (or other support/strategy) or environmental accommodation. Potential interventions supportive of the goals are written in the space provided on the form. When a new technology is being introduced to a person, it is better to work from an area of strength. Each item should be addressed, regardless if a professional believes it is relevant for this individual or not. You never know what connection will be triggered or what observations will be recollected that will impact later decision-making.

- **Step Two:** *History of Support Use* is used to identify supports used in the past, satisfaction with those supports, and why a new type of support may be better than alternatives. It is organized according to the same areas of functioning as the Initial Worksheet in Step One.

     Although steps one and two do focus on the "separate parts" of the individual, it is believed that unless each area is addressed, key barriers to optimal technology use may be missed. For example, when you focus on communication and are about to recommend a device that requires very go od vision, and that has not been assessed, there may be problems if the person does have significant vision loss. The goal is to emphasize the whole person and do a comprehensive assessment considering the whole person, environments of support use, and so on, but to achieve this by considering in turn the many parts that make up the whole and their relationship to one another.

- **Step Three:** *Specific Technology Matching.* The individual (person with a disability, family member, caregiver, or these separately) completes his or her version of the appropriate form depending on the type of technology under consideration. The modular nature of the assessments allows the use of one, two, or more forms –as well as and sections of forms. The individual versions of the Assistive Technology Device Predisposition Assessment and Cognitive Support Technology Device Predisposition Assessment have the option for computerized scoring with interpretive guidelines.

  - General:
  Survey of Technology Use—Individual
  Survey of Technology Use—Professional
     A 29-item checklist that inquires into the respondent's present experiences and feelings toward technologies. The questions ask individuals to list all of the different technologies they use and feel comfortable using, the idea being that the introduction of a new technology should build upon and capitalize on existing comfort and skill. Individuals are also asked to provide information about areas regarding their general mood, preferences, and social involvement that have been found in research to cause a favorable predisposition toward technology use. The professional version is identical to the consumer version.

  - Assistive:
  Assistive Technology Device Predisposition Assessment—Individual
  Assistive Technology Device Predisposition Assessment—Professional
     The ATD PA inquires into individuals' subjective satisfaction with key body functions (9 items), asks individuals to prioritize aspects of their lives in which they desire the most positive change (12 items), profiles individuals' personal factors and psychosocial characteristics (33 items), and asks for individuals' opinions regarding their expectations regarding the use of a particular type of assistive device (12 items). The scales are labeled view of capabilities, subjective quality of life, family support, support from friends, mood and temperament, autonomy and self-determination, self-esteem, and readiness for technology use. The final section allows for the comparison of competing devices and rates the device and person match. The ATD PA (professional form) allows the professional to determine and evaluate incentives and disincentives to the use of the device by a particular person.
  Ages 0–5, Matching Assistive Technology & CHild (MATCH—Early Intervention)
  Ages 6–21, Matching Assistive Technology & CHild (MATCH—School Version)

  - Cognitive Support:
  Cognitive Support Technology Device Predisposition Assessment—Individual
  Cognitive Support Technology Device Predisposition Assessment—Professional
  The CST PA is structured like the ATD PA, but it has an additional six items in body functions focused on specific mental functions:
  Paying attention, not getting distracted

TABLE 6.1 (CONTINUED)

Matching Person and Technology (MPT) Assessment Process and Forms

> Remembering information about people or events
> Remembering where I put things
> Managing appointments and doing things on time
> Solving problems that come up in daily life
> Reading

- Educational:
  Educational Technology Device Predisposition Assessment—Student
  Educational Technology Device Predisposition Assessment—Teacher
  The ET PA is a 43-item form designed to assess student and educator perspectives in four key areas: (1) educational goal and need, (2) particular educational technology under consideration, (3) psychosocial environments in which the technology will be used, and (4) student learning style and preferences.

- Workplace:
  Workplace Technology Device Predisposition Assessment—Individual
  Workplace Technology Device Predisposition Assessment—Employer
  The 28 items in the WT PA address key characteristics of the technology being proposed, the person or employee, and the workplace.

- Healthcare:
  Healthcare Technology Device Predisposition Assessment—Professional
  The 42-item HCT PA is a checklist addressing characteristics of the particular health problem, healthcare technology, likely consequence of HCT use, personal issues, and attitudes of significant others toward the course of treatment.

  Each of the individual forms may serve as a guide for an oral interview, if that seems more appropriate for the situation. The professional completes the professional version of the same form and identifies any discrepancies in perspective between the professional's and the individual's responses. These discrepancies then become a topic for discussion and counseling.

- **Step Four:** The professional discusses with the individual those factors that may indicate problems with his or her acceptance or appropriate use of the technology.

- **Step Five:** After problem areas (barriers, limitations) have been noted, the professional and individual work to identify specific intervention strategies and devise an action plan to address the problems.

- **Step Six:** The strategies and action plans are committed to writing because experience has shown that plans that are merely verbalized are not implemented as frequently as written plans. Written plans also serve as documentation and can provide the justification for any subsequent actions such as requests for funding or release time for training.

- **Step Seven:** A follow-up assessment is conducted to determine any adjustments to or accommodations needed for the technology and to inquire into realization of benefit, goal achievement, and whether the individual consumer has changed priorities. The measures in step three are used at baseline/initial assessment and then again at follow-up to determine change over time for a particular person.

6.6 Case Study

6.6.1 A Real-Life Example of a Vocational Rehabilitation Counselor's Solution-Seeking for James, Who Has Early Onset Alzheimer's Disease

James is a 53-year-old Caucasian male with early-onset Alzheimer's disease. He is currently functioning in stage 5 of the disease. He is a high-school graduate with two semesters of college. He is a very intelligent man and takes pride in the fact that most of his education was self-taught and he continues to take a proactive approach to learning. His overall physical health is good, but he does have other medical conditions such as diabetes and high blood pressure, but these conditions have been stable for the past five years. He had a pacemaker implanted two years ago without complications. He also has a diagnosis of major depression, which has been very unstable in the past but has improved in the last few months. He has never been hospitalized for depression. A neuropsychological evaluation in December 2009 revealed that his short-term memory and delayed short-term memory are severely impaired. He is on several medications appropriate to his medical conditions and he takes them regularly with the assistance of a medication daily/weekly planner device. He no longer drives a car, but he has a support system for his transportation needs for both work and leisure activities.

The goal is to help him maintain employment and independence with daily living skills and leisure activities. His primary hobby is reading. He is still coping with the loss of his major interests of participating in professional and community theater and his former profession of radio announcer/news director. Within 6 months of his diagnosis, he could no longer cope with the high stress and pressure of constant deadlines associated with the radio business. Within three weeks of resigning from this position he began working part-time at the ibrary. The activity he misses the most is acting in theater and films as well as directing plays. There were times in his life where his primary income came from this line of work; however, he can no longer remember lines or stage directions. Giving up the radio business and theater also represented a loss of notoriety in the community where he made personal appearances and donated his time for charitable organizations. The only exception to this was when he decided to "go public" with his diagnosis two years ago and has acted as a spokesperson for the local chapter of the Alzheimer's Association. He has made a TV commercial for them, raised funds, made personal appearances to "put a familiar face" on the disease, and volunteered his time to do general office work for the association.

James has significant limitations, but he also has important talents he can use to help others and to remain actively involved in life. Although he is currently employed, as the disease progresses over time he will need more assistance to maintain a level of functioning and as much independence as possible. Introducing simple-to-learn, low-tech AT will probably suit him best and it will be easier for him to learn how to use it now to help him sustain his level of functioning for a longer period of time.

6.6.2 MPT Survey Results and Assessment Analysis

The most important incentive to use AT is to prolong his independence and in some ways improve his current level of independence. Two specific issues were identified as problematic areas of his life. He is currently very dependent on others in that he has developed the habit that it is easier just to ask someone questions repeatedly rather than attempt to remember it on his own. If he could write down the instructions on how to check his voicemail messages on his cell phone, he would not have to repeatedly ask for assistance for this task or write down appointments on a calendar that he could refer to when he has a question about his commitments. These simple measures have the potential to go a long way in preserving relationships with co-workers and supervisors, as well as family members, who may lose their patience with him. The second identified issue is losing valuable and important items, such as his cell phone or eye glasses. Whenever he loses or even temporarily misplaces items of value, he quickly becomes depressed, expressing feelings of being worthless and a burden to those around him. Aside from repeated replacement costs, he cannot see to read without his glasses. If a locator device could be modified to fit his glasses without interfering with balance or line of vision, this would be a major financial incentive for his family and help with his self-esteem. This locator device could help this consumer locate his glasses before anyone else even knows they are missing, saving him this personal battle with his self-esteem and embarrassment in front of family and friends.

The only identified disincentive is that eventually the disease will rob him of his ability to use these low-tech devices. There will come a time when he will not remember what the locator device remote is for or how it works or he will forget to write things down, or even if he does write them down, he will not remember to look at the device. He may even lose these AT devices. All of these scenarios represent another loss of function in his life and during moments of clarity in cognition, he may realize yet another loss in his life. Conversely, even after he can no longer remember how to use the locator device, it could still be of assistance to his family to help them locate items he has misplaced. However, until that day comes, this consumer has the potential to be successful with these easy-to-use low-tech devices to improve his quality of life at work and at home.

The Initial Worksheet for the MPT model and History of Support Use was used and it covered the basics and promoted discussions questioning if those areas were applicable.

The Assistive Technology Device Predisposition Assessment (ATD PA) was the most helpful in revealing good information that may not have been divulged in the course of a conversation or counseling session. It appeared easier for this consumer to own these issues and feelings through this form without having to verbally admit to them. The computer-generated ATDPA results provided good feedback so everyone could clearly see his areas of importance, strength, and weakness. He identified participation in desired activities; freedom to go where desired; and fitting in, belonging, and feeling connected as his three most important quality-of-life issues. The results of the survey also concluded that he may have difficulty accepting and learning new devices and may not be ready to accept significant new challenges, stressing the importance of a slower introduction of devices and pacing to learn or incorporate their use. The device comparisons for potential successful use of the selected AT devices was very encouraging. The biggest hindrance to successful implementation at this point is the lack of availability of an appropriate product.

6.6.3 Research, Implementation, and Recommendations

All of the AT devices explored are assistive daily living devices to enhance short-term memory. All of these devices would be applicable to both the James' personal and professional life. In the course of the initial conversations several items were discussed, including a Palm Pilot Pre, Blackberry, iPhone 3G, various calendars including a day planner book, notebooks (8.5 × 11 and 8.5 × 5.5), and a locator device for lost items.

Professionals provided their personal Palm Pilot Pres, Blackberries, and iPhones, respectively. They worked with James to determine if he could learn to use the items, feel comfortable with them, and could remember how to use them. We met on two different days to judge his retention from one day to the next. James was not comfortable with any of these items, and they appeared to intimidate and overwhelm him. He found the Blackberry and Palm Pilot Pre particularly frustrating. The tiny keys for texting were particularly frustrating because his fingers kept hitting multiple keys. He also had difficulty remembering the commands, which buttons to push, or how to navigate within the system of each of these devices. Of the three devices, the iPhone 3G was the most user-friendly for him. Having the largest flat surface with the apps readily available with easily recognizable icons and the ease of accessing and moving the apps with the stroke of a finger appeared to lesson his anxiety; however, on the second attempt to use the iPhone the next day, he could not remember how to manipulate the apps or even how to access the most basic commands of answering the phone, checking voicemail messages, making and retrieving notes/calendar notations, or accessing the Internet. It was as if he had never seen an iPhone before. He literally could not remember how to do any of the functions. James admitted that he was never very technologically savvy and has never fully embraced or kept abreast of computer technology development.

Because of the diagnosis of early-onset Alzheimer's disease in which he has difficulty learning and retrieving new information, we decided to delve more into items that were a part of his past as a younger man or child. This approach led us to various types of paper/hard-copy notebooks and calendars.

Research has shown that even in the most advanced cases of Alzheimer's disease, keeping a calendar readily visible and marking off each day is vital to helping keep people with this disease oriented to time and date. James chose to use a basic wall calendar by the kitchen door that has simple, mostly unadorned squares to write his work schedule and medical appointments. For use of a notebook, he chose a smaller notebook 8.5 × 5.5 with a discrete black binder. He stated he will not use this AT device at work because of his specific work duties, he does not feel it is necessary, but he has agreed to use it at home for daily tasks and important instructions.

We have also been working on modifying existing technology to fashion a locator device for smaller objects such as eye glasses and a cell phone. The currently available products are based on a remote control locater that is synced with a receiver tag, about the size of a nickel or quarter, which can be hung on a key ring or the receiver can be attached with double-sided tape to a smoother surface like an eye-glass case. This has the potential to work fine if James remembers to replace his glasses in their case, which most of the time he does not. Both of these receiver devices are too large to attach to the actual eye glass frames or too bulky to attach to a cell phone. In researching the currently available products, most got mixed reviews at best. The main problems included that the audible signal (beeping) was not loud enough or did not work until you were within a couple of feet of the lost item (even when they were advertised to work within 25 feet) or the item was too complicated to program or set up. In working with the engineer member of our technology team, he suggested and did some research on RFID (radio frequency identification tag) technology. This is the same system that is used in large department stores to prevent shoplifting. Inventory is tagged with an RFID label that is deactivated by scanning during the checkout and what triggers the door alarm when the label is not deactivated properly. This technology is promising for this application because the labels can be made very thin and small; however, cost-effectiveness is an issue. The smallest labels are relatively inexpensive at less than $5 each, but they are made by a different company than that which makes the receivers, which can run as much as $20,000.

James appeared to be comfortable with the general process. He did appear to experience stress and was easily overwhelmed with some of the individual products during the AT exploration process. This made the professionals involved more aware of the importance of James' feelings and comfort with devices and choosing devices appropriate not only to the task at hand, but to the James' preference and not their own preferences.

Since this began, James has had mixed success with the chosen AT devices. He has begun using a basic wall calendar. He decided to only write the hours, such as 5:00—9:00 p.m., and leave the day he is off blank. This minimizes the appearance of clutter for him and he can tell at a glance whether or not he even works that day. He initially still had trouble figuring out which day it was, so he began crossing off the previous day first thing the next morning. On days when he forgets to cross of the days and he is confused as to which day it is, I have been working with him to check the display on his cell phone, which clearly shows this information on the LED screen.

He has also used the notebook at home to write important tasks and instructions, but he does not always remember to refer to it. It has worked well for noting daily chores. He is able to scratch off the chores as he completes them, giving him a greater sense of accomplishment. Another application for the notebook, which has been met with less success on the initial tries, is writing down instructions on how to do things that are important to him. For instance, how to retrieve his voicemail messages from his cell phone and how to get rid of the little red light that is displayed on the cable TV box indicating the cable company has sent a message about a special offering. These are two things that tend to agitate him until they are cleared. I assisted James by walking him through the steps for both of these tasks as he wrote down the directions. This AT application has been tested twice with the cable box red message light. During the first attempt, we discovered the written instructions did not work because he had thrown away the instructions when he threw out a completed task list. With assistance, he rewrote the instructions, adding in large letters across the top of each sheet what the instructions are for (Cell Voicemail and Cable Red Light) and placed them in the inside pocket of the binder separate from his daily task list. The one attempt at using this device since he has rewritten them worked minimally because the directions he wrote were very sketchy and not clear enough. Since then, I have written the instructions in simple, clear steps, but with more specific details. Because James has continued to try to use this device, it is promising that he will be able to successfully integrate it into his routine.

6.7 Conclusions

The cognitive therapist has multiple responsibilities, but one key fundamental role is the assessment of cognitive functioning and deriving means of ensuring that individuals achieve enhanced functioning, performance of activities, and successful participation in desired life roles and situations. Assistive and cognitive support technologies can greatly facilitate this achievement, but only if the selected technologies are well-matched to the individual's preferences, priorities, and needs.

Summary of the Chapter

Consistent with the biopsychosocial approach and the ICF framework, the role of the cognitive therapist focuses on the totality of cognitive, emotional/behavioral, and psychosocial functioning of the individual to enhance that person's functioning, community living, and social participation. Testing and measurement are key elements, as is behavioral cognitive therapy. Personal assistance and support from technologies, as well as environmental restructuring and the use of cognitive and behavioral strategies, are all important resources, but they require a selection process to facilitate appropriate matching of person and support.

References

Altman, I. M., Swick, S., Parrot, D., and Malec, J. F. (2010). Effectiveness of community-based rehabilitation after traumatic brain injury for 489 program completers compared with those precipitously discharged. *Archives of Physical Medicine and Rehabilitation, 91*(11), 1697–1704. doi:10.1016/j.apmr.2010.08.001

Arthur, A. R. (2003). The emotional lives of people with learning disability. *British Journal of Learning Disabilities, 31*(1), 25–30. doi:10.1046/j.1468-3156.2003.00193.x

Beck, A. T. (1976). *Cognitive Therapy and the Emotional Disorders.* New York: International Universities Press.

Beck, A. T., Emery, G., and Greenberg, R. L. (1985). *Anxiety Disorders and Phobias: A Cognitive Perspective.* New York: Basic Books.

Beck, A. T., Rush, A. J., Brian, F. S., and Emery, G. (1979). *Cognitive Therapy of Depression.* New York: Guilford Press.

Bharucha, A., Anand, V., Forlizzi, J., Dew, M. A., Reynolds III, C. F., Stevens, S., et al. (2009). Intelligent assistive technology applications to dementia care: Current capabilities, limitations, and future challenges. *American Journal of Geriatric Psychiatry, 17*(2), 88–104. doi:10.1097/JGP.0b013e318187dde5

Bickenbach, J. E. (2009). Disability, culture and the UN Convention. *Disability and Rehabilitation, 31*(14), 1111–1124. doi:10.1080/09638280902773729

Bocchi, G., and Ceruti, M. (Eds.). (1985). *La Sfida della Complessità.* Milano, Italy: Feltrinelli.

Bowlby, J. (1979). *The Making and Breaking of Affectional Bonds.* London: Routledge.

Bowlby, J. (1988). *A Secure Base: Clinical Applications of Attachment Theory.* London: Routledge.

Braddock, D., Rizzolo, M. C., Thompson, M., and Bell, R. (2004). Emerging technologies and cognitive disability. *Journal of Special Education Technology, 19*(4), 49–56.

Bruner, J. S. (1990). *Acts of Meaning.* Cambridge, MA: Harvard University Press.

Cicerone, K. D., Dahlberg, C., Kalmar, K., Langenbahn, D. M., Malec, J. F., Bergquist, T. F., et al. (2000). Evidence-based cognitive rehabilitation: Recommendations for clinical practice. *Archives of Physical Medicine and Rehabilitation, 81*(12), 1596–1615. doi:10.1053/apmr.2000.19240

Cicerone, K. D., Dahlberg, C., Malec, J. F., Langenbahn, D. M., Felicetti, T., Kneipp, S., et al. (2005). Evidence-based cognitive rehabilitation: Updated review of the literature from 1998 through 2002. *Archives of Physical Medicine and Rehabilitation, 86*(8), 1681–1692. doi:10.1016/j.apmr.2005.03.024

Cicerone, K. D., Langenbahn, D. M., Braden, C., Malec, J. F., Kalmar, K., Fraas, M., et al. (2011). Evidence-based cognitive rehabilitation: Updated review of the literature from 2003 through 2008. *Archives of Physical Medicine and Rehabilitation, 92*(4), 519-530. doi:10.1016/j.apmr.2010.11.015

Cicerone, K. D., Mott, T., Azulay, J., and Friel, J. C. (2004). Community integration and satisfaction with functioning after intensive cognitive rehabilitation for traumatic brain injury. *Archives of Physical Medicine and Rehabilitation, 85*(6), 943–950. doi:10.1016/j.apmr.2003.07.019

Cionini, L. (1991). *Psicoterapia Cognitiva* [Cognitive Psychotherapy]. Rome: Carocci.

Cionini, L. (Ed.). (1998). *Psicoterapie. Modelli a Confronto.* Rome: Carocci.

De Pompei, R., Gillette, Y., Goetz, E., Xenopoulos-Oddsson, A., Bryen, D., and Dowds, M. (2008). Practical applications for use of PDAs and smartphones with children and adolescents who have traumatic brain injury. *NeuroRehabilitation, 23*(6), 487–499. Retrieved from http://www.ncbi.nlm.nih.gov/pubmed/19127002

Durlak, J. A., Fuhrman, T., and Lampman, C. (1991). Effectiveness of cognitive-behavior therapy for maladapting children: A meta-analysis. *Psychological Bulletin, 110*(2), 204–214. doi:10.1037//0033-2909.110.2.204

Ellis, A. (1962). *Reason and Emotion in Psychotherapy.* New York: Lyle Stuart.

Ellis, A. (2003). Reasons why rational emotive behavior therapy is relatively neglected in the professional and scientific literature. *Journal of Rational-Emotive and Cognitive-Behavior Therapy, 21*(3/4), 245–252. doi:10.1023/A:1025842229157

Engel, G. L. (1977). The need for a new medical model: A challenge for biomedicine. *Science, 196*(4286), 129–136. doi:10.1126/science.847460

Gillette, Y., and De Pompei, R. (2004). The potential of electronic organizers as a tool in the cognitive rehabilitation of young people. *NeuroRehabilitation, 19*(3), 233–243. Retrieved from http://www.ncbi.nlm.nih.gov/pubmed/15502256

Gonzalez, J. E., Nelson, J. R., Gutkin, T. B., Saunders, A., Galloway, A., and Shwery, C. S. (2004). Rational emotive therapy with children and adolescents: A meta-analysis. *Journal of Emotional and Behavioral Disorders, 12*(4), 222–235. doi:10.1177/10634266040120040301

Guidano, V. F. (1987). Complexity of the Self: A Developmental Approach to Psychopathology and Therapy. New York: Guilford Press.

Guidano, V. F. (1991). The Self in Process: Toward a Post-Rationalist Cognitive Therapy. New York: Guilford Press.

Guidano, V. F., and Liotti, G. (1983). Cognitive Processes and Emotional Disorders: A Structural Approach to Psychotherapy. New York: Guilford Press.

Hart, T. (2010). Cognitive rehabilitation. In R. G. Frank, M. Rosenthal, and B. Caplan (Eds.), *Handbook of Rehabilitation Psychology* (2nd ed., pp. 285–300). Washington, DC: American Psychological Association.

Heerkens, Y. F., Bougie, T., and de Kleijn-de Vrankrijker, M. W. (2010). Classification and terminology of assistive products. In J. Stone, and M. Blouin (Eds.), *International Encyclopedia of Rehabilitation* (pp. 1–12). Buffalo, NY: Center for International Rehabilitation Research Information and Exchange (CIRRIE). Retrieved from http://cirrie.buffalo.edu/encyclopedia/en/article/265/

Heyvaert, M., Maes, B., and Onghena, P. (2010). A meta-analysis of intervention effects on challenging behaviour among persons with intellectual disabilities. *Journal of Intellectual Disability Research, 54*(7), 634–649. doi:10.1111/j.1365-2788.2010.01291.x

High, W. M., Sander, A. M., Struchen, M. A., and Hart, K. A. (2005). *Rehabilitation for Traumatic Brain Injury.* New York: Oxford University Press.

Hurley, A. D., Tomasulo, D. J., and Pfadt, A. G. (1998). Individual and group psychotherapy approaches for persons with mental retardation and developmental disabilities. *Journal of Developmental and Physical Disabilities, 10*(4), 365–386. doi:10.1023/A:1021806605662

International Standards Organization (ISO). (2007). ISO 9999:2007: Assistive Products for Persons with Disability—Classification and Terminology. Geneva, Switzerland: ISO.

Liotti, G. (1991). Il significato delle emozioni e la psicoterapia cognitiva [The meaning of emotions and the cognitive psychotherapy]. In T. Magri, and F. Mancini (Eds.), *Emozione e Conoscenza [Emotion and Knowledge]* (pp. 227–244). Roma: Editori Riuniti.

Liotti, G. (1999). Disorganized attachment as a model for understanding dissociative psychopathology. In J. Solomon, and C. George (Eds.), *Attachment Disorganization* (pp. 291–317). New York: Guilford Press.

Liotti, G. (2001). Le Opere della Coscienza. Psicopatologia e Psicoterapia Nella Prospettiva Cognitivo-Evoluzionista [The Labours of Consciousness]. Milan, Italy: Cortina Raffaello.

Liotti, G. (2005). La Dimensione Interpersonale Della Coscienza [The Interpersonal Dimension of Consciousness] (2nd ed.). Rome: Carocci.

Mahoney, M. J. (1980). Psychotherapy and the structure of personal revolutions. In M. J Mahoney (Ed.), *Psychotherapy Process: Current Issues and Future Directions* (pp. 157–180). New York: Plenum Press.

Mahoney, M. J. (1991). *Human Change Processes: The Scientific Foundations of Psychotherapy.* New York: Basic Books.

Maturana, H. R., and Varela, F. J. (1980). *Autopoiesis and Cognition: The Realization of the Living.* Boston: Reidel.

Maturana, H. R., and Varela, F. J. (1987). The Tree of Knowledge: The Biological Roots of Human Understanding. Boston: Shambhala.

McGinn, L. K., and Sanderson, W. C. (2006). What allows cognitive behavioral therapy to be brief: Overview, efficacy, and crucial factors facilitating brief treatment. *Clinical Psychology: Science and Practice, 8*(1), 23–37. doi:10.1093/clipsy.8.1.23

Olivetti Belardinelli, M. (1973). *La Costruzione della Realtà* [The Construction of Reality]. Torino, Italy: Boringhieri.

Olivetti Belardinelli, M. (1976). Prospettive dell'odierna psicologia scientifica. [Perspectives of Todays Scientific Psychology]. *Comunicazioni Scientifiche della Cattedra di Psicologia Generale IV*(1), 7–18.

Rait, S., Monsen, J. J., and Squires, G. (2010). Cognitive behaviour therapies and their implications for applied educational psychology practice. *Educational Psychology in Practice, 26*(2), 105–122. doi:10.1080/02667361003768443

Reda, M. A. (1986). *Sistemi Cognitivi Complessi e Psicoterapia* [Complex Cognitive Systems and Psichoterapy]. Roma: Carocci.

Sablier, J., Stip, E., and Franck, N. (2009). Remédiation cognitive et assistants cognitifs numériques dans la schizophrénie. [Cognitive remediation and cognitive assistive technologies in schizophrenia]. *Encephale, 35*(2), 160–167. doi:10.1016/j.encep.2008.02.010

Schalock, R. L., and Luckasson, R. (2004). American Association on Mental Retardation's *Definition, Classification, and System of Supports* and its relation to international trends and issues in the field of intellectual disabilities. *Journal of Policy and Practice in Intellectual Disabilities, 1*(3–4), 136–146. doi:10.1111/j.1741-1130.2004.04028.x

Scherer, M. J. (1986). Values in the Creation, Prescription, and Use of Technological Aids and Assistive Devices for People with Physical Disabilities. Doctoral Dissertation, University of Rochester and final report to the National Science Foundation. (University Microfilms No. ADG87-08247) Retrieved from http://worldcat.org /z-wcorg/

Scherer, M. J. (1998). Matching Person & Technology. A Series of Assessments for Evaluating Predispositions to and Outcomes of Technology Use in Rehabilitation, Education, the Workplace & Other Settings. Webster, NY: The Institute for Matching Person & Technology, Inc.

Scherer, M. J. (2005). Living in the State of Stuck: How Technologies Affect the Lives of People with Disabilities (4th ed.). Cambridge, MA: Brookline Books.

Scherer, M. J. (2012). Assistive Technologies and Other Supports for People with Brain Impairment. New York: Springer.

Scherer, M. J., Hart, T., Kirsch, N., and Schulthesis, M. (2005). Assistive technologies for cognitive disabilities. *Critical Reviews™ in Physical and Rehabilitation Medicine, 17*(3), 195–215. doi:10.1615/CritRevPhysRehabilMed.v17.i3.30

Scherer, M. J., Jutai, J., Fuhrer, M., Demers, L., and Deruyter, F. (2007). A framework for modelling the selection of assistive technology devices (ATDs). *Disability and Rehabilitation: Assistive Technology, 2*(1), 1–8. doi:10.1080/17483100600845414

Scherer, M. J., and Sax, C. L. (2010). Measures of assistive technology predisposition and use. In E. Mpofu and T. Oakland (Eds.), *Rehabilitation and Health Assessment. Applying ICF Guidelines* (pp. 229–254). New York: Springer.

Semerani, A. (2002). *Storia, Teorie e Tecniche Della Psicoterapia Cognitiva* [Cognitive Therapy: History, Theories and Techniques]. Bari, Italy: Laterza.

Taylor, J. L. (2005). In support of psychotherapy for people who have mental retardation. *Mental Retardation, 43*(6), 450–453. doi:10.1352/0047-6765(2005)43[450:ISOPFP]2.0.CO;2

Taylor, J. L., Lindsay, W. R., and Willner, P. (2008). CBT for people with intellectual disabilities: Emerging evidence, cognitive ability and IQ effects. *Behavioural and Cognitive Psychotherapy, 36*(06), 723. doi:10.1017/S1352465808004906

Tsaousides, T., and Gordon, W. A. (2009). Cognitive rehabilitation following traumatic brain injury: Assessment to treatment. *Mount Sinai Journal of Medicine, 76*(2), 173–181. doi:10.1002/msj.20099

United Nations (UN). (2006). *Convention on the Rights of Persons with Disabilities.* (A/RES/61/106). New York: UN. Retrieved from http://www.un-documents.net/a61r106.htm

United Nations Economic and Social Commission for Asia and the Pacific (ESCAP). (2010). *Training Manual on Disability Statistics*. Retrieved January 5, 2011 from http://www.unescap.org/stat/disability/manual/Chapter2-Disability-Statistics.asp

von Bertalanffy, L. (1968). General System Theory: Foundations, Development, Applications. New York: G. Braziller.

von Foerster, H. (1984). *Observing Systems*. Seadide, CA: Intersystems Publications.

von Glasersfeld, E. (1984). An introduction to radical constructivism. In P. Watzlawick (Ed.), *The Invented Reality: How Do We Know What We Believe We Know? (Contributions to Constructivism)* (pp. 17–40). New York: Norton.

Whitehouse, R. M., Tudway, J. A., Look, R., and Kroese, B. S. (2006). Adapting individual psychotherapy for adults with intellectual disabilities: A comparative review of the cognitive-behavioural and psychodynamic literature. *Journal of Applied Research in Intellectual Disabilities, 19*(1), 55–65. doi:10.1111/j.1468-3148.2005.00281.x

Willner, P., and Hatton, C. (2006). CBT for people with intellectual disabilities. *Journal of Applied Research in Intellectual Disabilities, 19*(1), 1–3. doi:10.1111/j.1468-3148.2006.00300.x

World Health Organization. (WHO). (2001). *International Classification of Functioning, Disability and Health (ICF)* Vol. 2010). Retrieved from http://www.who.int/classifications/icf/en/

7

The Special Educator

S. Zapf and G. Craddock*

CONTENTS

7.1 The Role of the Special Educator in Assistive Technology Assessment

The World Health Organization and the United Nations Global Disability report estimates that individuals with disabilities account for 15% of the world population, and there are approximately 150 million children with disabilities in the world (WHO 2010). The definition of special education varies worldwide because many countries use a social classification system similar to the International Classification System addressing the child's ability to participate across the educational domain, whereas other counties focus on a medical model for education that is based on specific categories of impairment or disabilities. Assistive technology (AT) has long been recognized as a tool for enabling independence and access for individuals with disabilities (Bowe 1995; Østensjø et al. 2005; Watson et al. 2010). Although changes in legislation have provided a positive shift to include the consideration of AT in the student's educational plan/setting, there still remains a deficiency in many developing countries for children with disabilities to have access to needed AT to assist with meeting their educational plan and participation in daily activities. The World Health Organization reports that only 5–15% of individuals with disabilities have access to AT in many developing countries. The United Nations Standard and World Health Organization Rule 4 (WHO 2010) promotes the training of personnel at various levels in AT to improve access for technology. The special educator can play a vital role in providing technology access and implementation of tools to be used with students in the educational setting.

---

* The views expressed by Dr. Ger Craddock are his own and are not of his employer, the National Disability Authority. ·

AT in the educational setting is individualized to the students' needs and is supported by the use of an individualized education plan (IEP). With the national trend of including children in special education in regular education classrooms, 75% of children with disabilities are spending at least 49–80% of their time in regular education classes, a significant increase over the past ten years (Swanson 2008). It is essential that teachers design classrooms to allow for curriculum access [e.g., the student can obtain information (written, oral, and graphic)] and provide information in a suitable and appropriate manner for all children. Although curricular access is paramount, it is also important that children have the opportunity to perform various social, academic, and personal care tasks/activities that impact functional participation in the educational setting. AT can be the bridge to successful participation for many children with disabilities.

The special educator is a crucial member on the AT team in the educational setting. Special educators work with students on a daily basis and are able to identify the student's strengths and needs in the area of academic performance. A needs assessment is the first step in the AT process. The special educator is in the best position to identify a student's area of need related to specific academic performance and can assist in determining the student's predisposition and personal characteristics related to the successful integration of AT. Working with students on a daily basis, special educators have the opportunity to become familiar with the personal characteristics of students and can help to identify predispositions that can support or hinder the student's use of AT.

An important responsibility of special educators is to develop an IEP for each student who requires learning support. The IEP is a collaborative process that focuses on the abilities of each individual student and their desired goals and is tailored to that student's individual needs and abilities. The consideration for AT devices or AT services should be embedded within the IEP (TATN 2007). The Texas 4-Step model is a process that can guide the special educator through the consideration process of AT aligned with the development of the student's educational plan. The first step is to identify the student's current academic achievement and functional performance level aligned to the national standards. This step aligns with the needs analysis step in an AT assessment to identify areas of strength for the student and areas of need that may require an AT solution. The second step is to identify the goals and objectives, i.e., what is expected that the student can achieve. The third step is to determine if any of the tasks involved in the students education plan will be difficult for the student to achieve and to subsequently decide if an AT solution or AT service is needed. The final step is to determine if AT solutions/services are needed; this step can be accomplished through gathering needed information in the assessment process and a trial of AT solutions.

AT evaluations are crucial because they identify if there is a need for an AT device and/or services that will allow the child to increase in quality, quantity, or independence in activities defined in the IEP (Bowser and Reed 1995; Lahm and Sizemore 2002). The AT evaluation should involve a comprehensive individualized assessment of the child's progress on current goals, the child's tasks, the environment in which the AT will be used, past experiences with the use of AT and other supports, and the child's predisposition to the use of alternative or additional supports (Scherer et al. 2005). Each child has a "predisposition" that can influence the use of AT. Such predispositions depend on personality characteristics; subjective well-being; and views of physical capabilities, experience, future expectations, social acceptance, and financial and environmental support for technology use (Louise-Bender Pape et al. 2002; Scherer 2005). In addition, assessing and conceptualizing the patterns and degree of the child's disability become crucial components. Special educators can help the AT team identify the student's predisposition, specific skills, past technology use, and abilities that can support the use of AT for the student.

The importance of a "good match" between the student and the technology has been found to be an essential element to the successful use of AT. One specific assessment process that has been effective in identifying predisposition characteristics and AT tool characteristics that influence and impact a person's general AT use is the Matching Person and Technology (MPT) model and assessments (Scherer 1998, 2005; Scherer and Craddock 2002). The MPT consists of measures validated for use by both young people and adults with disabilities. The Matching Assistive Technology to Child (MATCH) was developed under the theoretical framework of the MPT and uses similar constructs, but it is designed for the pediatric population in the educational setting (Scherer 1997; Scherer and Zapf 2008). Lenker and Paquet (2003) found that the MPT model had a framework that identifies potential predictive traits of AT users and nonusers through predisposition scores and uses a client-centered approach that is based on grounded research. Using the MPT evaluation forms in the assessment of 45 students, Craddock (2006) found that the MPT model guided the process. It ensured that the assessment procedure was user-focused and involved the student in all elements in the identification, selection, and acquisition of AT.

In tandem with the MPT, the IEP is a collaborative process that focuses on the abilities of each individual student and their desired goals and is tailored to that student's individual needs and abilities. It is based on a client-focused social and participatory service delivery model in AT (Craddock and McCormack 2002) that emphasises the active participation of the service user in the selection of appropriate equipment and in the ongoing evaluation and decision-making processes. It supports a bottom-up approach enabling the core personnel to define the complex issues involved in a service delivery system (Scherer and Craddock 2002). Person-centred planning begins by establishing individual's prioritized needs in collaboration with a team that consists of the individual's support network, family, close friends, teachers, and AT specialists.

The success of students with disabilities using AT is related, amongst other factors, to the AT knowledge and skills of special education teachers (Scherer and Craddock 2002; Scherer and Zapf 2008); however, findings indicate that AT training at the teacher training level may not be adequately addressed. Approximately one-third of undergraduate special teacher licensure programs, 28% of initial postbaccalaureate licensure programs, and less than 25% of master's degree programs require AT coursework. Many graduates are leaving special education teacher preparation programs without the critical knowledge, skills, and dispositions necessary to address the AT needs of their students (Judge and Simms 2009).

A significant change in the approach to technology within education is required if AT is to be included as an essential tool for students with disabilities. Information and communication technologies (ICT) is considered to be a ubiquitous tool within the classroom, and AT is considered to be a tool for students with disabilities to fit into the existing structures. New technologies can vastly increase access and learning opportunities; however, new media have yet to be exploited within the educational setting, talking books, descriptive video, and instructional environments where students are consistently supported in learning how to learn. An educational system is needed in which there is not one 'typical' learner but various learners each provided with adequate supports. Change can occur at many levels, but in particular, in the classroom setting where the teacher could view technology as a means for creating a collaborative learning environment.

7.2 Teaching Alternatives Using AT

One of the more significant findings in research on the use of ICT in education is the extent to which ICT can support the inclusion of students with special educational needs (British Educational Communications and Technology Agency (Becta 2003). Currently, in many countries the predominant practice is to withdraw pupils from the classroom for supplementary teaching with a support teacher. However, this reliance on individual supplementary classes on a withdrawal basis has been criticized as contrary to the principle of integration in teaching and learning and an inclusive system of education (Markussen 2004).

AT has long been recognized as a tool for enabling independence and access for individuals with disabilities. With the changes in legislation to include consideration of AT in the student's educational plan, there has been a positive shift in using more AT in educational settings (U.S. Department of Education 1998). Special education programs are required to be accountable for the use or nonuse of AT for each child; however, insufficient training, knowledge, and the inability of service providers to integrate AT into the learning environment continues to contribute to device discontinuance and underutilization (Dalton 2002; Copley and Ziviani 2004; Judge 2010).

In a study conducted with postprimary school students over a 2-year period, Craddock (2006) found that ICT and AT played critical roles in augmenting participation of the students at both a social and educational level. The use of these technologies acted as an important catalyst in the educational process and environment for students with disabilities and was one of the factors that led to the fulfilment of the students' goals. In particular, the students reported that the AT gave them the opportunity to show that they had the ability and the skills that they knew they had but had not previously had the means to demonstrate. In general, the students reported that AT increased their skills, their capacity, and their quality of communication. They were able to work better and faster and cover more of the curriculum. They felt that the technology enabled them to complete their education on an equal status with their peers. Craddock also found several factors that are associated with a student's successful use of technology, including

- *Early intervention:* The earlier the student is exposed to the technology, the more adept the student is in its use and the more comfortable the student is with technology association;
- *Formal supports:* The support of, primarily their teachers, but also the principals and the whole school ethos, both in its inclusive, support and understanding of disability but also the schools' engagement with technology;
- *The comfort level:* The comfort level of the school and the teachers in using the technology;
- *Education:* Educating teachers in using technology;
- *Informal supports:* The support of family and friends, in particular the mother played a crucial role in obtaining the AT devices and also supporting the use of AT in the home.

Similarly Dalton (2002) addressed issues concerning the need for teachers to be educated in the use of technology, especially special education teachers working with students with disabilities. A study completed on the level of competency for special educators on 35 core skills from the 1997 Council for Exceptional Children identified low levels of competence (ranging from barely adequate to inadequate) in the following areas: technology implementation with students with disabilities, use of technology in professional development plans, and use of technology to enhance the management of resources and appropriate application of technology to classroom learning. Lahm and Sizemore (2002) also identified a comprehensive list of essential AT knowledge and skill competencies for all special educators that included characteristics of learners, assessment, diagnosis and evaluation, instructional content and practice, planning and managing the environment, managing student behavior, communication and collaborative partnerships, and professional and ethical practices. Copley and Ziviani (2004) identified a lack of suitable training as a major barrier in effective AT implementation. A lack of follow-up support for teachers and students was also identified as a reason for nonuse of AT in the classroom.

Teacher comfort level with AT is a critical factor in continued use and support for AT use among students. Craddock (2006) found that important factors to emerge in the satisfaction of student AT use were

- The provision of supportive educational classrooms that included more imaginative layouts of classroom furniture versus the traditional column/row;
- Low-tech AT such as pencil grips and wedges, book stands, and magnifiers; and
- The integration of mainstream technology with AT, such as the use of laptops with specialized software uploaded onto all systems that linked remotely to electronic interactive white boards.

Craddock also identified human factors that were critical, such as having classroom assistants working closely with the students and the teacher. In many instances it was the support given by individual teachers that materialized as a critical factor in the successful use of AT. A recent study by Zapf and Scherer (2011) found a significant correlation ($p = 0.023$) between the variables of teacher/parent comfort and student motivation in AT use, indicating that teacher/parent comfort may affect student motivation in the use of AT. This finding supports the importance of using an assessment scale to assess the comfort level of the teacher/parent scale and its effect on the outcome use of AT. A study by Sze (2009) revealed that one of the most important predictors of successful integration of students with disabilities in the regular classroom is the attitude of general education teachers. The results confirmed the existence of a significant link between preservice teacher attitude and instructional practice. The success of instructional practice requires that general education faculty be prepared to work with students with disabilities. Preservice special education courses have benefited preservice teachers in gaining an understanding of students with special needs, thus increasing their comfort level with diverse learners overall. In studies on the attitudes of general education teachers, it was also revealed that a lack of knowledge of disabling conditions affected the ability of these teachers to accept not only students with disabilities but also other students with special needs.

Finally Craddock (2006) found that unsuccessful AT users reported many reasons for nonuse, including a desire to "fit in" that may be threatened by AT use, for example, being less inclined to use communication devices although they can improve communication because of the perceived stigma. Assistive devices may effectively improve mobility, communication, or accessibility, but if the device has a negative connotation because it brings unwanted attention and threatens the sense of "fitting in," this sense of "fitting in" may be more important to the user than independence and/or sense of control.

7.3 Outcome Studies of Assistive Technology in the Educational Setting

Assistive technology devices and tools are designed to improve a child's performance and to remove barriers that can exist towards independence. A recent study by Watson and colleagues (2010) found a significant effect in IEP goal improvements in 13 children who received AT devices and services from a trained multidisciplinary team based on pre- and post performance scores. These authors also found the AT intervention provided positive contributions to the subjects improvement in IEP mastery as compared with relative and supportive services and specific modifications to curricular tasks. The AT used in this study included written communication hardware and software, speech-generating devices, curriculum support software, and computer access.

Increased independence in students functional abilities should be a primary focus when developing IEP. Assistive technology can be a catalyst in achieving independence to prepare students towards functional life goals. Østensjø and colleagues (2005) analyzed the effects of environmental modifications and assistive devices on 95 children diagnosed with CP. These authors found a substantial reduction in the need for caregiver assistance with indoor and outdoor mobility and the self-care skill of eating. They also found a strong association between the child's independence and caregiver demands, indicating AT that supported independence could affect the amount of care needed for the child.

Various studies on product based research also support the use of AT in the educational setting. The use of word prediction software, such as CoWriter, was found to increase scores on spelling, improve general writing mechanics, and increase the number of correct word sequences for children with learning disabilities (Staples et al. 1995; Erikson, 2006; Mirendo et al. 2006). Text reader software products, such as Kurzweil, have also been found to support reading and writing skills in children with disabilities. Student's identified as Tier Level 1 in the state of Iowa used the Kurzweil program for reading and writing. Their scores improved significantly over time in the area of reading comprehension when using a text reader compared to reading from paper (Iowa Department of Education 2007).

The use of augmentative and alternative communication (AAC) interventions has been found to be beneficial for children with disabilities in the educational setting. A meta-analysis done by Millar and colleagues (2006) analysed 23 studies that involved 67 subjects using various types of AAC. Thirty-one percent of the studies used non-electronic-aided systems and 4% of the studies used electronic devices. The remaining 61% of the studies used manual signs. The outcome goals of the studies analyzed were to teach expressive communication in and they found that 82% of the subjects increased in speech production and only 7% decreased using these types of AAC. Results from single subject studies analyzing the use of electronic AAC devices also supports the use of these devices to enhance communication for children with disabilities in the areas of requesting items, responding to questions, and making social comments during play and snack routines (Schepis et al. 1998; Sigafoos and Drasgrow 2001).

7.4 Environmental Factors to Promote AT in the Classroom

Technology can play an important role in creating an inclusive classroom. The combined use of ICT and AT in the classroom can facilitate inclusive practises in education. Significant changes can be made to curriculum content, delivery and organisation of mainstream programmes through the effective use of technology. An example of the ubiquitous use of technology can be found within the Inclusive Learning through Technology (ILT) which involved the integration of technology in four schools, two mainstream and two special schools. This was achieved through the provision of a range of hardware and software technology, including

- The provision of laptop computers for each student;
- Interactive whiteboards;
- Assistive technology provision for individual students;
- Wireless broadband access;
- Microsoft Office Suite;
- Inspiration (mind mapping software);
- Video Conferencing Facilities;
- MP3 Players for each student.

Classrooms were provided with laptop computers equipped with wireless network capability and the latest technology and software to provide easier communication and exchange of information. The interactive whiteboards facilitated alternative teaching methodologies and supported teachers to move to a more interactive approach. The whiteboards also allowed for synchronised teaching between the schools and direct interaction between teachers and students across schools via a virtual learning environment. A variety of software resources were provided with the whiteboards, including Internet access, Kidspiration and access to the Atomic Learning site. Concept mapping software was introduced in order to scaffold students' thinking process. In addition to the technological inputs teachers were provided with training in the thinking skills developed by Edward De Bono and more specifically the CoRT (Cognitive Research Trust) Thinking Techniques for use in the classroom. The thinking skills programme aimed to provide students with tools to improve their learning strategies in a move away from a unidimensional or whole group instruction to a more differentiated and learner centred approach. The objective was to develop the students' ability to think critically, to apply their learning and to enable more creativity and flexibility. In addition, teachers were introduced to the use of mind mapping as a learning tool and to theories that support differentiated instruction. Differentiated instruction requires personalizing the curriculum in order to meet the individual learning needs of students, to capitalize on their strengths and enhance their capabilities. Teachers were trained to take recognition of the wide range of learning styles/ teaching styles used in differentiated instruction in acknowledgement of the significant effect that learning styles have on the learning and teaching process.

Teacher training was a crucial feature of the ILT project based on the belief that each teacher involved had unique talents and potential that could be nurtured, with the ultimate aim of improving teaching and learning. All professionals involved in the project attended CPD (continuous professional development) training. All new teachers were provided with a copy of the ILT summer course, there were a variety of small group sessions about the thinking methodologies used in the project for all teachers involved and technical support was offered in small group or on a one to one basis.

For students to become proficient in AT use, a teacher needs to have the skills and comfort using technology to provide opportunity for use and success. As with all subject areas, certain students exhibit different levels of proficiency. In a study by Craddock (2006) on the use of AT with teenage students; three discernable groups of students emerged, distinguishable by the type of technology they used, how they used it, and how satisfied and comfortable they were with it. They were typified as the novice, transition and power users. The power users were using high-end technology, such as voice recognition, screen readers and other voice output systems. They exhibited more than just a pragmatic adaptation to the technology; they displayed an emotional attachment evidenced by how the students defined themselves in relation to their technology. Their technology released in them hitherto hidden beliefs and abilities. The students described the devices as inextricably associated with their self-image, recognising that the technology changed their self-identity. Their "cultural capital" was increased, with the use of high-end portable technologies that enabled them first to "fit in" and second to compete and, in a number of cases, outperform their non-disabled peers. A key factor in becoming a power user was the length of time they were using technology; often starting its' use as a young child, from the ages of five or six.

The picture emerged quite differently for the students of the novice users group. They had little formal support outside of the curriculum. Their first introduction to high technology came much later. Surprisingly, none of these students had any experience of AT or knowledge that technology could have provided easier access to the curriculum. For the novice users, timing was a critical issue; it was difficult for them to assimilate new technology a few months before one of the most important examinations of their careers. However, a number of the novice group did achieve a competence with the technology. These students are characterized as "transition users." They incorporated the technology at a pragmatic level, but the lack of identification with the technology left them in a transitionary period that perhaps with time and consideration could lead them to become power users of the technology.

Craddock (2006) study supports the need for the special education teachers to become familiar with the students' needs matched to AT throughout the educational continuum. The special education teacher needs to become familiar with the roles of AT in the student' environments, including transitional stages between educational environments (elementary-to-high-school-to college). The goal of education is to prepare a student to function successfully in the world, including the home, social settings, and the work environment. The special educator should become familiar with technologies that can enhance the student's success in these settings. Transitional planning meetings are crucial to assure the AT needed for success is in place to optimize the student's success. Special educators need to understand the transitional process and act as facilitators to assure the student continues to receive the needed AT when transitioning into these new environments.

7.5 Going Forward: Universal Design for Learning (UDL)

A model of framing the integration of technology in the school context is Universal Design. Universal design is a strategy, which aims to make the design and composition of different environments and products accessible and understandable to, as well as usable by, everyone, to the greatest extent in the most independent and natural manner possible, without the need for adaptation or specialised design solutions. The main thrust of the UDL model is to support teachers in creating and adapting lessons in order to increase access and participation for all students. One of the main ideas is that of "flexibility," i.e., offering multiple means of presentation and participation to students and offering them different ways to show their understanding. In other words, getting the pupils to read a book and write answers into a workbook only reaches a certain percentage of pupils. Many students do not perform well with narrow parameters, but may work well when work is presented in a different way. Although UDL is not technology-driven per se, technology does offer some of the flexibility that benefits all learners. For example, text-to-speech software, such as ReadPlease, will help the pupil who is struggling to read. In addition, text can be enlarged and colours changed to help a student who finds it hard to distinguish text.

7.6 Case Evaluation

Craddock (2003) discussed nine stages in the service delivery process of AT:

1. Outreach;
2. Initiative;
3. Assessment;
4. Typology of the solution;
5. Selection;
6. Authorisation for financing;
7. Delivery;
8. Training;
9. Management and follow-up.

By applying the above model to students, we can observe how the key elements of the Matching Person with Technology (MPT) model—personal characteristics, Milieu and AT solution- combine to enable clients to fully participate in school, family life, and community. Our case studies will look at two students; Zoey, a young female student entering the pre-school program and followed though into the intermediate school; and John, a secondary student with plans to transition to college.

7.6.1 First Case Study: Zoey

Zoey is a 21-month-old female toddler who presents with neurological delays secondary to hypoxic-ischemic encephalopathy. She has a diagnosis of congenital quadriplegia. She was born at 41 weeks, distocical birth, and vacuum was applied to assist with delivery. Zoey was born with serious medical complications. Her Apgar score was 1. She was reanimated, incubated, and moved to the pediatric intensive care unit, where she received neurorehabilitative care for 40 days. She was discharged home to parents, and therapy services continued through an early childhood service program. The case for this chapter jumps to Zoey at age 36 months, at her transitional IEP meeting, because she is to begin educational services through the Pre-School Program for Children with Disabilities (PPCD) under the Individuals with Disabilities Act (IDEA).

During Zoey's transitional IEP meeting, her occupational and physical therapist from her early childhood intervention (ECI) program met with the school educational team [special education (SE) teacher, school administration, diagnostician, occupational therapist (OT), physical therapist (PT), and speech and language pathologist (SLP)] to discuss her current strengths, needs, and plans for education. Zoey's current level of performance and participation in the home is described as follows:

> Zoey is an attentive young girl and motivated to learn. She has a very supportive family and a good relationship with the health professionals she has worked with. She is able to sustain attention and learns best through visual model/representation versus kinetic learning because of her physical impairments. Zoey has paralysis in both her upper and lower extremities (severe motor impairment) and relies on primitive reflexes to illicit motor movement. She is able to sit supported in her wheelchair, and the therapists have been working on finding the best access position for her so she can control her environment and engage in tasks. She has tried using a wobble switch with upper extremity reflexive movements (arm reaching out to hit the switch), but she then moves her head away from the visual field. Her therapists are working on increasing her head control because they feel eye movement may be the best option for access as she gets older. Her vision acuity/convergence is mild impairment, but it is corrected with glasses. She is able to use track using visual scan and sustain attention visually. Zoey is delayed in language; however, her receptive skills are more intact (mild impairment) compared with her expressive (complete impairment) language skills. She demonstrates interest in engaging in interactions and likes to be in the middle of the action.

Her occupational and physical ECI therapists discussed the current AT that they have been using in the home setting, which includes a manual wheelchair with adapted seating and a mounted switch to access her toys during her playtime. She loves music and is engaged in computer-based learning tasks that use music as a positive reward. She has tried some built-up handles, but she seems to do better with a universal cuff when using materials.

Zoey's parent's main concern is her communication. They feel that she would be able to engage more independently if she could talk. The team has tried a mid-tech AAC with step scanning using a head switch; however, she still had limited endurance with head control and movement at that time. The team felt she was able to navigate through a dynamic screen and the static screen was limiting to her. Zoey is in the stage of novice user moving toward transitional user at the age 36 months through five years of age. As she becomes more independent, she moves into a power user stage with success at 10 years of age. This case will look at Zoey at the age of 36 months and then at ten years using her AT in the educational setting (Table 7.1).

7.6.2 Second Case Study: John

John is a young man with athetoid cerebral palsy. He attended his local mainstream primary school for seven years, then moved to a mainstream secondary college and progressed then to third-level education. The case study introduces John at age 7 and a novice user of technology. The case study jumps to when John is a young man of 17 and a power user of technology. Power and novice users refer to a study of students transitioning from the second to third level education conducted by Craddock (2006). Three discernable groups of students emerged from the study distinguishable by the type of technology they used, how they used it, and how satisfied and comfortable they were with it. They were typified as the novice and power users with students progressing between the two stages characterized as

TABLE 7.1

Stages of AT Service Delivery: Zoey, Age 36 Months to 5 Years, Novice User

Stages of the AT Service Delivery Model	Zoey, Age 36 months to 5 Years Novice User	Zoey, Age 10 years Power User of AT
Outreach	The educational team (SE Teacher, OT, PT, and SLP) attend regional meeting to stay abreast on current AT available, they are part of the school's AT team. Information on possible solutions is shared at Zoey's IEP meeting.	Seven years later, Zoey is in the fourth grade inclusion classroom. Zoey has taken ownership of her AAC device. She has asked her parents to make sure they program in her weekend activities and pictures of her new dog so she can share with her friends. As she has grown, it is more difficult to illicit arm movement using the ATNR reflex patterns because she tires easily because of increased exertion. She told her SE teacher and parents that she thinks that the head mouse or eye-gaze system could be more beneficial because she is not able to communicate as fast as with her wobble switch. She would also like her device to access the computer so she can E-mail and type.
Initiative	The educational team discusses with ECI team and parent the need to do an AT assessment to help identify Zoey's need for AT aligned to her current goals/objectives and to identify best solution for communication.	Zoey, the SE teacher, and Zoey's parents attend the regional AT center to look at the current technology available. The SE teacher meets with the AT team to discuss issues that have arisen with Zoey's access (because physical demand is decreasing her output) and interest in a new device (her current device is 6 years old).
Preassessment and assessment	The AT team (SE teacher, OT/PT/SLP) observe Zoey in the PPCD classroom and have identified the area of need related to Zoey's IEP. They have identified key predisposition factors of AT use in Zoey: high motivation, flexibility, comfort of AT, and support in the home/school setting.	The AT team (including the SE teacher) observes Zoey in her classroom. They meet at her reassessment planning meeting and discuss her current skill level and progress on the IEP with use of AT. At the meeting, her parents discuss an interest in using a grant to purchase a newer device that has the capability for head/eye tracking because she has improved greatly with head control and eye gaze. They also ask about the need for connecting her device to a computer for her writing because this is a high-focus area for next year. The team identifies Zoey's current success with AT and feels that she is capable of achieving more; an AT reassessment is recommended.
Typology of the solution	AT assessment team assess Zoey using the MATCH-ACES (a child version of the MPT process). A number of devices are tried using both switch access and head control.	The AT team uses the previous MATCH-ACES assessment to update Zoey's current area of need related to the IEP and her overall performance. They discuss possible solutions. The OT/PT provide recommendations for supporting head control so the head tracker and eye-gaze systems would be effective. Two device systems are tried.

(Continued)

TABLE 7.1 (CONTINUED)

Stages of AT Service Delivery: Zoey, Age 36 Months to 5 Years, Novice User

Stages of the AT Service Delivery Model	Zoey, Age 36 months to 5 Years Novice User	Zoey, Age 10 years Power User of AT
Selection	Arrangement agreed between Zoey's teacher and the regional AT loan center to loan two dynamic screen devices for trial. The team found at this time that Zoey did best with visual scan on a 20-icon display and was able to move to three dynamic pages. At this time her head control was limiting. She was able to use scanning with wobble switch (hand access with extensor pattern), but motor delay was an issue, so the scanning speed had to be decreased. The educational team assessed that she had difficulty maintaining her head upright for long periods and this affected her stamina for head control/eye gaze but is a potential for future plans. Switch access software using music and academic learning was also recommended. Universal-cuff-adapted classroom materials (paint-brush, music instrument) were also recommended so that Zoey could participate in all classrooms.	Arrangement was made, through the AT company that Zoey's first device was purchased from, to trial the next level of high-tech AAC device that had computer and ECU access and is compatible with a head/eye tracker. Another similar device owned by the district (AT storage) was also tried. Zoey had progressed from an initial 20-icon to a 60-icon page and is able to navigate through dynamic pages. The eye-gaze and tracker pro were on loan from the AT center. The team tried the tracker pro with infrared and an eye-gaze tracking system. Both AAC devices were compatible with the school's current network/computer system. The eye-gaze system had some software issues with connecting to the classroom computer, but the tracker pro could be connected and the SE teacher felt that it was more compatible. After a 4-week trial of each device, the team felt that there was a need to upgrade Zoey's AAC device because she was more successful with connecting to the computer. Zoey was also successful with the head/eye tracker pro to scan; the AT team recommended this option. The parents discussed that the eye-gaze system seemed effective because less movement was needed; however, in the AT meeting, the SE director stated that for the purpose of the IEP plan the team felt the head tracker pro was sufficient and a better solution than the previous access method. The AT team and SE director expressed concern about the eye-gaze system because of high-cost, software issues with compatibility on the school computer and technical needs of the staff. The IEP team agreed with the current recommendations.
Authorization for financing	The IEP team agreed that the AAC device was essential for Zoey to meet her IEP goals. The smaller/light AAC device was chosen because of size/mounting needs and the device capability matching Zoey's needs. The SE teacher contacted the AT team, and the team sent the request for the device and mount to the director for purchase.	The school owned the previous AAC device. The AT team and AAC vendor discussed with Zoey's parents that there was an available grant that they may want to pursue if they wanted to purchase the AAC device personally or the district would provide the device (and it would be owned by the school). The AT team had the device in storage, because a previous student had used it. The parents discussed options and wanted to try for the grant device first and an interim use of the district's device. The SE director ordered the tracker system.

TABLE 7.1 (CONTINUED)

Stages of AT Service Delivery: Zoey, Age 36 Months to 5 Years, Novice User

Stages of the AT Service Delivery Model	Zoey, Age 36 months to 5 Years Novice User	Zoey, Age 10 years Power User of AT
Delivery	The AT team met with the SE teacher to deliver the switches, computer software activities, and universal cuff for classroom materials. The device was delivered within 3 weeks, and the AC loan was returned to the regional center.	The AT team met with a funding agency and Zoey's parents and completed the grant information for the AAC device. While the grant was waiting for approval, the AT team, SE teacher, Zoey's parents, and Zoey set up the other device for use with the tracker pro (which arrived within 3 weeks). The grant process took 3 months for approval and delivery.
Training	The SLP and OT met with the SE teacher, regular-education teacher, Zoey, and her parents to set up the device and training. The OT/PT worked together with the SE teacher on positioning and mounting of the device. The OT/PT also met with the teacher to discuss strategies to build endurance in head control for Zoey for future possibilities of using other access points for her device. The SE teacher was responsible for carryover of the AT implementation and to contact AT team for maintenance. The SE teacher attended regional training on switch access and using AAC devices in the classroom to facilitate communication.	The SLP and OT met with SE teacher, the regular-education teacher, Zoey, and her parents to set up the new device when it arrived. The OT/PT worked together with the SE teacher on positioning and mounting of the new device with the tracker device. The head tracker device was also hooked up with the computer in the laboratory so that Zoey could complete assignments there. The SE teacher continued to be responsible for carryover of the AT implementation and also for contacting the AT team/parents for maintenance. The SE teacher attended regional training on switch access and using AAC devices in classroom to facilitate communication
Management and follow-up	The SE teacher and regular-education teacher (Zoey will be going into re-ed kindergarten with support) meet periodic to discuss Zoey's progress. The AT team will follow-up quarterly through E-mail. The team's OT/PT have met with the SE teacher/parents and they are looking at a head support system for the wheelchair that could help with using a head/eye tracker system. The SLP continued with follow-up on communication programming needs with the SE teacher. The SE teacher and aids continue to do activities to increase endurance of head control and eye gaze. The SE teacher contacts the team if needed. AT considerations are discussed annually at the IEP meeting. At this time Zoey is moving into transitional user and the current AT is successful.	The SE teacher documented the AT modifications that were needed for state testing. The SE teacher documented the equipment within the IEP for transition to the next school. The OT/PT continued to meet with the SE teacher and the regular-education teacher for access and positioning needs. The SLP continued with follow-up on communication programming needs with the SE teacher. At this time, Zoey is successfully using the device and tracking system and is able to complete her assignments. She is also able to navigate the computer to complete written assignments. She is 4 times faster than with previous the setup and tires less. She uses her device in all of her activities, and the device has become part of her persona. Her parents and SE teacher are very supportive and make sure that the device is available. Her parents have looked into other funding options for eye-gaze system and hope to receive a grant through the local CP foundation that would purchase the eye-gaze system.

TABLE 7.2

Stages of AT Service Delivery: John, Age 7, Novice User of AT

Stages of the AT Service Delivery Model	John Age 7 Novice User of AT	John, Age 17 Power User of AT
Outreach	Teacher visits travelling road show of assistive technology. Sees technology that may be suitable for one of her students. Collects contact information from the local technology liaison officer (TLO).	Ten years later, John is now in second-level education, keeping up to date with new technology by searching the Web and communicating with users on an online national user discussion forum.
Initiative	Teacher discusses with John's parents about having an assessment for AT. Parents agree and fill out a preassessment form with the support of the local TLO.	John finds the eye-gaze technology and shows the information to his teacher, who in turn contacts the local SENO (special educational needs officer).
Preassessment and assessment	TLO visits the school to see the teacher and observe John in the classroom and how he participates. TLO demonstrates and trials a selection of AT devices with John. Being only 7 years of age, the teacher, parents, and TLO invite an AT assessment team to assess John in school.	John is frustrated with current slow speed of his technology and feels an Eye Gaze system would help him speed up with his writing
Typology of the solution	The AT assessment team assess John using the MPT. A number of devices are tried, but John, having seen a number of the devices previously, is most interested in the round head switch that easily attaches to his wheelchair. He is delighted when he can type his own name for the first time on the computer screen.	Liaising with his teacher, the SENO, and local TLO, John gets to trial the portable eye-gaze system. The discussion is about the cost of this new equipment and the use of his existing system as a backup and portable device for movement between classes in school.
Selection	Arrangement agreed upon between John's teacher and the TLO to have a loan of a desktop computer with the switch and the special software to trial for 1 month. The TLO visits once a week to show the teacher and John some more features of the software. At the end of the month, the TLO and teacher discuss with John and his parents and all feel this is a very good solution for John.	Trial of the eye-gaze system is arranged with the local TLO, but John has to wait a number of months before getting access to the device. Because of the expense of the device, there are very few available on loan. Finally, John gets a 1-month trial of the system and finds that his typing speed has doubled.
Authorization for financing	The TLO liaises with the rest of the assessment team and a recommendation is forwarded to the parents and the teacher for the school to submit to the Department of Education for funding. In the meantime, the loan period of the equipment is extended until the new equipment arrives. At the review, John is assessed using the MPT model and the results show a good match.	The SENO, with technical support from the TLO, makes a recommendation for the new eye-gaze equipment to the Department of Education. The recommendation is turned down because of the high cost. The trial equipment is also returned. An alterative solution is investigated, the less expensive head tracking system is considered, and the trial equipment is organized. A recommendation is made to the Department of Education, and funding is agreed upon.

TABLE 7.2 (CONTINUED)

Stages of AT Service Delivery: John, Age 7, Novice User of AT

Stages of the AT Service Delivery Model	John Age 7 Novice User of AT	John, Age 17 Power User of AT
Delivery	Three months later, the new equipment arrives, and the teacher, with support from the local TLO, assembles and tests that the equipment is working. The loan equipment is returned.	The equipment is delivered to the school, and John supports the teacher in installing the system on his laptop computer.
Training	The TLO works closely with John's teacher to show how the new system works, and once a month for a half-year period the TLO spends an hour with the teacher on demonstrating new educational software that the teacher can use with John and the rest of the class.	John, being a power user of technology, trains himself in using the new equipment and finds YouTube videos of other users of the technology to help him speed up his writing. He is now 6 times faster typing using his new system and is now looking forward to going to third-level education.
Management and follow-up	The teacher works with John, and on a 6-month basis over the next couple of years liaises with the TLO on new software and some maintenance issues such as the switch, computer interface, and the ink cartridges for the printer.	John now uses Skype to contact the TLO if there are any maintenance issues. John works with the TLO and SENO on producing a SON specified to his AT needs and requirements for successful transition to third-level education.

transition users. The study also determined that students progressed to being power users of technology when they were introduced to technology at primary level, had teachers who were comfortable with the technology, and had a supportive home environment.

John attended his local primary school, which is in a rural part of Ireland. He was introduced to AT at the age of 7 by his teacher and the local technology liaison officer (TLO). He took to AT "like a duck to water" from the first time he pressed the head switch that was attached to his wheelchair (Table 7.2).

The STATEMENT (Systematic Template for Assessing Technology Enabling Mainstream Education) project was funded under the European Horizon initiative (2006). Its purpose was to produce a Statement of Need specific to AT for students progressing from second level to postsecond-level education.

7.7 Conclusions

This chapter outlined the important role of the special educator in provision of AT within education. It proposed that unless the special educator is "comfortable" in the use of technology, the successful use of AT in the classroom may be compromised. It purported that a successful assessment for AT use must include an understanding of the personal characteristics of the person and their predisposition for technology use. Furthermore, it is the responsibility of the special educator to bring AT to the attention of the interdisciplinary assessment team. To achieve teacher comfort in technology, training is essential and outlines the ILT as an example of technology integration and teacher training. The chapter also provides insight into the successful and unsuccessful users of technology and outlines the factors that can determine use or nonuse of AT. Finally, as technology advances and AT is increasingly supported within the mainstream market, the authors outline the next stage of technology provision within the classroom—UDL. Ultimately, providing an educational environment where classrooms are designed to cater for all types of students regardless of their disability or special need is optimal. It is imperative for teachers to recognize that all students have varying ability, and it is a measure of their ability, not disability, that should determine how their education is supported. The classroom should provide a range of supports for any student who may have issues in accessing the curriculum—from reading difficulties to writing to understanding. A special educator should have the knowledge, skills, and competence backed up with the support of technologies to support all within the education environment.

Summary of the Chapter

This chapter describes the importance of assistive technology in education and the role of the special educator in the process of integrating assistive technology for students with disabilities into the educational system. The special educator is a crucial team member, providing knowledge of the students' educational capabilities and their daily interaction in the use of assistive technology. Assistive technology can provide many children and adolescents with disabilities the tools necessary to be more successful in school, at work, and at achieving independence in daily living. Unfortunately, many special educators do not receive training in the application of assistive technology nor do they have adequate resources to effectively assess, implement, and follow-up on the use of assistive technology in the classroom. This chapter will identify the special educator's role in the assessment and implementation of AT. Recommendations for future training needs for special educators will also be discussed.

References

Bowe F. G. (1995). The political and economic issues that drive and derail assistive technology development. *Generations, 19*(1), 37–40.

Bowser, G., and Reed, P. (1995). Education TECH points for assistive technology planning. *Journal of Special Education Technology, 12*(4), 325–338.

British Educational Communications and Technology Agency (Becta). (2003). What the research says about ICT supporting special educational needs (SEN) and inclusion *What the Research Says Series*. Retrieved from Education.gov.uk website: https://www.education.gov.uk/publications/eOrderingDownload/15009MIG2791.pdf

Case, D., and Lahm, E. A. (2003). *The Essential Elements of an Assistive Technology Assessment and Assessment Report*. Paper presented at the CSUN Technology and Persons with Disabilities Los Angeles, CA, US.

Copley, J., and Ziviani, J. (2004). Barriers to the use of assistive technology for children with multiple disabilities. *Occupational Therapy International, 11*(4), 229–243. doi:10.1002/oti.213

Craddock, G. (2003). Statement of Need (SON) in assistive technology service delivery system-implications for policy and practice in an Irish context. In G. M. Craddock, L. P. McCormack, R. B. Reilly and H. T. P. Knops (Eds.), *Assistive Technology—Shaping the Future* (pp. 385–388). Amsterdam, The Netherlands: IOS Press.

Craddock, G. (2006). The AT continuum in education: Novice to power user. *Disability and Rehabilitation: Assistive Technology, 1*(1–2), 17–27. doi:10.1080/09638280500167118

Craddock, G., and MacKeogh, T. (2004). *Inclusive Learning through Technology—the ILT Project,* Paper presented at the History of Education Society Conference, October 7–8, Trinity College, Dublin, Ireland.

Craddock, G., and McCormack, L. (2002). Delivering an AT service: A client-focused, social and participatory service delivery model in assistive technology in Ireland. *Disability and Rehabilitation, 24*(1–3), 160–170. doi:10.1080/09638280110063869

Craddock, G., and Scherer, M. J. (2002). Assessing individual needs for assistive technology. In C. L. Sax and C. A. Thoma (Eds.), *Transition Assessment: Wise Practices for Quality Lives.* Baltimore, MD: P.H. Brookes.

Dalton, E. M. (2002). Assistive technology in education: A review of policies, standards, and curriculum integration from 1997 through 2000 involving assistive technology and the Individuals with Disabilities Education Act. *Issues in Teaching and Learning, 1*(1). Retrieved from http://www.ric.edu/itl/volume_01_articles.php#section10

Erickson, K. (2006). What works for all students. Unpublished research outcome. Retrieved from http://www.donjohnston.research.com

Iowa Department of Education. (2007). Summary of Iowa Text Reader Longitudinal Study 2006–2007. Unpublished. Retrieved from http://www.kurzweiledu.com/content/documents/Iowa%20Text%20Reader%20Study%20Final%20Report.pdf

Judge, S., Floyd, K., and Wood-Fields, C. (2010). Creating a technology-rich learning environment for infants and toddlers with disabilities. *Infants and Young Children, 23*(2), 84–92. doi:10.1097/IYC.0b013e3181d29b14

Judge, S., and Simms, K. A. (2009). Assistive technology training at the pre-service level: A national snapshot of teacher preparation programs, teacher education, and special education. *Teacher Education and Special Education, 32*(1), 33–44. doi:10.1177/0888406408330868

Lahm, E. A., and Sizemore, L. (2002). Factors that influence assistive technology decision-making. *Journal of Special Education Technology, 17*(1), 15–26.

Lenker, J. A., and Paquet, V. L. (2003). A review of conceptual models for assistive technology outcomes research and practice. *Assistive Technology, 15*(1), 1–15. doi:10.1080/10400435.2003.10131885

Louise-Bender Pape, T., Kim, J., and Weiner, B. (2002). The shaping of individual meanings assigned to assistive technology: a review of personal factors. *Disability and Rehabilitation, 24*(1–3), 5–20. doi:10.1080/0963828011006623 5

Markussen, E. (2004). Special education: Does it help? A study of special education in Norwegian upper secondary schools. *European Journal of Special Needs Education, 19*(1), 33–48. doi:10.1080/0885625032000167133

Millar, D. C., Light, J. C., and Schlosser, R. W. (2006). The impact of augmentative and alternative communication intervention on the speech production of individuals with developmental disabilities: A research review. *Journal of Speech, Language, and Hearing Research, 49*(2), 248–264. doi:10.1044/1092–4388(2006/021)

Mirenda, P., Turoldo, K., and McAvoy, C. (2006). The impact of word prediction software on the written output of students with physical disabilities. *Journal of Special Education Technology, 21*(3), 5–12.

Østensjø, S., Carlberg, E. B., and Vøllestad, N. (2005). The use and impact of assistive devices and other environmental modifications on everyday activities and care in young children with cerebral palsy. *Disability and Rehabilitation, 27*(14), 849–861. doi:10.1080/09638280400018619

Schepis, M. M., Reid, D. H., Behrmann, M. M., and Sutton, K. A. (1998). Increasing communicative interactions of young children with autism using a voice output communication aid and naturalistic teaching. *Journal of Applied Behavior Analysis, 31*(4), 561–578. doi:10.1901/jaba.1998.31–561.

Scherer, M. (1997). *Matching Assistive Technology and Child: A Process and Series of Assessments for Selecting and Evaluating Technologies Used by Infants and Young Children.* Webster, NY: Institute for Matching Person & Technology.

Scherer, M. J. (1998). *Matching Person & Technology. A Series of Assessments for Evaluating Predispositions to and Outcomes of Technology Use in Rehabilitation, Education, the Workplace & Other Settings.* Webster, NY: The Institute for Matching Person & Technology, Inc.

Scherer, M. J. (2005). Assessing the benefits of using assistive technologies and other supports for thinking, remembering and learning. *Disability and Rehabilitation, 27*(13), 731–739. doi:10.1080/09638280400014816

Scherer, M. J., and Craddock, G. (2002). Matching Person & Technology (MPT) assessment process. *Technology and Disability, 3*(14), 125–131. Retrieved from http://iospress.metapress.com/content/g0eft4mnlwly8y8g

Scherer, M. J., Sax, C. L., Vanbiervliet, A., Cushman, L. A., and Scherer, J. V. (2005). Predictors of assistive technology use: The importance of personal and psychosocial factors. *Disability and Rehabilitation, 27*(21), 1321–1331. doi:10.1080/09638280500164800

Scherer, M. J., and Zapf, S. (2008). Poster 50: Developing a measure to appropriately match students with disabilities and assistive technology devices. *Archives of Physical Medicine and Rehabilitation, 89*(10), e21-e22. doi:10.1016/j.apmr.2008.08.077

Sigafoos, J., and Drasgow, E. (2001). Conditional use of aided and unaided AAC: A review and clinical case demonstration. *Focus on Autism and Other Developmental Disabilities, 16*(3), 152–161. doi:10.1177/108835760101600303

Staples, A., Heying, K., McLellan, J. (1995). A study on the effects of Co:Writer word prediction Software on the writing achievement of students with learning disabilities. Retrieved from http://www/donjohnston.com/djlearning/lftfrm.htm

Swanson, C. B. (2008). *Special Education in America: The State of Students with Disabilities.* Bethesda, MD: Editorial Projects in America.

Sze, S. (2009). A literature review: Pre-service teachers' attitudes toward students with disabilities. *Education, 130*(1), 53–56.

Texas Assistive Technology Network (TATN). (2007). *Considering Assistive Technology in the IEP Training Module and Resource Guide Supplement.* Retrieved from http://www.texasat.net and http://techaccess.edb.utexas.edu

U.S. Department of Education Office of Special Education and Rehabilitative Services (OSERS). (1998). *20th Annual Report to Congress on the Implementation of the Individuals with Disabilities Education Act.* Retrieved from http://www2.ed.gov/offices/OSERS/OSEP/Research/OSEP98AnlRpt/index.html

Watson, A. H., Ito, M., Smith, R. O., and Andersen, L. T. (2010). Effect of assistive technology in a public school setting. *The American Journal of Occupational Therapy, 64*(1), 18–29. doi:10.5014/ajot.64.1.18

World Health Organization. (2010). *Disabilities & Rehabilitations.* Geneva, Switzerland: WHO. Retrieved from http://www.who.int/disabilities/media/events/idpdinfo031209/en/index.html

Zapf, S. A., and Scherer, M. J. (2011). Matching assistive technology to child assessment: A pilot study. Manuscript submitted for publication.

8

The Psychologist

F. Meloni, S. Federici, A. Stella, C. Mazzeschi, B. Cordella, F. Greco, and M. Grasso

CONTENTS

8.1 The Languishing Psychologist's Role in Assistive Technology Assessment

Psychology itself is dead. Or, to put it another way, psychology is in a funny situation. My college, Dartmouth, is constructing a magnificent new building for psychology. Yet its four stories go like this: The basement is all neuroscience. The first floor is devoted to classrooms and administration. The second floor houses social psychology, the third floor, cognitive science, and the fourth, cognitive neuroscience. Why is it called the psychology building? (Gazzaniga 1998, pp. xi–xii)

Together with the neuroscientist Gazzaniga, we ask why is the model called the bio-*psycho*-social model, one of the classifications of the International Classification of Functioning, Disability, and Health (ICF; WHO 2001), when it contains nothing psychological? We do not believe that psychology has ended, but surely (clinical) psychologists risk not finding its location if the World Health Organization's disability model does not build a "floor" for psychology. Maybe it would not be so bad if the problem were just circumscribed to the (clinical) psychologists' occupation in the world. It is very bad if psychology perhaps has the tools to prevent the abandonment of assistive technology (AT) (Philips and Zhao 1993; Zimmer and Chappell 1999; Riemer-Reiss and Wacker 2000; Lenker and Paquet 2004; Scherer et al. 2005; Verza et al. 2006; Waldron and Layton 2008; Söderström and Ytterhus 2010), to guarantee an AT assessment (ATA) "user-driven *process* through which the selection of one or more technological aids for an *assistive solution* is facilitated by the comprehensive utilization of clinical measures, functional analysis, and psycho-socio-environmental evaluations that address, in a specific context of use, the personal *well-being* of the user through the best *matching* of user/client and assistive solution." (see Conclusions, Section I this volume.)

Searching "psychologist role" and "disab*" or "rehabil*" in the "abstract" field of the main databases of the scientific indexes, such as Cambridge Scientific Abstracts (CSA), PubMed, Medline, PsyArticle, PsyInfo, Eric, and Ebsco, from 1900 to date, the findings are astonishing: 56 products between 1973 and 2010. By eliminating studies referring to school psychologists or related only marginally to the (clinical) psychologist's role in rehabilitation and AT assignation, the number of products is reduced to 36, comprising eight chapters in books and monographs and 28 journal articles. Twenty-three of them were published in the 26 years between 1973 and 1999, and the remaining 13 were published in the last 11 years. We found just two conference papers (Mitani et al. 2007; Nihei et al. 2007) in the Association for the Advancement of Assistive Technology in Europe (AAATE) conference proceedings by searching "psycholog*" in the title or in the abstract.

The international scientific literature has never given a clear definition of the role and competencies of the psychologist in the rehabilitation field. In the ATA process, the psychologist's role is given but it usually seems to be narrowed down to the testing and diagnostic phases.

The professional skills of psychologists and their usefulness in the following are all issues of minor relevance in the AT scientific literature (Barry and O'Leary 1989; Scherer 2000):

- Advocating the user's request in the user-driven process through which the selection of one or more technological aids for an assistive solution is reached;
- Acting as mediator between users seeking solutions and the multidisciplinary team of a center for technical aid;
- Team facilitating among members of the multidisciplinary team; and
- Reframing the relationship between the client and his or her family within the framework of the new challenges and limitations and restrictions they face.

Nevertheless, the recent advance of the bio-psycho-social model in the social and scientific communities (Plante 2005); the integration of objective and subjective measures in the diagnostic process (Ueda and Okawa 2003; Uppal 2006; Federici and Meloni 2010; Kayes and McPherson 2010); the recognized relevance of contextual factors and, particularly, the personal ones affecting the long-term success of AT matching (Nair 2003); and the increasing attention to the "imbalance of power" (Brown and Gordon 2004) in the relationship between professionals and users all require a change of attitudes and practices concerning the role of the psychologist in the whole ATA process.

It is reasonable to assume that the deafening silence on the psychologist's role in the ATA process is largely due to the absence of personal factor codes in the ICF.

8.2 Nothing about "Psycho" without Psychologists: The ICF and the Need for Its Revision

The second part of the ICF covers "contextual factors" and is divided into two components: environmental factors and personal factors. The latter are not actually coded in the ICF framework but are involved in the process of functioning and disability and are comprised in the conceptual background of the classification (Geyh et al. 2011). Personal factors are defined in the ICF as "the particular background of an individual's life and living and comprise features of the individual that are no part of a health condition or health states" (WHO 2001, p. 23). They include

> gender, race, age, other health conditions, fitness, lifestyle, habits, upbringing, coping styles, social background, education, profession, past and current experience, overall behaviour pattern and character style, individual psychological assets and other characteristics, all or any of which may play a role in disability at any level. (WHO 2001, pp. 23–24)

They encompass one domain (internal influences on functioning and disability) and one construct (impact of the attributes of the person) (Table 8.1). The domain is "what" the ICF classifies in each of its components at the highest semantic level (e.g., mental functions, structures of the nervous system, learning and applying knowledge, etc.). The construct refers to "how" each category is weighed in an operational way by means of specific qualifiers. For example (WHO 2001, p. 217 Annex 2), the performance of a person (positive aspect: functioning qualifier to weigh) who lost his leg [body structure domain (cod. s750); negative aspect: impairment qualifier (cod. s750.4)] in a work-related accident and since then has used a cane [environmental factor construct (cod. e1201); positive aspect: facilitator qualifier (1201. + 3)] but faces moderate difficulties in walking around [activity and participation construct; negative aspect: activity limitation qualifier (cod. d4500.2)] because the pavements in the neighborhood are very steep and have a very slippery surface [environmental factors construct; negative aspect: barriers qualifier (cod. e2100.-3)] is classified as "moderate restriction in performance of walking short distances": cod. d4500.2.

According to a previous vignette, the use of the aid, the cane, reduces the impact of the physical impairment and the environmental barriers on the individual's performance, although the individual's capacity without assistance and/or in a standardized environment might be considered more limited (e.g., cod. d4500.2 3). This entire assessment process may be carried out by a multidisciplinary team, in which a (clinical) psychologist professional might not be necessary because competence in human cognition, emotion, behavior, and social relations systems are not essential for classifying the person in the example or for assigning him the aid (the cane). According to such biosocial perspectives on functioning and disability classification, "psycho" remains just a prefix to a word to say that the internal influences and the impact of attributes of the person on functioning

TABLE 8.1

An Overview of ICF

	Part 1: Functioning and Disability		Part 2: Contextual Factors	
Components	Body functions and structure	Activities and participation	Environmental factors	Personal factors
Domains	Body functions Body structures	Life areas (tasks, actions)	External influences on functioning and disability	Internal influences on functioning and disability
Constructs	Change in body functions (physiological) Change in body structures (anatomical)	Capacity Executing tasks in a standard environment Performance Executing tasks in the current environment	Facilitation of hindering impact of features of the physical, social and attitudinal world	Impact of attributes of the person
Positive Aspect	Functional and structural integrity	Activities and participation	Facilitators	Not applicable
	Functioning			
Negative Aspect	Impairment	Activity limitation Participation restriction	Barriers/ hindrances	Not applicable
	Disability			

Source: World Health Organization (WHO). *ICF: International Classification of Functioning, Disability, and Health*, Geneva, Switzerland: WHO, 2001.

and disability are not considered, so preventing the cultural and professional development of (clinical) psychologist figures even in the field of the ATA process. Universally, in a center for technical aid the clinical psychologist does not belong to the center's multidisciplinary team of professionals, often being present just as an external consultant. Engineers, physiotherapists, and specialists in rehabilitation (e.g., speech language pathologists, audiologists, optometrists, special educators, and occupational therapists) usually make up the internal team of a center for technical aid and outline the current biosocial outlook on disability.

The ICF imputes the lack of codes for the personal factors to "the large social and cultural variance associated with them" (WHO 2001, p. 9). However, the real novelty of the bio-psycho-social model compared with the previous medical and social ones is precisely the presence of the "psycho" prefix between "bio" and "social." The failure in coding such an important component of the contextual factors 10 years after the ICF edition, given also the distinctive value for the whole classification, creates a disturbing parallel between the International Classification of Impairments, Disabilities, and Handicaps (ICIDH) of 1980 (WHO 1980) and the ICF because ICIDH aimed to describe and represent disability in terms of the social model but ended up revealing a substantial consistency with the medical model: So the ICF seems to ignore the call to complexity, implied in the bio-psycho-social model, to be only, literally, an integration between the medical and social models without a comparatively real qualitative leap. The psychological variables included in the ICF personal factors can make substantial differences to the rehabilitation process and, particularly, they play a central role during the ATA process. The lifestyle, the coping style, the social and cultural background, or the character style really determines the success of matching the person with technology. An appropriate psychological evaluation or a precise clinical intervention with the user/client and/or their significant human context over the course of the whole AT assignment process may prevent, for example, the abandonment or the discard of the assistive solution provided and is a big problem in the matching outcome. It is reasonable to assume that the lack of importance given to the "systemic" skills of the psychologist in the process of matching the person with technology is largely due to the noncoding of personal factors in the ICF.

The ICIDH needed to be revised because it needed to include environmental factors into the coding scheme (Pfeiffer 1998); today we claim that the ICF needs to be revised because there is an urgent need to develop personal factors (see also Steiner et al. 2002). Moreover, as Geyh and colleagues remark, concluding a recent literature review on the conceptualization of the personal factors component of ICF, personal factors "have not been studied extensively or are undervalued (Lehman 2003; Threats 2007; Cruice 2008; Weigl et al. 2008) […]. It is suggested that one aim of further research should be the development of PF categories within the ICF (Khan and Pallant 2007)" (2011, p. 1097).

8.3 The Personal Factors of Functioning and Disability

The recent literature review, already cited in the previous paragraph—carried out by Geyh along with other eminent scholars of the ICF Research Branch and Classifications, Terminology, and Standards Team of the WHO (Geyh et al. 2011) on the conceptualization of the personal factors component of the ICF—yielded 353 citations in 79 papers. Five hundred and thirty-eight statements about personal factors were classified. In addition to conceptual statements, authors have identified personal factors (Verbrugge and Jette 1994; Fougeyrollas et al. 1999; Ueda and Okawa 2003; Badley 2006; Viol et al. 2006). Authors maintain that there is a need for standardization, pointing to "the potential of PF [personal factors] in enhancing the understanding of functioning, disability and health, in facilitating interventions and services for people with disabilities, and strengthening the perspective of individuals in the ICF" (Geyh et al. 2011, p. 1089). An outline list of personal factors is already provided by the ICF and the ICF-CY: "gender, race, age, other health conditions, fitness, lifestyle, habits, upbringing, coping styles, social background, education, profession, past and current experiences, overall behavioural pattern and character style, individual psychological assets" (WHO 2001, pp. 23–24; 2007, pp. 15–16). A more comprehensive list of 238 examples of personal factors not named in the ICF definition is created by Geyh and colleagues (2011) by collecting all of those named in 23 papers of the 79 reviewed. 199 factors out of 238 are found only one time and each one just in a single paper. Of the 39 remaining concepts, the consensus of more than five papers converges on only three concepts: self-efficacy (13), motivation (7), and personality (7). These findings push authors to claim "a need for further standardisation in relation to personal factors as part of the ICF" (Geyh et al. 2011, p. 1099).

The contexts in which personal factors are most frequently mentioned are the rehabilitation of communication disorders and musculoskeletal conditions. In any event, there is universal agreement on the role of personal factors in all stages of the rehabilitation process (Geyh et al. 2011; Gutenbrunner et al. 2007; Steiner et al. 2002) especially "when the ICF was introduced as a framework for comprehensive, holistic and multidisciplinary assessment in a clinical context" (Geyh et al. 2011, p. 1097). But what about personal factors and assistive devices?

8.4 Personal Factors and Assistive Solutions

According to the authors of the above-mentioned reviewed literature (Geyh et al. 2011), personal factors are prevalently mentioned in papers related to occupational and vocational rehabilitation, psychiatric rehabilitation, rehabilitation counselling, and psychosocial care intervention, and in just four papers related to assistive devices (Barker et al. 2006; Cruice 2008; Henderson et al. 2008; Howe 2008). In addition to these four papers, Stephen and Kerr (2000), Pape et al. (2002), Scherer and colleagues (Scherer et al. 2004; Scherer 2005, 2011; Scherer and Dicowden 2008, 2005), and Jahiel and Scherer (2010) pointed out that relevant personal factors affect the use and abandonment of assistive devices, consistent with Philips and Zhao's findings in 1993 in their famous research to determine how technology users decide to accept or reject assistive devices: Three of four factors significantly related to abandonment—lack of consideration of user opinion in selection, easy device procurement, and change in user needs or priorities—were related to personal factors (Philips and Zhao 1993).

Notwithstanding the scarcity in the attention given in international scientific literature to the role and competencies of the psychologist in the ATA process, it is universally ascertained that personal factors are an essential and unavoidable dimension for the best matching of user/client and device. This outlook has pushed scholars in the AT field to reword AT as assistive solution to stress that it is more than a technological device for a technical fix or to overcome a disablement (Roulstone 1998); it involves "something more than just a device, it often requires a *mix* of mainstream and assistive technologies whose assembly is different from one individual and another, and from one context to another" (AAATE 2003).

A useful tool for identifying personal factors that might play a decisive role in successfully matching user/client and AT is provided by the paper of Pape and colleagues (2002). In this review article, 81 publications are considered to individualize meanings assigned to AT and how these personal meanings influence the integration of AT into daily activities (p. 5). In addition to each personal factor code retrieved from the literature reviewed, the paper offers a novel tool for seeking which meanings are ascribed to AT by individuals. A topic guide implemented by questioning routes makes up a worksheet for exploration of personal factors. The questions are classified under two main criteria: disability types and variation factors. The first relates to four disability types: disability due to aging, acquired disability, congenital disability, and disability due to progressive disorder. The variation factors relate to the type and morbidity of impairment, namely the peculiarities referable to the body factors: impairment type and degree, illness type and severity, origin and diagnosis of disability, and functional improvements. The authors then transformed the personal factor concepts emerging from the 81 papers reviewed using operationally probative questions. These probative questions involve psychological, cultural, and adaptation issues (Pape et al. 2002, p. 12).

Despite the scarcity of scientific works focusing on the relations between personal factors and the assignment of suitable AT according to a bio-psycho-social perspective, the personal factors emerge as central to successful matching. Therefore, the most skilled professional profile in the knowledge of individual features and behavior is definitely that of the psychologist.

8.5 The Psychologist in a Center for Technical Aid: The Specialist in Personal Factors

As stated by Scherer, Craddock, and MacKeogh,

> People's predispositions to, expectations for, and reactions to ATD [assistive technology device] use are highly individualised and personal. These predispositions, expectations and reactions emerge from such influences as varying needs, abilities, preferences and past experiences with and exposures to technologies. Importantly, predispositions to use support (as well as realised benefits from use) also depend on one's sense of well-being and satisfaction with current performance of activities and participation in daily life events (2011, p. 812).

Of all of the professionals making up the multidisciplinary team, the psychologist is the one who, in terms of curriculum and training, is the greatest expert in personal factors as they are conceptualized by ICF, expertise that he or she only partly shares with the psychotechnologist (see Chapter 9). The psychotechnologist's skills are more focused on the technological side of matching the person with technology and are less oriented to clinical and psychological dimensions of human-technology interaction:

> The psychotechnologist is an expert of Information and Communication Technologies (ICT), in particular in Human-Computer Interaction (HCI) and human factors and he or she analyses the relations emerging from the person-technology interaction by taking into account: a) all the psychological and cognitive components [...]; b) the possibilities of adapting and designing eSystems and eServices in an adaptable and accessible manner (eAccessibility) (Chapter 9 of this text, p. xxx).

Division 22 of the American Psychological Association, by reporting Scherer and colleagues' entire entry of *The Corsini Encyclopedia of Psychology and Behavioral Science* (2004), remarks that the "rehabilitation psychologist works with the individual with a disability to address personal factors impacting on the ICF domains of activities and participation" (2004, p. 802). Moreover, it illustrates most of the issues that should be investigated by a psychologist in a center for technical aid:

> Neurocognitive status, mood and emotions, desired level of independence and interdependence, mobility and freedom of movement, self-esteem and self-determination, and subjective view of capabilities and quality of life as well as satisfaction with achievements in specific areas such as work, social relationships, and being able to go where one wishes beyond the mere physical capability to do so. (Scherer et al. 2004, p. 802)

Because the psychologist works on the adaptive changes on the human side of the person-environment polarity, he or she should take care to know the features and properties of the personal factors. One of the most relevant categorizations focuses on which personal factors are changeable and which are not (Threats 2003, 2007; Howe 2008; Geyh et al. 2011). Ethnicity, language, cultural background, gender, age, developmental level, sexual orientation, and sexual identity are all unchangeable personal factors that highly affect, in a given context, the relation of the user/client with technology (Threats 2003, 2007; Howe 2008; Geyh et al. 2011). This distinction plays a central role because the psychologist, according to the humanistic and cross-cultural psychology principles (Olkin 1999), promotes the user/client's awareness of the individual resources on which he or she can operate to obtain the best person-technology matching and empowers user/client well-being. In other words, the team of the center for technical aid operates not only to turn environmental barriers into facilitators but also to motivate the user/client to do the same on his or her adjustable individual resources. The psychologist encourages the user/client to explore his or her individual features and to leverage on all of his or her personal factors that can disclose an adaptive potential in a given context.

Another main distinction within personal factors concerns the difference between objective and subjective factors. As reported by Wade, "the focus of rehabilitation is the patient's activities, their behavior" (2000, p. 115), but "the nature of a patient's beliefs and expectations can influence the extent and nature of disability, and indeed may on occasion be the primary cause" (p. 117). The subjective dimension of functioning has been described by Ueda and Okawa (2003) as a combination of negative and positive subjective experiences situated at a "psychological–existential level" (Ueda and Okawa 2003, p. 599). The subjective dimension is strictly linked with the objective one, interrelated and interacting but also strongly independent of each other. Ueda and Okawa (2003) make a distinction between personal factors and the subjective dimension because they put almost all of the traits proposed in literature as belonging to personal factors within the objective level. Aside from whether or not any consideration of the subjective dimension of functioning is gathered by the personal factors of the ICF and the extent to which they overlap, there is no doubt that the "psychological-existential level" should be held in high consideration by the psychologist. In other words, objective and subjective dimensions are concerned with the different point of view of individual functioning: On the side of the professional, most of the ICF's dimensions can be viewed as objective dimensions, for a codifiable and measurable individual functioning; on the side of the user/client, most of the ICF codes are relevant insofar as these are elements of subjective individual functioning or disability experience. Because the goal of the ATA process is user/client well-being, by providing the best match of user/client and assistive solution, with human well-being as an outcome of a subtle equilibrium between the subjective and objective dimension of health (Sen 2002; Federici and Olivetti Belardinelli 2006; Chapter 2 of this text), the psychologist then should pay significant attention to balancing the subjective and objective factors by mediating between the user/client's request and the multidisciplinary team's assistive solution provision.

The psychologist should give special attention to the difference between body functions and personal factors. As reported by Threats (2007), there has been some confusion in the literature between those two components and it is really important to make the right attribution, especially during the assessment stage. In a center for technical aid this distinction may become particularly relevant when the professional measures the predisposition of the user/client to the use of technology. Technology use was found to be influenced not only by factors associated with the user's environment and technology characteristics, but also by nature, characteristics of the purpose of use, and by personal characteristics of the user (Scherer 1998, 2002). Properly encoding the predisposition to the use of the technology allows for the identification of the best-matching solution. For example, if a client with palsy due to a car accident indicates that he was not confident with technology prior to the incident and that he continues to lack confidence, this trait may be considered a personal factor. However, if he reports that his confidence reduced coinciding with the onset of his palsy, this factor may be categorized within the body function component (Howe 2008). From this point of view, the Matching Person and Technology (MPT) series of assessments (Scherer 1998) is a useful measure to make the right attribution concerning the technology predisposition of the user/client:

> The MPT model and accompanying assessment instruments address three primary areas to assess as follows: (a) determination of the milieu/environment factors influencing use; (b) identification of the consumer's needs and preferences; and (c) description of the functions and features of the most desirable and appropriate technology (Scherer and Cushman 2001, p. 127).

Two instruments within the MPT tool kit are particularly suitable for the psychologist's use: the Assistive Technology Device Predisposition Assessment (ATD PA) and the Survey of Technology Use (SOTU). The ATD PA is a self-report questionnaire with items on a five-point scale and yes/no questions that measure an individual's predisposition to and readiness for AT device (ATD) use. The follow-up version assesses the realization of benefit from the selected ATD and reasons for situations of nonuse. The ATD PA was developed to help reduce inappropriate ATD recommendations and the frustration that often accompanies a poor match of person and device (Scherer et al. 2011). In addition, some of the areas investigated by ATD PA (section B: Well-Being, QOL, and section C: Psychosocial factors) offer insights for further investigations of the personal traits of the user/client (Scherer 2005). The SOTU is another MPT instrument designed for professionals considering providing an individual with any kind of technology but who suspect that the individual may be reluctant to use it. The purpose of the psychologist in administering SOTU is both to detect if the user/client feels that the use of technology threatens his/her well-being or self-esteem and to help him/her to discover the positive aspects (Scherer 1998).

Concluding this section, we hold that the psychologist's profile in a center for technical aid is that of the specialist in personal factors, who, more than a rehabilitator, is an enhancer and an "empowerer" of personal awareness and a mediator and defending counsel of personal and subjective factors in the multidisciplinary team of professionals.

8.6 Outlining the Psychologist's Role in the ATA Process

Although we do not believe that psychology has ended, as we held above in contradiction to Gazzaniga's statement, modern psychology has assumed a paradoxical attitude toward disability not facilitating the formation of a clear role for the psychologist in the field of disability. On the one hand, Finkelstein's autobiography assertion about the risk of psychology imprisoning disabled people in their bodies "as being *not*-able" when he was "introduced to the concept of mental deficits in brain functioning" (1998, p. 31) is certainly true if that little mention of disability is raised only during the study of neurophysiology. What is proved otherwise is that a defense of a discipline as "abnormal psychology" does not resolve Finkelstein's assertion when it is claimed that

> the distinctions of normal and abnormal are not synonymous with good or bad. Consider a characteristic such as intelligence. A person who falls at the very upper

end of the curve would fit under our definition of abnormal; this person would also be considered a genius. Obviously, this is an instance where falling outside of the norms is actually a good thing. (Cherry 2010)

It does not sound very convincing, but it almost says *excusatio non petita, accusatio manifesta*.* On the other hand, modern psychology has grounded its theory in the "school of suspicion" (Ricœur 1976) of Freud. Abnormality reveals the structures and dynamics of human behavior. As an anachronistic anticipation, clinical and developmental psychology is founded on the basis of a universal model of abnormality. The cases of hysteria and neurosis gave Freud not only an insight for developing a new therapeutic methodology but, much more, for creating an ontogenetic human theory. Whereas cognitive neurosciences observe the abnormal behavior of people with brain injury to understand the normal nervous representation of mental processes, so that abnormality remains an exception in the human normal functioning (see the section *Cognitive Neural Science Integrates Five Major Approaches to the Study of Cognitive Function* in Kandel 2000, p. 384), clinical and dynamic psychology conversely generalize the abnormal behavior because the mechanisms below, highlighted by mental illness, are shared by the whole human race. What Zola did in the 1990s, by promoting a demystification of the "specialness" of disability (1989) and assuming a conception of disability that is fluid and contextual, modern clinical psychology had done 100 years before. As a contemporary master of suspicion, Zola indeed reaffirmed what was an acquired theory of clinical psychology—that the dichotomy between normal and abnormal "is not a human attribute that demarks one portion of humanity from another [...]; it is an infinitely various but universal feature of the human condition" (Bickenbach et al. 1999, p. 1182; see also Zola 1989; WHO and World Bank 2011). The issue of disability for individuals "is not *whether* but *when*, not so much *which one*, but *how many* and in *what combination*" (Zola 1993, p. 18, italics in the original). The clinician psychologists well know that it is not the basal mechanisms (i.e., body structures and functions) that make the difference among individuals, but the degrees and combinations of individual functioning.

So, in outlining the psychologist's role in the ATA process, we do not want to pour "new wine into old wineskins," namely, to create a new psychologist's profile from a psychology that is past. We would recover that which is owned by modern psychology: a hermeneutic suspicion toward all assessment processes that transform users/clients "as objects to code rather than human beings to support" (Duchan 2004, p. 65). We would like to outline a psychologist's role that is grounded in the psychology's assumption that the goal of any psychological support is not the technical fix of an abnormal functioning individual, but personal well-being. In plain words, the psychologist in the ATA process will answer for a person-centered evaluation through which the selection of one or more technological aids is facilitated by the (self) awareness of the user/client and his/her milieu in which the assistive solution provided is only for the personal well-being of the user.

8.6.1 When the Psychologist Role in the ATA Process Is Required

According to the ideal model of an ATA process in a center for technical aid proposed by Federici and Scherer, the phases in which the clinical psychologist's competencies are specifically used may be divided into six steps (follow in Figure 8.1 the three blue hexagons with "ψ"):

---

* An excuse that has not been sought [is] an obvious accusation.

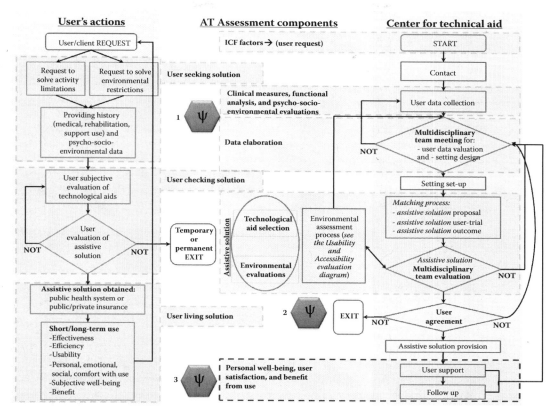

FIGURE 8.1

Flow chart of the ATA process in a center for technical aid: the ATA process can be read both from the perspective of the user/client or from the perspective of the centre for technical aid. The central column indicates the ATA components. The three blue hexagons with a "ψ" point out where the clinical psychologist's competencies are specifically requested.

1. Acceptance and evaluation of the user's request (ψ hexagon 1)

a. *User data collecting*: When the user provides data to the center for technical aid, data are collected; then, the case is opened and transmitted to the multidisciplinary team. All of the clinical measures, functional analyses, and psycho-socio-environmental evaluations provided by the user/client are analyzed by the clinical psychologist to: (i) profile, within the limits of the data collected, the user/client according to a bio-psycho-social and holistic perspective; and (ii) draw up a psychological report for the following multidisciplinary team evaluation.

b. *Meeting with the multidisciplinary team*: The multidisciplinary team evaluates the user's request and data. The clinical psychologist's tasks at this stage are (i) to emphasize the unique and peculiar aspects of the case represented by the user/client in terms of personal factors and of his or her human and relational context of life; (ii) to advocate the user/client's request in the multidisciplinary team; and (iii) to facilitate team members' communications and solution-seeking in the interest of the user/client.

2. Promoting the assistive solution (ψ hexagon 2)

    a. *Assistive solution multidisciplinary team evaluation*: The multidisciplinary team arranges a suitable setting for the matching assessment and, along with the user/client, assesses the assistive solution proposed, tries the solution, and gathers outcome data. After the matching process the multidisciplinary team evaluates the outcome. If successful, the team proposes an assistive solution to the user/client and schedules a new appointment. If not successful, the process restarts. In this step the clinical psychologist advocates the user/client's request guaranteeing a user-driven assignation process through which by selecting one or more technological aids an assistive solution is reached. Active listening, empathy, and ability to reformulate in a shared language the user/client requirements are the main instruments used by the clinical psychologist in this step. Furthermore, the psychologist might offer the opportunity to reframe the relationship between the user/client and his or her family within the framework of the new challenges, limitations, and restrictions they face with the introduction of a new AT.

    b. *User/client agreement*: The multidisciplinary team proposes the assistive solution to the user/client, who evaluates whether or not the technological aid proposed by the professionals is a suitable solution. If yes, the user/client then goes ahead with the process; if no, the user/client exits the process without a solution for their request or waits for new technological products or professionals' solutions. The clinical psychologist may play a central role in this step (e.g., by requesting that the user/client explores the reasons for rejection, especially if they are related to personal factors or factors depending on the context of human relationships). Although the main objective of the ATA process is the best assistive solution for the user/client, it is equally true that often a sufficiently good solution is better than no solution.

3. User support and follow-up (ψ hexagon 3)

When the technological aid is delivered to the user/client, a follow-up and ongoing user support are activated. The clinical psychologist works to promote the well-being of the user/client by regularly monitoring the good quality of matching achieved in terms of impact on his or her personal empowerment.

8.6.2 How a Psychologist Facilitates the Awareness of the User/ Client's Context and Multidisciplinary Team Perspectives

8.6.2.1 Methodology

In the model we propose here, we suggest that the person with disability should be the focus of intervention, being the real "protagonist" of the overall process. Some specifications are otherwise requested, depending on the specific features of the subject, by which we mean macrofeatures that can be used as guidelines to orient the methodology of working "with" the subject. These features are the age of the disabled subject and the type of disability. These variables overlap with other variables connected with the "time" and thus with when the clinical psychologist operates, whether during the assessment phase, the evaluation of the user's request, the phase of promotion of the assistive solution, or, in the third moment, the phase of support and follow-up (see Section 8.6.1). From the methodological point of view, the clinical psychologist has tools specific to his or her profession: the clinical interview and psychological tests (personality tests, performance-based personality tests, questionnaires, rating scales, etc.), tools that belong to the realm of psychological assessment for evaluating personality function in the case of disability.

The psychological assessment, having the specific aim to investigate and know the personal factors (psychological ones) that can mediate the choice and, then, the efficacy of the use of the AT chosen, will be conducted in a multimethod way (e.g., Hunsley and Meyer 2003), thus by using a multimethod assessment battery, to maximize the validity of individualized assessments (Meyer et al. 2001).

Moreover, in the area of psychological assessment, a relatively new way of conducting evaluation has recently emerged that has also been applied in different fields (e.g., McInerney and Walker 2002; Tharinger et al. 2009). It is called collaborative assessment and is mainly based on collaboration between the subject(s) and the psychologist. According to Finn and Fischer (1997; see also Finn 2003), in the collaborative approach to the assessment the psychologist and the client work together to develop productive understanding, ensuring that patients will get the most out of their assessment. In the last few years in the field of therapeutic research a new paradigm called collaborative assessment has been devised. This approach, first devised in 1982 by Fischer in the United States, is based on the assumptions of collaboration between the psychologist and the client starting from the testing session. Its major features are collaboration, individualization of the assessment procedure (in the choice of assessment tools), and flexibility (different pathways for different clients). In the assessment conducted with a collaborative approach, the client is directly engaged: The psychologist asks for client feedback on the assessor's integrated impressions. The findings are thereby tailored to the client's words (APA 2010). A recent meta-analysis shows that psychological assessment procedures—when combined with personalized, collaborative, and substantial test feedback—have positive, clinically meaningful effects on treatment, especially regarding treatment processes, and improve the impact (Poston and Hanson 2010).

We believe that this method of conducting assessment could guide the work of the clinical psychologist in the ATA center with different clients.

- *Phase 1. Acceptance and evaluation of the user's request (see Figure 8.1, ψ hexagon 1):*
  - *Children*: Children with disabilities do not arrive at the ATA center alone but with their parents or caregivers. For this simple but important reason, it will be necessary to involve the parents (caregivers) in the evaluation process because they mediate the information with the child and because they will be responsible for guaranteeing the sustainability and the use of the chosen assistive solution. For this reason we think that, with children, the search for a suitable assistive solution is a task that should involve the entire family (see Chapters 5 and 13 of this text). The clinical psychologist will meet the parents together in a clinical interview, separately from the child, to give them the necessary time and space for freedom of expression without reciprocal influence. After the clinical interview and on the basis of what arises at that stage, tests will be used for better understanding and objectively acknowledging aspects of the parenting function that can support, or hinder, the ambition of the ATA center for the child with a disability. In general, the use of psychological tests in this phase will concern both parents and the child. This psychological assessment phase, conducted with the use of a few tests and thus constituting a multimethod approach (e.g., Hunsley and Meyer 2003), has the specific aim of investigating and ascertaining the personal factors (psychological ones) that can mediate the choice and consequently the efficacy of the technical aid.

- *Preadolescents and adolescents*: What is stressed for children's and parents' (or caregivers') involvement in the assessment phase is also true for this age group, but, because the main goal of this age is the construction of self-identity in terms of self-autonomy, the involvement of the subject in the assessment phase is particularly important and delicate. Because self-efficacy is central to the adolescent's psyche, the clinical psychologist will evaluate through the use of the clinical interview and psychological tests—administered in a collaborative way—the active participation of the subject to ensure that the adolescent is engaged in the process of evaluation of the technical aid, also considering the impact it could have, especially as it regards his or her self-esteem and self-image. Parents will also be involved and evaluate if and how their functioning facilitates or hinders the development of the adolescent in the presence of the technical aid.

- *Adults*: The adult subject with a disability has to be treated as a person. Depending on the specificity of his or her disability, the assessment of his or her personal factors (psychological assessment) will be done with the use of the clinical interview and of psychological tests (in a multimethod approach), also using in this case a collaborative approach, which enhances his or her active engagement and participation in the process to choose the best technical aid. Through the clinical interview(s), the psychologist will be allowed to observe the personal and interior experience of the subject with respect to the disability and to investigate his or her representations of self with respect to the disability, his or her expectations of the technical aid, his or her availability regarding the use of the aid, the best choice of aid, his or her wish for autonomy, and his or her self-efficacy. The use of psychological tests—proposed in a collaborative way and according to a multimethod approach—will allow the psychological assessment to focus better on aspects of his or her psychological functioning (personal and relational) that can hinder or support the use of the shared choice of the technical aid.

- *Elderly people*: Assessment of personal factors depends on his or her level of cognitive and affective autonomy. If the subject is autonomous and self-sufficient, he or she will be regarded as if they were an adult. With regards to the older person, we must consider his or her life perspective and the impact of the technical aid on this in terms of improving his or her quality of life. If the subject is not autonomous or self-sufficient, the psychologist will consider and carefully evaluate the subject's context (caregivers). In this sense personal factors will not be separate from the contextual ones.

- *Phase 2. Promoting the assistive solution (see Figure 8.1, ψ hexagon 2)*: In this phase, the clinical psychologist, by the use of the clinical interview and, if needed, tests, will observe the suitability of the choice in light of what happened in phase 1. Working with the subject with the disability (and with the family in the cases described above), the clinical psychologist gives psychological support to the subject and, as in an assessment phase, detects the presence of obstacles to the use of the chosen technical aid, difficulties in its acceptance by the subject (or by his or her context), and aspects of his or her functioning that could interfere with the use of the aid. The clinical psychologist observes, from the point of view of the subject with disability (e.g., efficacy, autonomy, mood, self-esteem, and satisfaction), the impact the aid has on his or her life (and life context) in a positive sense (increment) and in a negative sense (e.g., depressive mood, isolation, withdrawal, etc.). Active listening, empathy, and the ability to reformulate in a shared language user/client requirements are the main instruments used by the clinical psychologist in this stage within the interview. Furthermore, the psychologist might offer the opportunity to reframe the relationship between the user/client and his or her family within the framework of the new challenges, limitations, and restrictions they face with the introduction of a new AT.

- *Phase 3. User support and follow-up (see Figure 8.1, ψ hexagon 3)*: In this phase the clinical psychologist assesses the match between the subject and the aid together with the client. If phase 1 has been conducted rigorously with the psychologist listening carefully to the subject, it is probable that this third phase will be a good outcome to the process. It is also possible that in this phase events (external or internal) in the life of the subject may occur that require a "revision"—a new assessment phase—to reframe the first choice of aid. Factors of change can also result from developmental facts (e.g., children with technical aids for learning disabilities). Through the use of the clinical interview and tests, the psychologist will conduct this phase as a follow-up step in the process. We expect that particular attention will be paid to the satisfaction of the subject as a measure of the efficacy of the matching intervention that the psychologist and the client have conducted together. Quality of life will also be a measure to be taken into account.

8.6.2.2 Goals

The role of the clinical psychologist within the ATA center is mainly linked to his or her diagnostic competencies and skills and the planning of the intervention. These are clinical competencies: assess to know (in our model, assessing and knowing together) and to intervene if convenient, useful, and necessary.

The first goal then is the identification of those aspects of psychological functioning (personal factors) that promote and sustain the awareness of the subject with a disability and that are supposed to mediate (1) the choice of a certain technical aid, (2) the acceptance of the aid, (3) its use, (4) its use over time, and (5) the possibility to change it (for another or none) if personality changes occur in the person and in case the that the aid is no longer useful or suitable. In this context, another aspect on which the clinical psychologist will work—compatibly with the cognitive psychological functioning of the subject with disability—is the possibility to improve the reflective functioning of the subject with the aim of identifying aspects of the self (of the present and of the future) that mediate the use and acceptance of the technical aid. The clinical psychologist will also detect and assess clinical conditions significantly connected to the deficit that could hinder the intentional use of the aid (e.g., depression in a boy affected by injury to the legs after a traumatic accident. The boy does not accept the wheelchair that could help him to improve his autonomy because he does not accept the limitation and he is ashamed and feels different from his friends. He withdraws, does not go outside of his home and does not accept the aid wheelchair because it makes him feel different from others).

Tools used in the assessment phase can be used again in the follow-up phase as measures of the efficacy of the intervention. Other specific measures, such as the perceived quality of life, will be used to verify the efficacy of the intervention, including measures directly taken by the subject with disability (and/or by the caregivers) and measures taken by the psychologist him/herself (or by an external member of the team). Other measures concern the global evaluation of the subject's autonomy and more specific measures assess the change of the psychic function with respect to the technical aid used.

8.6.2.3 What a Psychologist Should Do in Promoting a User/Client Request

To conclude this section on the psychologist's role in the ATA process, we remark, in a guidelines style, what a clinical psychologist should do in promoting a user/client request.

- Be an expert in the relational field that is able to listen, receive, and understand others.
- Be aware of the idiographic approach and sensitive to individual differences in psychological functioning.
- Have expertise and dynamic comprehension of the bio-psycho-social variables of functioning, so that the hyphen between "bio-," "psycho-," and "social" will not be a separator but a connector. The perspective is that of interaction, something less valued by the ICF model.
- Have a developmental perspective, not only when working with children but also with adults and elderly people. This allows him/her to appreciate the change always present in life (decremental or incremental; continuous or discontinuous).
- Be able to actively involve the subject in the psychological assessment process with the aim of improving his or her awareness of the personal factors that mediate the choice and use of the technical aid.
- Be able to work with, depending on the subject, the different people that belong to his or her life, respecting their roles and competencies.
- Have clinical competencies: evaluation and planning of the intervention. He or she should be able to conduct an early assessment but also be able to evaluate the course of the process and to test its efficacy. We consider as intervention the process of the choice of a specific aid, done together with and for a specific person with a disability, which has the specific features of psychological-personal –functioning.
- Be able to use psychological tests and conduct a psychological assessment through the use of tests in a multimethod way (using not just one instrument but several to ensure the incremental validity of the evaluation to appreciate the psychological functioning of the subject). Working in a team that includes the neuropsychologist, clinical psychologists with such competencies will orient their evaluation to the axis of psychological functioning with regard to relational functioning and emotional-affective functioning, being aware of their strong connection.

8.7 Psychologist "Know Thyself": Psychologist and Professional's Representations of the Disabled Users/Clients and Assistive Technologies

The perspective that takes into account human complexity and its mutability better than others is the biopsychosocial one. The possibility of carrying out this perspective, usefully combining the contribution of professionals working in the team, needs to acknowledge the specificity and the asset value of interdisciplinary work (Telfener 2011) despite literature showing how the physicians' and social workers' identities are better defined than the psychologists'. In fact, the psychologist's professional identity tends to follow the physician or social worker's model depending on the context (Grasso 2001), as has been highlighted in a recent study (Cordella et al. 2011) carried out by the Dynamic and Clinical Psychology Department of the Medicine and Psychology Faculty at Sapienza University in Rome.

8.7.1 Professionals' Representation of Disability

Research has been performed in an Italian vision rehabilitation center that serves the central and southern areas of the country and has worked in the field for almost one and a half centuries. It provides many services, including rehabilitation for blind and visually impaired people of all ages, with a multidisciplinary approach carried out by a variety of professional figures making up the team. The aim of the study was to explore professionals' identity by using their narrations (Freda 2009) of their professional experiences in the rehabilitation of people with visual disability.

Interviews were integrally audiotaped, transcribed, and underwent a text analysis performed with a computer software package, T-Lab (Lancia 2004). T-lab performed a correspondence analysis and a cluster analysis to identify groups of lemmas having high variances within and between clusters. This analysis allows for the identification of revealing words that characterize the way professionals represent their professional function, their impaired patients, and the rehabilitation process.

The results show four different clusters characterizing professionals' accounts that reflect the richness of professionals' skills and experiences. They highlight the professionals' ability to deal with a large variety of problems connected with disability. Management, prevention, training, and advocacy seem to be the goals of the rehabilitation process carried out by the interaction of the multidisciplinary team. Moreover, professionals working at the vision rehabilitation center represented four groups: physicians, paramedics, psychosocial workers, and vision rehabilitation professionals (Table 8.2), and the cluster distribution in each group was ascertained to explore how it characterizes each group (Figure 8.2).

TABLE 8.2

Profession Groups

GROUP	N°	PROFESSION	N°
A: PHYSICIANS	6	Neuropsychiatrist	4
		Ophthalmologist	1
		Psychiatrist	1
B: PARAMEDICS	12	Logotherapists	2
		Music therapist	1
		Nurses	2
		Occupational therapist	1
		Optometrists	2
		Physiotherapist	1
		Psychomotricity therapists	3
C: PSYCHOSOCIAL WORKERS	3	Psychologists	2
		Social worker	1
D: VISION REHABILITATION PROFESSIONALS	13	Typhlo-therapists	13

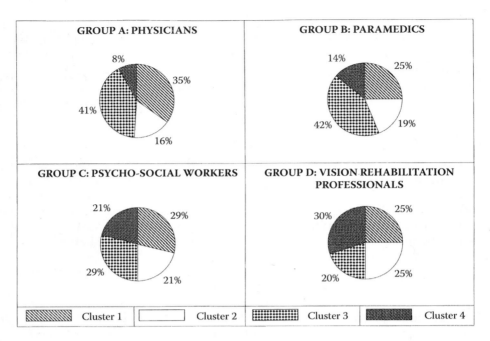

FIGURE 8.2
Clusters distribution in four groups of professionals.

The management cluster mostly characterizes physicians and refers to the need to manage the working team. Their accounts seem to have contributed particularly to this cluster construction. Working in a multidisciplinary team determines the necessity to consider different needs and points of view for these professionals. A comprehensive vision rehabilitation service seems to imply the necessity to work on professionals' interactions. Therefore, working together is not just a resource because it produces an additional job that overcomes problems caused by multidisciplinarity. In addition, in this cluster the target is the team itself and the professional function is focused on management and coordination. Moreover, this representation of the rehabilitation process is not vision-specific. This representation of the professional function focuses on problematic situations and puts aside the visual center specificity. Therefore, it targets the team of professionals working on interventions' definition rather than the person with disability needs.

Accounts of paramedics and physicians have particularly contributed to the construction of cluster 3 (prevention). In fact, cluster distribution in the paramedics' group is similar to that of the physicians', although it does not overlap with it. In fact, cluster 3 characterizes both of these groups, but for paraprofessionals it seems to be the most important one. These professionals seem to focus on disabilities associated with visual disability, giving particular attention to multihandicapped children who need a multidisciplinary approach. Therefore, professional function is focused on a particular aspect of disability, especially intellectual, losing visual specificity. The patient is represented as multihandicapped and the professional function does not deal directly with visual disability.

It was interesting to note that psychologists have an almost equal distribution in all clusters not being particularly characterized by any of them, suggesting that these professionals do not have professional function specificity. Nevertheless, clusters 1 and 3 are slightly more represented. Hence, probably like physicians and paramedics, these professionals focus their attention on the plurality of disability affecting the young person that necessarily needs a multidisciplinary approach.

Accounts of vision rehabilitation professionals contribute mostly to clusters 2 (training) and 4 (advocacy), which characterize this group. They represent their professional function more like training (cluster 2). The process is focused on the professional intervention of teaching specific solutions through professional training and experience. The process is considered morally right and attention is not directed to the relationship with someone but on the professionals' performances. Although this representation refers to specific tools, no attention is given to the employment of tools. Therefore, it suggests that rehabilitation is focused on professional performance rather than on the person with disability needs.

These professionals are also characterized by advocacy (cluster 4), aiming to support people in the development of knowledge. Visual disability implies behavioral limits that could hinder the learning process. Therefore, the intervention is directed to young students and aims to support their learning as a way to emancipate them from disability. It is for this reason that the professional's function is to replace their patient's deficient one. Whereas the rehabilitation process seems to be focused on a particular moment in life, this cluster does not take into account the possibility of building new abilities. Substitution seems to be the only possibility to help the disabled person, but it implies a high personal involvement for these professionals.

Therefore it is interesting to observe the following:

- Disabled people's representations focus on their deficiencies rather than on the resources enhancing them. They are not represented as independent, productive, self-effective, or able to solve problems. This representation does not help professionals to motivate their patients or help them to assume an active role. A few recent studies suggest that taking responsibility for managing their own conditions with support and advice from health-care professionals is an important factor in the rehabilitation process for patients with chronic conditions (Holman and Lorig 2000; Bodenheimer et al. 2002; Girdler et al. 2010). This is different from the professional teaching particular solutions or making changes to the patient's home environment. Hence, to assume an active role in the process, people with disability need to be motivated. This new paradigm in health care aims to provide the patients with skills and resources to manage the practical, social, and emotional consequences of their disabilities and to seek specialist support when needed.

- Professionals often address children and young people, whereas the ability to deal with disabled adults of working age seems to be unexplored. In fact, restrictions related to disability often result in loss of independence, which is often associated with a loss of social and economic status, which also implies a cost to society.

- Those who train in the use of ATs do not wonder what these aids represent for the disabled person and how they will be used.

- Finally, psychosocial workers seem to have less professional function specificity. In fact, the psychological professional's function seems to find its specificity particularly when it overlaps with psychotherapeutic specificity (Carli 1993; Cordella et al. 2001). Nowadays, in the disability area, psychological function aims to support disabled people to face the emotional difficulties that arise from the loss of an ability. Nevertheless, this is not the only function psychologists can carry out, although it remains useful in the rehabilitation context.

Considering psychological professional expertise as the ability to seize, interpret, and make more functional the representations that mediate the relationship between individuals and their contexts would allow the widening of the psychologists' area of intervention. In this approach, psychologists could facilitate the work of professionals and the multidisciplinary team, making the rehabilitation process of the disabled person more effective.

8.7.2 New Approach in Psychological Practice

To understand how psychological practice could be useful in the ATA process in a center for technical aid, it is important to introduce the concept of representation. According to cognitivism, individuals categorize reality not only on the basis of their perceptions, but also on beliefs related to the perceived object, which makes some similarities more important than others (Neisser 1989). Therefore, there is a connection between culture and human cognition, in which the context influences the individuals' perception, attitudes, and behaviors (Ugazio 1989).

According to Moscovici (Moscovici 1961; Farr and Moscovici 1984), representation is a system of ideas, values, and practices that provides individuals with a code for social exchange and for categorizing and naming various aspects of their world. Therefore, it facilitates communication and orientates individuals in their social world, allowing them to master it. Representations are an approach to the interpretation and social sharing of knowledge. They are learned from the social context and, at the same time, are discursively constructed by individuals belonging to the context itself. Therefore, representations are the process and the result of social construction, constantly converted into a social reality while continuously being reinterpreted, rethought, and re-presented.

Finally, Matte Blanco (1975) suggests that individuals categorize reality not only by means of a cognitive process but also through an emotional one. Individuals facing reality categorize it emotionally and cognitively, which allows them to perceive the context as intentioned. For example, the child that bumps against the corner of a table and strikes it back attributes a negative intention to the table. Therefore the child recognizes the object (table) because of his or her ability to categorize it cognitively and, at the same time, he or she sets his or her behavior (striking the table back) through his or her ability to categorize it emotionally, representing it. Hence, each time individuals relate with an object (person, thing, service, technical aid, etc.) they categorize it cognitively and represent it emotionally depending on their own culture. Therefore, representations determine behaviors that can be more or less effective in achieving goals.

According to this perspective, psychological expertise is the ability to identify individuals' emotional representations, helping them to eventually understand how they can hinder goal achievement (Carli 1993; Grasso et al. 2003; Grasso and Salvatore 1997; Grasso 2010). For example, a child's ability to avoid the table's impact is granted by his or her ability to pay attention to barriers surrounding him rather than striking back the table. Therefore, working on individuals' representations allows for intervention in the problem (avoid bumping against the table) rather than on the behavior (striking back the evil table) or directly on the object perceived by the individual as responsible for the problem (the evil table). Moreover, it helps individuals to relate effectively with their context adapting to it.

8.7.3 Psychological Professional Practice Guidelines in the ATA Process

As claimed previously, psychologists have the skill to work on representations by making them more functional. Therefore, some guidelines about the psychological approach in the

ATA process is drafted here to better understand how to set the practice according to the target. In fact, psychologists can usefully contribute to the professional team during the six steps of the ATA process, working on representations and thereby improving service effectiveness.

8.7.3.1 The User

The user who comes to a center for technical aid has his or her own representation of the center and of the service provided, which sets his or her requests, behavior, attitudes, and expectations. This representation will influence his or her relationship with the professionals of the center, hindering or facilitating their work. Hence, the psychologist could start his or her work from the incoming user request for technical aids. He or she should explore which needs pushed the disabled user to ask for technical aid at that particular moment of his or her life. If the professionals take for granted the answer to the user's request, the intervention will be focused on the user's disability rather than on the representation he or she has of his or her problem. Accordingly, only the "bio" and "social" dimensions of disability are focused on, omitting the "psycho" dimension, which influences the way that the user builds his or her own relationships.

The user's representation of the service provided by the center determines his or her request. In fact, two users with the same disability can differently represent their problems and expect a different reaction (service) from the center. Therefore, one of them could focus on the right he or she has to obtain the technical aid because of his or her disability, setting his or her request as a claim for damages and pretending reparation from the professionals. The other could focus on his or her passive and dependent role because of his or her inability, limiting extremely his or her participation and complaining and distrusting professionals. Both of these users would not benefit entirely from the service and the professionals would probably face difficulties in working with them, being limited in their effectiveness by the users' representations.

Integrating the ATA process with psychologists that are trained to seize, interpret, and make representations more functional could facilitate the professionals' work and make it more effective. In fact, psychologists can work on users' representations of the center for technical aid and of the disability, promoting a functional development of their representations so as to facilitate their active participation in the process.

8.7.3.2 The Family

Families also have their representations of the center and of the disability, which can hinder or facilitate the disabled user and increase or decrease center effectiveness and the professionals' work. Some families are overprotective whereas others are less protective. They might have expectations overestimating or underestimating the outcomes, which will condition their relationship with the disabled user and the professionals.

In fact, relatives' representations of disability can help or limit the disabled person's independence, influencing their expectations of his or her abilities. In some rehabilitation centers performing ATA, a day's role play session has been set up to put relatives in the same condition as the person with the disability, helping them to face the same challenges (Greco in press). At the end of the day, participants have an interview with a psychologist aiming to reorganize their representations of disability. This process helps relatives to develop a more functional representation, overcoming their fears about disability.

Furthermore, it helps them to cooperate with the disabled user and with the professionals to solve problems related to disability.

8.7.3.3 *The Professionals' Multidisciplinary Team*

Psychologists can also work on professionals' representations of the center and of the disabled users because they can hinder or facilitate the process and the achievement of goals. In fact, as has been highlighted in the previously presented study, if the representation of the user is passive, user abilities are not taken into account, hindering the user's active participation in the process. This representation does not help professionals to motivate their users in assuming an active role. To be effective, the process needs the users' collaboration; they should take responsibility for managing their own conditions and use support and advice provided by professionals to become independent. For instance, assigning a long cane to a disabled user and teaching him to walk with it does not imply that once the process is over, the disabled person will use the cane to get out of his or her home. There is a difference between obtaining or being trained in the use of a technical aid and using it in everyday life.

Because of the psychological difficulties people face in adapting to disability, it is up to the professionals to promote a change in the users' attitudes (Hayeems et al. 2005; Godshalk et al. 2008). To achieve this goal, it is important for professionals to perceive the user as able to state his or her needs and solve his or her problems, representing him as independent, productive, and self-effective. This is why passive user representation does not help professionals in being effective. Moreover, the incoming user may not have an active representation of himself or herself.

Users' passivity is not negative in all cases. Sometimes it is important for a person to rely upon the professionals' ability to take care of them (e.g., when it is not possible to act directly in relation to the problem, as when it is necessary to undergo surgery). In fact, passivity can solicit professionals' care, and it is useful because intervention relies upon their performance. Nevertheless, in the ATA process, users have to rely upon professionals' performance, but participate actively, because it helps them to collaborate effectively with professionals.

Moreover, a team of professionals implies different representations that have to be combined. As shown in cluster 1 (management) of the research, this does not facilitate the work and needs extra effort to manage it. The difficulty faced in combining types of professional expertise can lie within the professionals' different representations of the process and of the user.

Finally, the possibility to understand and reorganize the representations of all of the participants in the ATA process (users, professionals, relatives) would allow for the improvement of the service provided by professionals, thus making it more effective for the disabled user in the short and long term. Furthermore, the center could become a real reference for the disabled user if further problems should occur.

8.8 Conclusions

This chapter deals with the professional skills of the psychologist and the way in which they are applied in a center for technical aid. This chapter also provides an original contribution to the study of the representations that psychologists and other professionals endorse of disabled people and AT.

As Meloni, Federici, and Stella demonstrated in a recent study (2011), and as is reported and discussed in Sections 8.1–8.3, the international scientific literature pays very little attention to the role and skills of the psychologist in the field of rehabilitation and, in particular, in the process of matching people with AT. One of the likely causes of this neglect could be that the real novelty of the biopsychosocial model, constituted by the presence of the prefix "psycho" between "bio" and "social," has been largely disregarded through the noncoding of personal factors in the ICF. The psychologist in a center for technical aid is, first and foremost, an expert on personal factors because the predispositions and reactions of people to using AT are highly personal and individual. Only the psychologist has the appropriate curriculum and expertise to investigate personal factors, to identify which ones are critical in allowing or hindering the matching of person and technology, and to promote adaptive changes on the human side of the person-environment polarity. More specifically, the competencies of the psychologist are involved in some crucial phases of the ideal model of the ATA process: (1) accepting and evaluating the user's request, (2) promoting the assistive solution, and (3) providing support and follow-up.

In Section 8.6, Mazzeschi highlighted the psychologist's main professional goals in a center for technical aid, which we can summarize as follows: (1) to advocate the user's request in the user-driven process, through which the selection of one or more technological aids for an assistive solution is made; (2) to act as a mediator between users seeking solutions and the multidisciplinary team of a center for technical aid; (3) to facilitate team-building among the members of the multidisciplinary team; and finally (4) to reframe the relationship between the client and his or her family or caregivers within the framework of the new challenges, limitations, and restrictions that they are faced with. To achieve these goals, the psychologist should be an expert in handling the main diagnostic and assessment tools and in using his or her relationship with the user/client to promote personal awareness, growth, and the development of human potential and to maximize empowerment.

In the last section, Cordella, Greco, and Grasso developed another important point in outlining the psychologist's role in a center for technical aid that concerns the representations that the psychologist and other multidisciplinary team members endorse of disability and the functions of AT. The quality of life and well-being of a disabled person depend largely on the ability of professionals, relatives, and caregivers to imagine a range of existential alternatives and not to nail the prevailing social stereotypes and cultural prejudices onto the disabled person. For this reason, the psychologist should be engaged in promoting (both in the multidisciplinary team and in the broader sociocultural context) the diffusion of a complex, multidimensional, universal, and holistic approach to disabled people that is firmly founded on the biopsychosocial model of disability.

In conclusion, we have noted the need for a change in attitude and practice in relation to the role of the clinical psychologist in the ATA process, spurred on by the recent advance of the biopsychosocial model in the social and scientific communities, the integration of objective and subjective measures into the diagnostic process, the recognized relevance of contextual factors and, in particular, the personal factors affecting the long-term success of AT matching, and the increasing interest in the "imbalance of power" in the relationship between professionals and users. We are convinced that a revision of the ICF is urgently needed to develop those personal factors that can make a substantial difference during the rehabilitation process and, in particular, during the ATA process.

Summary of the Chapter

This chapter deals with the role and the competencies of the psychologist in a center for technical aid. The lapse of the psychologist's role in ATA is probably due to the noncoding of personal factors in the ICF. In viewing the psychologist as the "specialist" on personal factors, the authors call for a revision of the ICF so that in the biopsychosocial model, the "psycho" does not remain as just a prefix. The psychologist in the center has the goals to support the user's request in the user-driven process as well as to act as a mediator between users seeking solutions and the multidisciplinary team. He or she also acts to build a team spirit and enhance the relationship between the client and his or her home environment. Finally, an original study closes the chapter, focusing on psychologists and professionals' representations of disabled users/clients and ATs.

Acknowledgments

Fabio Meloni, Stefano Federici, and Aldo Stella contributed equally to this study, except for Section 8.6, which was edited by Claudia Mazzeschi, and Section 8.7, which was edited by Barbara Cordella, Francesca Greco, and Massimo Grasso.

References

AAATE. (2003). *AAATE Position Paper: A 2003 View on Technology and Disability.* Retrieved from http://www.aaate.net/

American Psychological Association (APA). (2010). *Ethical Principles of Psychologists and Code of Conduct.* Retrieved from http://www.apa.org/ethics/code/index.aspx

Badley, E. M. (2006, June 5–7). *More than Facilitators and Barriers: Fitting the Full Range of Environmental and Personal Contextual Factors into the ICF Model.* Paper presented at the 12th annual North American Collaborating Centre Conference on ICF, Vancouver, Canada.

Barker, D. J., Reid, D., and Cott, C. (2006). The experience of senior stroke survivors: Factors in community participation among wheelchair users. *Canadian Journal of Occupational Therapy, 73*(1), 18–25. doi:l 0.2182/cjot.05.0002

Barry, P., and O'Leary, J. (1989). Roles of the psychologist on a traumatic brain injury rehabilitation team. *Rehabilitation Psychology, 34*(2), 83–90. doi:10.1037/h0091712

Bickenbach, J. E., Chatterji, S., Badley, E. M., and Üstün, T. B. (1999). Models of disablement, universalism and the International Classification of Impairments, Disabilities and Handicaps. *Social Science and Medicine, 48*(9), 1173–1187. doi:10.1016/S0277-9536(98)00441-9

Bodenheimer, T., Lorig, K., Holman, H., and Grumbach, K. (2002). Patient self-management of chronic disease in primary care. *Journal of the American Medical Association, 288*(19), 2469–2475. doi:10.1001/jama.288.19.2469

Brown, M., and Gordon, W. A. (2004). Empowerment in measurement: "Muscle," "voice," and subjective quality of life as a gold standard. *Archives of Physical Medicine and Rehabilitation, 85*(Suppl. 2), S13–S20. doi:10.1016/j.apmr.2003.08.110

Carli, R. (1993). *L'Analisi Della Domanda in Psicologia Clinica* [Demand Analysis in Clinical Psychology]. Milan, Italy: Giuffré.

Cherry, K. (2010). What Is Abnormal Psychology? Retrieved from http://psychology.about.com/

Cordella, B., Cardarelli, L., and Pizzi, E. (2001). L'identità professionale dello psicologo: Competenze specifiche/capacità di orientarsi [The professional identity of psychologist: Specific skills/professional orientation abilities]. In M. Grasso (Ed.), *Modelli e Contesti dell'Intervento Psicologico* (p. 352). Rome: Kappa.

Cordella, B., Greco, F., and Grasso, M. (2011, May 17–20). *Strategies of Development of a Vision Rehabilitation Service*. Paper presented at the 16th International Association of Psychology and Psychiatry for Adults and Children Conference: APPAC '11, Athens, Greece.

Cruice, M. (2008). The contribution and impact of the International Classification of Functioning, Disability and Health on quality of life in communication disorders. *International Journal of Speech–Language Pathology, 10*(1–2), 38–49. doi:10.1080/17549500701790520

Duchan, J. F. (2004). Where is the person in the ICF? *International Journal of Speech–Language Pathology, 6*(1), 63–65. doi:10.1080/14417040410001669444

Farr, R. M., and Moscovici, S. (1984). *Social Representations*. Cambridge, MA: Cambridge University Press.

Federici, S., and Meloni, F. (2010). WHODAS II: Disability self-evaluation in the ICF conceptual frame. In J. Stone, and M. Blouin (Eds.), *International Encyclopedia of Rehabilitation* (pp. 1–22). Buffalo, NY: Center for International Rehabilitation Research Information and Exchange (CIRRIE). Retrieved from http://cirrie.buffalo.edu/encyclopedia/en/article/299/

Federici, S., and Olivetti Belardinelli, M. (2006). Un difficile accordo tra prevenzione e promozione. [Hard-won agreement between prevention and promotion]. *Psicologia Clinica dello Sviluppo, 10*(2), 330–334.

Finkelstein, V. (1998). Emancipating disability studies. In T. Shakespeare (Ed.), *The Disability Reader: Social Science Perspectives* (pp. 28–49). London: Cassell.

Finn, S. E. (2003). Therapeutic assessment of a man with "ADD." *Journal of Personality Assessment, 80*(2), 115–129. doi:10.1207/S15327752JPA8002_01

Finn, S. E., and Fischer, C. T. (1997, Aug 15–19). *Therapeutic Psychological Assessment: Illustration and Analysis of Philosophical Assumptions*. Paper presented at the American Psychological Association Convention, Chicago, IL.

Fischer, C. T. (1982). Intimacy in assessment. In M. Fisher, and G. Stricker (Eds.), *Intimacy* (pp. 443–460). New York: Plenum.

Fougeyrollas, P., Cloutier, R., Bergeron, H., Cote, J., and St-Michel, G. (1999). *The Quebec Classification: Disability Creation Process*. Québec, Canada: International Network on the Disability Creation Process.

Freda, M. F. (2009). *Narrazione e Intervento in Psicologia Clinica. Costruire, Pensare e Trasformare Narrazioni tra Logos e Pathos* [Narration and Intervention in Clinical Psychology. Building, Thinking and Transform Narratives Between Logos and Pathos]. Napoli, Italy: Liguori Editore.

Gazzaniga, M. S. (1998). *The Mind's Past*. Berkeley, CA: University of California Press.

Geyh, S., Peter, C., Müller, R., Bickenbach, J. E., Kostanjsek, N., Üstün, B. T., et al. (2011). The personal factors of the International Classification of Functioning, Disability and Health in the Literature—A systematic review and content analysis. *Disability and Rehabilitation, 33*(13–14), 1089–1102. doi:10.3109/09638288.2010.523104

Girdler, S. J., Boldy, D. P., Dhaliwal, S. S., Crowley, M., and Packer, T. L. (2010). Vision self-management for older adults: A randomised controlled trial. *British Journal of Ophthalmology, 94*(2), 223. doi:10.1136/bjo.2008.147538

Godshalk, A. N., Brown, G. C., Brown, H. C., and Brown, M. M. (2008). The power of hope: Being a doctor is more than relying solely on the numbers. *British Journal of Ophthalmology, 92*(6), 783–787. doi:10.1136/bjo.2008.141663

Grasso, M. (2001). *Modelli e Contesti dell'Intervento Psicologico* [Models and Contexts of Psychological Intervention]. Rome: Kappa.

Grasso, M. (2010). *La Relazione Terapeutica* [The Therapeutic Relationship]. Bologna, Italy: Il Mulino.

Grasso, M., Cordella, B., and Pennella, A. R. (2003). *L'Intervento in Psicologia Clinica: Fondamenti Teorici* [Intervention in Clinical Psychology: Theoretical Foundations]. Roma, Italy: Carocci.

Grasso, M., and Salvatore, L. (1997). *Pensiero e Decisionalità. Contributo alla Critica della Prospettiva Individualista in Psicologia* [Thinking and Decision-Making. A Contribution to the Critique of the Individualist Perspective in Psychology] (Vol. 134). Milan, Italy: Franco Angeli.

Greco, F. (in press). *Resoconto Clinico di un Processo di Rieducazione in un CRPM di Parigi* [Clinical Report of a Rehabilitation Process in a CPMR in Paris]. Rome: Nuova Cultura.

Gutenbrunner, C., Ward, A. B., and Chamberlain, M. A. (2007). White Book on Physical and Rehabilitation Medicine in Europe (Revised November 2009). *Journal of Rehabilitation Medicine, 45*(Suppl), 1–48. doi:10.2340/16501977-0028

Hayeems, R. Z., Geller, G., Finkelstein, D., and Faden, R. R. (2005). How patients experience progressive loss of visual function: A model of adjustment using qualitative methods. *British Journal of Ophthalmology, 89*(5), 615–620. doi:10.1136/bjo.2003.036046

Henderson, S., Skelton, H., and Rosenbaum, P. (2008). Assistive devices for children with functional impairments: Impact on child and caregiver ffunction. *Developmental Medicine and Child Neurology, 50*(2), 89–98. doi:10.1111/j.1469-8749.2007.02021.x

Holman, H., and Lorig, K. (2000). Patients as partners in managing chronic disease. Partnership is a prerequisite for effective and efficient health care. *British Medical Journal, 320*(7234), 526–527. doi:10.1136/bmj.320.7234.526

Howe, T. J. (2008). The ICF contextual factors related to speech–language pathology. *International Journal of Speech–Language Pathology, 10*(1–2), 27–37. doi:10.1080/14417040701774824

Hunsley, J., and Meyer, G. J. (2003). The incremental validity of psychological testing and assessment: Conceptual, methodological, and statistical issues. *Psychological Assessment, 15*(4), 446–455. doi:10.1037/1040-3590.15.4.446

Jahiel, R. I., and Scherer, M. J. (2010). Initial steps towards a theory and praxis of person-environment interaction in disability. *Disability and Rehabilitation, 32*(17), 1467–1474. doi:10.3109/09638280802590637

Kandel, E. R. (2000). From nerve cells to cognition: The internal cellular representation required for perception and action. In E. R. Kandel, J. H. Schwartz, and T. M. Jessell (Eds.), *Principles of Neural Science* (4th ed., pp. 381–403). New York: McGraw-Hill.

Kayes, N. M., and McPherson, K. M. (2010). Measuring what matters: Does 'objectivity' mean good science? *Disability and Rehabilitation, 32*(12), 1011–1019. doi:10.3109/09638281003775501

Khan, F., and Pallant, J. F. (2007). Use of the International Classification of Functioning, Disability and Health (ICF) to identify preliminary comprehensive and brief core sets for multiple sclerosis. *Disability and Rehabilitation, 29*(3), 205–213. doi:10.1080/09638280600756141

Lancia, F. (2004). *Strumenti per l'Analisi dei Testi. Introduzione all'Uso di T-LAB* [Tools for the Analysis of Texts. An Introduction to the Use of T-LAB]. Milan, Italy: Franco Angeli.

Lehman, C. A. (2003). Idiopathic intracranial hypertension within the ICF model: A review of the literature. *Journal of Neuroscience Nursing, 35*(5), 263–269. doi:10.1097/01376517-200310000-00004

Lenker, J. A., and Paquet, V. L. (2004). A new conceptual model for assistive technology outcomes research and practice. *Assistive Technology, 16*(1), 1–10. doi:10.1080/10400435.2004.10132069

Matte Blanco, I. (1975). *The Unconscious as Infinite Sets: An Essay in Bi-logic*. London: Gerald Duckworth & Co.

McInerney, R. G., and Walker, M. M. (2002). Toward a method of neurophenomenological assessment and intervention. *Humanistic Psychologist, 30*(3), 180–193. doi:10.1080/08873267.2002.9977034

Meloni, F., Federici, S., and Stella, A. (2011). The Psychologist's Role: A Neglected Presence in the Assistive Technology Assessment Process. In G. J. Gelderblom, M. Soede, L. Adriaens & K. Miesenberger (Eds.), *Everyday Technology for Independence and Care: AAATE 2011* (Vol. 29, pp. 1199–1206). Amsterdam, NL: IOS Press. doi:10.3233/978-1-60750-814-4-1199

Meyer, G. J., Finn, S. E., Eyde, L. D., Kay, G. G., Moreland, K. L., Dies, R., et al. (2001). Psychological testing and psychological assessment: A review of evidence and issues. *American Psychologist, 56*(2), 128–165. doi:10.1037/0003-066X.56.2.128

Mitani, S., Fujisawa, S., Mima, A., Shiota, H., Yanashima, K., Takahara, M., et al. (2007). The importance of measuring medical and psychological characteristics in visibility measurement of persons with low visual capability. In G. Eizmendi, J. M. Azkoitia, and G. Craddock (Eds.), *Challenges for Assistive Technology: AAATE 07* (pp. 331–335). Amsterdam: IOS Press.

Moscovici, S. (1961). *La Psychanalyse, son Image et Son Public* [Psychoanalysis: Its Image and Its Public]. Paris: Presses Universitaires de France.

Nair, K. P. S. (2003). Life goals: The concept and its relevance to rehabilitation. *Clinical Rehabilitation, 17*(2), 192–202. doi:10.1191/0269215503cr599oa

Neisser, U. (1989). *Concepts and Conceptual Development: Ecological and Intellectual Factors in Categorization.* Cambridge, MA: Cambridge University Press.

Nihei, M., Inoue, T., Kaneshige, Y., and Fujie, M. G. (2007). Proposition of a new mobility aid for older persons: Reducing psychological conflict associated with the use of assistive technologies. In G. Eizmendi, J. M. Azkoitia, and G. Craddock (Eds.), *Challenges for Assistive Technology: AAATE 07* (pp. 80–84). Amsterdam: IOS Press.

Olkin, R. (1999). The personal, professional and political when clients have disabilities. *Women and Therapy, 22*(2), 87–103. doi:10.1300/J015v22n02_07

Pape, T. L.-B., Kim, J., and Weiner, B. (2002). The shaping of individual meanings assigned to assistive technology: A review of personal ffactors. *Disability and Rehabilitation, 24*(1–3), 5–20. doi:10.1080/09638280110066235

Pfeiffer, D. (1998). The ICIDH and the need for its revision. *Disability and Society, 13*(4), 503–523.

Philips, B., and Zhao, H. (1993). Predictors of assistive technology abandonment. *Assistive Technology, 5*(1), 36–45. doi:10.1080/10400435.1993.10132205

Plante, T. G. (2005). *Contemporary Clinical Psychology* (2nd ed.). New York: Wiley & Sons.

Poston, J. M., and Hanson, W. E. (2010). Meta-analysis of psychological assessment as a therapeutic intervention. *Psychological Assessment, 22*(2), 203–212. doi:10.1037/A001s679

Ricœur, P. (1976). *Interpretation Theory: Discourse and the Surplus of Meaning.* Fort Worth, TX: Texas Christian Press.

Riemer-Reiss, M. L., and Wacker, R. (2000). Factors associated with assistive technology discontinuance among individuals with disabilities. *Journal of Rehabilitation, 66*(3), 44–50.

Roulstone, A. (1998). Researching a disabling society: The case of employment and new technology. In T. Shakespeare (Ed.), *The Disability Reader: Social Science Perspectives* (pp. 110–128). London: Cassell.

Scherer, M. J. (1998). *Matching Person & Technology. A Series of Assessments for Evaluating Predispositions to and Outcomes of Technology Use in Rehabilitation, Education, the Workplace & Other Settings.* Webster, NY: The Institute for Matching Person & Technology, Inc.

Scherer, M. J. (2000). *Living in the State of Stuck: How Technologies Affect the Lives of People with Disabilities* (3rd ed.). Cambridge, MA: Brookline Books.

Scherer, M. J. (Ed.). (2002). *Assistive Technology: Matching Device and Consumer for Successful Rehabilitation.* Washington, DC: American Psychological Association.

Scherer, M. J. (2005). *Cross-Walking the ICF to a Measure of Assistive Technology Predisposition and Use.* Paper presented at the 11th Annual North American Collaborating Center (NACC) Conference on the International Classification of Functioning, Disability and Health (ICF), Rochester, NY.

Scherer, M. J., Blair, K. L., Banks, M. E., Brucker, B., Corrigan, J., and Wegener, S. (2004). Rehabilitation psychology. In W. E. Craighead and C. B. Nemeroff (Eds.), *The Concise Corsini Encyclopedia of Psychology and Behavioral Science* (3rd ed., pp. 801–802). Hoboken, NJ: John Wiley & Sons.

Scherer, M. J., Craddock, G., and MacKeogh, T. (2011). The relationship of personal factors and subjective well-being to the use of assistive technology devices. *Disability and Rehabilitation, 33*(10), 811–817. doi:10.3109/09638288.2010.511418

Scherer, M. J., and Cushman, L. A. (2001). Measuring subjective quality of life following spinal cord injury: A validation study of the assistive technology device predisposition assessment. *Disability and Rehabilitation, 23*(9), 387–393. doi:10.1080/09638280010006665

Scherer, M. J., Cushman, L. A., and Federici, S. (2004, Jun 2). *Measuring Participation and the Disability Experience with the "Assistive Technology Device Predisposition Assessment."* Paper presented at the American Collaborating Center (NACC) Conference on ICF: Advancing a Research Agenda for ICF. Retrieved from http://www.icfconference.com/downloads/Marcia_Scherer.pdf.

Scherer, M. J., and Dicowden, M. A. (2008). Organizing future research and intervention efforts on the impact and effects of gender differences on disability and rehabilitation: The usefulness of the International Classification of Functioning, Disability and Health (ICF). *Disability and Rehabilitation, 30*(3), 161–165. doi:10.1080/09638280701532292

Scherer, M. J., Sax, C. L., Vanbiervliet, A., Cushman, L. A., and Scherer, J. V. (2005). Predictors of assistive technology use: The importance of personal and psychosocial factors. *Disability and Rehabilitation, 27*(21), 1321–1331. doi:10.1080/09638280500164800

Sen, A. (2002). Health: Perception versus observation. *British Medical Journal (Clinical Research Edition), 324*(7342), 860–861. doi:10.1136/bmj.324.7342.860

Söderström, S., and Ytterhus, B. (2010). The use and non-use of assistive technologies from the world of information and communication technology by visually impaired young people: A walk on the tightrope of peer inclusion. *Disability and Society, 25*(3), 303–315. doi:10.1080/09687591003701215

Steiner, W. A., Ryser, L., Huber, E., Uebelhart, D., Aeschlimann, A., and Stucki, G. (2002). Use of the ICF model as a clinical problem-solving tool in physical therapy and rehabilitation medicine. *Physical Therapy, 82*(11), 1098–1107.

Stephens, D., and Kerr, P. (2000). Auditory disablements: An update. *Audiology, 39*(6), 322–332. doi:10.3109/00206090009098013

Telfener, U. (2011). *Apprendere I Contesti. Strategie Per Inserirsi in Nuovi Ambiti Di Lavoro* [Learning the Contexts. Strategies to Fit into New Contexts of Work]. Milan, Italy: Raffaello Cortina.

Tharinger, D. J., Finn, S. E., Gentry, L., Hamilton, A., Flower, J., Matson, M., et al. (2009). Therapeutic assessment with children: A pilot study of treatment acceptability and outcome. *Journal of Personality Assessment, 91*(3), 238–244. doi:10.1080/00223890902794275

Threats, T. T. (2003). The conceptual framework of ASHA's new scope of practice for speech–language pathology. *Speech Pathology Online*. Retrieved from http://www.speechpathology.com

Threats, T. T. (2007). Access for persons with neurogenic communication disorders: Influences of personal and environmental factors of the ICF. *Aphasiology, 21*(1), 67–80. doi:10.1080/02687030600798303

Ueda, S., and Okawa, Y. (2003). The subjective dimension of functioning and disability: What is it and what is it for? *Disability and Rehabilitation, 25*(11–12), 596–601. doi:10.1080/0963828031000137108

Ugazio, V. (1989). *La Costruzione della Conoscenza: l'Approccio Europeo alla Cognizione del Sociale* [The Construction of Knowledge: The European Approach to Social Cognition]. Milan, Italy: Franco Angeli.

Uppal, S. (2006). Impact of the timing, type and severity of disability on the subjective well-being of individuals with disabilities. *Social Science and Medicine, 63*(2), 525–539. doi:10.1016/j.socscimed.2006.01.016

Verbrugge, L. M., and Jette, A. M. (1994). The disablement process. *Social Science and Medicine, 38*(1), 1–14. doi:10.1016/0277-9536(94)90294-1

Verza, R., Carvalho, M. L. L., Battaglia, M. A., and Uccelli, M. M. (2006). An interdisciplinary approach to evaluating the need for assistive technology reduces equipment abandonment. *Multiple Sclerosis, 12*(1), 88–93. doi:10.1191/1352458506ms1233oa

Viol, M., Grotkamp, S., van Treeck, B., Nuchtern, E., Hagen, T., Manegold, B., et al. (2006). Personal contextual factors, Part I—A first attempt at a systematic, commented listing of personal contextual factors for sociomedical expertise in the German-speaking region. *Gesundheitswesen, 68*(12), 747–759. doi:10.1055/s-2006-927328

Wade, D. T. (2000). Personal context as a focus for rehabilitation. *Clinical Rehabilitation, 14*(2), 115–118. doi:10.1191/026921500672636483

Waldron, D., and Layton, N. (2008). Hard and soft assistive technology: Defining roles for clinicians. *Australian Occupational Therapy Journal, 55*(1), 61–64. doi:10.1111/j.1440-1630.2007.00707.x

Weigl, M., Cieza, A., Cantista, P., Reinhardt, J. D., and Stucki, G. (2008). Determinants of disability in chronic musculoskeletal health conditions: A literature review. *European Journal of Physical and Rehabilitation Medicine, 44*(1), 67–79.

World Health Organization (WHO). (1980). *ICIDH: International Classification of Impairments, Disabilities, and Handicaps. A Manual of Classification Relating to the Consequences of Disease.* Geneva, Switzerland: WHO.

World Health Organization (WHO). (2001). *ICF: International Classification of Functioning, Disability, and Health.* Geneva, Switzerland: WHO.

World Health Organization (WHO). (2007). *ICF-CY: International Classification of Functioning, Disability, and Health—Children and Youth Version.* Geneva, Switzerland: WHO.

World Health Organization (WHO), and World Bank. (2011). *World Report on Disability.* Geneva, Switzerland: WHO.

Zimmer, Z., and Chappell, N. L. (1999). Receptivity to new technology among older adults. *Disability and Rehabilitation, 21*(5–6), 222–230. doi:10.1080/096382899297648

Zola, I. K. (1989). Toward the necessary universalizing of a disability policy. *Milbank Quarterly, 67*(Suppl. 2 Pt. 2), 401–428. doi:10.2307/3350151

Zola, I. K. (1993). Disability statistics, what we count and what it tells us: A personal and political analysis. *Journal of Disability Policy Studies, 4*(2), 9–39. doi:10.1177/104420739300400202

9

The Psychotechnologist: A New Profession in the Assistive Technology Assessment

K. Miesenberger, F. Corradi, and M. L. Mele

CONTENTS

9.1 Introduction

In 1991 the Canadian sociologist Derrick De Kerckhove coined the term "psychotechnology" to define "any technology that emulates, extends, or amplifies sensory-motor, psychological or cognitive functions of the mind" (De Kerckhove 1991b, p. 132). According to De Kerckhove, underlying this definition there is a reflection about the emerging aspects of person-technology interaction, which evolves into the constitution of electronic sensory extensions of our central nervous system and externalizes cognitive functions able to extend the human mind. In this way, any technology is an object able to externalize a property of the body and it represents the amplification and the extension of the human mind connecting to other people's cognitive processes (De Kerckhove 1990, 1991a, 2001).

According to a biopsychosocial perspective, a psychotechnology could better be defined as a "technology that emulates, extends, amplifies and *modifies* sensory-motor, psychological or cognitive functions of the mind" (Federici 2002). By borrowing what Olivetti Belardinelli (1973) claims, Federici's definition of psychotechnology affirms that intrasystemic relation is not to be considered simply as an addition of the objective component—the artifact—with the subjective components—the user—of the interaction: The object cannot be considered per se because it always falls out of the human experience. The introduction of the "modification" factor into De Kerckhove's definition of psychotechnology highlights the dynamic and mutual nature of the human-technology interaction and also allows for overcoming the current cause/effect perspective by considering human behavior as the result of the interaction between personal, environmental, and social features. As Bruner highlights (1977), the human being specializes his or her abilities by means of technologies, which allow a consequent evolution of the species. In fact, any kind of artifact can be conceived both as an amplifier transporting in itself systems of symbols organized by rules, restrictions, and knowledge possibilities and a way to guide users to a cognitive and cultural readaptation. In this way, psychotechnology has a double function: By one side, it permits the human being's adaptation to the environment-system; on the other side, it forces users to a cognitive and cultural modification and adaptation (Federici et al. 2010).

Furthermore, the modification function of psychotechnology is permitted by increasing the information conveyed by the human-technology interaction process. In fact, the interaction with an artifact enhances and enriches the information flow and modifies the knowledge stored in the long-term memory. In this light, information systems (e.g., sensory and cognitive extensions) directly take part in the working memory processes. Following this perspective, the artifact is not to be considered only as an object of which affordances emerge during the user-technology interaction (Gibson 1979), but it is also a psychotechnology that shares and modifies the features and the functions of the mind. During the interaction with psychotechnologists, the object becomes a part and an extension of the subject while he or she is interacting. In this way, psychotechnologists allow a different synthesis of the information and provide the reorganization of the relations between the elements constituting the experience.

Following this perspective the artifact becomes, at the same time, structure of knowledge and mental representation and has the function of reconfiguring and restructuring the problem by enriching and recodifying information or decreasing constraints. In other words, psychotechnology is not only a cause of the insight process—as the concept of affordance can be interpreted—but it also takes an active part in the insight process becoming a "place" of a whole synchronous perception of a meaningful *gestalt* (Koffka 1935).

Starting with this theoretical perspective, this chapter will illustrate and discuss the role of the psychotechnologist with regard to

- The analysis and the evaluation of the ***user-assistive technology*** matching, conducted by taking into account the three dynamic components of the interaction system—the person-system, the technology-system, and the socioenvironment-system—to analyze both barriers and facilitators occurring within the interaction system (WHO 2001, 2007).
- The field of assistive technologies, eAccessibility, or eInclusion, which allows for overcoming limitations and disabilities by enabling interfacing and interacting mainstream information and communication technologies (ICT)-based systems and services by using assistive (psycho)technology.

We will discuss outline the profession of the psychotechnologist by analyzing the following: (1) the psychotechnologist and the assistive technology (AT) assessment process; (2) a case example of the application of the model and measurements; (3) the AT assignation process in a center for technical aid and the psychotechnologist; and (4) an example of psychotechnology education.

9.2 The Psychotechnologist and the AT Assessment Process

The psychotechnologist is an expert in ICT, in particular in human-computer interaction (HCI) and human factors, and he or she analyzes the relations emerging from the person-technology interaction by taking into account

- All of the psychological and cognitive components which, according to De Kerckhove (1990, 1991a, 1991b), are directly involved in the technological system as a fundamental and dynamic part of it.
- The possibilities of adapting and designing eSystems and eServices in an adaptable and accessible manner (eAccessibility). eAccessibility defines the mechanisms and concepts of how eSystems and eServices, in particular at the level of HCI, have to be designed so that people with disabilities and the aging population can seamlessly interact with mainstream ICT, using the embedded adaptability and flexibility features of the general ICT/HCI, or using AT. To "interface the interface" (Crombie et al. 2004) and to access mainstream eSystems and services, both in terms of AT and eAccessibility, is a key component of the work of the psychotechnologist.

The role of the psychotechnologist is to

- Evaluate the pertinence of one or more technological aids selected for an assistive solution in a user-driven assessment process during a "setting set-up" phase arranged by a multidisciplinary team (see Section 9.4). For the evaluation of the user and technology matching, the psychotechnologist makes use of direct and participant observation methods such as Cognitive Walkthrough (Wharton et al. 1994) combined with Thinking Aloud (Lewis 1982) or integrated models

(Federici, et al. 2003, 2005, 2011; Federici and Borsci 2010) by using validated measures, such the Matching Persons and Technology assessment tools (Scherer 1998) or the Quebec User Evaluation of Satisfaction with Assistive Technology (QUEST) (Demers et al. 2000, 2002).

- Evaluate the environment if and how eAccessibility is taken into account and how to affect the redesign for accessibility using related guidelines, methodologies, tools, and laws (e.g., W3C/WAI 2011). A key role of the psychotechnologist is to influence the mainstream population to take up eAccessibility as a fundamental human right in information society.

The multidisciplinary team—along with the user—assesses the proposed AT and seeks an assistive solution in a specific context of use. During the observation, the psychotechnologist checks if the AT matches the user's needs during the evaluation trial (AT efficacy) and in prospect of the AT introduction within the end-user's environment (AT effectiveness). Moreover, the psychotechnologist supervises the reorganization of relations between user and the assigned AT solution within the interaction environment by following a biopsychosocial perspective. In this way, the psychotechnological approach allows for measuring both postural and cognitive changes resulting from the user-assistive technology matching. The psychotechnologist analyzes the components emerging from the person-technology, matching the cognitive apparatus developing through the relationship between the space and time dimensions (De Kerckhove 1990, 1995). He goes beyond the person-environment-centered adaptation and reaches out to support a general implementation of eAccessibility as a sociopolitical and economic issue.

To better understand the focus of the measurement and assessment process in which the psychotechnologist is involved, it is important to clarify the distinction between the role of the ergonomist and the role of the psychotechnologist. The cognitive ergonomist analyzes the effects arising from the user-technology interaction and the resulting mental model of the system (Halasz and Moran 1983), and he or she points out the necessary strategies to evaluate all of the responses related to an artifact or to a specific interaction contest. In particular, the ergonomist analyzes the following components of the human-technology interaction:

- The effects of technologies on health, performance, and human behavior; and
- The implementation of working settings by taking into account the related needed activities and the potential skills of final users to improve the productivity and avoid both cognitive and physical load.

In this way, the main purpose of ergonomics is to evaluate and focus each implementation and design phase on the cognitive processes (perception, attention, memory, etc.) involved in the user-technology interaction system. As Donald Norman stated (1983), ergonomics recognizes three typologies of mental models taking part in the user-technology interaction system:

1. The user's mental model,
2. The image of the system, and
3. The conceptual model of the system.

Starting from these three typologies—which are related to the person-system and the technology-system—the psychotechnologist introduces a new feature—the socioenvironment-system—by following the biopsychosocial perspective (Figure 9.1). In this way, the psychotechnologist aims to analyze both barriers and facilitators occurring within the interaction system to obtain the best combination among all of its components (WHO 2001, 2007).

According to the International Classification of Functioning, Disability, and Health (ICF) perspective, it is important to follow a systemic approach in which aid becomes a part of a complex system composed of the user and his or her caregivers in a specific environment to allow him or her better autonomy (Scherer 2005). In this way, the psychotechnologist overcomes the ergonomic approach, which analyzes only the user system-technology system interaction, by also taking into account the user's needs to evaluate the related goals contextualized within the user's environment and his or her reached autonomy degree.

By following an integrated or intrasystemic model (Federici et al. 2005, 2011; Federici and Borsci 2010), the psychotechnologist investigates the three person, aid, and environment dimensions as a whole and complex system in which object (system) and subject (user) are a part of a composite and dynamic empirical observation process within a specific environment. For this reason, the evaluation process of the system is based on a combination of top-down and bottom-up evaluation methodologies (Federici et al. 2005). The top-down methodologies are used to verify the accordance of the specific environment to standard rules and guidelines, e.g., the specifications suggested by the International Standard Organization (ISO) and the World Wide Web Consortium (W3C, WAI). These kinds of methodologies could mainly be applied to the evaluation process to identify the accessibility parameters of the related interface. On the other hand, the bottom-up methodologies are used to evaluate the way in which the final user interacts with the interface in the specific environment of use. The evaluations are conducted by observing the user's behavior and giving psychometric analytic trials. These kinds of methodologies are mainly addressed to observe the user's behavior while interacting with the interface and measure satisfaction levels. In this way, the bottom-up methodologies measure the usability levels of a user-technology-behavior system.

That being so, the psychotechnologist's role is to investigate and verify the dynamic and complex user-technology-behaviour system by integrating top-down and bottom-up methods to highlight the empowerment offered to the user by the assistive solution (Federici et al. 2003, 2005, 2011; Federici and Borsci 2010).

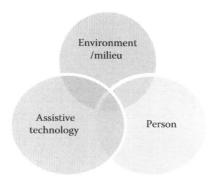

FIGURE 9.1
The interaction system according to the biopsychosocial model.

9.3 Case Example: Application of Models and Measurements

This section describes the application of the assessment process to a case example shared by the authors of Sections II and III of this handbook. Taking as example the case of S.A. (Table 9.1), the psychotechnologist will investigate whether the environmental expectations (family, health, and educational operators) meet the actual user's possibilities to use the AT to communicate; moreover, the psychotechnologist will also analyze all of the related clinician material, and once he or she individualizes the real user's needs, he or she will seek the appropriate assistive solution in cooperation with the entire multidisciplinary team by using different tools (e.g., the Vineland scale). During the checking trials of the

TABLE 9.1

Medical Case of S.A.

Name: S. A.

Age: 37.6 years

Beginning of disease: 35.4 years

Diagnosis: ICD-10-CM: I69 Sequelae of cerebrovascular disease // ICD-9-CM: 438 Late effects of cerebrovascular disease

ICF at arrival:

B110 – 0	S110 – 9	D110 – 0.2	E110 - + 4
B114 – 0	S730 – 4	D140 – 0.0	E115 - + 4
B117 – 0	S750 – 4	D145 – 0.0	E120 - + 4
B144 – 0		D150 – 0.0	E310 - + 4
B210 – 2		D315 – 0.0	E355 - + 2
B710 – 4		D330 – 4.4	E410 - + 4
B765 – 4		D335 – 1.1	E455 - + 2
B310 – 0		D350 – 0.3	
		D430 – 4.4	
		D510 – 4.4	

Barthel index

Nourishment: 0

Bath/shower (to wash himself): 0

Personal care: 0

Dressing: 0

Intestine continence: 2

Urinary continence: 8

Use of toilet: 0

Transfer bed ←→ wheelchair 8

Deambulation: 0

Stairs: 0

Use of the wheelchair: 5

Total scores: 25

SPMSQ

Mistakes total scores: 1

S.V.A.M.A.

Language (comprehension): 3

Language (production): 1

Hearing: 3 (no hearing aid)

Sight: 1 (no use of spectacles and contact lenses)

matching process, the psychotechnologist will lead the team by monitoring critical issues, strengths, and possible problems.

9.3.1 Medical Case

At the age of 35 years and four months, apparently without any relevant symptoms, Mr. S.A. was struck by a bulb-pons intraparenchymal cerebral hemorrhage with a consequent comatose state. The computed tomography (CT) scan, conducted on the same day, emphasized the presence of a "voluminous intraparenchymal hematoma next to the bulb-pons with tetra-ventricular hemorrhage." The following day the patient underwent a neurosurgical operation. The coma lasted for approximately three months, during which a trachea-stomachic cannula (removed at the age of 37 years) and percutaneous endoscopic gastrostomy (PEG) tube (still present) was positioned.

The patient currently presents with marked dysarthria, serious dysphagia (he can only be nourished through PEG), sialorrhoea, and open bite. Eye motility is possible only in bilateral lagophthalmos vertical look. A noticeable lowering of the hearing standard is present in the left ear.

9.3.1.1 Motor Evaluation

The subject presents hypotonic tetraparesis with serious control deficit of the pelvis, trunk, and head. He cannot autonomously maintain a sitting position because of marked kyphosis of the trunk, retroverted pelvis, head noticeably placed before the scapular cingulum, and lower limbs positioned in extra rotation. The right upper limb presents a residual mobility at the proximal level, but no functional activity is possible because of serious movement hindrance. The left upper limb presents both residual proximal mobility and sufficient movement capability. The patient is able to index, but there is serious dysmetria: With this limb the patient can reach his face to clean the mouth; he can beat, grasp, pull, and press; and the left hand is used to produce an alphabetic gestural code by using the thumb and the index and middle fingers.

The lower limbs are used to cooperate during the transfers (e.g., from wheelchair to bed) by using the right leg as a pivot. On request, the patient is able to move the head in any direction but through very laborious and extremely difficult movements. The transfers can be realized either through a hand-pushed wheelchair or an electric wheelchair, which can be driven by a joystick handled by the left hand. S.A. is enlisted in an physiokinesitherapy rehabilitation program, which aims to improve control of the trunk, head, and pelvis by reducing as much as possible the kyphosis and the dysmetria. The patient is also undergoing phoniatric and respiratory therapy.

9.3.1.2 Neuropsychological Test

The neuropsychological test was performed one year and nine months after the lesion. Because of the marked motor and communicative limitations, a standardized evaluation and most verbal and nonverbal tests could not be done. A rough evaluation of verbal memory capabilities was made through a codified alphabetic code. Notwithstanding the unfavorable conditions, in a prose memory test S.A. showed good capabilities of storing the material in the short term, and he was able to recall it without substantial loss information. Logical-deductive reasoning capabilities, which were evaluated by means of nonverbal material, are perfectly preserved. Finally, an overview of the analyses made through the tests, conversation, and medical observations shows no large deficits in upper cognitive functions. In any case, the patient was enlisted in cognitive therapy to improve and generalize his own communicative strategies.

9.3.1.3 Communication Strategy

At the moment the patient uses, with the help of his brother, a codified gestural alphabet that is very difficult to understand by other people. Through an alphabetic paper chart, he can compose words by pointing at the letters, but in an extremely slow and difficult way because of his serious dysmetria.

9.3.1.4 Evaluation of Visual, Perceptive, and Motor Functions

The patient can evaluate after having bandaged his right eye (RE) to counterbalance diplopia and without wearing the glasses prescribed for a slight myopia and astigmatism. There is a vertical nystagmus movement more evident in the RE at the beginning of the evaluation that successively also appeared in the left eye (LE). The patient can only follow horizontal movements by completely moving his head, but he can more easily follow vertical movements without needing to move the head too much. A least eye movement can be observed in the direction of the nasal region. There is no great difference between the RE and LE. The monocular sight evaluation was 1/10 for the RE and 3/10 for the LE both at a distance and from a proximal point. However, we recommend not using characters smaller than 5 mm. There is a slow convergence movement. It is not possible to elicit efficient saccadic movements, although in this case the patient can compensate for them with his head movements. The patient can correctly scan stimuli adequately segregated in a target. The peripheral awareness of stimuli is normal.

9.3.1.5 Aids and Assistance

At the moment, Mr. S.A. has neither aids nor assistance to communicate. In the past he was able to learn how to use a computer and acquired a good knowledge of its main functions. He still uses the computer to browse on the Internet, although he needs help. He has never used either a videogame or multimedia instruments (such as an encyclopedia on a CD).

9.3.1.6 Request

Communication assistance and access to a computer (Macintosh) have been requested. The request concerning the computer is specified as follows: "use of keyboard and mouse and facility to visualize the contents of a monitor" to allow the patient to read, write, and manage the Internet and his e-mail.

9.3.2 The ATA Process

The psychotechnologist acts in the following six steps.

9.3.2.1 Multidisciplinary Team Meeting

- User data valuation
- Setting design

In this step, the psychotechnologist analyzes all of the related clinician material (user data) and through instruments such as Matching Person and Technology model he or she set the framework assessment agreement together with the multidisciplinary team by highlighting any environmental, personal, and technological issues. In agreement with the multidisciplinary team, the psychotechnologist analyzes the medical case of S.A. by detecting the individual predisposition to the assistive solutions by considering his previous experiences with AT, the current motivation to use an AT, and all of those environmental factors that may affect the matching process [SOTU and ATD-PA of the Matching Persons and Technology tests by Scherer (1998)]. More specifically, the psychotechnologist

- Checks if the social environment will support the solution ("His brother can help him?");
- Checks the equipment that will be part of tests during the assessment to select some ATs, such as keyboard supports, mouse emulators (based on motor detection), and communication software (e.g., a word prediction program); and
- Selects a hand-held communicator designed for wheelchair use.

9.3.2.2 Setting Set-Up

In this step, the psychotechnologist prepares the setting and checks that all of the selected technologies are correctly working. In the case of S.A., the psychotechnologist tests different types of keyboards targeted for him, e.g., keyguards (i.e., a shield with holes over the keys) or mouse emulators (such a switch-based system) compatible with Macintosh systems along with a word prediction software (i.e., a portable alphabetical QWERTY communicator with at least one shield).

9.3.2.3 Matching Process

- Assistive solution proposal
- Assistive solution user trial
- Assistive solution outcome

Together with the occupational therapist, the psychotechnologist directly offers S.A. the previously tested technologies by explaining their functioning and features. Then, supported by the occupational therapist, S.A. tests the proposed assistive solutions while the psychotechnologist supervises his interaction by collecting any critical situation to subsequently apply the better solutions to optimize the AT use. If it is possible, any customization and/or configuration of the tested instruments will be applied by following the results of any trial performed by S.A. through the use of a direct and participant observation methods, such as the Cognitive Walkthrough (Wharton et al. 1994) combined with Thinking Aloud (Lewis, 1982) or integrated models of evaluation (Federici et al. 2005; Federici and Borsci 2010) such the Matching Persons and Technology tools (Scherer 1998).

9.3.2.4 Assistive Solution Multidisciplinary Team Evaluation

In this phase, the psychotechnologist discusses the observations made during the interaction of S.A. with the ATs with the multidisciplinary team, highlighting the strengths and weaknesses. The team decides whether tests are altogether satisfactory or not and

.communicates the results of the whole session to S.A., showing him the potential and the limits of the proposed solutions.

9.3.2.5 User Support

After the evaluation process, the psychotechnologist meets S.A. and his brother to inform them about the potential and limits of any proposed technology and to collect information about any issues raised during the use of the given AT solutions.

9.3.2.6 Follow-Up

The psychotechnologist periodically gets through to S.A. to ask him information about his experience of use with the solution and his needs by using tools such as QUEST (Demers et al. 2000, 2002). If necessary, the psychotechnologist asks S.A. to return to the center for technical aids to perform a new evaluation process.

9.4 The AT Assignation Process in a Center for Technical Aid and the Psychotechnologist

The following two flow charts show the phases within the assistive technology assessment (ATA) process in which the psychotechnologist is involved. As is shown in Figure 9.2, the psychotechnologies specialist plays a role within the user-driven processes by working in concert with the occupational therapist, the architect, and the engineer.

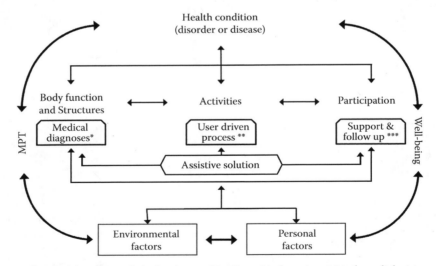

*   the physician, the psychologist, the cognitive therapist, the optometrist, the audiologist, the pediatric specialist, the geriatrician

**   the psychotechnologist, the occupational therapist, the architect, the engineer

*** the therapist, the special educator, the occupational therapist, the psychologist, the consumer support, speech language pathologist, the physiotherapist

FIGURE 9.2
The Assistive Technology Assessment process under the lens of the ICF biopsychosocial model.

In Figure 9.3, a brown button sign shows the phases of participation for the psychotechnologist intervention.

The psychotechnologist, along with the multidisciplinary team, evaluates the data and user's request.

- If the data provided by the user are not sufficient for a "matching process," the user is requested to convey more information and the process returns to "user data collection."

- If the data provided by the user are sufficient for a "matching process," the psychotechnologist, in accordance with the multidisciplinary team, proceeds by setting and scheduling an appointment for a meeting with the user.

The psychotechnologist, because his or her principal skill is technological and psychological competency, receives from the multidisciplinary team the commitment to arrange a suitable setting for the matching assessment. Then, the multidisciplinary team, along with the user, assesses the assistive solution proposed, tries the solution, and gathers outcome data.

The psychotechnologist, according to the multidisciplinary team, evaluates the outcome of the matching assessment.

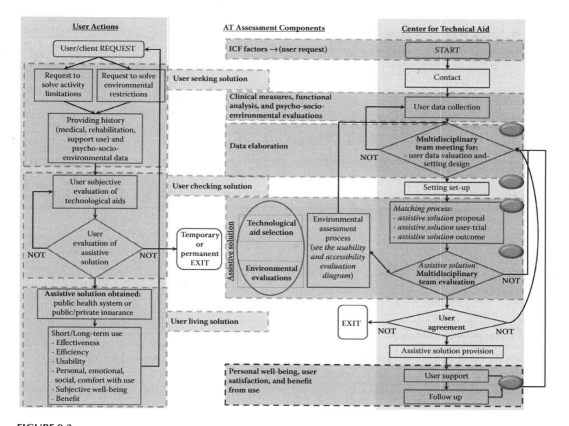

FIGURE 9.3
The Assistive Technology Assessment process flow chart. Button signs show the phases of participation for the psychotechnologist intervention.

- If successful, the team proposes an assistive solution to the user and schedules a new appointment.
- If not successful, the team restarts the "matching process."

When the assistive solution proposed requires an environmental evaluation, the team initiates the environmental assessment process and orients toward possibilities of influencing the mainstream to respect eAccessibility requirements.

9.5 Psychotechnology Education: An Example

The concept of disability is basically integrated into the psychotechnological framework. Disabilities or functional limitations are preconditions that enter into the profile of adaptive systems or services with widened system boundaries. Nevertheless, it has to be underlined that psychotechnology for the user group of people with disabilities is of much higher importance for allowing access to and interaction with the mainstream population by overcoming functional limitations. Presenting efficient or fancy alternatives for the average person, people with disabilities using ICT and AT often gain their first independent access to and participation in systems and services and thereby to the mainstream population.

For people with disabilities, psychotechnology offers new possibilities for overcoming sensory-motor limitations and pushes adaptation or "normalization" to a new level that is known today as (e)Inclusion. Most important, the general ICT forces societal contexts to change by making them modifiable, adaptable, and more fluent. This ICT revolution leads to a process of ongoing adaptations of societal contexts to better meet the requirements of users. This fundamentally changes the understanding of disability because it can no longer be defined as a pure individual phenomenon defined by sensor-motor-cognitive conditions against a fixed environmental context, but much more as a social phenomenon defined by the environmental settings and designs allowing, supporting, or hindering interaction and participation. It is no longer only asking how to best match an individual with AT into an environment; it is more and more how to design and adapt the environment to best match the needs of users with a widened diversity of skills and requirements (Miesenberger 1998, 2004, 2009a). From an individual/medical over an environmental model, we reach a social model of disability (Gustavsson and Zakrzewska-Manterys 1997). The plasticity of ICT includes the demand toward the mainstream population to respect the needs and requirements of AT users—eAccessibility—into the assessment and matching process and complements the scope of tasks of the psychotechnologist.

9.5.1 The Context of the Profession "Psychotechnologist"

A psychotechnologist is a person/profession who fixes persons with technology to become social and interactive with the mainstream population. Usability and sometimes accessibility experts call themselves a "psychotechnologist" (http://restrictionisexpression.com/post/43184264/am-i-a-psychotechnologist-now). In the context of AT, this outlines the "intentional" character of the profession. The psychotechnologist supports inclusion and participation in established contexts by providing access to mainstream systems and services. eAccessibility and eInclusion are two-folded: AT should enable people with disabilities to interact with mainstream systems and services. As outlined above, AT permits a human being's adaptation to the environment-system and also asks users to a cognitive and cultural modification and adaptation (Federici et al. 2010).

Further on, eAccessibility asks for a general societal adaptation and for respecting and implementing the mentioned accessibility standards to allow AT-powered interaction with mainstream systems and services as a prerequisite for participation (Darzentas and Miesenberger 2005; Miesenberger, 2009a, 2009b). This brings a wide and complex scope to the psychotechnologist because it is not only the user and their personal technological framework which is at discussion; with eAccessibility, ICT in general is addressed. The technological infrastructure, developments, and changes affect our communities and thereby the possibility and quality of participation. Because of the accepted need to overcome the traditional separation and exclusion of people with disabilities, a more intense interaction and communication with mainstream processes is a key objective.

This of course expands the number of potential contexts and in particular the complexity of changing external opinions, procedures, and processes to suit the needs of AT federated participation. AT users live and act in diverse contexts, and most of the time they address inclusion in mainstream contexts; therefore, AT assessment and the psychotechnologists inherit an according complexity from both the "internal," person-centered AT and the "external," eAccessibility context. "Making AT social" in this wide contextual sense is the core challenge of AT psychotechnologists.

9.5.2 Psychotechnologist—The Need for Education

This multilevel complexity underlines the need for a broad set of skills and qualifications. Analyzing and watching the state of the art (Matausch et al. 2006; Miesenberger, 2006; Miesenberger et al. 2010) showed that by far no appropriate training and qualification programs are available. Traditional professions such as ergotherapists, rehabilitation specialists, or special/inclusive teachers are still very reluctant to take AT (in particular ICT-related AT, which is a key enabler for inclusion today) and eAccessibility on board. Education is more or less still oriented toward an "internal" context of a medical, therapeutical, special educational, or technological approach. The ICT, AT, eAccessibility, and "Design for All" revolution seems not to have touched ground with traditional disciplines and the according education.

On the other hand, the last few years are characterized by a constantly growth of awareness toward aging and disability, also leading to the associated legal framework demand for eAccessibility and eParticipation (W3C/WAI 2006). Demographic developments clearly show an increase in older adults and people with disabilities in general (Lifetool 2004). Several economic sectors already reacted to these developments by starting to produce apparatuses especially for older adult people that respect and follow the concepts of eAccessibility and Design for All. Not only are technical apparatuses for a convenient life of interest for older adults, but so too are support systems to gain independence through life because this population group is more likely to be affected by a disability. Surveys show that older adult people aim for autonomy in their lives. People with disabilities and older adults are able to gain greater control over their own life through the use of ATs. ATs allow for participation and more contribution to activities at home, school, work, leisure time, or other communities.

The current educational offer in the field is inconsistent. Expertise is developed through both learning –by doing and single seminars. Different enterprises that work in the field of ATs offer seminars, each lasting at most a couple of days. Another offering was SART (1999), a summer academy on rehabilitation technologies, which took place in 1999. Beyond the local context at the European and international level there is still a lack of appropriate possibilities. The TELEMATE (TeleMate 2011) network, online lectures in Italian language (SIVA 2011), and CSUN's AT Training Programme (CSUN 2011) are some of the few examples that take AT, eAccessibility, and this complex matching process into account, at least in part. All of this motivated work toward a more holistic and comprehensive course for experts (psychotechnologists) in this field (Matausch et al. 2006; Miesenberger 2006; Miesenberger et al. 2010).

The need for education is rising, expressed first as a need for "training on the job" that experts can cope with eAccessibility. Step by step this should lead to an increasing demand for more comprehensive and formal educational settings. To satisfy the growing demand, more and well-educated experts in AT and eAccessibility will be necessary. To make full use of the potential of AT and eAccessibility, it is again not only the technological background that matters; it is the whole context that the psychotechnologist must take into account and manage that defines the frame of skills and competencies required. This gap between a growing need for professionals and the lack of education motivated work toward a new academic course aimed at providing a holistic curriculum for the profession we call here "psychotechnology," which is aimed at matching people with AT to make systems and service social and inclusive. The Assistec program aims at decreasing the gap between the growing need for and lack of education by creating experts able to manage this complex, multidimensional process of eAccessibility and eInclusion.

9.5.3 The Assistec Program

In the following, we will outline the set-up of the university course (Matausch et al. 2006; Miesenberger 2006; Miesenberger et al. 2010). The duration of the university course encompasses four terms. The first course started in the winter term 2006 and the course language is German. The Assistec course is offered as an online eLearning application with a certain amount of mandatory attendance hours. The course can be referred to as in-service training. Intentions for this kind of realization are a high temporal and regional flexibility for participants, especially for employees. However, it also supports lecturers because they save time and it was easier to involve experts from different regions. The course graduates will be awarded an academic degree entitled "Expert on Assistive Technologies."

The university course aims to educate people from different vocational and academic backgrounds in the outlined complexity of AT provision and eAccessibility. Graduates will be experts in the area of AT, especially concerning assortment of appropriate AT, usability of AT, environmental and social contexts, funding, application, adaptation, management and service, and counselling. Practical experiences show that these professionals also have a strong need, in addition to technical and personal skills, for expertise in demand analysis, environmental and social analyses, finances, funding, and more. Moreover, the course stresses concentrated and goal-oriented transfer of knowledge according to the up-to-date state of the art in a multidisciplinary environment. One major feature and goal is that the course substantially emphasizes practical training and application of the theoretically gained knowledge. Another major intention is to enhance quality in the practical treatment regarding the profession fields of health care and support and services of people with disabilities. In addition, the implementation of the university course aims to improve and foster product development of ATs.

The course is intentionally appealing to people from different vocational and educational backgrounds. Therefore, the target groups addressed by the university course are multifaceted and could be summarized as follows:

- *Vocational field of rehabilitation, therapy, and welfare:* Within this vocational field, the course especially addresses people employed in the field of "people with disabilities" and "integration of people with disabilities" dealing with counselling, care, support, service, and accompaniment of people with disabilities.
- *Vocational field of health care:* People who are working in the fields of rehabilitation, nursing, and care and support of people with disabilities and older adult people are approached in particular.
- *Vocational field of education:* Within this target group, we appeal to teachers of standard schools and adult education as well as special school teachers and pedagogues dealing with children with disabilities.
- *Vocational field of AT:* Especially addressed are people who are engaged in the areas of production, distribution and trading, maintenance, training, and research and development of AT.
- *(Emerging) vocational field of eAccessibility and Design for All:* In particular, the course addresses the still small but growing number of people focusing on eAccessibility and Design for All in their job, be it in mainstream (e.g., software/web developers) or specialized fields such as the AT industry of service provision for people with disabilities.

To be in accordance with the idea of equal access to education, Assistec encourages in particular people with disabilities to participate. Being disabled and having experiences in this context is seen as a benefit. Entering into the field of Assistive Technology Service provision is also seen as a contribution too enhance the vocational chances of people with disabilities in the open labor market and the course wants to support this.

9.5.4 The Curriculum

The university course's curriculum consists of four modules. Each of the modules is composed of single seminars. As a whole, the university course comprises four modules and a total of 17 seminars. Figure 9.4 outlines the university course's contents.

Module one focuses on imparting fundamental knowledge concerning medicine, physiology, psychology, and classification of disability; legal foundations regarding disability and funding facilities; ATs; and Design for All and eAccessibility. As the module's name already implies, the contents constitute fundamentals for the course as a whole and especially for the following subject.

The teaching contents of module two emphasize the special knowledge of ATs, including practical training units regarding AT products and their application. Therefore, this module disposes of a central position in the whole curriculum. This also includes the referral of AT to eAccessibility and the requirements of mainstream systems and services to allow AT-facilitated interaction and participation.

Module two allows students to specialize in AT for a specific target group, including a first phase for working on concrete practical examples. Module three deals with the management and realization of the process of assortment and provision of ATs, and a goal could be described as "to educate counsellors and process/case managers." Hence, pivotal issues are needs

```
                                                            Contents of "Assistec"

   module 1: Fundamentals
      eLearning
      Medical and physiological fundamentals
      Legislative framework and funding
      Design for all
      Fundamentals AT & Reha-Technology

   module 2: Assistlve technologies special knowledge
      Aids for specific learning difficulties
      Aids for hearing impaired
      Aids for vision impaired
      Mobility aids
      Augmentative or alternative communication
      ATs in different areas (work, home, education, leisure time)
      Practical experience

   module 3: Process of assortment and provision of AT & leT
      Assessment and demand analysis
      Environment analysis in technical area, sociological area, economical area
      AT-management and mediation

   module 4: Assistive technologies in practice and application
      Practical course and thesis
      Research in the field of AT and future developments
```

FIGURE 9.4
Contents of the university course "Assistec." The mentioned components accord to the contents and do not exactly reflect the whole seminar title.

assessment; analysis of the environment of people with disabilities in respect of technical, sociological, and economical areas; and mediation. It is this module treating with the outlined complexity of the field of psychotechnology in its technological, medical, and psychological aspects in diverse social, political, and other environmental contexts. A particular emphasis, as outlined, is given on how to cooperate with and influence the mainstream population with respect to the eAccessibility needs of AT users.

During the fourth module, participants must undergo practical experience by managing and documenting a process of assortment and provision of AT by means of composing a scientific thesis. This kind of work placement/secondment can also be completed while holding down a job because the whole university course is organized as an in-service training. On the basis of an understanding of AT provision taking into account both the user and the environment, a special emphasis is given to the practical problems of covering the whole complexity of AT provision.

This shows that the developed curriculum is a composition of different professional subjects and contents of teaching taking the complex nature of AT provision, as outlined in Chapter 4, into account. The range of subjects highlighted covers medical, legal, technical, economical, management, sociological, and psychological aspects. In addition, crucial elements of the course are the cooperation and networking with enterprises in the field of AT as well as dealing with eAccessibility as a mainstream requirement.

9.5.5 eLearning System

The design of the course is characterized by a blended learning system, which "combines face-to-face instruction with computer-mediated instruction" (Bonk and Graham 2006).

According to this definition, blended learning is used regarding the university course Assistec as a combination of online learning and presence learning elements.

Because the university course should be equally open for all people, regardless of a possible disability, the issue of accessibility must be raised. Because a fully accessible system is not to be found in the market, the idea occurred to adapt an already existing eLearning system. An open source course management system (CMS) called "Moodle" (2011) was chosen because of its good results according to a first accessibility evaluation following the Web Content Accessibility Guidelines published by the Web Accessibility Initiative (Chisholm et al. 1999). The used eLearning system has been evaluated several times by people with specific needs. Nevertheless, the fact is that the evaluation and the gathered experiences using and testing this system still show deficits concerning full accessibility. Great attempts are being undertaken to achieve a fully accessible version until the start of the course. The eLearning system acts both as a communication platform and a platform in which all study materials are available in accessible formats.

Although the eLearning system Moodle plays a crucial role within the blended learning settlement, the phases of personal attendance are also of great significance. Mandatory presence is planned for an average of three times per term with a duration of two days. The phases of presence are used to initiate social contacts and formation of groups as well as to demonstrate and present practical and theoretical contents.

Overall, the blended learning settlement enables a high level of regional and temporal flexibility for the participants, and this is especially beneficial for people with disabilities with respect to access to the course itself and mobility issues.

9.5.6 Graduates—Psychotechnologists

The qualification profile of the graduates is characterized by the following features:

- Graduates gain comprehensive and scientific specialist knowledge in the area of ATs and eAccessibility and their application in diverse and complex societal settings.
- Graduates have the ability to provide people with disabilities and older adults with adequate ATs and to support them through the process of assortment and provision of AT, taking the diverse environmental settings into account.
- Graduates gain skills and competencies in implementing eAccessibility and mediating the process of changing design and development processes toward eAccessibility. They have profound knowledge in related guidelines, laws, evaluation, repair, design, and development methods and tools.
- Graduates are qualified to perform self-contained organization, coordination, management, and handling of the whole process of assortment and provision of ATs.
- Graduates open up of a new field of the profession because of their interdisciplinary knowledge concerning the social, technical, medical, and rehabilitation areas.
- Graduates are highly aware of the societal context of disability, aging, and AT.
- Graduates have knowledge regarding the legislative framework and funding possibilities with respect to the issue of disability associated with AT.
- Graduates have an increased sensibility and social competence in interacting and dealing with people using ATs.
- Graduates acquire a verifiable degree.

Keeping in mind this profile of qualifications, the graduates of Assistec gain during their education the vocational title of psychotechnologist or "Expert on Assistive Technologies," which can be specified by some criteria. First of all, they are the one central contact person for clients and users of ATs. Having one main contact person arranging all aspects of the assortment and provision of AT is a crucial advantage for people provided with AT. The experts are independent counsellors who are not sales-oriented but do have a detailed overview of the whole range of AT products and choose the most adequate device for the clients. Furthermore, AT experts are process managers; that is to say that they are empowered to organize and coordinate the provision process of AT, taking into account juridical, medical, psychological, technical, economical, and sociological aspects. Obviously not experts in all domains, they are able to make available the resources and expertise needed for individual provision. Because of this, they have leadership and management skills. Moreover, they are a representative of the user group of AT as well as of the economy, referring to AT organizations producing and distributing AT. In addition, these experts act as multipliers in their vocational field because they fulfil the task of awareness raising and sensitization for eAccessibility and eInclusion. Finally, a significant aspect of the expert's vocational field is the use of mediation and conflict management skills if conflicts and difficulties emerge during the process of assortment and provision of AT. Figure 9.5 summarizes the influence and impact of the developed Assitec university course and its graduates on wider society.

9.5.7 Impact

Assistec is seen as an example of education for the emerging field of psychotechnology in the AT and eAccessibility domain. The course is a contribution toward current efforts on the eInclusion of people with disabilities by reducing the gap between the growing need and the lack of offers in education. Graduates have competencies to manage a process of assortment and provision in complex and diverse settings from the very beginning through required trainings and maintenance relating to all categories of ATs. They orient toward eAccessibility and its application in mainstream eSystems and eServices. This should help to improve the quality of service provision for people with disabilities and

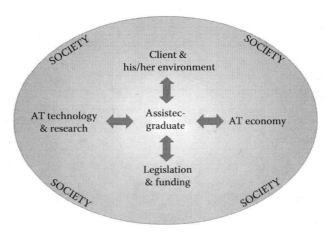

FIGURE 9.5
Fields of expertise of Assistec graduates.

eAccessibility implementation in the mainstream. This should also allow for incentives to product development because of an intensive communication between clients and psychotechnologists.

9.6 Conclusions

In this chapter we introduced the meaning and background of psychotechnology, and we explained the role of the psychotechnologist within the matching people with disabilities and AT process. In particular, we described some applicative examples in different contexts, from the traditional context, focused on the interaction between persons with disabilities and ATs within their everyday life environments, to the ICT context, in which eAccessibility is a fundamental requirement to allow for participation, independence, and inclusion of people with disabilities. Starting from a theoretical background, we described the evolution of the meaning of psychotechnology, "a technology that emulates, extends, amplifies and *modifies* sensory-motor, psychological or cognitive functions of the mind" (Federici 2002). The interaction between user and technology is a dynamic intrasystemic relationship in which the artifact has the role of amplifier, transporting rules and knowledge possibilities and permitting both the adaptation to the system and a cognitive and cultural modification (Federici and Borsci 2010). In this light, we have shown the role of the psychotechnologist by focusing on two different fields of application: the AT assignation process in a center for technical aid and the psychotechnologist education field, concerning ICT-based systems and services.

The role of the psychotechnologist is to investigate the psychological and cognitive components involved into the interaction environment—be it either a physical environment or a ICT environment—by analyzing and evaluating the following issues: (1) the pertinence of one or more technological aids selected for an assistive solution in a user-driven assessment process by means of different tools such as, for example, the Matching Persons and Technology model (Scherer 1998); and (2) if and how eAccessibility is considered in an ICT environment and how to affect the redesign for accessibility using related guidelines, methodologies, tools, and laws (e.g., W3C/WAI 2011). To better explain the role of the psychotechnologist, we have shown two case examples. First, we described the role of the psychotechnologist within the assessment process by showing as a case example the case of S.A., shared with Sections II and III of this handbook. We then focused on an example of an educational project, the Assistec program, which aims at lowering the gap between the growing need for and lack of education by forming experts able to manage this complex, multidimensional process of eAccessibility and eInclusion.

Summary of the Chapter

This chapter focuses on explaining the concept behind the term "psychotechnology" and the role of the "psychotechnologist" within the matching people and AT process. According to a biopsychosocial perspective, a psychotechnology is defined as any "technology that emulates, extends, amplifies and modifies sensory-motor, psychological or cognitive functions of the mind" (Federici 2002), highlighting in this way the intrasystemic relation between the artifact and the user. Starting from these suggestions, the primary role of psychotechnologist is to follow a systemic approach to allow users a better autonomy (TeleMate 2011). This goal is only possible by taking into account the users' needs, their reached autonomy degree, and the environment in which they live. In this work, we have explained in more detail two fields of application of this new professional figure: the AT assignation process in a center for technical aid and the ICT-based systems and services, i.e., *e*Systems and *e*Services.

References

Bonk, C. J., and Graham, C. R. (2006). *The Handbook of Blended Learning: Global Perspectives, Local Designs*. San Francisco: Pfeiffer.

Bruner, J. S. (1977). *The Process of Education: A Landmark in Educational Theory*. Cambridge, MA: Harvard University Press.

Chisholm, W., Vanderheiden, G., and Jacobs, I. (1999). Web Content Accessibility Guidelines 1.0—W3C Recommendation. Retrieved from http://www.w3.org/TR/WAI-WEBCONTENT/

Crombie, D., Lenoir, R., McKenzie, N., and Miesenberger, K. (2004). Interfacing the interface: Unification through separation. In C. Stary and C. Stephanidis (Eds.), *User-Centered Interaction Paradigms for Universal Access in the Information Society* (Vol. 3196, pp. 125–132). Berlin: Springer. doi:10.1007/978-3-540-30111-0_10

CSUN. (2011). AT training program. Retrieved from http://www.csun.edu/cod/training/index.php

Darzentas, J., and Miesenberger, K. (2005). Design for all in information technology: A universal concern. In K. V. Andersen, J. Debenham, and R. Wagner (Eds.), *Database and Expert Systems Applications* (Vol. 3588, pp. 406–420). Berlin: Springer. doi:10.1007/11546924_40

De Kerckhove, D. (1990). *La Civilisation Vidéo-Crétienne*. Paris: Retz/Atelier Alpha Blue.

De Kerckhove, D. (1991a). *Brainframes. Technology, Mind and Business*. Utrecht, The Netherlands: Bosch & Keuning.

De Kerckhove, D. (1991b). Communication arts for a new spatial sensibility. *Leonardo, 24*(2), 131–135. doi:10.2307/1575281

De Kerckhove, D. (1995). *The Skin of Culture: Investigating the New Electronic Reality*. Toronto, Canada: Somerville.

De Kerckhove, D. (2001). *The Architecture of Intelligence*. Berlin: Birkhäuser.

Demers, L., Weiss-Lambrou, R., and Ska, B. (2000). Item analysis of the Quebec User Evaluation of Satisfaction with Assistive Technology (QUEST). *Assistive Technology, 12*(2), 96–105. doi:10.1080/10400435.2000.10132015

Demers, L., Weiss-Lambrou, R., and Ska, B. (2002). The Quebec User Evaluation of Satisfaction with Assistive Technology (QUEST 2.0): An Overview and Recent Progress. *Technology and Disability, 14*(3), 101–105. Retrieved from http://iospress.metapress.com/content/b23egtty2mph84b0/

Federici, S. (2002). *Linee-Guida di Psicotecnologie [Guidelines on Psychotechnology]*. Graduate course on Psychotechnology for learning. Department of Psychology. Sapienza University of Rome. Rome, Italy. Retrieved from http://www.psicologia1.uniroma1.it/cgilocal/didattica.cgi?FileManager = 60

Federici, S., Corradi, F., Mele, M. L., and Miesenberger, K. (2011). *From cognitive ergonomist to psychotechnologist: A new professional profile in a multidisciplinary team in a centre for technical aids*. In G. J. Gelderblom, M. Soede, L. Adriaens and K. Miesenberger (Eds.), Everyday Technology for Independence and Care: AAATE 2011 (Vol. 29, pp. 1178–1184). Amsterdam, NL: IOS Press. doi:10.3233/978-1-60750-814-4-1178

Federici, S., and Borsci, S. (2010). Usability evaluation: models, methods, and applications. In J. Stone and M. Blouin (Eds.), *International Encyclopedia of Rehabilitation*. Buffalo, NY: Center for International Rehabilitation Research Information and Exchange (CIRRIE). Retrieved from http://cirrie.buffalo.edu/encyclopedia/article.php?id = 277&language = en

Federici, S., Borsci, S., Mele, M. L., and Stamerra, G. (2010). Web Popularity: An Illusory Perception of a Qualitative Order in Information. *Universal Access in the Information Society, 9*(4), 375–386. doi:10.1007/s10209-009-0179-7

Federici, S., Micangeli, A., Ruspantini, I., Borgianni, S., Corradi, F., Pasqualotto, E., et al. (2005). Checking an integrated model of web accessibility and usability evaluation for disabled people. *Disability and Rehabilitation, 27*(13), 781–790. doi:10.1080/09638280400014766

Federici, S., Scherer, M. J., Micangeli, A., Lombardo, C., and Olivetti Belardinelli, M. (2003). A Cross-cultural analysis of relationships between disability self-evaluation and individual predisposition to use assistive technology. In G. M. Craddock, L. P. McCormack, R. B. Reilly and H. T. P. Knops (Eds.), *Assistive Technology—Shaping the Future* (pp. 941–946). Amsterdam: IOS Press.

Gibson, J. J. (1979). *The Ecological Approach to Visual Perception*. Boston: Houghton Mifflin.

Gustavsson, A., and Zakrzewska-Manterys, E. (1997). *Social Definitions of Disability*. Kraków, Poland: Wydawnictwo "Żak."

Halasz, F. G., and Moran, T. P. (1983). *Mental Models and Problem Solving in Using a Calculator*. Paper presented at the Proceedings of the SIGCHI Conference on Human Factors in Computing Systems, Boston, MA.

Koffka, K. (Ed.). (1935). *Principles of Gestalt Psychology*. New York: Harcourt, Brace.

Lewis, C. (1982). *Using the "Thinking Aloud" Method in Cognitive Interface Design*. (RC-9265 (#40713)). Retrieved from http://www.watson.ibm.com/index.shtml

Lifetool. (2004). *Informations- und Kommunikationstechnologie für Menschen im Alter*. Retrieved from http://www.lifetool.at/rte/upload/6_Fachforum/IKT_studie_2004_Endbericht.pdf

Matausch, K., Hengstberger, B., and Miesenberger, K. (2006). "Assistec"—A university course on assistive technologies. In K. Miesenberger, J. Klaus, W. Zagler, and A. Karshmer (Eds.), *Computers Helping People with Special Needs* (Vol. 4061, pp. 361–368). Berlin: Springer. doi:10.1007/11788713_54

Miesenberger, K. (1998). *Informatik für Sehgeschädigte, Soziale Aufgabenstellung einer Technischen Disziplin*. Doctoral Dissertation, Universität Linz, Linz, Austria.

Miesenberger, K. (2004). Equality = e-quality. "Design for all" und "accessibility" als Grundlage für eine demokratische, offene und inklusive Gesellschaft. In E. Feyerer and W. Pammer (Eds.), *Qual-I-Tät und Integration. Beiträge Zum 8. Praktikerinnenforum* (Vol. 16, pp. 405–416). Linz, Austria: Universitätsverlag Rudolf Trauner.

Miesenberger, K. (2006, Sep 13–15). *BFWD and Assistec: Two University Degrees Relevant to Design for All: Accessible Web Design and Assistive Technologies*. Paper presented at the International Design for All Conference, Rovaniemi, Finland. Retrieved from http://dfasuomi.stakes.fi/EN/dfa2006/rovaniemi/

Miesenberger, K. (2009a). Best practice in design for all. In C. Stephanidis (Ed.), *The Universal Access Handbook* (p. 58). Boca Raton, FL: CRC Press.

Miesenberger, K. (2009b). Design for all principles. In C. Sik Lányi (Ed.), *Principles and Practice in Europe for e-Accessibility* (pp. 15–25). Veszprém, Hungary: EDeAN Publication 2009, Panonia University Press.

Miesenberger, K., Hengstberger, B., and Batusic, M. (2010). Web_Access: Education on Accessible Web Design. In K. Miesenberger, J. Klaus, W. Zagler and A. Karshmer (Eds.), *Computers Helping People with Special Needs* (Vol. 6179, pp. 404–407). Berlin: Springer. doi:10.1007/978-3-642-14097-6_64

MOODLE. (2011). Open Source Course Management System. Retrieved from http://moodle.org/

Norman, D. A. (1983). Some observations on mental models. In D. Gentner and A. L. Steven (Eds.), *Mental Models* (pp. 7–14). Hillsdale, NJ: Lawrence Earlbaum Associates.

Olivetti Belardinelli, M. (1973). *La Costruzione della Realtà* [The construction of reality]. Torino, Italy: Boringhieri.

SART. (1999). Sommerakademie für Rehabilitationstechnik. Retrieved from http://www.is.tuwien. ac.at/fortec/reha.d/projects/sart/sart.html

Scherer, M. J. (1998). *Matching Person & Technology. A Series of Assessments for Evaluating Predispositions to and Outcomes of Technology Use in Rehabilitation, Education, the Workplace & Other Settings.* Webster, NY: The Institute for Matching Person & Technology, Inc.

Scherer, M. J. (2005). *Living in the State of Stuck: How Technologies Affect the Lives of People with Disabilities* (4th ed.). Cambridge, MA: Brookline Books.

SIVA. (2011). Educational Activities. Retrieved from http://www.siva.it/eng/education/default. htm

TeleMate. (2011). TeleMate: Assistive Technology Devices. Retrieved from http://www.telemate. org/

W3C/WAI. (2011). Policies Relating to Web Accessibility. Retrieved from http://www.w3.org/ WAI/Policy/

Wharton, C., Rieman, J., Lewis, C., and Polson, P. G. (1994). The cognitive walkthrough method: A practitioner's guide. In J. Nielsen and R. L. Mack (Eds.), *Usability Inspection Methods* (pp. 105–140). New York: John Wiley & Sons.

World Health Organization (WHO). (2001). *ICF: International Classification of Functioning, Disability, and Health.* Geneva, Switzerland: WHO.

World Health Organization (WHO). (2007). *ICF-CY: International Classification of Functioning, Disability, and Health—Children and Youth Version.* Geneva, Switzerland: WHO.

10

The Optometrist

M. Orlandi and R. Amantis

CONTENTS

10.1 Introduction

The choice of the appropriate assistive technology is conditioned by the visual skills of the subject. Visual perception is a complex process in which various subprocesses participate and in which various anatomic structures are involved. It is therefore necessary that the assessment protocol used permits having a clear picture of all of the visual abilities and skills of the patient as well as his/her limits. A detailed analysis of the visual skills permits the assistive technology assessment (ATA) team to plan specific test settings to be used with the patient without having to make random attempts, which usually prove themselves not only to be useless, but also to be frustrating for the patient and the family.

This chapter is not intended to be an optometry manual, but it will provide the reader with some guidelines on the protocols that can be implemented that have been developed by the authors over the years. Procedures will be described in details that significantly diverge from the normal optometric clinical practice once they are modified to adapt to patients with neurologic diseases.

In conclusion, the general theoretical framework of this chapter aims at reintegrating the role of the optometrist when it comes to supporting and providing follow-up in the possibilities of visual recovery, which is possible to attain when visual training is combined with the correct use of assistive technologies.

The chapter will be divided into five subsections—vision, base protocol, additional tests, clinical analysis of the example cases, and visual training—along with an introduction and conclusions.

A final important consideration: Although this chapter deals with optometry, it should also and above all be read by nonoptometrists. It is fundamental that each operator knows what is meant by a visual problem and that all operators share a common specific language with the optometrist working in the team.

10.2 Vision and the Role of the Optometrist in ATA

The assessment of the visual functions, because of the various aspects they entail, can theoretically be extremely long and complex. Peripheral aspects can be assessed, which are linked to eye function, both in the perceptional as well as in the motor area, central perceptional processes mainly linked to the quality of the detection, and analysis processes of the visual stimulus, as well as to the skills of binocular fusion. Superior processes will also be assessed, such as recognition, access, and use of visual memory processes, perceptional styles, and the analysis of the abilities of integration with other cognitive or motor processes.

It is therefore evident that all of this flow of information is not entirely necessary for its preliminary assessment at the assistive technology center, but as for all diagnostic activities, it is necessary to focus and, when required, to study the parameter that is of more significance in detail. Knowing the clinical history of the patient will lead the operator to correctly determine the series of tests to be submitted, always having on hand the alternative methods that could be necessary during the exams.

10.2.1 The Complexity of the Visual Process from Eye to Brain

A precise knowledge of the eye structures permits understanding some of the statements about the visual process. Everybody knows that the eye is usually compared to a camera, with its dark room, objective lenses, and a very sensitive film that captures light (Figure 10.1).

Less known are those aspects concerning the motor and accommodative skills of the eye, not to mention the particular processing process that takes place already in the retina.

An efficient eye, with no refraction problems, is called emmetropic and it perfectly focuses to infinite. In the optical approximation, a proper focus can be obtained beyond 5 m. When an eye watches an object at a closer distance, the optical system of the eye modifies its dioptric power through the ciliary muscle, which makes the crystalline lens curvature vary (Figure 10.2).

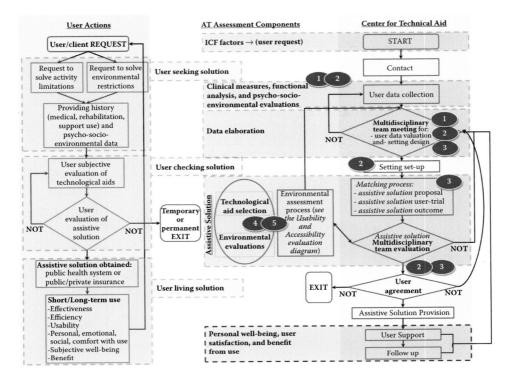

FIGURE I.1
Flow chart of Assistive Technology Assessment (ATA) process in a Centre for technical aid: The ATA process can be read both from the perspective of the user/client or from the perspective of the Centre for Technical Aid. In the central column are indicated the ATA components. Numbered button signs refer to the chapter in Section I. Their position in the flow chart show an ideal matching with the ATA process.

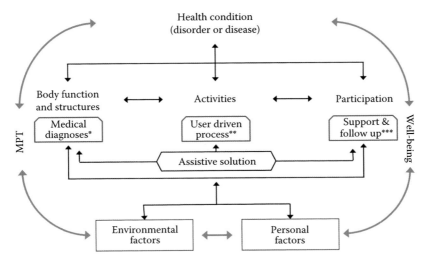

* The physician, the psychologist, the cognitive therapist, the optometrist, the audiologist, the pediatric specialist, the geriatrician
** The psychotechnologist, the occupational therapist, the architect, the engineer
*** The therapist, the special educator, the occupational therapist, the psychologist, the consumer support, speech language pathologist, the physiotherapist

FIGURE 1.1
Assistive technology assessment under the lens of the ICF biopsychosocial model.

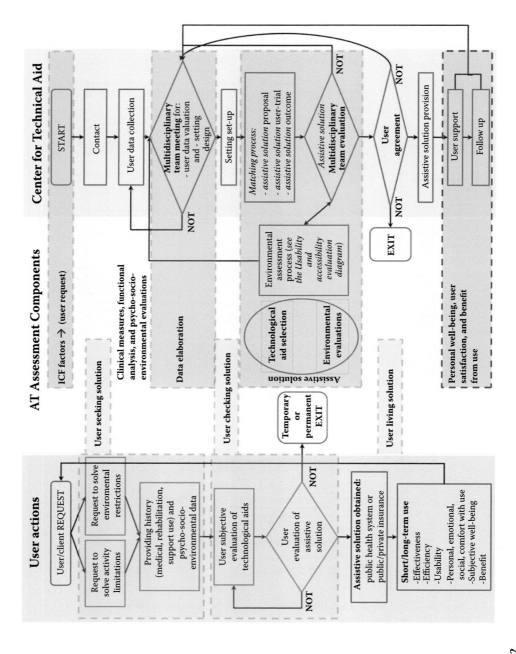

FIGURE 1.2
The assistive technology assessment process flow chart.

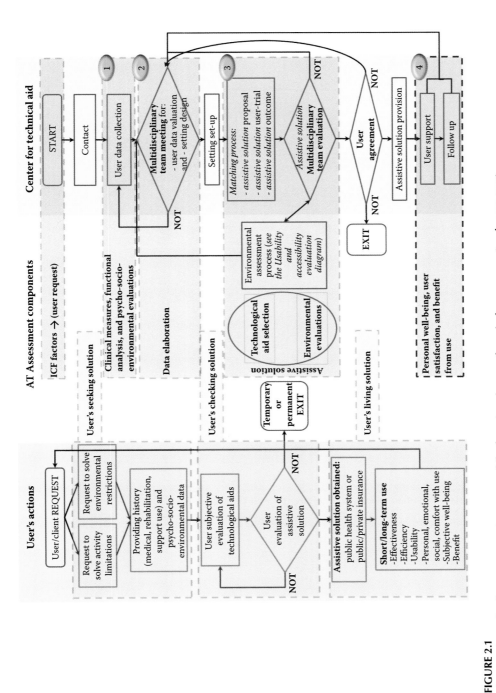

FIGURE 2.1

The assistive technology assessment process and the four steps (orange shapes) of measurement and assessment.

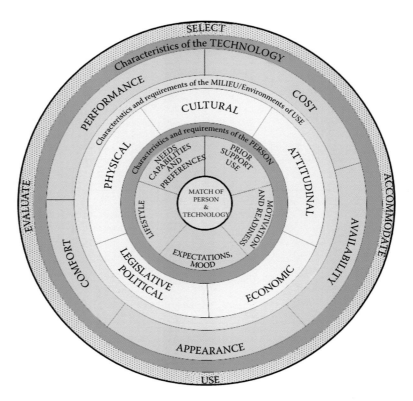

FIGURE 3.1
The matching person and technology model (Scherer, 2005). The "Match of Person and AT" (the smallest circle) equals the assistive solution when quality of life and well-being raise from.

Universal design
Sustainability
Accessibility

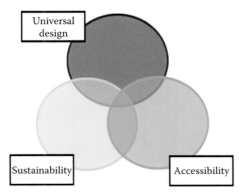

FIGURE 4.1
The intersection model of conceptual dimensions of accessibility, sustainability, and universal design.

Maximal access
Accessibility
No access
No impact/ high efficiency
Sustainability
High impact/ low efficiency
Intuitive/ flexible/integrated
Universal design
Specialized/ technical/segregated

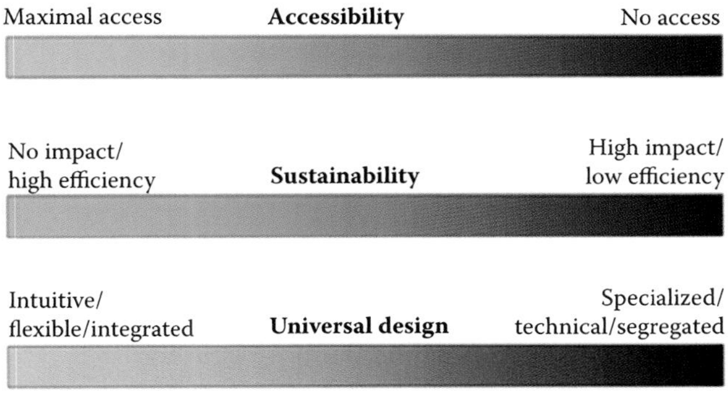

FIGURE 4.2
The continuum model of conceptual dimensions of accessibility, sustainability, and universal design.

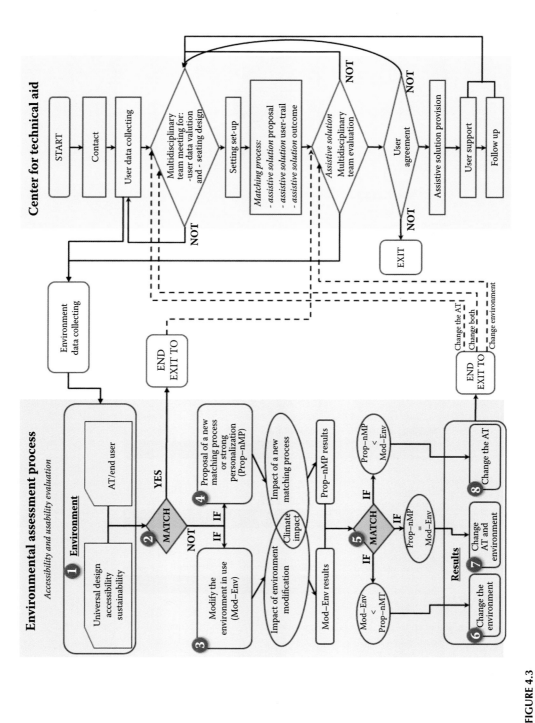

FIGURE 4.3
Environmental assessment process and interaction with the center for technical aid model.

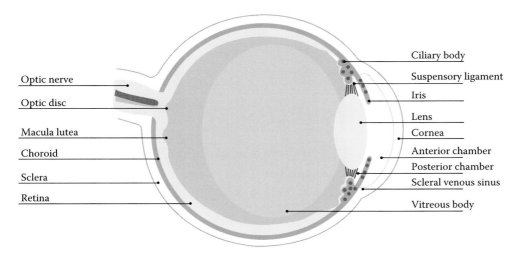

FIGURE 10.1
The structure of the eye.

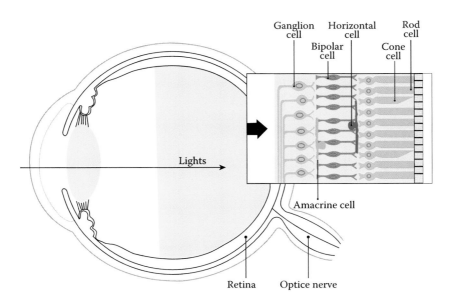

FIGURE 10.5
Structure of the retina.

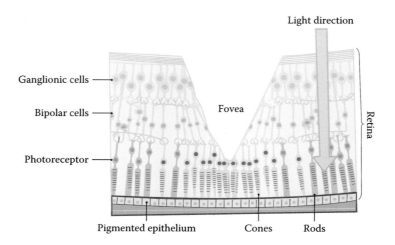

FIGURE 10.7
Histological characteristic of the retina.

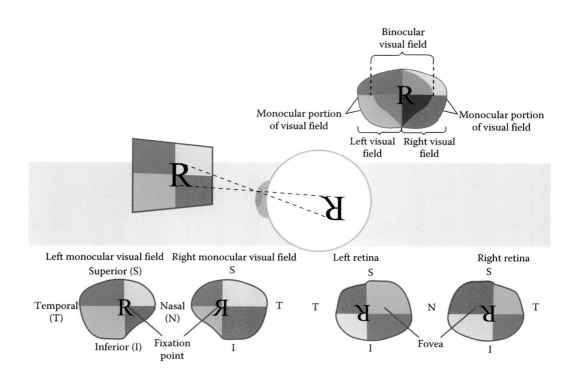

FIGURE 10.8
Projection of the visual fields onto the left and right retinas. Projection of an image onto the surface of the retina. The passage of light rays through the optical elements of the eye results in images that are inverted and left-right reversed on the retinal surface. Retinal quadrants and their relation to the organization of monocular and binocular visual fields as viewed from the back surface of the eyes. Vertical and horizontal lines drawn through the center of the fovea define retinal quadrants (bottom). Comparable lines drawn through the point of fixation define visual field quadrants (center). Color coding illustrates corresponding retinal and visual field quadrants. The overlap of the two monocular visual fields is shown at the top.

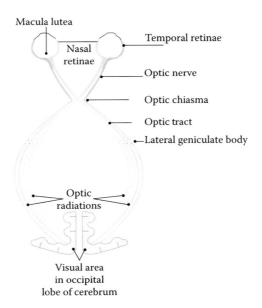

FIGURE 10.9
The optic chiasm and the optic nerves and their pathway.

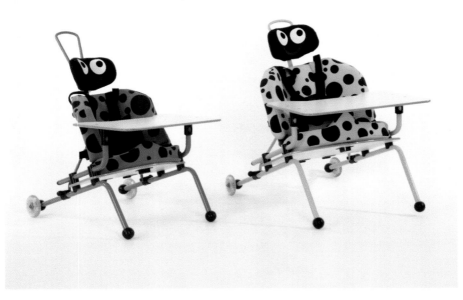

FIGURE 12.1
Special chair to help the child sit and use upper limbs.

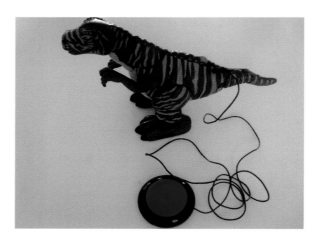

FIGURE 12.2
Electronic toy with adapted switch.

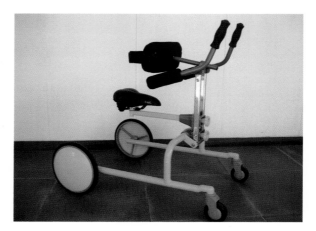

FIGURE 12.3
Device for independent locomotion.

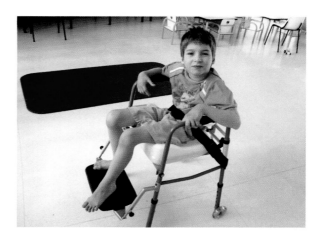

FIGURE 12.4
Customized toilet seat.

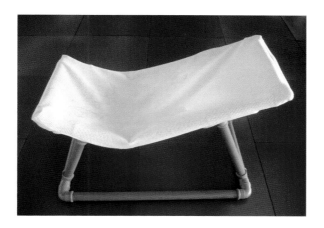

FIGURE 12.5
Bathing chair.

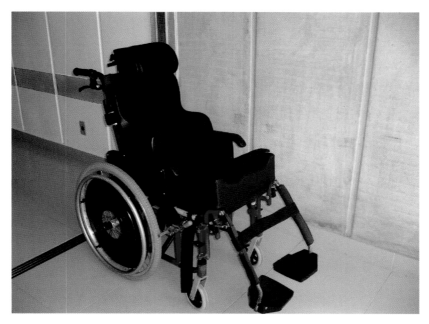

FIGURE 12.6
Pediatric wheelchair with anatomical seat and backrest.

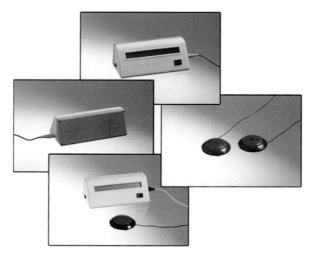

FIGURE 12.7
Talker that uses simple switches to scan letters for forming words.

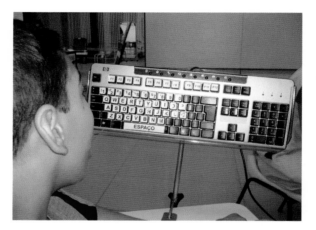

FIGURE 12.8
Rod for holding a conventional keyboard for better positioning and viewing.

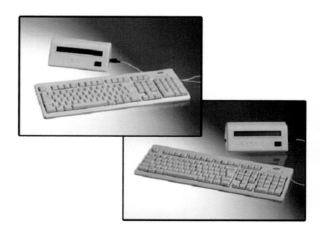

FIGURE 12.9
Talker with keyboard

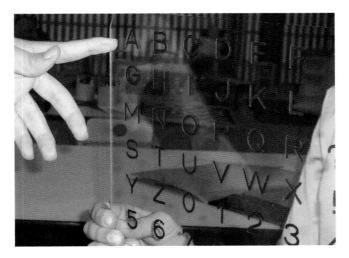

FIGURE 12.10
Acrylic board for communication in the pool.

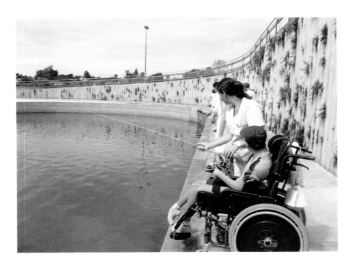

FIGURE 12.11
AT resources that facilitate social interaction.

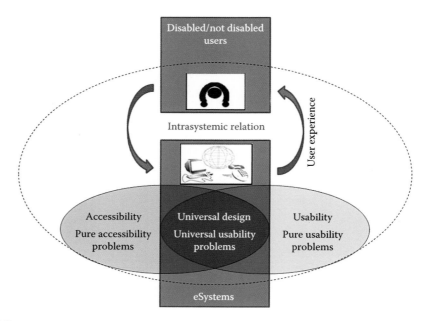

FIGURE 15.2
The intrasystemic relation between users and eSystems. UX is represented as the user perspective in the intrasystemic relation of action and feedback with the eSystem (Federici et al. 2005; Federici and Borsci 2010). The universal design properties that make up the eSystem are obtained by the intersection of the accessibility and the usability of the eSystem. By following Petrie and Kheir (2007), the universal usability problems represent interaction problems of usability and accessibility that are found by all kinds of users in a bad intrasystemic relation because of a bad UX (universal design problems). When the problems affect mostly disabled people's interaction, we may use the term "pure accessibility problems," when the problems do not pertain to disabled users' interaction, we may use the term "pure usability problems." However, between these two extremes there are many different degrees of interaction problems that affect the UX of disabled and nondisabled users.

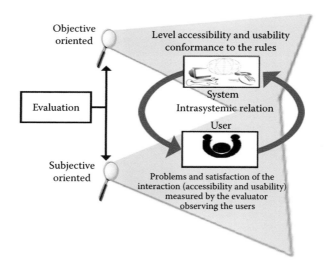

FIGURE 15.3
The possible evaluation perspectives during the evaluation of the intrasystemic dialogue between user and system: the objective-oriented and the subjective-oriented perspectives. The interaction evaluation has to take into account not only the properties of a single dimension (the accessibility or the usability), but also the relations that bind the objective part of the interaction to the subjective one (and vice versa). In this context, accessibility and usability are considered as necessary steps for the evaluation of the intrasystemic relation between interface and user.

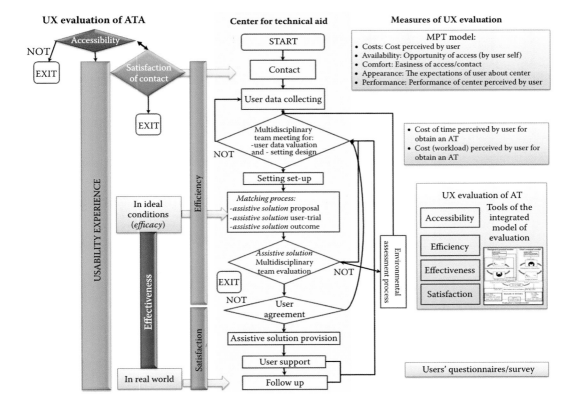

FIGURE 15.6
The dimensions and the measures of the UX evaluation of the model's functioning of the ATA process of a center for technical aid. In this schema, the UX evaluation of the AT, with its dimensions, is part of the efficiency and efficacy evaluation of the relationship between the user and the center for technical aid.

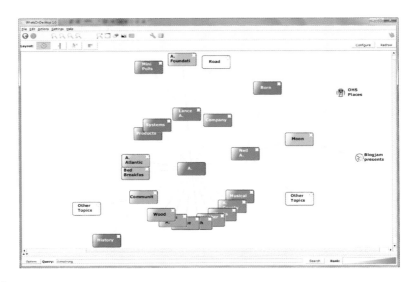

FIGURE 16.2
Example of diagrammatic interface that reduces the search commands to be executed when accessing a page on the Web.

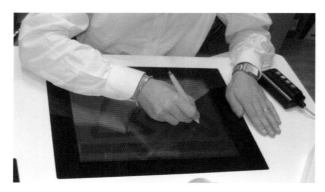

FIGURE 16.3
Nu!Reha Desk example of writing or "pre-graphism" exercise.

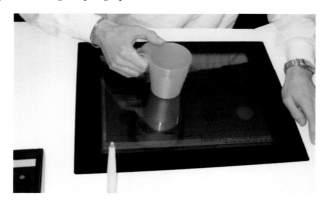

FIGURE 16.4
Nu!Reha Desk example of physical contextual activities exercise.

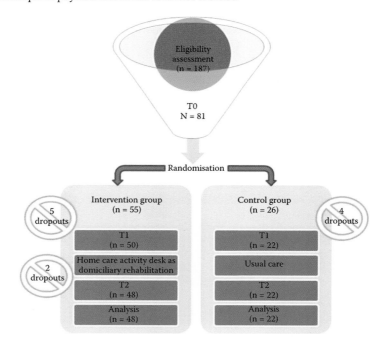

FIGURE 16.5
Flow chart of the experimental design for the clinical evaluation of the Nu!Reha Desk

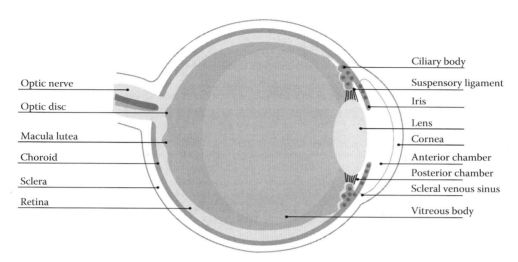

FIGURE 10.1
(See color insert.) The structure of the eye.

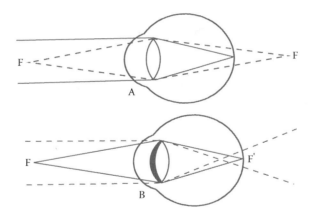

FIGURE 10.2
Accommodation.

The ciliary muscle is a smooth muscle, innervated by the parasympathetic system, and it acts when an image is unfocused. This process is closely related to convergence, which keeps centering and focus synchronized (Figure 10.3).

This implies that the skills of a patient may sensibly vary as the distance at which the assessment is carried out changes.

Another less known element that should always be considered is the functional characteristics of the retina (Liuzzi and Bartoli 2002). The retina is made up of two types of receptors: the cones, which are divided into three different groups that each detect one primary color, and the rods, which likewise all react to the different wavelengths of the light (Figure 10.4).

The receptors are connected to bipolar first-order cells and ganglion second-order cells. Their axons unite in the blind spot to form the optical nerve (Figure 10.5).

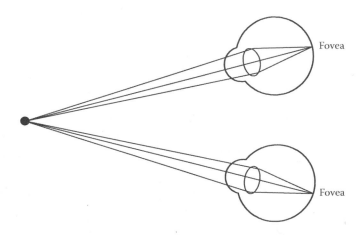

FIGURE 10.3
Convergence.

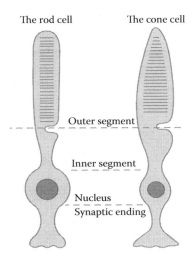

FIGURE 10.4
Cone and rod cell.

Not everybody notices that in the retina the receptors are covered with neurons, except for the fovea, where the neurons are laterally shifted to avoid any interference on the optic pathway of the light.

It is anatomically possible to distinguish three different areas in the retina (Figure 10.6):

1. The blind spot, where the optic nerve emerges;
2. The macula, with the fovea in the middle, the area where the maximal visual acuity can be detected; and
3. The periphery, defined in function as the angular distance from the fovea.

For the histological characteristics of the retina and for the connections between rods and cones and the first- and second-order neurons, the resolution capability of the retina is different in the various areas (Figure 10.7).

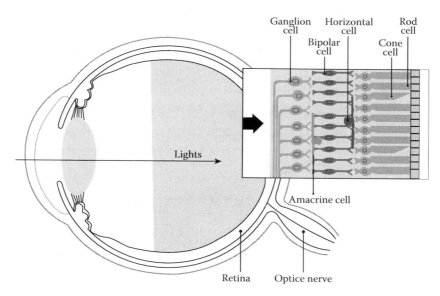

FIGURE 10.5
(See color insert.) Structure of the retina.

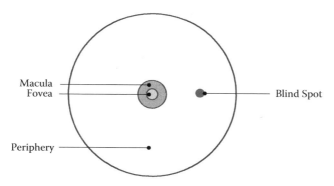

FIGURE 10.6
Functional division of the retina.

The resolution is at its highest point at the fovea level, rapidly diminishes in the first 10°, and then stabilizes in the peripheral retina. This peculiarity of the retina is the reason why we perform eye movements; that is to say, they are activated by the need for letting the image of the interested object to be projected on the fovea, where it will be possible to analyze its tiniest details. The peripheral retina, with its convergent connections, is really sensitive to light and insufficiently able to spatially segregate. The primary function of the retina is then to receive the changes that can occur in the environment around the subject and to trigger the foveation.

The eye movements are carried out by six muscles that are innervated by three cranic nerves. We can see how the contraction of the medial recti induced a synergic contraction in the ciliary muscle. The activation of the accommodation, as an effect of hypermetropy or induced with negative lenses, can also trigger a convergence movement. This can lead to a wrong alignment of the converging visual axes, which can be noticed in the

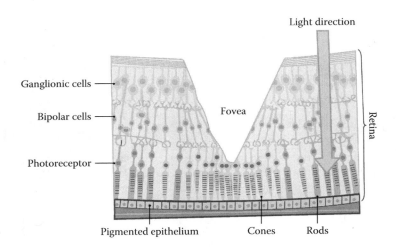

FIGURE 10.7
(See color insert.) Histological characteristic of the retina.

so-called accommodative strabismus (Griffin 1982). In minor, physiological hypermetropy this movement will not be manifest, but it will remain latent, because fusion, a central analysis process, contrasts it, activating the lateral recti. The simple apparently static fixation requires a fair coordination of various couples of agonist and antagonist muscles; striated, voluntary muscles; and of the accommodative system muscles, smooth, involuntary muscles (Traccis and Zambardieri 1996).

The image forming on the retina is made up of a central component, in a retinal sense, foveal, and a peripheral component. This one can be divided between the information in the right perceptual hemispace and the left perceptual hemispace. As an effect of the dioptric convergence of light, rays place themselves on the left and on the right hemiretina, respectively (Figure 10.8).

The visual information travels along the ganglion axons and reunites on the blind spot to form the optic nerve. The nerve, coming out from the bulb, is myelinated, and it proceeds via the orbit to the foramen; the nerve then converges and crosses in the optic chiasm (Figure 10.9).

This is a rather critical structure because here is where the information from both eyes' inherent homologous perceptual hemispace is first integrated. After this crossing, any information from what is in the left visual space, and has reached the left or the right eye, travels in the same bundle of fibers of the right optic tract, and vice versa on the other side.

The fibers in the optic tract reach the lateral geniculate nucleus (LGN), a thalamic nucleus (Hubel 1995). At this level the pathway of the peripheral fibers differentiates from the one of the foveal fibers. Two different pathways can be individuated, one for WHERE the object is and one for WHAT the object is. The fibers, which are already differentiated because of the retinal level, in this tract are also spatially segregated. From the LGN, the fibers, called optic radiation, reach the occipital cortex. In this area called 17 or V1, all processing that allows the extraction of the elementary characteristic of the images takes place. We thus find a columnar organization, separated for each eye, as well as neurons that can detect light only if surrounded by dark (on center) or vice versa (off center), or lines of a certain length or angular orientation, moving toward a direction or its opposite,

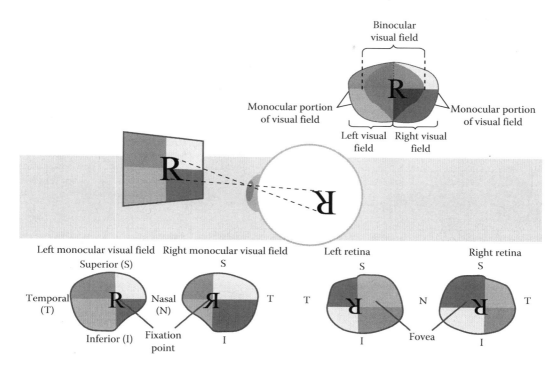

FIGURE 10.8
(See color insert.) Projection of the visual fields onto the left and right retinas. Projection of an image onto the surface of the retina. The passage of light rays through the optical elements of the eye results in images that are inverted and left-right reversed on the retinal surface. Retinal quadrants and their relation to the organization of monocular and binocular visual fields as viewed from the back surface of the eyes. Vertical and horizontal lines drawn through the center of the fovea define retinal quadrants (bottom). Comparable lines drawn through the point of fixation define visual field quadrants (center). Color coding illustrates corresponding retinal and visual field quadrants. The overlap of the two monocular visual fields is shown at the top.

and so on. All of these pieces of information are still separate and require further processing in area 18 or V2, where the single elements are united to build up the perception of the object. One part of the fibers coming from area 18 or V2 moves toward the temporal cortex, where further analysis of the superior characteristics of the visual information is carried out. All of those lines, with their own information on length, color, topologic relations, etc., are classified with a verbal tag and memorized. In this moment, the "What is it?" is identified. Other fibers proceed toward the parietal cortex, where spatial visual information is processed, allowing detection of where the object is in relation to us. In conclusion, these two pieces of information must go together to form one perception so that we can perceive, localize, and recognize the object. This will make us interact with the object itself, grasping it, manipulating it, using it, and having an immediate feedback on the quality of our actions. This further and crucial integration occurs at the prefrontal and frontal cortex level (Hubel 1995).

This concise overview of the visual process, which is not at all complete, is aimed at underlining the complexity of what happens during one simple gaze. Later in this work, the importance of every point discussed will be analyzed to understand some of the responses of our patients and to allow us to be able to adapt suitable instruments to every single patient.

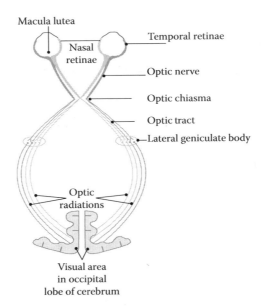

Macula lutea
Temporal retinae
Nasal retinae
Optic nerve
Optic chiasma
Optic tract
Lateral geniculate body
Optic radiations
Visual area in occipital lobe of cerebrum

FIGURE 10.9
(See color insert.) The optic chiasm and the optic nerves and their pathway.

A short closing remark. What has been described here is the so called retino-geniculate cortex pathway. However, not all of the fibers rising from the optic nerve follow this path. Approximately 20% follow a retino-collicular-cortical path, involved in space localization. However, this particular kind of fiber does not permit identification of the object and is apparently responsible of the blind-sight phenomenon.

10.2.2 The Visual Abilities in Behavioral Optometry

The precedent description underlined that the visual process is something much more complex than a good visual acuity. The well-known 10/10 (20/20 in the United States, 6/6 in the United Kingdom) represents just one among the visual abilities, which is not even the most important one, although this parameter is usually used to distinguish those having a good sight from those who do not. In this section, object of analysis will be the main visual ability that must be assessed in patients who require assistive technology (Bardini 1982; Birnbaum 1985, 1993; Sabbadini et al. 2000).

10.2.2.1 Visual Acuity

Visual acuity represents the ability to recognize two points as separate, and it is mainly conceived as an angular measurement. It does not directly indicate the dimension of the object, the details of which can be recognized, but only their angular dimension. Under the same visual acuity, the dimensions are modified by distance (Figure 10.10).

Visual acuity is not only an indication of the correct focus of the eye's optical system, but it is also a consequence of the transparency of the means, not to mention the integrity of the nerves and of the superior cortical areas.

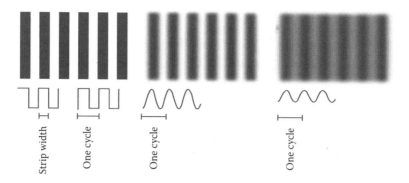

FIGURE 10.10
Types of grating stimuli used to measure acuity and contrast sensitivity, including a high-contrast (from the left to the right) square-wave grating, a high-contrast, sine-wave grating, and a low-contrast, sine-wave grating. The graph to the right of each grating illustrates its luminance profile.

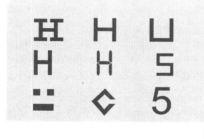

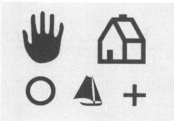

FIGURE 10.11
Optotype symbol examples. From left top: Snellen, Green, Danielle, Monoyer, Dennett, digital numbers, by resolution, variation of Landolt C, and targeting generic (DIN). On the right: Types of grating stimuli used to measure acuity and contrast sensitivity, including a high-contrast, square-wave grating (from the left to the right), a high-contrast, sine-wave grating, and a low-contrast, sine-wave grating. The graph to the right of each grating illustrates its luminance profile.

Various instruments are clinically used to assess visual acuity, usually consisting of tables with symbols, letters, or numbers with a definite dimension and for which single elements are separated by a specific angle at the examined distance (Figure 10.11).

With noncooperative patients, black/white gratings are used, presenting precise angles of separation at the distance examined (Figure 10.12).

The parameters used to measure the visual acuity are usually expressed in the form of a fraction, the numerator of which indicates the distance at which the subject must be kept so that he/she can properly identify the distance, and the denominator of which indicates

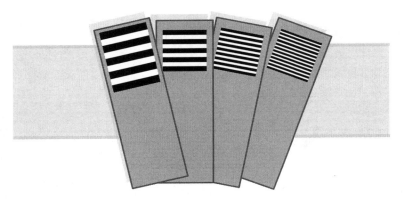

FIGURE 10.12
Teller acuity card.

the distance at which a given symbol must be recognized. For instance, 5/10 indicates that the subject can read at a distance of 5 m what he/she should read at a 10-m distance. In research, cycles/degree are usually used as unit of measurement. They indicate the number of black/white cycles in a grating. Knowing the subject's visual acuity is of utmost importance because it provides for information in the dimension of the letters, icons, or objects that have to be used.

10.2.2.1.1 Methods

The assessment of visual acuity in patients is generally performed by requesting the patient to identify letters on a table appropriately set at the examined distance. The usual procedure cannot be practiced with our patient, although they are able to recognize the presented letters, because of simple problems in verbalization. The problem can be slightly reduced using illustrations. Again it may happen that the name pronounced can be wrong because of difficulty accessing vocabulary. The image of a bicycle was named "car" by some patients because this is the prototypical word for a means of transport. In such situations, the exam must therefore be repeated a few times, and it is better to continue, even if mistakes are made.

An expedient we frequently use with our patients with fixation disorders, both for strictly visual problems and for poor head postural control, is to always present single stimuli and avoid tables with more than one symbol because, after a loss of fixation, it is much easier for the subject to get back to that single object instead of having to reorganize his/her sight to find the symbol indicated by the operator among the others. This is why the presentation on cardboard is preferred, instead of techniques involving projection, because it is possible to place them in the exact point where the patient finds it easier to set his/her look. It can thus be shifted up, down, or laterally as we wish. Particular attention is given to the requested modality of response. As already indicated above, verbal response can sometimes be inappropriate or unreliable. Usual praxis is to make the patient name the images, presenting the bigger ones, generally 1/10, at a 30-cm distance from the patient, and noting the name that the patient spontaneously uses. We will not say "This is a house" and "This is a flower": The patient must use those words that are easily evoked to him/her by the images. Further tests are performed through coupling techniques. A few charts will be submitted to the patient at a distance so that he/she is able to touch them. The charts represent images presented at an exam distance. In this case, the number of images must be adapted to the motor abilities of the patient: the lower the motor control is, the fewer are the images he/she is called to pick. Generally, the number of images ranges from a minimum of two to a maximum of six. The fewer the alternatives presented, the more tests that must be formed for every single visual acuity level to avoid false positives. In some patients affected by a serious motor situation impairment (e.g., severe tetraparesis), the indication of the gaze has been successfully used as a response. Visual acuity is generally evaluated at a distance because in the nonpresbyotic patients, it is exactly correlated with the visual acuity at a proximal distance. However, this is true if an appropriate accommodation is present. If accommodation deficiency occurs during the test, the visual acuity must also be reassessed at a proximal distance.

Visual acuity values can be then related to known dimension of fonts (Figure 10.13).

In the case of noncooperative patients, the preferential look and the optokinetic reflex techniques are used. In the first case, a grating is placed in front of the subject on a plain background and the test is based on whether the patients uses his/her gaze to find his/her way on the grating.

On the other hand, the optokinetic nystagmus is elicited through cylinders or monitors on which grids are reproduced with a definite dimension. They are then slowly moved in front of the patient only when the resolution system of the eye perceives the bands as separate. Of course, such a technique cannot be used with a subject that is affected by pathologic nystagmus and with patients affected by epilepsy.

10.2.2.2 Fixation

The visual system acquires information during the so-called fixation period, a short period in which the eyes remain still after a saccade. Some subjects cannot keep their eyes completely still, and some spurious movements occur that reduce visual ability (Phillips and

Visus	Visus	Visus	Cycles/degree	Ex. of fonts
20/20	6/6	10/10	30	Labels insurance policies
20/22	6/6,7	9/10	27	Bible, dictionary
20/25	6/7,5	8/10	24	Economic announcements
20/28	6/8,6	7/10	21	Phone book
20/32	6/10	6/10	18	Newspaper
20/40	6/12	5/10	15	Cheap books
20/50	6/15	4/10	12	Books
20/66	6/20	3/10	9	Children's book
20/10	6/30	2/10	6	Children's book
20/20	6/60	1/10	3	Books for low vision

FIGURE 10.13
Visus font. (Data partially from Rossetti, A. and Gheller, P. *Manuale di Optometria e Contattologia*, Zanichelli, Bologna, Italy, 1997.)

Edelman 2008). In particular, erratic looks and nystagmus can be found. The first case is characterized by a fluid and continuous movement, not aimed at a particular object and that never completely blocks. This picture can be found in patients affected by severe vision impairment. Nystagmus is a continuous alternating of a slow sliding phase and a rapid saccadic recuperation (Traccis 1992). Nystagmus can have a physiologic origin, as when we look at the landscape out of the window of a moving train or during vestibular stimulations, or a pathologic origin. Various forms of nystagmus have been identified and are differentiated by their metrics, duration, age of onset, and various other causes. Nystagmus produces a reduction of visual acuity, sometimes rather severe, and a difficulty in performing all eye movements, such as pursuit eye movements and saccadic movements. Often, but not always, nystagmus can decrease and be reduced to particular gaze positions. There is no effective therapy against nystagmus; a few optical, surgical, or postural expedients can be used to limit its effects.

Some subjects cannot keep a stable fixation on a particular point because they cannot inhibit the orientation reflex that is activated as soon as the peripheral field changes. These subjects do not show altered metrics, but rather reduced fixation timings, which are usually mistaken for attention deficiencies.

10.2.2.2.1 Methods

Testing the fixation is apparently the easiest thing to be done. A target is placed in front of the subject, and the position of the eyes is observed. If the eyes cannot remain focused on the target, the contrast is deepened, lowering the environmental light and setting light on the target until an absolute contrast of 100% is reached. If stable fixation still does not occur, red targets can be used because they can be better perceived by foveal receptors in comparison with peripheral receptors. In particularly severe cases, the target must be passively put in front of the eyes, and operators will check whether fixation occurs.

Another element that proved to be of major importance was posture, which may variably affect the stability of this visual component. Some children with no apparent fixation ability managed to keep an acceptably stable gaze in the supine position. This shows that it is often recommended to try the less proficuous ways to solve situations of impasse.

10.2.2.3 Slow Pursuit

Slow pursuit movements are the movements performed in an attempt to maintain fixation on a moving object. Pursuit movement requires a high level of attention on the task and adequate oculomotor skill (Contreras, Ghajar, Bahar, Suh 2011). These movements are performed to keep the image of the object impressed on the fovea. In little children, pursuit movements are aided and integrated with head movement. As the children grow up, they progressively learn how to only move their eyes and not their head. In situations of retardation in development, the head movement is still present. Pursuit movements are the movements that the eyes use to follow the mouse cursor, for instance, and performing them properly leads to continuous loss of fixation and consequent saccadic leaps to recuperate.

10.2.2.3.1 Methods

In testing pursuit movement, parameters must be considered such as the ability to perform them without involving the head, fixation stability, automaticity (i.e., the possibility of performing a second interfering task), the consistency of the performance over time, and the integration with hand movement. There are various tests through which the performance can be quantified under these parameters. They are also useful to facilitate a rapid comprehension of the patient's skills. However, it is important to emphasize in particular the part of automaticity, which is seldom taken into account in the tests. We often obtain good performance from the patients, a continuous, stable pursuit that is often carried out together with rotations, but when the patient is asked to perform even a slight gesture, such as clapping hands, or a simple verbal request, such as counting to ten, it is possible to observe an evident loss in performance quality. This indicates that the subject needs to use his full attention to control the visual performance and that the slight interference breaks this control. This reproduces the effect of a realistic behavior during a visual pursuit as might occur in real life or during the use of an assistive device.

10.2.2.4 Saccadic Movements

Saccadic movements represent the most frequent eye movement. These movements are used during the visual exploration of the environment, when we read, and when we look distractedly without really looking at something. Saccades are characterized by a very rapid movement that shifts the eye to a target identified through peripheral vision. During this movement, a phenomenon known as saccadic masking occurs by "blocking" the visual process to avoid the unfocused and blurred images that are observed. At the end of this movement, a phase of stillness occurs, namely fixation, during which the information is acquired (Traccis and Zambardieri 1992). The quantity of information acquired mainly depends in this case on central factors. Saccades cannot provide for a continuous feedback: Verifying the correctness of the movement can be done only after the movement is completed, and in case of error, the only possible thing to do is to perform a new corrective movement (Figure 10.14).

Programming and performing saccades is a very complex task because the movement must be calculated in advance, during the central foveal fixation, using peripheral information filtered on the basis of minimal shape and movement indicators. Any deficiency in each of the above-mentioned passages can lead to inaccurate or insufficient saccade. We can observe dysmetric saccadic movements, as well as hypometric and hypermetric saccades, slightly elicited, with reduced shifting speed or an insufficient level of visual information acquisition.

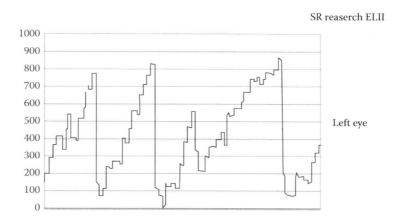

FIGURE 10.14
Eye movements during reading text (Centro Ricerche sulla Visione Roma, www.crvisione.it).

10.2.2.4.1 Methods

Saccades are tested with the same parameters used for pursuit: the possibility of performing them without involving the head, the quality of the metrics, the automaticity, the consistency of the performance over time, and the integration with a hand movement. Saccades can be reflected, induced by changes in the peripheral visual space, or voluntary. During the evaluation, the presence of the reflex skill is first tested using single stimuli presented behind masking grids as well as stimuli with alternating illumination or stimuli in tachistoscopic presentation on a computer.

10.2.2.5 Binocular Vision

During fixations, pursuits, and saccades, both eyes must point at the same object. In this way, the images, slightly different from eye to eye, are mixed together into one visual perception, providing for a tridimensional perception of space (stereopsis). Any alignment error prevents the development of such skill. The absence of eye alignment is called heterotropy or strabismus, which can be triggered by various causes. Muscular paralysis, innervation deficiencies, structural alteration of the orbit, and focus deficiencies can trigger various kinds of strabismus of various levels. Strabismus implies a fixating eye, except in the cases in which there is an alternating fixation between the right and left eye; in this case, the functional tests on fixation and movement must be performed in the function of the fixating eye.

There are forms of inaccurate binocular alignment that can be kept under control by the central system using a fusional process. These kinds of latent strabismus, the correct term for which is heterophoria or phoria, do not manifest themselves with the deviation of an eye, if not in particular stress/decompensation, usually because of weariness. However, even if not revealed, heterophorias produce effects on posture, effectiveness, correctness, and the rapidity of other visual skills.

10.2.2.5.1 Methods

A preliminary test is performed on steroacuity. To carry out such a test, both a stereotest and the Titmus can be used; in this case polarizing glasses are required (Figure 10.15), as with tables such as Lang, which do not require any glasses. As in younger children, it is possible to obtain a direct verbal response instead of a motor response with attempts at grasping.

Detecting a stereoacuity informs us of the presence of a sufficient binocular integration and of an accurate perception of depth, especially at a proximal distance. With cases of strabismus it is important to detect the fixating eye, even observing corneal reflexes. It is also important that the stability of the fixating eye is tested in different gaze positions and width of the eye movement.

As far as the phorias are concerned, they are physiologically present in all of the population at a very slight level. High levels of phorias can produce rapid weariness, especially when working at close distances, and if not appropriately compensated for they can manifest themselves into heterotropias. The methods that allow for the assessment of phorias are varied and can also be used with noncooperative patients (e.g., the covertest) or to obtain more accurate minimal values the tests often require a high level of cooperation from the patient.

10.2.2.6 Convergence

Convergence is the simultaneous movement of both eyes when objects at a close distance are observed (Figure 10.3). This movement is also triggered to maintain single binocular

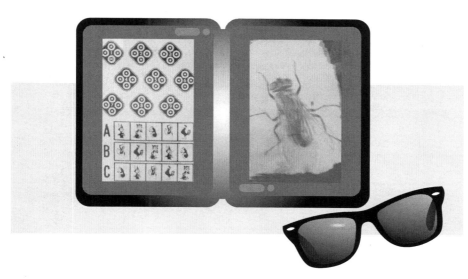

FIGURE 10.15
Titmus stereo test.

vision with foveation of both eyes on the same object. Convergence becomes critical in the actions performed at a proximal distance, such as manipulation, reading, and writing. Difficulties in convergence, with loss of alignment and subsequent adjustment, slow down all of the other pursuit and saccadic eye movements. A particularly critical situation is when there is a rapid request of shifting the fixation from the blackboard to the exercise book.

Convergence, activated to maintain binocular vision of close objects, is strictly linked to adjustment. It is often clinically observed how the two processes can mutually interfere, sometimes being an obstacle for each other, but also involving mutual strengthening.

10.2.2.6.1 Methods

Convergence movement can be assessed in terms of the most proximal point that can be singularly seen (Figure 10.16) and in terms of shifting the speed of binocular vision. This parameter becomes particularly critical when the patient is asked to shift the gaze from points at different distances in space.

An excessive slow-down will indicate the use of systems for which the stimuli and instruments are coplanar. No particular expedients are needed to assess convergence. It is therefore important to create a double testing channel with stimuli requiring accommodation, such as a stick presenting writings or images, and stimuli that do not require accommodation, such as a ball or a toy. This is because accommodation can favor better convergence efficiency.

10.2.2.7 Accommodation

The optical system of an emmetropic eye, that is to say without optic deficiencies such as myopia, hypermetropia, and astigmatism, in a relaxed state allows for perfect focus of the images placed at the optic infinite, approximated at 5 m (Figure 10.2). The rays of light from any object coming closer to the eye focus on the back of the retina, creating a blurred image. This problem has been solved for cameras, shifting the lenses in the objective; the

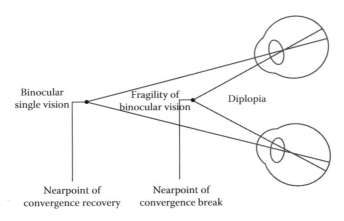

FIGURE 10.16
Near point of convergence.

human eye modifies the conformation of the crystalline lens as an effect of ciliary muscle contraction. This allows for bringing the image back onto the retina. As was mentioned above, accommodation is strictly connected to convergence in a synergy that is used especially to compensate for some specific deficit. Accommodation can result as reduced in its width, often because of inhibitory interferences triggered by vergence, and sometimes also slowed down in its response. The total accommodation width available tends to increase with age, and at approximately 40 years of age the values no longer allow for reading comfortably at a close distance.

10.2.2.7.1 Methods

Accommodation is also assessed with both the width and the shifting speed of the focus. The methods of assessing the accommodation width are based on the use of negative lenses or approaching the target to the subject. It should not be assumed that a deficiency in accommodation width can only occur in subjects over 40 years of age with manifest presbyopia. Our experience showed that there can also be an incidence of such cases in children and in subjects who are not affected by neurologic or malformative diseases. The shifting speed of the focus can similarly occur using lenses that are alternatively positive-inhibiting/negative-excitatory or by asking the patient to read at two different distances. In noncooperative patients, it is possible to assess if there is a sufficient accommodative response using retinoscopy, which objectively assesses the focus error residue at various distances from the stimulus. The next step is then verifying how the response changes if an object on which the attention of the patient is drawn is shifted closer or further from the patient. Although this test is not completely accurate on a quantitative point of view, it permits verification of the focus stability or variations when an object is fixated.

10.2.2.8 Refraction

The eye's optical system can be affected by some focusing errors caused by a nonadequate balance between the anterior/posterior length of the eye and the total dioptric power because of alterations in the shape and/or in the position of the eye lenses (Saunders et al. 2010; Rossetti and Gheller 1997).

There are three main ametropias (see Figure 10.17):

1. Myopia, in which the image is formed before the retina. The rays of light coming from objects at a proximal distance are focused correctly. Myopia is generally due to an excessive length of the bulb.
2. In hypermetropia, the image is placed behind the retina and there is no point in space where the rays are focused on the retina. Hypermetropia is generally due to a small length of the bulb.
3. In astigmatism, the images look doubled, and they can be placed both before and behind the retina. This also implies that, even in this case, there is no point in space where all rays are focused on the retina.

Hypermetropia is a physiologic condition at birth. It is spontaneously compensated for by means of an accommodating system. Hypermetropic patients can therefore have a normal visual acuity at all distances, until they are supported by an adequate accommodation system, although this requires a continuous muscular contraction. Accommodation also triggers convergence movements and this often implies esophoria. The perfect visual acuity of a hypermetropic patient therefore requires a higher muscular effort, especially in proximal vision.

Ametropias can be compensated for through different ophthalmic lenses for each ametropia. The positive, convex, converging lenses are used to compensate for hypermetropia, whereas negative, concave, diverging lenses are used for myopia (Figure 10.17). Compensating astigmatism requires toric lenses.

It is also important to note that the unit of measurement of the dioptric power of the lenses is the diopter (D), which can be defined as the reciprocal of the focal distance (f) in

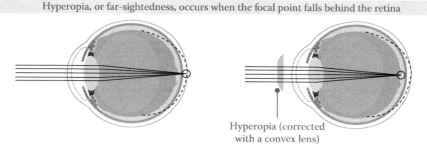

Hyperopia, or far-sightedness, occurs when the focal point falls behind the retina

Hyperopia (corrected with a convex lens)

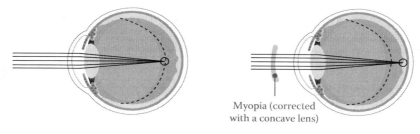

Myopia, or near-sightedness, occurs when the focal point falls in front of the retina

Myopia (corrected with a concave lens)

FIGURE 10.17
Ametropie. From the top: far-sighted eye and near-sighted eye.

meters, or $D = 1/f$ (Catalano 2006). This is a physical indication and it does not provide any information about the visual acuity of the patient.

10.2.2.8.1 Methods

The methods that can be used to quantify an ametropia and to determine the ophthalmic prescription are numerous and they are very well known by all optometrists.

It is useful to recall some simple precautions. However, the use of a phoroptor is not recommended in patients affected by nystagmus because this instrument forces a posture that often does not allow patients to reach their own blockage point.

The most important evaluation in particularly severe clinical pictures is that obtained in binocular conditions, in which interferences and mutual accommodations may produce unexpected results. In situations of low cooperation of the patient, it may be that we only are able to determine an ophthalmic correction by means of objective methods, but it must be verified with test glasses whether the other visual abilities benefit or whether a deterioration of such abilities occurs. This is the case with medium-high myopia; test glasses allow a perfect vision at a proximal distance, but once they are corrected, the use of proximal vision is made difficult although long-distance visual ability is improved.

10.2.2.9 The Field of Vision

The field of vision is the part of the space that provides the visual information to the patient.

The binocular field of vision has a wider horizontal range than the vertical one, both for anatomical reasons and for the sum of the single monocular fields of vision (Figure 10.8).

The field of vision is divided into a central area and a peripheral area in which the visual ability gradually decreases depending from the distance from the fovea.

In many retinal diseases and in central or visual tract diseases, defects in the field of vision may occur. At a monocular level, this only happens in a few meridians, but there could also be defects in the whole periphery of the field of vision so that the tubular vision is limited to the central area where an adequate visual ability is preserved. The opposite can be said for some maculopathies, in which the central visual ability is diminished, whereas the peripheral vision is preserved.

In severe myopias or in other ocular diseases there can be scotomas, blind areas of various extensions but always limited, in various parts on the retina. When the damage occurs in the area from the chiasm toward the LGN, losses in the field of vision may affect both eyes.

There also could be both homonymous or contralateral hemianopsies and quadrantopsies (Figure 10.18).

Lesions of cortical area V1 cause blindness in the area topographically linked to the retina. The presence of damages in the field of vision affects the choices that have to be made about the possible assistive technologies to be used with the patients, their features, and their positioning.

10.2.2.9.1 Methods

The assessment of the field of vision is performed through various instruments that are usually computerized. These instruments require a high attention level, a good knowledge of the task, and sufficient manual skills.

For many of our patients the test is performed through behavioral methods by using the orientation reflex toward objects appearing in the peripheral area. These techniques do not

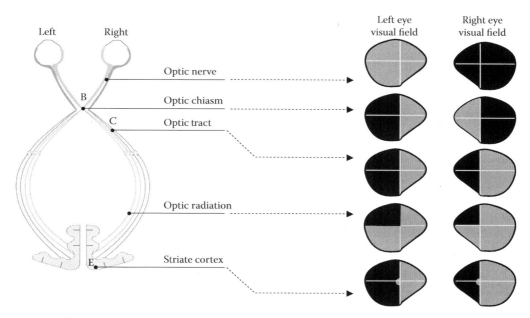

FIGURE 10.18
Visual field deficits resulting from damage at different points along the primary visual pathway. The diagram on the left illustrates the basic organization of the primary visual pathway and indicates the location of various lesions. The right panels illustrate the visual field deficits associated with each lesion. From the top: loss of vision in right eye. Bitemporal (heteronomous) hemianopsia. Left homonymous hemianopsia. Left superior quadrantanopsia. Left homonymous hemianopsia with macular sparing.

allow for a detailed measurement of all of the areas with a diminished field of vision, but they are able to show us field asymmetries and the most serious reductions.

10.2.2.10 Superior Perceptive Abilities

Several superior perceptive abilities can be examined during an optometric evaluation. The most important ones are the skills of recognition of a target in a range of conditions of crowding with interfering stimuli, with rotations and modifications to the enlarging modulus, against a more or less confounding background; the short and long-term span visual memory; and the spatial relationship among the target and between the targets and the perceptual space (Denes and Pizzamiglio 1996). The perceptual span is also important. It is the amount of space containing all of the information that can be acquired through a single fixation (Greene, Pollatsek, Masserang, Lee, Rayner 2010). Sensitivity to perceptual crowding is the degrading of the recognition of peripheral stimuli when surrounded by other elements (Levi Dennis 2008; Nisha, Yeotikar, Sieu Khuu, Asper, Suttle 2011).

All of these skills and many others can be critical in some clinical cases. However, their impact on the significance of the test is often reduced.

10.2.2.10.1 Methods

Most of these tests have a standardized procedure, but they often have to be carried out with nonstandardized procedures to adapt them to the needs of the patient. This prevents the use normative data; however, it is useful to receive important indications about the skills of the patients, at least in qualitative terms. An accurate choice of tests should be made on a case by case basis by discussing with the entire team and depending on the actual objectives.

To conclude, some fundamental considerations should be made. In patients with neurological deficiencies of all kinds that are subject to an assessment of visual function, we have to remember that their performances during the evaluation are not constant in all postures. Often, huge changes can be observed in performance with changes in the patient's posture, in the control of the head, and even in shifting from being seated to a laying position.

Obviously it is necessary to be perfectly aware of the changes that may occur, both for a proper organization of the location of use of assistive technologies and to be able to plan a possible preparation period with a specific visual training.

10.3 The Role of Optometrists in the ATA Process

The description made in the previous paragraphs was aimed at giving a summary explanation of vision and of the specific skills that help create efficient vision. This is true in every clinical situation, but in the specific case of the ATA process it is necessary to use a specific approach so that the work of the whole team can be enhanced. An optometrist should always provide some basic information (Leslie 2004), however important the disability of the patient is, and he/she must do so in a way that allows other ATA team specialists to adapt their interventions.

The main question we are asked is, "Can the patient use vision to control and interact through assistive technologies?" If the answer is affirmative we have to answer the next question: "What are the operational limits of the patient?" For example, in our team it is a consolidate practice to indicate not only the visual acuity of a patient, but also to what equivalent stimulus dimension his/her visual acuity corresponds at different working distances. Limitations to the saccadic movements will bring us to recommend the use of systems with reduced scanning and with target positioned so as to minimize the effect of the visual deficiency on the whole performance.

For every function listed above, precise indication can or, more appropriately must, be given. This indication does not need to be an absolute value. For example, a patient affected by strabismus whose deviated eye is bandaged will not be evaluated on the basis of the residual functions of this eye because the aim is not to carry out a visual rehabilitation, but to help the patient in the choice of the appropriate assistive technology. The team will be told that that patient is not functionally using the deviated eye and that every reference to the evaluated skills is to be considered only in relation to the fixating eye.

The exchange of information between the optometrist and his/her team must be continuous and bidirectional (Figure 10.19).

The team should inform the optometrist about the various working hypotheses and should provide enough information about the visual abilities of the patient and the optometrist, who in turn will provide them with information in the concrete framework of these hypotheses.

It is unnecessary to carry out detailed measurements of the field of vision if we already plan to work in a system with minimal spatial extension.

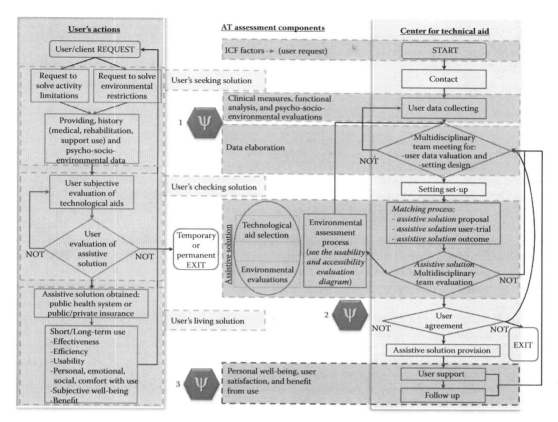

FIGURE 10.19
The ATA process.

On the other side, the optometrist must be competent in the existing assistive Sttechnologies that allow him/her to formulate their alternative hypothesis to those that have to be tested by the ATA team.

The information provided should be related to a real environment and should not be limited to a list of numerical data that are scientifically irreproachable but difficult to interpret and to use.

That is why it is less useful to state that a patient has a visual ability of 1/10 at 50 cm instead of communicating that a patient is able to recognize objects, symbols, and letters at a 50-cm distance and can differentiate details of 7-mm size.

The indications concerning the width of the saccadic movements or of the pursuit, in which a sufficient performance is held, must be provided in reference to a monitor's dimensions, instead of to an angular width.

The speed needed to make a pursuit movement without any losses of fixation should be binding a key element to consider in determining the velocity of the movement of the mouse cursor.

The stability of the fixation and the quality of the saccadic movement will be critical in determining effective interfaces when a software or printed texts and tabs are used (Orlandi 2003).

If the optometrist actually becomes a part of the team, he represents a fundamental asset for the enhancement of the evaluations and for the achievement of the optimal results, which otherwise will be slower and based on attempts and errors.

The optimal result may not be achieved starting from the assumption that better results cannot be reached. This assumption may be generated from the lack of information, for example, if no one told the team that a patient with a certain limitation in his/her field of vision could make marked progress by positioning a horizontal monitor on the bottom-left side of the patient. (This example comes from an actual examination.)

From his/her side, the optometrist who enters this kind of structure for the first time has to make two important professional efforts. The first one, which is also the easiest one, is to study all of the various available assistive technologies, work closely with the other operators, and think of how his/her knowledge can be applied in this kind of scenario, which is impossible to standardize. The second effort is very complex as well as fascinating and is linked to the idea that every single patient is special, therefore the whole team has to make available every possible variation in the standard assessment procedure, getting ready to approach every case in the appropriate way, learning from the patients, and being flexible in the procedures but at the same time rigid in the objectives. There are not and there should never be patients who do not cooperate: This is just a simple excuse for hiding our limitations because every single patient can give us important clues on his/her visual skills as long as we observe him/her with the right instruments.

10.4 Evaluation of Visual, Perceptive, and Motor Functions: Clinical Case 1

The child presents a symmetric corneal reflex. At the cover test the answer is ortho. The child is able to follow slowly by using a normal movement of the head while lying. While sitting, the child is able to follow even vertically, but she is conditioned by the control of the head. The evaluation of the refractive state shows hypermetropia that is in the physiological range of age. While fixing proximal objects, an adaptive reaction during the retinoscopy and a sporadic vergence are noticed. The saccadic movements are metrically correct, but there is a latency of reaction that is higher than the standard. The metric is adequate until a saccadic width of 20°. The visual acuity, evaluated both through optokinetic reflex elicitation and preferential look, is 6 c/g.

The young age of the child and the serious neuromotor disease do not allow for a subjective evaluation of the visual functions. It is therefore necessary to elicit all of the possible visual answers with variations in dimension and target contrast, even associated with tactile stimuli or sounds.

The first evaluation made on the child was her fixation ability. The examination of the corneal reflex of the lightened fixation target was symmetric and centered in both eyes. Nystagmic movements or lateral shifts were not observed (Traccis 1992). This could support the hypothesis of binocular vision, not necessarily bifoveal. A further confirmation of the absence of important phorias or tropias resulted from the cover test. This examination only requires keeping fixation on a point in space and it was repeated both with the short- and the long-distance target. In both cases the answer was ortho. This term means that the shift of the occlusion both in the left eye (LE) and the right eye (RE) did not cause adaptive movements in the fixating eye or in the bandaged eye. These results confirm the absence of strabismus.

Once the first level of visual skills was completed, after noticing a sufficient fixation ability, the evaluation of the eye's slow pursuit movements was carried out. Horizontal movements were made fluently with a postural accommodation of the head in the most extreme positions. This answer is absolutely physiological in smaller children, but as they grow up, a progressive segregation of the eye movement from the movement of the head can be observed. The vertical pursuit movement is generally more complex because of the anatomical structure of the extraocular muscles and because of the lower frequency of this kind of movement.

The patient shows she can move vertically, but she cannot properly control her head and this leads to a loss of fixation. This element should suggest the use of visual stimuli with less vertical expansion and paying special attention to posture.

The next examination concerned the refractive state and was carried out through retinoscopy. Various precautions were used to lead the child keep her fixation at a distance. If the parents were present, they were asked to reach a 3-m examination distance, call to the child, and show her some toys, maybe even colorful and loud ones. An alternative tool is represented by cartoons on the computer. Without a strong distant stimulus, the flashlight of the instrument attracts the attention of the child, causing her to turn her gaze to the operator. To neutralize the movement of the corneal reflex, lens racks (long guides on which there are found many progressive power lenses) were often used, although they are sometimes very cumbersome and can scare the children. For this reason, we instead use single lenses from the test box, although this option requires more time for the test to be completed.

The child showed a slight hypermetropia that was in the physiological range of age. The greatest accuracy is not necessary, but it is critical that the anisometropias are recognized, i.e., the differences in the refractive state between the LE and RE.

The same test was repeated by placing the fixation target at the matching distance, and a change in focus was observed, thus indicating that the accommodating system had been activated.

Moreover, placing the target closer produced unstable convergence movements. This kind of unstable convergence movement can often occur and is generally linked to factors such as visual attention, which may be shifted to the peripheral area and is often not linked to a convergence deficiency.

It is also necessary to note that very often hypermetropia is associated with esophoria, which favors convergence movements. The saccadic movements showed an adequate metric until a width of 20°, but with too much latency of response. This parameter can be observed through single stimuli. A slight increase of the latency of response was not very important in this case because the metrics were adequate. The visual acuity was tested with two different methods with the aim of integrating and confirming the obtained data. The first method consisted of the elicitation of the optokinetic nystagmus. This technique was executed using a wide band with a square-wave grating printed on it that was slowly moved from left to right and vice versa, rather than using the usual drum. Indeed, it was observed that if a wider part of the field of vision was covered by the grating, the nystagmus was favored.

The second examination method was the preferential look. The results showed us that the child responded up to 6-c/g gratings. This dimension corresponds approximately to 2/10, which is the font size of children books.

10.5 Evaluation of Visual, Perceptive, and Motor Functions: Clinical Case 2

The patient can evaluate after having bandaged his RE to counterbalance diplopia and without wearing the glasses prescribed for a slight myopia and astigmatism. There was a vertical nystagmus movement more evident in the RE at the beginning of the evaluation that successively also appeared in the LE. The patient could follow horizontal movements only by completely moving his head, whereas he could more easily follow vertical movements without needing to move his head too much. A least eye movement was observed toward the nose direction. There was no great difference between the RE and LE. The monocular sight evaluation was 1/10 for the RE and 3/10 for the LE both at a distance and from a proximal point; however, we recommend using characters 5 mm or larger.

There was a slow convergence movement, and it was not possible to elicit efficient saccadic movements, but, even in this case, the patient could compensate by using the movement of his head. He could perform a correct scanning of stimuli adequately segregated in a stimulus. The peripheral awareness of the stimuli was normal.

The global framework of the patient was quite complex. The brain damage caused a variable-angle strabismus and a vertical nystagmus in both eyes, more evident in the RE. This implies a diplopia, which during the evaluation was not compensated for by bandaging of the nondominant eye. In cases such as this one, patients complain mainly about diplopia, which is even more disturbing than possible blurred or unfocused images because of ametropias. In this case it was not possible to use compensatory prismatic lenses because of the variability of the deviation angle; therefore, the only possible solution was to bandage the LE to enhance the remaining vision.

The patient used an ophthalmic correction for a slight myopia and astigmatism. During the evaluation the usual glasses were taken off to favor focusing at a test distance of 50 cm.

It is useful to consider that in the range of age of the patient (37.6 years of age), it is possible to observe the first signs of presbyopia.

The patient was only able to perform horizontal pursuit movements with complete involvement of his head. This shows a sufficient foveal functionality that stimulates motor responses, first of all ocular and then also compensatory, such as the movement of the head and the trunk, to keep the image inside of the macula region. However, in this particular case this causes the performance to slow down. The vertical pursuit was less difficult, and the patient could perform it with a smaller movement of his head. The convergence movements were possible, but slow. This led us to use a single working distance where we placed all of the objects that the patient should see.

The evaluation of the visual acuity showed a marked reduction in the RE (1/10) and the LE (3/10) from a long and a short distance. Regarding the RE, these results showed an ability to recognize 3-mm letters at a 50-cm distance. This figure was obtained in the best possible conditions with isolated stimuli and without any pressure. The suggestion was therefore to use a character size of at least 5 mm to make the recognition easier even when the fixation was not perfectly centered on the letter itself. At the same time, the letter was not too big and the patient was not forced to shift his look when scanning.

It was impossible to elicit a saccadic movement oriented toward a definite stimulus because the patient even in this case compensated with his head by turning toward the significant element in his perceptual space. These movements obviously result slower than a saccadic movement and they are not adequate to read fluently and with continuity. Even the accuracy of the movements was very low, and it is extremely easy to point on an unnecessary stimulus when the movements are very close to each other. To increase the accuracy of the gaze, the stimuli should therefore be less frequent by increasing the distance between each other. This suggestion is in contrast with the previous one, relating to the difficulty to perform horizontal movements; therefore, in this case the best combination of separation and collocation must be assessed empirically.

10.6 Visual Training

These short notes illustrate one of the possible alternative solutions offered by optometry. In many patients the limited visual skills may be improved through special techniques that stimulate the vision and are reunited under the denomination of visual training (Adler 2002; Gallaway 2002; Shainberg 2010). Visual training is not only a specific training for the eyes, it is also an integrated sequence of procedures that increase the efficiency of vision, especially through multichannel stimulation protocols (sight, hearing, touch, proprioception, balance, etc.) and through the integration of cognitive aspects (Martinoli and Delpino 2009).

The reason to mention this opportunity is that many patients have been observed who show such a low visual ability that the range of alternative choices in the assistive technologies is very limited but also show a relevant potential. To obtain even the slightest improvement can allow for the use of more efficient instruments with a positive feedback in addition to the improved vision, so that a positive cycle is triggered. This can be true in cases in which marked difficulties in slow pursuit while sitting can be reduced in a supine position.

Evidently the interferences induced by the need for postural control eliminate every possibility of working efficiently when sitting. For these children the use of a computer provided with a cursor would not be possible because they would not be able to follow the trajectory and would be forced to search for the cursor every time they lost fixation. Alternatively, a large cursor, so that it could be easily recuperated, or an excessively slow cursor should be used, but a great part of the interactive functions would be lost. These children should be asked to follow some visual training programs that are aimed at enhancing their pursuit function in different postures. The description of the techniques used is not related to the aim of this book, but in short we can state that we act starting from the situations at a minimum visual and postural load and then we gradually increase the interfering elements in the most ecologic perspective (Padula 1996, Sabel and Kasten 2000).

The use of instruments that cause unnatural alterations, as well as the use of stereoscopic and polarizing systems is limited, except for the twin prisms. This kind of lens produces a distortion in the perceived environment that induces a reflex of posture adjustment. As long as the child develops even a minimal pursuit skill, his/her ability to use more efficient assistive technologies can be verified.

10.7 Conclusions

This chapter aimed at showing the role of the visual process, conceived as a complex skill involving both peripheral and central aspects, when choosing the appropriate assistive technology. Some procedural and technical aspects have been purposefully omitted because they are too complex to be integrated in this project. We tried anyway to provide some simple operative advice to the optometrists who are approaching the world of the ATA.

The importance of the role played by vision must be understood by all operators. We usually tend to interfere with the visual abilities of the patient, observing him in a non-structured environment, during interviews or during functional assessments. In each of these conditions, the response we expect from the visual system may vary consistently, although there is no clear evidence of this happening. Observing the patient as he/she comfortably explores objects in a room should not lead us into believing that a similarly appropriate scanning pattern can reproduce the same situation as the patient is asked to explore images on a piece of paper at a 30-cm distance from his/her face. This situation often proves to be correct, but this is not always the case. If not, we run the risk of blaming a more central limitation to create some constraints that could be avoided using a targeted approach.

The other point that deserves our attention is that we never have to rely on the functional assessment of vision. Experience shows that even in the worst cases, except the blindness cases, the visual residue can be used, no matter how big or small it is, to undertake all activities and to use all of the instruments suggested. Sometimes it will be necessary use very specific technical tools, such as twin prisms; other times it will be necessary to use unorthodox solutions, which usually prove themselves to be effective.

As far as the skill of the optometrist is specifically concerned, we underline the importance of experiencing the environment of the assistive technologies. The professional role of an optometrist needs to mix with the requests of the operators, who want the optometrist to tell them which path to follow. Optometrists must be also able to recognize their limits when it comes to suggesting certain solutions, as in clinical case 2. Although the functioning of the vision and the limits of the patients are clear to the professional, only an empirical assessment will permit determining the best solution.

In conclusion, the optometrist has various tools to assess each aspect of the vision. However, in this sector we will usually find ourselves in the condition of literally having to reinvent tools for very special cases. We always have to take into account the present function and not just the quantification of the patient's deficiency.

Summary of the Chapter

Vision is a complex process that combines several subprocesses and involves various anatomical structures. The analysis of visual abilities made by the optometrist should always provide some basic information in a way that allows other ATA team specialists to adapt their interventions. In the first of the five sections of the chapter, the anatomical structures and physiology of the visual pathways are briefly described. The second section describes the basic visual skills that contribute to efficient vision and the methods used to investigate it. The third section examines the importance of the optometrist as an expert who is able to select the information necessary for the implementation of the process of ATA. In the fourth section, two clinical cases are described and the assessment procedures used in the cases are explained. In the last section special techniques of visual training are briefly described.

Acknowledgments

The authors thank Loreti Alessandra for figure drawings.

References

Adler, P. (2002). Efficacy of treatment for convergence insufficiency using vision therapy. *Ophthalmic & Physiology Optics, 22*(6), 565–571.

Bardini, R. (1982). *La Funzione Visiva Nell'analisi Optometrica.* Società Italiana d'Optometria. Asti.

Birnbaum, M. H. (1985). Nearpoint visual stress: Clinical implications. *Journal of the American Optometric Association, 56*(6), 480–490.

Birnbaum M. H. (1993). *Optometric Management of Nearpoint Vision Disorders.* Oxford, UK: Butterworth Heinemann.

Catalano, F. (2006). *Elementi di Ottica Generale.* Bologna, Italy: Zanichelli.

Contreras, R., Ghajar, J., Bahar, S., and Suh, M. (2011). Effect of cognitive load on eye-target synchronization during smooth pursuit eye movement. *Brain Research,* 1398, 55–63.

Denes, G., and Pizzamiglio, L. (1996). *Manuale Di Neuropsicologia.* Bologna, Italy: Zanichelli.

Gallaway, M. (2002). Optometric vision therapy. *Binocular Vision & Strabismus Quarterly, 17*(2), 82.

Greene, H. H., Pollatsek, A., Masserang, K., Lee, Y. J., & Rayner, K. (2010). Directional processing within the perceptual span during visual target localization. *Vision Research, 50*(13), 1274–1282.

Griffin, J. (1982). *Binocular Anomalies Procedures for Vision Therapy.* Oxford, UK: Butterworth-Heinemann.

Hubel, D. H. (1995). *Eye, Brain and Vision.* Scientific American Library, No. 22. New York: WH Freeman.

Leslie, S. (2004). The optometrist's role in learning difficulties and dyslexia. *Clinical and Experimental Optometry Journal, 87*(1), 1–3.

Liuzzi, L., and Bartoli, F. (2002). *Manuale di Oftalmologia.* Torino, Italy: Minerva Medica.

Martinoli, C., and Delpino, E. (2009). *Manuale di Riabilitazione Visiva per Ciechi ed Ipovedenti.* Milan, Italy: FrancoAngelo.

Orlandi, M. (2003). I Deficit Visivi nella Dislessia. *Acta Phoniatrica Latina, XXV,* 85–95.

Padula V. W. (1996). *Neuro-Optometric Rehabilitation,* Santa Ana, CA: Optometric Extension Program.

Phillips, M. H., and Edelman, J. A. (2008). The dependence of visual scanning performance on search direction and difficulty. *Vision Research, 48*(21), 2184–2192.

Rossetti, A., and Gheller, P. (1997). *Manuale di Optometria e Contattologia.* Bologna, Italy: Zanichelli.

Sabbadini, G., Bianchi P. E., Fazzi E., and Sabbadini M. (2000). *Manuale di Neuroftalmologia dell'età Evolutiva.* Milan, Italy: Franco Angeli.

Sabel, B. A., and Kasten, E. (2000). Restoration of vision by training of residual functions. *Current Opinion in Ophthalmology, 11*(6), 430–436.

Saunders, K. J., Little, J. A., McClelland, J. F., and Jackson, A. J. (2010). Profile of refractive errors in cerebral palsy: Impact of severity of motor impairment (GMFCS) and CP subtype on refractive outcome. *Investigative Ophthalmology and Visual Science, 51*(6), 2885–2890.

Shainberg, M. J. (2010). Vision therapy and orthoptics. *The American Orthoptic Journal, 60,* 28–32.

Traccis, S. (1992). *Il Nistagmo Fisiologico e Patologico.* Bologna, Italy: Pàtron Editore.

Traccis, S., and Zambarbieri D. (1992). *I Movimenti Saccadici.* Bologna, Italy: Pàtron Editore.

Traccis, S., and Zambarbieri D. (1996). *Le Interazioni Visuo-Vestibolari.* Bologna, Italy: Pàtron Editore.

Yeotikar, N. S., Khuu, S. K., Asper, L. J., and Suttle, C. M. (2011). Configuration specificity of crowding in peripheral vision. *Vision Research, 51*(11), 1239–1248.

Suggested Reading

American Academy of Ophthalmology. (2001). *Complementary Therapy Assessment: Vision Therapy for Learning Disabilities,* Retrieved from http://one.aao.org/CE/PracticeGuidelines/ Therapy_Content.aspx?cid=8021c013–7e4b-43f3-aa1a-698307ae526c

American Academy of Ophthalmology. (2004). *Complementary Therapy Assessment. Visual Training for Refractive Errors.* Retrieved from http://one.aao.org/asset.axd?id=2907836b-705a-4509-b86f-e2c493b7ca0

Bankes, J. L. (1974). Eye defects of mentally handicapped children. *British Medical Journal, 8*(5918), 533–535.

Barrett, B. T. (2009). A critical evaluation of the evidence supporting the practice of behavioral vision therapy. *Ophthalmic & Physiological Optics, 29*(1), 4–25.

Birnbaum, M. H., Soden, R., and Cohen, A. H. (1999). Efficacy of vision therapy for convergence insufficiency in an adult male population. *Journal of the American Optometric Association, 70,* 225–232.

Di Blasi, F. D., Elia, F., Buono, S., Ramakers, G. J, and Di Nuovo, S. F. (2007). Relationships between visual-motor and cognitive abilities in intellectual disabilities. *Perceptual and Motor Skills, 104*(3 Pt 1), 763–772.

Forrest, E. B. (1976). Clinical manifestations of visual information processing. *Journal of the American Optometric Association, 47*(1), 73–80.

Harris, J. M., Nefs, H. T., and Grafton, C. E. (2008). Binocular vision and motion-in-depth. *Spatial Vision, 21*(6), 531–547.

Jennings, J. A. M. (2000). Behavioral optometry: A critical review. *Optometric Practice, 1,* 67.

Judica, A., De Luca, M., Di Pace, E., Orlandi, M., Spinelli, D., and Zoccolotti, P. (1998). Dislessia superficiale in un soggetto adulto: Analisi del comportamento di lettura e trattamento riabilitativo. *Archivio di Psicologia Neurologia ePsichiatria, LIX,* 729–755.

Lavrich, J. B. (2010). Convergence insufficiency and its current treatment. *Current Opinion in Ophthalmology, 21*(5), 356–360.

Sabbadini, G., Bonini P., Pezzarossa B., and Pierro M. (1978). *Paralisi Cerebrali e Condizioni Affini.* Rome: Il Pensiero Scientifico Editore.

Scheiman, M. (2002). *Understanding and Managing Vision Deficits: A Guide for Occupational Therapists,* 2nd ed. Philadelphia: Slack Inc.

Scheiman, M., Mitchell, G. L., Cotter, S., Kulp, M. T., Cooper, J., Rouse, M., et al. (2005). A randomized clinical trial of vision therapy/orthoptics versus pencil pushups for the treatment of convergence insufficiency in young adults. *Optometry and Vision Science, 123*(1), 14–24.

Scheiman, M. M., and Rouse, M. W. (2006). *Optometric Management of Learning-Related Vision Problems,* 2nd ed. St. Louis, MO: Mosby Elsevier.

Scheiman, M., Rouse, M., Kulp, M. T., Cotter, S., Hertle, R., and Lynn, M. G. (2009). Treatment of convergence insufficiency in childhood: A current perspective. *Optometry and Vision Science, 86*(5), 420–428.

Skeffington, A. M. (1964). *Introduction to Clinical Optometry.* Optometric Extension Programme Continuing Education Courses, Vol. 37. Santa Ana, CA: Optometric Extension Program.

Solt, I. (2001). The representation of the egocentric space in the posterior parietal cortex. *Harefuah, 140*(6), 553–557.

Stein, J. F. (1989). Representation of egocentric space in the posterior parietal cortex. *Quarterly Journal of Experimental Physiology, 74*(5), 583–606.

U.S. Preventive Services Task Force. (2004). Screening for visual impairment in children younger than age 5 years: Recommendation statement. *Annals of Family Medicine, 2*(3), 263–266.

Vera-Diaz, F. A., Gwiazda, J., Thorn, F., and Held, R. (2004). Increased accommodation following adaptation to image blur in myopes. *Journal of Vision, 4*(12), 1111–1119.

Vora, U., Khandekar, R., Natrajan, S., and Al-Hadrami, K. (2010). Refractive error and visual functions in children with special needs compared with the first grade school students in Oman. *Middle East African Journal of Ophthalmology, 17*(4), 297–302.

Zoccolotti, P., Angelelli, P., Colombini, M. G., De Luca, M., Di Pace, E., Judica, A., et al. (1997). Caratteristiche della dislessia superficiale evolutiva nella lingua italiana. *Archivio di Neurologia e Psichiatria, LVIII,* 253–284.

11

The Occupational Therapist: Enabling Activities and Participation Using Assistive Technology

D. de Jonge, P. M. Wielandt, S. Zapf, and A. Eldridge

CONTENTS

11.1 Occupational Therapist's Perspective

Occupational therapists use a holistic approach in which they recognize the transaction among the person, the activities they need or want to engage in, and the environments in which these activities are undertaken. Occupation, or activity engagement and participation, is seen as playing an essential role in human life and influencing people's state of health (Kielhofner 2004). Disruption to occupation or activity engagement affects people's quality of life, restricts their development, reduces capacity, and leads to maladaptive reactions (Kielhofner 2004). In contrast, removing barriers to participation allows people to engage in necessary and desired occupations, which result in improved health (Kielhofner 2004).

Each person is seen as simultaneously fulfilling various roles that require them to perform a diversity of activities in a range of environments. Activities range from personal care and household activities to work, leisure, and social participation. People have personal preferences, interests, and expectations that influence their choice of activities and the way they undertake activities. Activities are invariably performed in and across a number of environments and each environment, whilst offering opportunities for participation, have physical, social, and cultural dimensions, which can provide additional challenges. Because circumstances rarely remain constant, the temporal aspect of the environment is also recognized as being important when selecting and using assistive technologies because the person's past experience with technology and their expectations for the future can have can also define their technology preferences and requirements. Increasingly, the virtual world of the Internet is an environment that people need to be able to operate in and it holds particular opportunities for people who have difficulty navigating and participating in the natural and built environments.

This transactive view of the person, activities, and the environment is supported by a number of occupational therapy models including the Person-Environment-Occupation model (Law et al. 1996) and the Person Environment Occupation Performance (PEOP) model (Christiansen and Baum 1997) and aligns well with assistive technology (AT) models such as the Human Activities and Assistive Technology (HAAT) model (Cook et al. 2002) and the Matching Person and Technology (MPT) model (Scherer 2005) as well as the International Classification of Functioning, Disability, and Health (ICF) (WHO 2001). Although the terminology and emphasis varies, the primary focus of each of these models is on optimizing activity and participation. Each model also recognizes the dynamic and reciprocal interaction among the person, activity, and the environment. All are founded on the notion of "goodness of fit," or match between the person's skills and abilities and the occupational and environmental affordances and demands. The models also reflect the values of the disability movement, in which the environment is viewed as an agent in creating disability and value (Brown 2009).

Given the complexity of each person's situation, occupational therapists use a client-centered approach in which each person's unique perspective is recognized and valued. Individuals are viewed as having distinctive personal attributes, capacities, and life experiences that influence their priorities and preferences. Evaluation methods focus on identifying the AT user's goals and specific concerns about the activities they seek to engage in and the environments where these are to be undertaken. Informal and standardized evaluation strategies are selected to ensure

- Occupational performance issues or problems are identified by the AT user and his or her family,
- The unique nature of each person's participation in occupations is recognized,
- Opportunities for both the subjective experience and the observable qualities of occupational performance are recorded,
- AT users (and relevant others) have a say in how the outcomes are evaluated,
- The unique qualities of the application environments are recognized, and
- AT users and their family are actively engaged throughout the process and afforded the opportunity to understand the perspective and concerns of each stakeholder involved in the process (Law and Baum 2005).

Once the individual's situation has been fully examined and articulated, occupational therapists then use and balance the art and science to creatively yet systematically address his or her specific goals.

11.2 Overview of Interventions Used by Occupational Therapists and the Place of AT within These

Activities are generally undertaken using a combination of strategies, tools, and social and physical supports in the environment (Dunn et al. 1994; Enders and Leech 1996). When engaging in any given activity, an individual uses a unique blend of these resources. Litvak and Enders (2001) described this support system for human accomplishment and similarly the function of people with disabilities as being variously supported by adaptive strategies (AS), assistive devices (AD) (tools), and personal assistance (PAS) or social support (see Figure 11.1).

Therapists seek to optimize activity engagement or performance by improving the fit between the person and their occupations and roles and pertinent environments. Working with the unique capacities, skills, preferences, and experiences of each individual, therapists examine how strategies, tools, and the social and physical environment are currently working to support activity engagement and how they might be modified to optimize performance. Therapists work with the client to ensure their capacities and skills have been optimized before introducing alternative strategies or tools. For example, if a therapist observes that the person is poorly positioned, he or she will examine the impact of

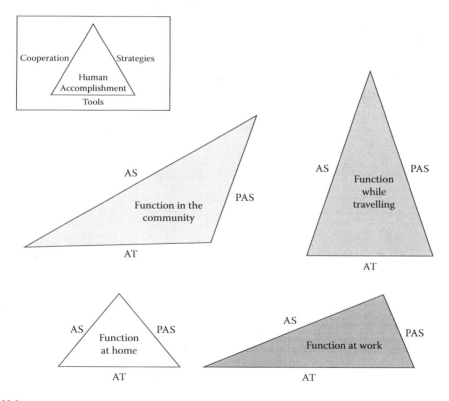

FIGURE 11.1
Generic support system for human accomplishment. (From Litvak, S. and Enders, A., *Handbook of Disability Studies*, Sage Publications, Thousand Oaks, CA, pp. 711–733, 2001.)

repositioning or supporting the person on performance before exploring assistive devices. Similarly, an individual with limited experience using a keyboard may benefit from skills training before looking to introduce an alternative access method.

Assistive technologies have long been considered an essential intervention strategy by occupational therapists (Ostensjo et al. 2005). Traditionally viewed as an accommodation for a loss of function, assistive devices were frequently prescribed by therapists on the basis of the individual's impairment. For example, a manual wheelchair would be recommended for someone with paraplegia because they could push the chair independently, whereas a motorized wheelchair would be recommended for someone with tetraplegia who was unable to use their arms to push. Little consideration would be given to the various activities the person wanted to engage in or the range of environments they sought to mobilize in. More recently, the enabling capacity of assistive technologies has been recognized and devices are selected with the aim of optimizing activities and participation in all relevant environments. With the focus on what the person needs to be able to do and where they need to do these activities, assistive technologies are being designed and selected to meet the activity and environmental demands. For example, the person with paraplegia, referred to previously, may need to move quickly across a university campus between classes and would therefore prefer a motorized chair so that they are not too exhausted from pushing a wheelchair to take notes on their laptop.

Although occupational therapists (OTs) routinely use AT to assist individuals to optimize their functional abilities, OTs also need to seek further training in AT and stay abreast on current research on AT assessment and device outcomes. The field of AT is ever changing with new technology devices added every year. In a study by Long and colleagues (2007), investigating competency levels of OTs in the area of AT, therapists were found to have decreased confidence in providing AT services in the educational setting. They found that 68% of OTs surveyed lacked confidence in evaluating an individual for AT device and service and 79% lacked confidence in selecting and matching AT to the individual needs. Long and Perry (2008) did a similar survey with pediatric physical therapists (PTs) and found that 62% of PTs surveyed lacked confidence in assessing an individual for AT and 79% lacked confidence in matching and selecting a device to needs. OTs are crucial members of the AT team because of their background in occupation performance and motor development. They can provide information to the assessment on a person's movement and function to access or position AT devices, identify key components of the whole person that can contribute or hinder the use of AT access, and identify functional performance skills and need matched to the specific features of the AT device. There is a need for more AT training for OTs to build confidence in AT assessment and delivery of services.

11.3 The Definition and Role of AT

AT is "an umbrella term for any device or system that allows individuals to perform tasks they would otherwise be unable to do or increases the ease and safety with which tasks can be performed" (World Health Organization 2004, p. 10). This definition recognizes both the physical device (hard technology) and the systems (soft technologies) that enable a person to use that technology (Cook et al. 2007; Waldron and Layton 2008).

Devices or hard technologies include equipment such as wheelchairs, seating and positioning systems, computer access technologies and specialized software, augmentative communication devices, and environmental control systems. AT ranges from simple low-tech options to sophisticated, high-tech devices (Cook et al. 2007). Low-tech options are generally simple and inexpensive devices such as bathboards, typing splints, or a communication board. High-tech options include expensive, sophisticated, dedicated technologies such as power wheelchairs, an onscreen keyboard, or an environmental control system. These devices are usually highly specialized and designed with a specific group in mind (e.g., people with tetraplegia or vision impairments). However, the devices alone are rarely enough to ensure the success of an AT intervention. Supports or soft technologies are generally required to ensure the effective use of AT. Soft technologies include customizing the device to suit the individual's specific requirements, training to enable the person to use the device, and providing support for the repair and maintenance of the device.

Many people who rely on AT use a number of devices together. People with significant impairments are often faced with complex positioning, mobility, access, and communication issues that require diverse expertise and extensive problem-solving. The AT team generally comprises rehabilitation engineers, physiotherapists, OTs, speech pathologists, educators, technicians, suppliers, and most importantly AT users. The success of the AT solution is dependent on each team member bringing their specialist knowledge and understandings to the table and working collaboratively to identify the components required and integrating these into the final solution.

11.4 Overview of the Process Involved in Selecting and Using AT

The AT user's quest for the most appropriate technology generally begins before they contact a professional, and the effective use of the device extends well beyond their encounter with an AT team. A number of steps are critical to the effective selection and use of AT, including (de Jonge et al. 2007)

- Visioning possibilities
- Establishing goals/expectations
- Identifying specific requirements
- Establishing device criteria
- Identifying potential technologies and resources
- Locating local resources and supports
- Developing a funding strategy
- Trying and evaluating options
- Purchasing the technology
- Setting up and fitting the technology
- Training
- Maintenance and repair follow-up
- Monitoring and evaluation

The process generally begins with someone envisioning doing something or anticipating the potential of technology (Alliance for Technology Access 2005). Some people come to the process with this vision, but this vision often evolves slowly throughout the process. Consequently, service providers need to embrace people's visions of what they want to be able to do and provide them with information on technologies that can enable them to realize these visions. For those who have not yet developed a vision, the OT works with them to imagine what might be possible by exploring the technology and introducing them to AT users who are using technology to achieve their goals (Baum 1998).

Once a vision has been created and the person's need and desire for technology have been identified, the potential of technology can be explored (Scherer and Galvin 1996). At this stage the therapist gathers information about the person's preferences, past experiences, and expectations of technology and examines if they are open to the use of technology and able to manage it. Further, the capacity of the application environment(s) to accept and support the technology is considered (Scherer and Galvin 1996). Although some AT users can have very clear and specific goals (Sprigle and Abdelhamied 1998) others require further assistance to develop and articulate their goals (Scherer 2000). Therapists often collaborate with other stakeholders (e.g., family, teachers, therapists, or employers) to develop specific goals and expectations if the AT user is uncertain or unable to articulate their gaols (Nochajski and Oddo 1995; Scherer and Galvin, 1996; Sprigle and Abdelhamied 1998; Cook et al. 2007).

Therapists commonly use informal interviews to develop an understanding of a person's goals; however, structured processes offered by tools such as the Canadian Occupational Performance Measure (COPM) (Law et al. 1994) can assist in developing an understanding of the person's current performance and priorities. This and similar tools such as Goal Attainment Scaling (GAS) (Malec 1999) and the Individualized Prioritised Problem Assessment (IPPA) (Wessels et al. 2002) also provide a mechanism for evaluating the effectiveness of the technology in addressing the person's goals. The MPT assessment process, specifically designed to examine a person's technology needs, has dedicated forms that provide a structure for exploring goals, preferences, and the person's view of technology (Scherer 2000). Once the person's overall goals have been determined, the specific requirements can be detailed.

The next stage of the process focuses on establishing the user's specific requirements (Bain and Leger 1997; Sprigle and Abdelhamied 1998; Kelker and Holt 2000; Cook et al. 2007). A clear understanding of the user's requirements is essential to identifying the best technology (Sprigle and Abdelhamied 1998). Therapists have traditionally focussed on anthropometric data such as the person's age, size, weight, etc. (Sprigle and Abdelhamied 1998) to determine the appropriate dimensions of the device. Further, the person's specific skills and abilities have been evaluated (Bain and Leger 1997; Sprigle and Abdelhamied, 1998; Cook et al. 2007). Many AT users with established impairments are able to provide a reliable report of their functional capacities that would be sufficient to enable the service provider to identify the type of technology options to explore without the need for further assessment. However, it is often more useful to examine the person's ability to access and use the technology to develop a clear understanding of the user's actual abilities because it is not always possible to predict how well someone will manage a piece of technology.

When establishing user's requirements, it is also necessary to define the requirements of the activity/activities to be undertaken. Valued activities identified by the AT user are examined in detail to understand how they want to engage in these activities and all of the tasks involved in full participation. By defining discrete tasks, the barriers to participation and performance can be examined for all aspects of the activity. For example, wheelchairs were traditionally designed to allow people with injuries and health conditions to mobilize on flat surfaces from one location to another. Today, our understanding of where and how people move within a community and the value of being at eye level with others has resulted in a number of features being incorporated into the design of wheelchairs that has substantially contributed to the wheelchair user's ability to actively participate in society.

Similarly, a thorough understanding of the environments in which the person wishes to participate now and in the near future also provides a richer and more accurate appreciation of the technology requirements (Bain and Leger 1997; Cook et al. 2007). Because OTs seek to extend rather than confine the AT user's participation, they seek to ensure that the technology can operate in and move between as many environments as possible. The potential demands of the environment, likely to affect technology, typically include the physical aspects (i.e., the topography, temperature, climate, sound, and lighting conditions) (Bain and Leger 1997; Cook et al. 2007), the milieu or psychological, social, and cultural aspects of the application environment (Scherer 2000; Cook et al. 2007). The technology also needs to work well with other technologies in the environment. The aesthetic appeal of the technology and its impact on other's perception of the user is increasingly being recognized as a critical consideration.

Once the requirements are clearly articulated, the device criteria/characteristics can be established (Bain and Leger 1997; Kelker and Holt 2000; Alliance for Technology Access 2005). The user's goals determine the nature of technology, whereas their preferences influence the style of device. A user's experience with technology often dictates the level of sophistication, whereas their skills and abilities would determine the interfaces and programming requirements. The range of activities and tasks dictates the specific features and functions required of the technology system(s) whereas the range of application environments determines the characteristics required of the technology to ensure it can manage and be managed in the application environments.

With an ever-expanding range of mainstream and specialized technologies available, it is increasingly difficult to distinguish between them (Alliance for Technology Access 2005). Therapists work with the AT user and other team members to develop a good understanding of the range of devices available and the features and characteristics that are best suited to the user, the activities he or she wishes to engage in, and the environments where the technology is to be used. During this stage it is imperative to trial the device and allow the user to review the aesthetics, comfort, and usability of the device. The trial further affords the user, the therapist, and other team members an opportunity to evaluate how each device meets the criteria and discuss the relative merits of each option (Scherer and Galvin 1996; Bain and Leger 1997; Sprigle and Abdelhamied 1998; Alliance for Technology Access 2005; Cook et al. 2007).

Therapists also assist the user to explore funding sources and navigate the administrative processes to secure the appropriate technology. Once the best device is selected (Nochajski and Oddo 1995; Alliance for Technology Access 2005), it is then purchased (Cook et al. 2007). Although many consider the purchase of the device to be the end of the process, for the AT user, there are an important number of stages they need to continue to manage.

After the device is purchased, it may need to be fitted to the specific requirements of the user (Nochajski and Oddo 1995; Scherer and Galvin 1996; Bain and Leger 1997; Kelker and Holt 2000; Alliance for Technology Access 2005; Cook et al. 2007) and set up by someone with appropriate expertise (Scherer and Galvin 1996; Cook et al. 2007) to ensure it is operating as intended and is integrated with other technologies (Nochajski and Oddo 1995). Many devices require further customization after purchase to ensure the device is adjusted to the specific requirements of the user when undertaking various tasks in a range of environments. The ongoing effectiveness of technology is dependent on the comfort and ease of the user when using the device for extended periods of time. Recently, research has raised concerns about the amount of pain and discomfort technology users experience and the long-term implications of this pain (Cowan and Turner-Smith 1999; Patterson et al. 2002). Technology interventions need to be adjusted to ensure that use does not result in discomfort and strain (Scherer and Vitaliti 1997).

Training in use of the device is also fundamental to the ongoing effectiveness of technology interventions (Nochajski and Oddo 1995; Kelker and Holt 2000; Cook et al. 2007). Without adequate training, the technology is likely to be abandoned (Cook et al. 2007). OTs, who are often responsible for training, ensure the effectiveness of this stage by establishing well-defined objectives (Cook et al. 2007). AT users need to develop both "operational and strategies competence" (Cook et al. 2007) for successful AT use. Operational competence ensures that the user is able to turn the device on and off, adjust the various features, understands the maintenance requirements, and can troubleshoot problems. "Strategies competence (Cook et al. 2007) enables the user to use the device to perform specific tasks. Although operational training can be provided soon after delivery, strategic training is most effective in situ (Nochajski and Oddo 1995) when the user can develop skills in using the device to complete activities in the application environment(s). AT users also need to know how to maintain the device and who to contact when it is in need of repair (Kelker and Holt 2000).

Periodic reevaluation is required because there are likely to be ongoing changes in terms of the user's skills and abilities, the activities they wish to engage in, and the application environments that will affect the effectiveness of the acquired technology. Scherer (2005) identified possible factors that were associated with nonuse of AT in adults with disabilities included unrealistic expectations, inappropriate needs assessment, poor device selection, lack of support from caregivers, changes in person's abilities, or any combination. These findings indicate the importance of reassessment and need for follow-up of AT to ensure that the AT solutions are effective and decrease the potential for AT abandonment. Further, as technologies continue to improve, the user may benefit from technological developments. Ongoing monitoring of the effectiveness of the technology and developments in the design of devices ensures that technology interventions are replaced and upgraded as required.

11.5 Overview of the Process Involved in Selecting and Using AT Case Studies

The case studies will use the PEO (Person, Environment, Occupation) format used by OTs in practice.

11.5.1 Case Study Number 1: ZA

11.5.1.1 Person

ZA is a 21-month-old female toddler who presents with neurological delays secondary to hypoxic-ischemic encephalopathy. She has a diagnosis of congenital quadriplegia and hypermetropia. She was born at 41 weeks, distocical birth, and vacuum was applied to assist with delivery. ZA was born with serious medical complications and an Apgar score of 1; she was reanimated, incubated, and moved to the pediatric intensive care unit, where she received neurorehabilitative care for 40 days. She was discharged home to parents, and therapy services continued through an early childhood intervention (ECI) service program. She has received occupational, physical, and speech therapy services through the ECI program since birth.

11.5.1.2 Current Status

This case will discuss the role of occupational therapy in the delivery of AT for ZA through the ECI program. The early intervention team's evaluation of ZA's current level of performance was discussed with her parents at their annual review plan meeting. The team used the ICF-CY model to assess her performance; her scores are as follows:

- *Psychosocial/emotional skills:* ZA is an attentive female toddler and motivated to learn. She has a very supportive family and a good relationship with the health professionals she has worked with. She is engaged in therapy sessions and appears to try her best even when she is frustrated. She enjoys social interactions with her siblings and peers. The speech–language pathologist (SLP) and OT have looked into various augmentive and alternative communication (AAC) devices and have tried some basic devices with switch selection. ZA is just learning to make choices among three items using visual scan.

- *Cognitive:* ZA is able to sustain attention and learns best through visual model/ representation versus kinetic learning because of her physical impairments. She understands cause and effect and seems to understand basic concepts with use of adapted toys during play and exploration. She is able to attend to task and sustain attention.

- *Visual-perceptual:* ZA has hypermetropia (but within physiological age-level) and a symmetric corneal reflex. She has a sporadic convergence and a latency delay with visual processing/fixating on target. She currently uses her visual system to scan items for communication.

- *Physical:* ZA has paralysis in both her upper and lower extremities (complete motor impairment ICF-CY: S-730-4, 750-4) and relies on primitive reflexes to elicit motor movement. She has increased tone (hypertonia) and still displays primitive reflexes. She is able to sit supported in her manual wheelchair with an adapted seating system and headrest, and the therapists have been working on increasing her head control. She does use an asymmetrical tonic neck reflex (ATNR) pattern to reach toward an item, but she is unable to grasp the item because of decreased functional hand use. She wears resting hand splints at night to facilitate a neutral hand position and decrease contractures. ZA also wears bilateral ankle-foot orthotics (AFOs) to decrease tone and maintain position to prevent contractures. She has been able to hit a wheelchair-mounted switch using her ATNR to activate her adapted toys with a wobble switch. She has decreased head control, but she does keep her head up when supported with an adapted headrest. The OT and PT have placed a head switch on her headrest, and she has been successful with using this to access her toys and computer. She is able to maintain visual fixation when her head is supported by an adaptive head collar for 10–15 min; this has greatly improved over the past year.

- *Spiritual:* ZA attends church with her family. They are engaged in church events and believe they have a strong support system within their church family.

11.5.1.3 Environment

ZA lives at home with her biological parents and one older sister, age 6. They have a family dog that ZA adores and ZA's parents have taught the dog to retrieve items that ZA has dropped. Her sister enjoys playing with ZA and will play the piano for her. The family is involved in their local church and enjoys being active in the community. Her parents have expressed concerns on how to adapt their home environment to optimize ZA's independence.

11.5.1.4 Occupation

- *Activities of daily living:* ZA is dependent with all dressing and hygiene needs. She will extend her arm using the ATNR to assist with dressing but relies on her parents for her self-care needs. She is dependent for all grooming and hygiene needs because of physical limitations. The OT and SLP are working on ZA using an eye gaze system to tell her mother the routine of her personal skills (teaching early self-advocacy skills). ZA is currently dependent with her feeding and does eat three meals; again the OT and SLP are encouraging parents to use eye gaze to make choices of preferred meal items. ZA enjoys making choices and smiles when she gets to choose dessert because she enjoys chocolate cake.
- *Play and leisure:* ZA is attentive and enjoys being engaged various activities in the playroom. Her occupational and physical therapists have been using switch access for play activities and functional learning skills. She is currently using a head switch to access computer early learning activities. She loves music and is engaged in computer-based learning tasks that use music as a positive reward. The OT also adapted the music stereo at ZA's church so she can access and play the music while attending church. ZA is currently using a manual wheelchair with adapted seating, and the PT is working on positioning need when in her wheelchair. She has tried some built-up handle items but seems to do better with a universal cuff when holding items/materials during art and play.
- ZA is in the stage of novice user at the age of 21 months as the family and therapists are becoming familiar with her skill level matched to skills needed for potential devices. The ECI team identified ZA's personal characteristic that can influence her use of AT solutions. The ECI team indicated that ZA is very motivated and determined to complete her tasks. She seems willing to learn new strategies and does not get frustrated despite her physical limitations. Her parents are very involved in her care and appear to be comfortable with technology.
- *AT plan of intervention:*
  - Set up home environmental modifications to enhance the ZA's independence through an environmental control system and toy adaptations using switch access.
  - *Mobility:* OT/PT will assess potential skills needed for ZA's ability to activate an electric wheelchair with a head switch to increase independence in mobility.

- OT and SLP will discuss with parents options for a communication device and skills needed for ZA to be successful in this area. The parents have expressed an interest in using a device, and ZA seems motivated by voice output.
- Complete AAC assessment with the SLP to determine the need for an AAC device.
- Trial the recommended AAC device and make a determination on the basis of the trial results. Discuss funding options with parents and AAC company.
- Training plan for AAC device to ensure optimal use in all settings.
- *Transitional needs*
  - ECI team to coordinate transitional AT needs when ZA is ready to attend the preschool program for children with disabilities offered through her local special education agency.
  - Training of others involved in the care of ZA.

11.5.2 Case Study Number 2: AB

11.5.2.1 Person

AB is a 59-year-old male who presented to the hospital with a left middle cerebral artery (MCA) ischemic stroke. He was having dinner with his wife when he suddenly slumped in his chair and was unable to move his right side and could not speak. The wife phoned EMS and the patient was admitted to the local hospital. Upon admission, the physician reported a facial droop, complete paralysis in arm and leg, flaccid in arm and leg, and global aphasia. The patient also appeared to have a visual field cut. The computed tomography (CT) scan showed early MCA regional changes indicative of a large ischemic stroke. The patient's NIHSS was 2.3, and he received tPA at 2.35 h poststroke with only minimal improvements noted. A referral was made to the rehabilitation team 24 h after tPA.

Upon assessment by the OT and PT, AB was able to make some incomprehensible words, understand gestures, and only inconsistently follow simple (one-step) commands. His wife was present and stated that he was healthy before admission, playing golf in the summer and indoor soccer during the winter. They have three adult children and two grandchildren and are a close family. AB always enjoyed spending time (on an almost-daily basis) with his grandchildren who live close by. AB works as a supervisor for a construction company and spends most of his day in the office, but at times he is required to drive to the various construction sites. His wife works part-time as an administrative assistant at a local school and cares for both grandchildren each Wednesday and Saturday. She appears to be having difficulty coping with her husband's illness and is worried about the future because they were both looking forward to retirement and spending more time with family.

A physical evaluation showed that AB had difficulty with a shoulder shrug, and upon testing the therapist was able to feel some resistance in the biceps, although the hand remained flaccid. On the Chedoke assessment, the patient scored arm = 2 and the hand = 1. With assistance, AB was able to roll to his right side by using the bedrail and only required assistance from one person. During moving from lying to sitting, AB required a two-person assist. He was unable to maintain his core sitting balance but once placed in midline he could maintain his sitting for approximately 30 s. During therapy, AB fatigued after approximately 10 min and was required to be transferred to a high-back wheelchair using a two-person assist. AB was then able to sit up in his wheelchair chair for approximately 1 h. His alpha FIM score was 7.

AB spent the next 19 days in acute care where the OT saw the patient 4–5 times per week and worked on his sitting balance, transfers, upper extremity training, and his grooming tasks. Upon arrival to the tertiary rehabilitation facility, AB seemed withdrawn and had limited eye contact with staff. Furthermore, he only answered questions put to him when staff offered a large amount of encouragement.

11.5.2.2 Current Status

Within the next 3 weeks AB will be discharged to home from rehabilitation, and his current status is thus:

- *Person:*
  - *Cognition:* AB is able to follow simple verbal commands and say some words accurately, although his speech remained mostly incomprehensible. He uses a lot of nonverbal language to get his message across. Because of his difficulties with language it has been difficult to fully assess all aspects of his cognition. The OT has observed that there may be difficulties with his executive functioning but has so far been unable to determine the extent of these difficulties.
  - *Emotional:* AB finds his difficulties with communication extremely frustrating. This has resulted in him lashing out at staff, his wife, and his children. This frustration has limited his progress in rehabilitation because he often finds it difficult to remain engaged in therapy tasks. AB has a supportive family and this has helped his progress in rehabilitation. His wife visited most days during his stay in rehabilitation. His children have also visited regularly, except when restricted by work or family commitments. He has been very focused on his discharge home, and at times he has used this as a motivator to continue to work toward his therapy goals.
  - *Physical:* AB continues to have a right facial droop. Because he failed his swallow assessment in acute care he has had a percutaneous endoscopic gastrostomy (PEG) tube inserted. Assessment revealed that AB does have a left visual field cut. His arm improved to a Chedoke score of arm = 4 and hand = 2. He started to develop tone in his right side and was seen daily by the therapist assistant for passive range of motion (PROM). His leg improved to a Chedoke score of leg = 4 and foot = 1. AB is now able to sit unsupported, but when displaced out of his base of support he loses his balance to the left. On the unit AB can transfer using a sask-a-pole and one-person assist. Within the therapy unit he is able to undertake various transfers with a one-person assist. He is now able to walk 3 × 5 m in the parallel bars using an AFO and assistance from the PT. Daily he is able to sit in his wheelchair for most of the day, taking a nap after lunch and before the 3:00 p.m. therapy session. He attends a 30-min exercise class with the therapy assistant in the morning, a 30- to 45-min therapy session with the OT in the morning, and a 30-min session with the PT in the afternoon. There was no therapy coverage on the weekends.

- *Spiritual:* Before his admission in hospital AB regularly attended mass at his local church, and his wife reported that this was an important part of his life. Attending church is a priority for him once he returns home.

- *Environment:* AB's wife visits him daily and she assists with his grooming tasks. She seems overwhelmed and is having difficulty coping with the situation. She has indicated on several occasions that between coming to the hospital and looking after things at home she feels extremely stressed. Previously AB had taken care of the family finances and his wife is now having difficulties with paying bills, etc. She is most reluctant to ask for assistance from her children and was referred to the social worker. Because AB will be unable to return to work for sometime, his wife is concerned about how this decrease in income will affect the family finances. AB and his wife live in a bungalow house with stairs to the basement in a small country town that is an approximate 2-h drive to a regional town. Previously AB was responsible for all of the yard work including lawn-mowing in the summer and snow-shoveling during the winter. His wife is primarily responsible for most of the instrumental activities of daily living (IADLs); however, AB used to drive his wife for their grocery shopping excursions to the nearest large town. His wife has always been reluctant to drive (especially during winter months) and will only drive on familiar routes and not long distances. AB's children have agreed to assist with driving while he is recovering; however, they will not always be available because of their own commitments. His three adult children live locally and are able to assist with chores and grocery shopping on the weekends; however, they cannot assist during the week because of their own work commitments. The grandchildren will visit regularly as they did before the stroke. His wife has decided that she can no longer cope with looking after the grandchildren during the week, and AB feels responsible for this.

- Occupation:

  - *Activities of Daily Living (ADLs):* AB is able to wash his face and upper body sitting in a wheelchair in front of the sink with objects placed within reach for him. He is able to brush his teeth (wife assists with putting the toothpaste on the brush), comb his hair, and shave using an electrical shaver. The tasks require extra time, but AB is able to accomplish them independently. AB can use the urinal and commode and has no continence issues. He moves around the unit propelling himself whilst sitting in a low-back wheelchair using his left arm and leg to mobilize. AB has not engaged in any instrumental activities of daily living while in the rehabilitation facility.

  - *Leisure:* Because of his current functional limitations AB is unable to participate in the previously valued activities of playing golf and indoor soccer. During rehabilitation the OT worked with AB to discover some new leisure activities that he can successfully participate in. AB has expressed interest in working toward continuing to participate in his prior leisure activities, but he stated he is also open to trying more "sedentary" pursuits, such as reading and top-based activities. He has yet to find an activity that he finds relaxing and enjoyable that he can complete independently, and this is an important goal for his recovery.

  - *Work/Productive Occupations:* At his current level of functioning AB will be unable to return to work. His job and his role as provider for his wife are very valuable to him, and being able to return to work in some capacity is one of AB's key goals after discharge from the rehabilitation facility.

- *Issues to be dealt with prior to discharge:*
  - Return to work/driving.
  - Transfers at home.
  - *Independent mobility:* Consider use of one-arm drive wheelchair or a powered wheelchair if endurance is an issue.
  - Environmental assessment for successful use of a mobility device in different environments (inside home, yard, work, church, etc.).
  - Environmental modifications (home environment as a priority, but others also).
  - Referral to a community domiciliary nursing organization to assist with ADL completion and to reduce some of the impact on AB's wife. Any prescribed equipment for ADL tasks should be compatible with assistance from a domiciliary nursing organization (e.g., shower chairs, etc.).
  - Communication device.
  - Once communication device has been prescribed, reattempt to assess cognition.
  - AT to be used at home, e.g., lower-limb dressing.
  - Plan developed for re-engagement in valued leisure activities or exposure to new activities that AB expresses interest in. May require a combination of task grading and AT.
  - Plan developed for re-engagement in church and church activities.
  - Investigate avenues of career support for AB's wife and family.

11.6 Conclusions

OTs use a holistic approach that supports the use of AT solutions for individuals with various disabilities. OTs are able to combine their knowledge of a person's psychosocial, cognitive, physical, and neurological skills and identify how these systems can affect the person's overall participation in functional and meaningful occupations. Understanding the person's area of need and current level of performance, OTs can identify AT solutions that best match the person's skill to device features. As the field of AT continues to evolve, OTs must stay abreast on current technology solutions utilizing current AT research, clinical experience, and patient values to make the best-practice decisions in AT solutions for the individuals they serve.

Summary of the Chapter

This chapter details the unique contribution of occupational therapists to the selection and utilization of assistive technologies. Occupational therapists use a holistic approach which recognizes the transaction among the person, the activities they need or want to engage in, and the environments in which these activities are undertaken. In doing so, they can identify the specific requirements of the technology and ensure that it is able to meet the goals and skills of the person as well as the demands of current and future activities and environments. A detailed understanding of these requirements also enables the therapist to customize the technology to ensure it can be used efficiently and effectively. Occupational therapists also work with the AT user to promote his or her understanding of the technology and its application so that he or she can monitor its ongoing utility.

References

Alliance for Technology Access. (2005). *Computer and Web Resources for People with Disabilities.* Berkeley, CA: Hunter House.

Bain, B. K., and Leger, D. (1997). *Assistive Technology: An Interdisciplinary Approach.* New York, NY, US: Churchill Livingstone.

Baum, C. M. (1998). Achieving effectiveness with a client centred approach: A person-environment interaction. In D. B. Gray, L. A. Quatrano and M. L. Lieberman (Eds.), *Designing and Using Assistive Technology* (pp. 137–147). Baltimore, MD: Paul H. Brookes.

Brown, C. E. (2009). Ecological models in occupational therapy. In E. B. Crepeau, E. S. Cohn, and B. A. Boyt Schell (Eds.), *Willard and Spackman's Occupational Therapy* (11th ed., pp. 435–445). Philadelphia: Wolters Kluwer Lippincott Williams & Wilkins.

Christiansen C. H., and Baum, C. M. (1997). Person-environment occupational performance: A conceptual model for practice, In C. H. Christiansen, and C. M. Baum (Eds.), *Occupational Therapy: Enabling Function and Well-Being* (2nd ed., pp. 46–71). Thorofare, NJ: Slack Inc.

Cook, A. M., Polgar, J. M., and Hussey, S. M. (2007). *Cook & Hussey's Assistive Technologies: Principles and Practice* (3rd ed.). St. Louis, MO: Mosby Elsevier.

Cowan, D., and Turner-Smith, A. (1999). The user's perspective on the provision of electronic assistive technology: Equipped for life? *British Journal of Occupational Therapy, 62*(1), 2–6.

de Jonge, D., Scherer, M. J., and Rodger, S. (2007). *Assistive Technology in the Workplace.* St. Louis, MO: Mosby Elsevier.

Dunn, W., Brown, C., and McGuigan, A. (1994). The ecology of human performance: A framework for considering the impact of context. *American Journal of Occupational Therapy, 48*, 595–607.

Enders, A. and Leech, P. (1996). Low-technology aids for daily living and do-it-yourself devices. In J. C. Galvin and M. J. Scherer (Eds.), *Evaluating, Selecting and Using Appropriate Assistive Technology* (pp. 30–39). Gaithersburg, MD: Aspen Publishers, Inc.

Kelker, K., and Holt, R. (2000). *Family Guide to Assistive Technology.* Cambridge, MA: Brookline Books.

Kielhofner, G. (2004). The development of occupational therapy knowledge. In G. Kielhofner (Ed.), *Conceptual Foundations of Occupational Therapy* (3rd ed., pp. 27–63). Philadelphia: F. A. Davis.

Law, M., and Baum, C. M. (2005). Measurement in occupational therapy. In M. Law, C. Baum, and W. Dunn (Eds.), *Measuring Occupational Performance: Supporting Best Practice in Occupational Therapy* (pp. 3–20). Thorofare, NJ: SLACK Inc.

Law, M., Baptiste, S., Carswell, A., McColl, M., Polatajko, H., and Pollock, N. (1994). *Canadian Occupational Performance Measure* (2nd ed.). Toronto, Ontario, Canada: Canadian Association of Occupational Therapists.

Law, M., Cooper, B., Strong, S., Stewart, D., Rigby, P., and Letts, L. (1996). The Person-Environment-Occupation Model: A transactive approach to occupational performance. *Canadian Journal of Occupational Therapy, 63*(1), 9–23.

Litvak, S. and Enders, A. (2001). Support systems: The interface between individuals and environments. In G.L. Albrecht, K. D. Seelman, and M. Bury (Eds.), *Handbook of Disability Studies* (pp. 711–733). Thousand Oaks, CA: Sage Publications.

Long, T. M., and Perry, D. F. (2008). Pediatric physical therapists' perceptions of their training in assistive technology. *Physical Therapy, 88*(5), 629–639. doi:10.2522/ptj.20060356

Long, T. M., Woolverton, M., Perry, D. F., and Thomas, M. J. (2007). Training needs of pediatric occupational therapists in assistive technology. *The American Journal of Occupational Therapy, 61*(3), 345–354. doi:10.5014/ajot.61.3.345

Malec, J. (1999). Goal attainment scaling in rehabilitation. *Neuropsychological Rehabilitation, 9*(3), 253–275. doi:10.1080/096020199389365

Nochajski, S. M., and Oddo, C. R. (1995). Technology in the workplace. In W. C. Mann and J. P. Lane (Eds.), *Assistive Technology for People with Disabilities* (2nd ed., pp. 197–261). Bethesda, MD: AOTA.

Ostensjo, S., Carlberg, E. B., and Vollestad, N. (2005). The use and impact of assistive devices and other environmental modifications on everyday activities and care in young children with cerebral palsy. *Disability and Rehabilitation, 27*(14), 849–861. doi:10.1080/09638280400018619

Patterson, D. R., Jensen, M., and Engel-Knowles, J. (2002). Pain and its influence on assistive technology use. In M. J. Scherer (Ed.), *Assistive Technology: Matching Device and Consumer for Successful Rehabilitation* (pp. 59–76). Washington, DC: American Psychological Association.

Scherer, M. J. (2000). *Living In a State of Stuck: How Technology Impacts the Lives on People with Disabilities* (3rd ed.). Cambridge, MA: Brookline Books.

Scherer, M. J. (2005). Assessing the benefits of using assistive technologies and other supports for thinking, remembering and learning. *Disability and Rehabilitation, 27*(13), 731–739. doi:10.1080/09638280400014816

Scherer, M. J., and Galvin, J. C. (1996). An outcomes perspective to quality pathways to the most appropriate technology. In J. C. Galvin and M. Scherer (Eds.), *Evaluating, Selecting, and Using Appropriate Assistive Technology* (pp. 1–26). Gaithersburg, MD: Aspen.

Scherer, M. J., and Vitaliti, L. T. (1997). Functional approach to technological factors and their assessment in rehabilitation. In S. S. Dittmar and G. E. Gresham (Eds.), *Functional Assessment and Outcome Measures for the Health Rehabilitation Professional* (pp. 69–88). Gaithersburg, MD: Aspen.

Sprigle, S., and Abdelhamied, A. (1998). The relationship between ability measures and assistive technology selection, design and use. In D. B. Gray, L. A. Quatrano, and M. L. Lieberman (Eds.), *Designing and Using Assistive Technology: The Human Perspective* (pp. 229–248). Baltimore, MD: Paul H. Brookes.

Waldron, D., and Layton, N. (2008). Hard and soft assistive technology: Defining roles for clinicians. *Australian Occupational Therapy Journal, 55*(1), 61–64. doi:10.1111/j.1440–1630.2007.00707.x

Wessels, R., Persson, J., Lorentsen, Ø., Andrich, R., Ferrario, M., Oortwijn, W., et al. (2002). IPPA: Individually prioritised problem assessment. *Technology and Disability, 14*(3), 141–145. Retrieved from http://iospress.metapress.com/content/2bm793b7pbdah9bw/

World Health Organization (WHO). (2001). *ICF: International Classification of Functioning, Disability, and Health.* Geneva, Switzerland: WHO.

World Health Organization (WHO). (2004). *A Glossary of Terms for Community Health Care and Services for Older Persons.* (WHO/WKC/Tech.Ser./04.2). Retrieved from http://whqlibdoc.who.int/wkc/2004/WHO_WKC_Tech.Ser._04.2.pdf

12

Pediatric Specialists in Assistive Solutions

L. W. Braga, I. L. de Camillis Gil, K. S. Pinto, and P. S. Siebra Beraldo

CONTENTS

12.1 Pediatric Specialists in the Process of Development and Rehabilitation

The development or neurorehabilitation process of the child with impairments requires an approach involving different areas of specialization because these children may present difficulties or challenges in various developmental domains (sensorial, motor, neuropsychological, communication, and socialization, among others). This generates the need for assessments and interventions by interprofessional teams of physicians (pediatricians, orthopedic surgeons, neurologists, geneticists, psychiatrists, and other specialists); nurses; physical, occupational, and speech therapists; psychologists; special educators; technologists such as engineers; and prosthetics/orthotics technicians.

A child's development is a process that is mediated by both family and sociocultural setting. It is the family's natural role to help stimulate and encourage children's development; teach them how to play, walk, talk, and think; and to help them become individuals and social beings part of a community. However, this role is often transferred to health-care professionals when a child is born with or acquires a brain injury and presents the attendant impairments this may bring (Braga et al. 2005). Once a diagnosis is made, the daily life of these children and their families is often transformed into a series of visits to medical facilities of various specialized professionals. This fact may often result in depriving the child and family of experiences specific to childhood, such as parks and places in which actions become significant to the child's development (Braga and Campos da Paz Jr 2006).

However, an approach to the child's rehabilitation goes beyond interventions from different areas of specialization. Human beings must integrate different abilities to engage in their activities. It is known that interprofessional teamwork is both a fundamental factor in rehabilitation and an essential element in rendering quality health assistance (Halper 1993; Bakeit 1996; King et al. 1998; Körner 2010).

The fact that a child is seen by many different professionals does not guarantee an integrated approach. Families often complain of a fragmentation in the health services they receive, which may often be due to a multidisciplinary (albeit nonintegrated) manner of treating the individual. The professionals work in a parallel or serial manner, with well-defined roles and tasks, focused on conducting their specific evaluations and interventions and assuming responsibility only for their particular aspect of development. Although the child is seen by an entire team, the professionals establish their own goals and treatment proposals for the child (Körner 2010). Poor communication and differing treatment courses commonly lead to this type of fragmented assistance, generating conflict and extra stress for the families insofar as it increases the risk of discrepancies or redundancies in treatment.

Teamwork is not defined by the isolated interventions of various specialties. The professionals' effective communication and cooperative action are among the most important characteristics of an interdisciplinary team approach (Bakeit 1996; Körner 2010). This model consequently requires that practitioners meet frequently to discuss, assess, and define coherent and consistent rehabilitation goals and plans and to conduct the child's treatment in a cooperative manner. Joint teamwork integrates knowledge and experience from practitioners in diverse areas of specialization (King et al. 1998; Braga 2006).

To be effective, teamwork has to be established so that the child is at the center of rehabilitation efforts. This unified approach is developed in conjunction with the family, who in turn is empowered to exercise their natural role of educators and co-collaborators in the child's stimulation (Braga 2009). This signifies that the joint assessments and discussions be done in partnership with those who care for the child, focusing on existent developmental and contextual needs (Braga 2000; Hinojosa et al. 2002; King et al. 2004; Braga 2006).

In this way, it is possible to construct a unique, individualized program that is based on functional, contextualized, child-centered activities that require the child to concomitantly use various skills. The program should be based on and guided by realistic, viable, long- and short-term goals depending on the child's potential and sociocultural setting. This effort by a team of pediatric specialists constitutes a context-sensitive, family-based approach to promoting the child's development (Braga and Campos da Paz Jr 2006).

Integrated teamwork incorporates the knowledge and experience that each professional from distinct fields brings to the rehabilitation program. It also fosters professional development and growth for the practitioner because intrateam communication promotes continued acquisition of knowledge across different areas. Furthermore, it enables more coherent communication between the team of practitioners and the family, thereby improving compliance with the treatment program.

In a child's infancy, families often consult a pediatrician before any other doctor. In a rehabilitation team, the pediatrician plays a broader role, such as establishing the diagnosis and prognosis, discussing and defining the treatment program with the rest of the team, and accompanying the child's development over time. In this first contact with the family, it is essential that the pediatrician be attentive to the various aspects of childhood development and aim toward an integrated approach with other pediatric specialists to guarantee a treatment plan targeting not only the child's clinical needs, but also his/her developmental necessities.

To this end, it is essential that the pediatrician's approach encompass, in addition to general pediatric knowledge and experience, broad knowledge including childhood development, psychology, neurology, orthopedics, genetics, and psychiatry. The aim is to trace, and, if possible, diagnose, any existent disorder in these areas. It is often necessary, in the process of defining a diagnosis, to integrate the various members of the neurorehabilitation team, which also includes other medical fields, to discuss the varied and complex developmental disorders in a way that fosters cooperation, mutual understanding, and consensus.

A comprehensive approach that addresses both the definition of the diagnosis and the treatment plans requires that the pediatrician and the rest of the team work in cooperation to develop increasingly effective rehabilitation programs. Pediatricians should acknowledge and understand that their role in the process of development and rehabilitation goes far beyond that of the clinical alone.

Another reason that the process of rehabilitating children with disabilities often involves a large number of practitioners is that many areas of development may be impacted (Campos da Paz Jr et al. 1996; Ylvisaker 1998). This can generate obstacles to an integrated approach between the family and the team in planning adequate, contextualized interventions. Effective teamwork does not mean that all of the practitioners must be present at every step of the treatment process. This process is dynamic. Some children may have predominantly motor disorders whereas others have more language or neuropsychological impairments. Depending on the significance of the main problems, the child may need closer follow-up from one or more practitioners, who end up becoming case managers, i.e., the team members closest to the family throughout treatment.

Case managers play the role of organizing and directing the rehabilitation process, integrating information and decisions among the team, child, and family (Braga 2006). Over the course of development, the case managers can be substituted by other practitioners working with the child depending on the treatment needs at that particular moment. For example, a child with cerebral palsy and acute involuntary movements (e.g., dystonia) who has significant pain and difficulties sitting will benefit from a joint collaboration between the pediatrician and the physical or occupational therapist. Together they can determine the best way to position the child by using assistive technology (AT) resources (e.g., adaptations to sit) and the need for pharmacological intervention. With adequate, comfortable positioning, alternative communication systems can be better implemented, with closer support and follow-up from other members of the team, such as speech therapists or special-needs educators.

On the other hand, in the case of children with predominantly neuropsychological or behavioral disorders [for example, caused by traumatic brain injury (TBI)], the pediatrician would work more closely with the psychologist and educator, who would be the case managers, to establish a diagnosis and determine the best treatment plan for these conditions. This incorporated teamwork then enables more effective communication, guidance, and support for the family, teachers, and school community, facilitating instruction about the best educational strategies and ways of handling the child's special needs and behavioral challenges.

Development is procedural; thus, the team's longitudinal follow-up of the child ensures that progress is being assessed and goals are being adjusted to his/her potential, interests, and the needs that change over time.

Every approach to rehabilitation should aim at promoting independence and expanding the child's ability to interact with the world. It is important to acknowledge (1) the child as an individual person in a process of development, with unique interests and potential; (2) the fundamental partnership and role of the family; and (3) the value of sociocultural contexts for the child's development and inclusion.

12.2 Pediatric Specialists in Assistive Solutions

Studies have shown that interdisciplinary team approaches are more effective in the rehabilitation process (Bakeit 1996; Körner 2010), especially with regards to the implementation of assistive solutions (Stoner et al. 2010). AT services and tools are important for fostering and maximizing the development and/or rehabilitation of children with impairments. For an effective assistive solution, this technology should be applied in a functional manner aimed at improving the child's abilities and expanding his/her potential for social interaction with surroundings and community (Scherer et al. 2011).

Children with disabilities in early childhood may have impairments that linger throughout life and change as the child grows and develops (Warzak et al. 1995; Cattelani 1998). These changes can be characterized by the learning of new skills as well as an early loss of performance when the child reaches adolescence or adulthood (Bottos et al. 2001; Strauss et al. 2004). Over time, the use of AT resources can also be valuable for helping people with disabilities acquire or maintain independence (Wilson et al. 2009).

Three aspects that should be highlighted when studying the application of assistive solutions are the participation of the interdisciplinary team; the solutions proposed in the context of the binomial child-family; and, particularly, these approaches in the child's learning process. Because of the importance of these aspects, their main characteristics will be described next.

12.3 Assistive Solutions and the Interdisciplinary Team Approach

Given the great variation of motor, cognitive, communication, and sensorial disorders that a child with disabilities may have, and the diverse social and cultural circumstances involved, it is evident that individualized goals should be adopted, avoiding fragmented and one-size-fits-all approaches. Therefore, a thorough assessment by the team of pediatric specialists should precede the introduction of any AT tools. It is important to investigate the child's potentials and/or limitations in various domains (motor, cognitive, language, etc.), in addition to developmental needs, special interests, social setting, and context of daily life (e.g., family, school).

The main focus of interdisciplinary intervention is to foster the child's development and social participation through activities geared toward acquiring as much autonomy as possible, often with the aid of AT resources.

The functional use of AT tools conjoins the interaction of motor, cognitive, emotional, and somatosensitive aspects. Thus, assistance in development and rehabilitation can be qualified by the joint action of rehabilitation, which favors the establishment of developmental priorities and permits a focus on contextualized activities that involve more than one area of development (Braga and Campos da Paz Jr 2006). In many instances, this joint action can be optimized through integrated sessions, in which more than one professional participates, contributing to the observation of the child's potential through the simultaneous perspective of different areas of specialization and the discussion of what they observed, thereby informing the decision-making process.

At times, difficulty performing a task, such as using an adaptation for drawing a design or using a walker to get around, can initially appear to stem from a motor disorder, but it may actually be caused by an attention deficit. In other words, a poorly designed drawing or problems getting around obstacles with a walker could be caused by attention or visuoconstructive disorders rather than actual coordination or balance impairments. In these cases, a team working in an integrated manner can program activities that ally motor and neuropsychological components on the basis of joint evaluations and discussions. In these cases, the rehabilitation professionals, working in an integrated manner, can design activities that associate motor and neuropsychological components, chosen after the team has jointly assessed and discussed the case. For example, the team can unite gait training with the demarcation of obstacles that need to be circumnavigated, establishing signs and techniques for the child to use and orienting the parents about verbal strategies that can be applied when the child's focus wanders from the task at hand.

The teamwork in the sphere of AT improves not only the approach to the child, but also enhances the team's effectiveness as a joint force and as individual practitioners: Interdisciplinary knowledge is constructed throughout the group discussions and course of treatment. Shared knowledge transforms and broadens the experience of each team member, making the evaluation and intervention processes more efficient. The team-based process has benefits for the teams, including the development of more specific and achievable technology goals, confidence of team members, and more effective teamwork to assist decision-making (Copley and Ziviani 2007).

As a result, the family also become part of the team. They bring knowledge about the child and daily life at home, routines, interests, likes, and dislikes, which enrich the clinically obtained information and constitute essential elements for the decision-making process (Braga 2000; King et al. 2004). A joint approach optimizes and enhances rehabilitation and how to proceed with the selection and implementation of AT tools. It also enables better coordination of technology use between home and school.

Some researchers in the field focus on studies about refining the assessment process and how to best select and implement resources; the goal is to help match technologies to the child on the basis of his/her needs, interests, characteristics, and the way each tool works (Scherer and Craddock 2002; Scherer 2004; Scherer et al. 2005). It is important to evaluate how well the child is able to understand the manner in which these tools function and what their purpose is and to assess the efficacy of the AT tools in day-to-day life. In other words, during the evaluation, the team should focus not only on observing the skills of the child and factors intervening in development but also formulate hypotheses about possible strategies or resources that can help foster their interaction and social participation.

Depending on the type of adaptation, more complex skills may be required. For example, children with cognitive disorders may have difficulties using tools that demand more complex movement sequences and more elaborate working memory and planning (Pueyo-Benito and Vendrell-Gomez 2002; Scherer 2005), such as handling a lever to control a self-propelling car with only one hand. Strategies like dividing the task into several stages and encouraging trial-and-error can help in the implementation of more complex AT resources. Also, getting to know the child's previous experiences with AT can be helpful when adding and adjusting AT resources (Scherer 2005; Murchland and Parkyn 2010).

In sum, the team's interdisciplinary work, together with the participation of the child's family, are fundamental to the planning, implementation, assessment, and follow-up of any assistive solutions for improving the child's performance and quality of life.

12.4 AT Resources Applied to the Daily Life of the Child and Family

The effective use of an AT tool is achieved through its functional application in daily life; in other words, when it is incorporated into the child's day-to-day routine, altering the possibilities and manner in which the child can interact in and with the environment (Lindsay and Tsybina 2011). Two aspects are essential to this process: (1) the active involvement of the family, which provides ongoing opportunities for practice; and (2) the effectiveness of the tool for helping the child improve performance in a given task.

Many of the activities in the child's daily life are centered around tasks that are culturally significant to the family. The more a family values a given resource, the more opportunities the child will have for practicing and using it (Kellegrew 2000). For example, some families will encourage their child to evolve in self-care activities, such as going to the bathroom alone and eating independently without needing the help of others. The tasks emphasized by the family reflect their beliefs and values about childhood and impairments, socioeconomic and educational views that influence their daily routines, and, consequently, the child's participation (or lack of participation) in certain activities. Depending on cultural values, the use of adaptations in performing daily life tasks can be either reinforced or ignored by the family (Ripat and Woodgate 2011).

In their interactions with the rehabilitation team, families often signal which tasks their child shows the most interest in or those they are trying to perform (Hinojosa et al. 2002). The pediatric specialist, on the basis of the team's assessment, aims at adjusting the rehabilitation goals to the child's potential. By helping the families understand the child's potential, as well as identify the needs and limitations brought on by the impairment, the specialist can help them direct their expectations and make changes in the family setting to maximize the child's development and progress.

The demands brought about by the child's need for assistance cause a number of changes in the family's daily routine. In addition to the importance of a joint assessment of the child by the interdisciplinary team, the amount of time that will be spent on the activity is relevant in the discussion about the team's involvement in training the child and family to use AT resources. One change includes giving the child as much time as needed (Ostensjo 2003). The time variable tends to wield a more profound impact in children whose functional abilities are more compromised or who are slower than independent children (Kellegrew

2000). The time spent on each activity should be evaluated to avoid excessive efforts by the child (Ostensjo 2003). The team should also be aware of the impact that time may have on the family's perception of the child's performance. They may feel anxious or concerned watching the child take too long to perform a task or use a given AT tool. It is important to help the family understand the challenges that the child is facing, as well as the resources that can help facilitate the child's performance; this may help family members feel more at ease. They can see that the child is using time more efficiently, even if it takes longer. Furthermore, the child will play a more active role when the activities are planned around the family's daily routines at home (Ketelaar et al. 2001). The situations that the child faces can also change depending on the setting. For example, at home the child may have more time to carry out a task than at school. In this sense, strategies need to change to ensure greater participation in activities, such as taking bite-size foods to school that do not require cutting, thereby reducing the amount of time needed for lunch and snack time.

Often, an AT tool may end up in disuse by the child and family because it lacks significance for their particular routine and setting. For example, when the team fails to work in conjunction with the family in the implementation of an AT tool, there is the risk that it will not be effective. This can occur because it is not directed toward the family's needs and environment, even if the device itself would have brought important benefits to the child. It is important to investigate how the AT tools are seen by the child, how the family perceives them, and how they can become part of the child's and the family's social context (Skär 2002).

The pediatric specialist should be attentive to the child's real potential and capacity for executing a given task so that the most effective assistance can be offered to the whole family (e.g., guiding the participation of others in the activity or introducing adaptations, when necessary). This type of intervention can most positively impact the quality of life of the child and family.

12.5 AT and Learning

The application of AT resources involves a learning process that grows as the child's skill at using the tools evolves. The use of a device implies the development of a functional ability that encompasses planning and executing organized movements through which the child achieves an objective or function. The capacity for developing a skill is, in part, determined by biological potential. Nevertheless, the development or reorganization of functional brain systems is promoted by social demands and depends on the lifestyle, beliefs, and values of each culture in accordance with the possibilities of the child's morphological substrate and chances for practice (Leontiev 1978; Vygotsky 1984, 1991). In other words, certain functional skills that evolve through the use of AT tools are achieved or honed according to the child's capacity and opportunity to develop them (McNaughton et al. 2008).

For example, the ability to use an alternative communication interface is achieved through the ability to control certain bodily movements or after attaining a level of cognitive development. However, it also depends on the child's chances to learn and improve the way in which the tool is used. What at first may appear to be a difficult or uncoordinated movement that demands a lot of time and effort can, with practice and incentive, become easier and more effective.

For example, the strategies used by the family for communicating or managing mealtimes (e.g., how they initiate and conduct conversations or how they encourage the child to eat) can significantly contribute to the development and improvement of skills that will gradually lead to greater functional independence. Allowing a child to experiment using a device for handling a spoon will contribute to the development of that functional skill. Communication can even be improved by AT devices in children and adolescents who have severe motor impairments and minimally intelligible speech (Puyuelo 2001; Pennington et al. 2004).

Augmentative and alternative communication (AAC) systems should be adjusted periodically throughout development and adapted to the child's communication needs and settings (McNaughton et al. 2008). The system may initially appear ineffective because the child will likely need time to express a communicative intention, and the interlocutor may have to adapt his/her conversational style to the child's new forms of self-expression. It is important to remember the benefits that communication will bring to the child's socialization and academic processes (Branson and Demchak 2009). Although AAC systems facilitate more autonomy in social interactions, they do not substitute speech nor do they guarantee real time in dialogue, thus demanding that interlocutors adapt to and respect the child's temporal dynamic. It is important that everyone involved be skillful at handling the devices so that they can be properly used and can come to effectively improve the child's competence (Murphy et al. 1996; Scherer 1996).

Furthermore, any AT resource that is indicated for and used by the child is much more than a simple mechanical aid. AT tools are integral to the child's body and impact self perception of functionality and appearance. Generally, the simpler and more functional the tool, the greater the chances that the child and family will regularly use it. When AT tools are truly incorporated into the child's daily life and activities, they can eventually be seen as extensions of the child's own body (Huang et al. 2009).

When dealing with a child who has the potential for attaining a greater level of independence, it is important to ensure that the family understands what their child is capable of achieving. It is also essential that they be aware of what can be done to promote the child's development through the application of AT resources and the planning of domestic routines.

In a longitudinal follow-up, the use of AT resources varies from very simple to more complex, depending on each child's abilities, potential, and developmental stage. In addition, changes in the child's interests and the consolidation of new functional skills can alter performance and possibilities, which in turn demand modifications of the tools being used over time (Jahiel and Scherer 2010).

Going back to the example of using an AAC system, throughout his/her life, a child can develop motor or cognitive skills and better emotional self-control, which may permit updating the AT tools to more complex ones. For example, using an interface with only one key requires a single motor action. However, as the child's motor skills develop, and coordination of movements increases, along with improved cognitive functions that allow for more elaborate mental planning involving sequential procedures, it is possible to use an interface with five keys and a semidirected search engine. A change such as this one permits greater communicative effectiveness by promoting speed in dialogues or written communication.

Furthermore, an alternative communication interface of a single key can have several uses throughout the child's development. Initially, it can be a resource used for playing with toys. As the child grows, it can be used for signaling "yes" or "no" and, later, it can be used for computer programs. Consequently, this tool can have more than one function at any given time in the child's development. If it is adjusted to the needs and potential of the child's specific stage, the same tool can be applied to achieve the main goal of expanding communication.

The strategy chosen for introducing an AT aid in the child's daily life should be adjusted to his/her current motor and cognitive potentials. For example, the construction and use of communication symbol boards enhances the vocabulary of children with unintelligible speech and improves their chances for self-expression. The child's level of mental representation will determine his choice of symbols; these can be photographs, drawings, graphic symbols, letters, words, and/or sentences. The rehabilitation team and family should explore the child's communicative needs and context, purposes of interactions, and choice of symbols (Fallon et al. 2001; 2003); the boards should be created according to the child's abilities, mode of selection, and scanning (Blackstone et al. 2007). Similarly, it is essential that everyone involved in the use of these tools be adequately instructed in their application, thereby facilitating, through a context-sensitive and family-based approach, their true integration in the child's daily life and improvement of everyone's quality of life (Jans and Scherer 2006).

Rehabilitation intervention is formative in nature. The aim is to understand a routine that already exists and gradually include new aspects in the most natural way possible, which changes and enriches the functioning of the real-world activities. An intervention program that focuses on function and on a context-sensitive approach facilitates carryover and transference of learning to other contexts (Ylvisaker 1998). In addition to the contextualization of proposed activities, it is important to anticipate the gradual decrease of proffered support as the child's self-sufficiency increases.

In sum, adequately selected AT resources are those that expand the child's ability to act, promote new learning, and foster development. By expanding the manner in which the child can interact and communicate with the world, these tools enrich his/her experiences and interactions, leading to changes in development and social participation.

12.6 Case Evaluation in an Interprofessional Team

Two case studies are presented to illustrate how the team of pediatric specialists selects and promotes the appropriate use of these tools, taking into account the child's setting and developmental needs. These cases are in longitudinal follow-up and are described according to the International Classification of Functioning, Disability, and Health (ICF) model and framework (Raghavendra et al. 2007; OPS/OMS 2008; McDougall et al. 2010, 2011).

12.6.1 Case 1—Michael (Cerebral Palsy)

12.6.1.1 Case History

Michael* presented tetraplegic choreoathetoid cerebral palsy (CP) caused by perinatal hypoxia. Today he is 11 years old and has been seen by an interprofessional team at the SARAH Network of Neurorehabilitation Hospitals since he was 10 months old. He was born with respiratory insufficiency due to prolonged labor and was intubated for 40 min immediately after birth, remaining in the intensive care unit (ICU) for two days on mechanical ventilation. He is the first child born of the couple (a geographer and an economist) and has a sister who is four years younger. He has no associated cognitive or sensorial deficits or seizure disorders.

12.6.1.2 Motor Evaluation

Michael evolved with neurodevelopmental delays. At admission to SARAH, he presented with involuntary movements of the four limbs and perioral muscles, which continue to this day and interfere with his coordination, handling of objects, postural control, and facial mimicry.

---

* Not the patient's real name.

At ten months, Michael had not yet attained any motor acquisitions and had no head control. There was persistence of some archaic movements, such as asymmetrical tonic neck reflex; placing and parachute were absent. He tried to reach and grasp objects but was unable to because of movement difficulties.

He currently exhibits regular trunk balance and is in a customized wheelchair that facilitates positioning and locomotion.

12.6.1.3 Neuropsychological Evaluation

Michael's cognitive development has always been compatible with his chronological age. At admission, he showed interest in social interaction and exploring objects. His attention was at the expected level for his age, but his concentration was impaired because of his involuntary movements. He could recognize familiar faces, persisted in reaching for objects, and tried to imitate ways of exploring them.

When he was five years three months old, he underwent a cognitive evaluation with the Columbia Mental Maturity Scale. He scored a total of 42 points, compatible with the 77th percentile and a maturity level of a six year old.

He currently attends regular school and his scores and performance are compatible with his age and grade.

12.6.1.4 Communication Strategy

Upon admission, Michael's means of communication were precarious. He had difficulties controlling the movements involved in gesturing and vocalizing. He communicated his basic needs by cries, social smiles, and by responding to visual contact. He had good contextual comprehension, but no conventional forms of expressing communication with his interlocutors, such as head nods, pointing, or "yes/no" signals.

Today, Michael is capable of independently communicating through alternative communication systems, although he still requires interlocutors familiar with his communicative signals.

12.6.1.5 Evaluation of Visual, Auditive, and Perceptive Functions

Michael does not present any associated sensorial deficits or convulsive disorders.

12.6.1.6 Neurorehabilitation Team Approach

The program for stimulating Michael's neurodevelopment at a young age comprised integrated activities to improve his neck and trunk balance, manual skills, joint attention, exploration of objects, vocabulary expansion, and conventionalization of nonverbal communication signals. At that time, the AT resource used was primarily a special chair that more adequately positioned Michael in a seated position, making it easier for him to choose and play with toys and sustain visual attention so that he could observe his surroundings and interact socially. Figure 12.1 shows a special chair that permits positioning the child in a manner that increases stabilization of the trunk, better visual contact, and allows him to use the upper limbs to handle toys.

As expected, his cognitive and linguistic development progressed more quickly than his motor development. Over time, the impact of his involuntary movements made it impossible for him to walk, speak intelligibly, or write manually.

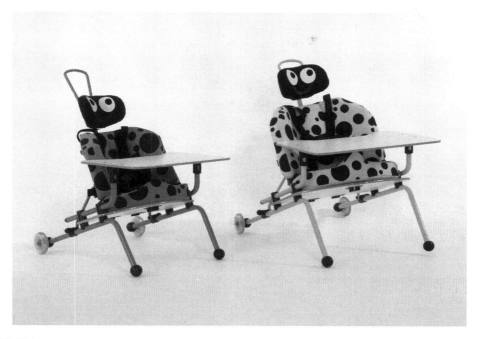

FIGURE 12.1
(See color insert.) Special chair to help the child sit and use upper limbs.

Michael currently exhibits regular trunk balance and can remain seated by using his hands. He gets around by dragging himself in a seated position. He can kneel without support, but only for a short time. Michael uses his left hand to grasp objects, albeit with significant lack of coordination. He is not capable of manual writing and is dependent in activities of daily living (eating, dressing, hygiene). He continues to use a customized wheelchair for positioning and locomotion.

Michael's cognitive development has always been compatible with his age, but the use of AT became necessary because of his learning disabilities and difficulties making new acquisitions. One of the main targets of AT use was the expansion of expressive communication and fostering of social interaction.

The concern was initially to create a consistent pattern of affirmative and negative responses by means of conventionalizing Michael's specific gestures, as well as to provide him with dialogical actions with his interlocutors so he could more actively participate in conversations. To this end, the interlocutors had to say question-like phrases, which also requires training. The themes chosen on this occasion were situations based on his routine, but in a make-believe manner, using AT aimed at fostering greater control of his environment, such as custom-made switches on electronic toys that allowed Michael to control them as if he were using a remote control. Figure 12.2 is an example of a custom-made switch on electronic toys that require a single movement of a hand, foot, or the head.

Another goal of the neurorehabilitation team was to help Michael attain more functional means of getting around because he was able only to drag himself about in a seated position with substantial balance deficits; he was usually transported in a conventional baby carriage. To this end, an alternative device for locomotion was introduced, such as the adapted flyer in Figure 12.3. This tool allowed Michael to get around more independently in controlled environments (e.g., home, school, and stores).

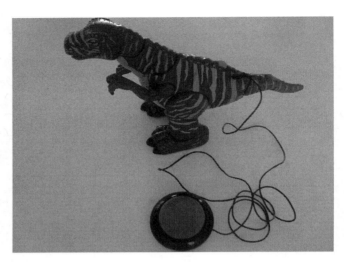

FIGURE 12.2
(See color insert.) Electronic toy with adapted switch.

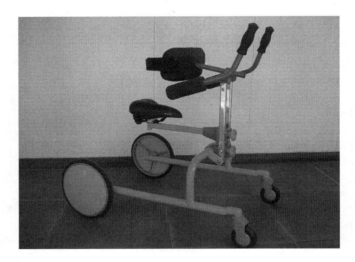

FIGURE 12.3
(See color insert.) Device for independent locomotion.

Because of Michael's dependence on others for his activities of daily life (eating, dressing, hygiene), his toilet seat was customized to allow him to remain sitting while using it (see Figure 12.4) In much the same way, the use of a customized bathing chair, such as the one in Figure 12.5, allowed for better positioning during bathtime.

The introduction of AT resources for better communication and learning gave Michael greater autonomy in his communication processes and daily school life. As Michael's symbolic development evolved, other devices were incorporated, such as communication boards to enhance learning and foster the construction of scholastic concepts. Digital accessibility was also enhanced by new AT resources. Because he was not able to use a conventional mouse and keyboards, switches to run software and attention and memory games (which were developed by the SARAH Network) were added to help stimulate

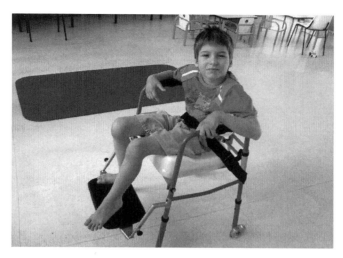

FIGURE 12.4
(See color insert.) Customized toilet seat.

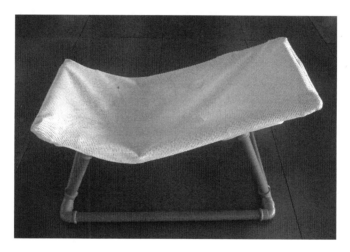

FIGURE 12.5
(See color insert.) Bathing chair.

voluntary attention and planning—neuropsychological skills necessary for using more complex systems in the future.

At that point, Michael began using a pediatric wheelchair. This aid was customized with anatomical seat and backrest, as well as a seatbelt, to provide better positioning, contributing to his head and trunk balance, manual function, and improved ability to grasp and explore objects. Figure 12.6 is an example of an adapted wheelchair. A table-board was adjusted across the armrests as a support for communication boards, which contained vocabulary words associated with daily life activities (eating, leisure, places, people) to expand his means of expression during conversations at home and in school.

The boards were enhanced with letters and numbers to aid in the activities of learning to read. Learning to read is an important acquisition for these children because mastering written language permits use of unlimited vocabulary, which in turn expands the child's means of expression and allows for the use of more complex AT, such as editing words and using talkers.

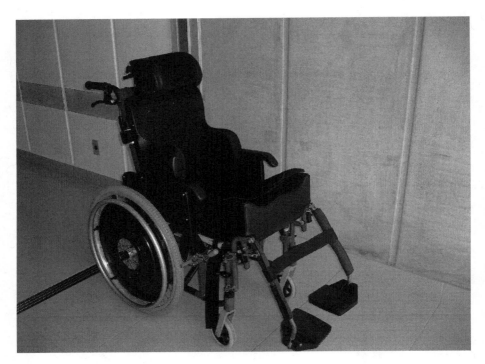

FIGURE 12.6
(See color insert.) Pediatric wheelchair with anatomical seat and backrest.

Michael's alphabetization was supported by boards with symbols and letters, which he selected by pointing with his thumb, a motion that he started to associate with this function. As he learned to read, more sophisticated AT resources were introduced, such as SKM software and activation switches for his left hand. Better control of the movements of his left hand made it possible for Michael to use a keyboard enhanced with a template, joystick, and switch for the mouse functions. Nevertheless, it is hard to safely transport a computer to parks, clubs, or children's parties. So a talker was also incorporated to help Michael communicate in these settings, allowing him to more fully partake of the social situations they entail.

Michael continues to study in regular school without any difficulties mastering the curriculum. He has a customized computer and printer in the classroom to help him complete his school activities and a board attached to his chair-top desk with symbols and letters as well as a switch, joystick, and talker. This permits Michael to communicate using agreed-upon gestures, boards, computer writing, and a talker according to the setting and how much his interlocutors know about the technological resources he uses. Figure 12.7 shows a talker developed by the SARAH Network that uses simple switches to scan letters for forming words.

Michael was longitudinally followed-up by the pediatric specialists team. In addition to using AT, Michael's process of school inclusion was facilitated by favorable Brazilian educational policies, although there are some moderate barriers existent in educational services. Within this context, the aid and participation of the family, integration among the educational and health-care professionals, and support in the classroom by a personal assistant hired by Michael's parents were indispensible to his development and success in school. This process is detailed in Table 12.1, in accordance with ICF.

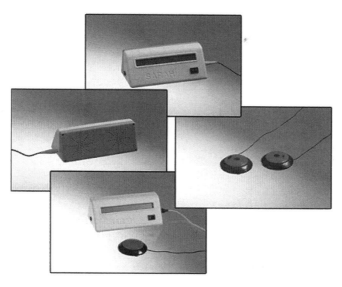

FIGURE 12.7
(See color insert.) Talker that uses simple switches to scan letters for forming words.

TABLE 12.1

Case 1. Michael

Bodily Functions	Activities and Participation	Environmental Factors	Assistive Technology
b117.0 b167.0 b210.0	d4103.4 (admission) d4103.2 (current)	e1151 + 3	– special chair – customized toilet seat – customized bathing chair
b230.0 b320.4 b7354.4 b7650.4	d4102.4 (admission) d4102.2 (current) d450.4 (admission and current)	e1201 + 3	– adapted wheelchairs – alternative device for locomotion (adapted "flyer")
	d335.4 (admission) d335.2 (current) d330.4 (admission) d330.3 (current)	e1251 + 3 e1301 + 3	– "yes/no" signs – communication boards – letter boards – game software – switches for running software – software keyboard mouse (SKM) – talker
	d440.4 (admission) d440.3 (current)	e1401 + 3	– toys with switch – customized remote control – digital books – virtual games
		e355 + 4 e415 + 4 e340 + 4 e5852 + 4 e5850 + 2	

Bodily functions were classified according to data obtained in the initial evaluation; activities and participation were classified according to performance at admission and currently; environmental factors reflect the procedural aspect of the application of AT resources, according to the needs of each developmental stage.

12.6.2 Case 2—John (Traumatic Brain Injury)

12.6.2.1 Case History

John*, currently 15 years old, sustained a TBI (Glasgow 8) in a serious car accident when he was 12. He was treated at a trauma center and remained in the ICU for 58 days. When he was admitted to the ICU, he underwent a computed tomography (CT) scan of the brain, which revealed various cranial fractures and mild to moderate brain swelling. He was tracheostomized for 19 days and experienced seizures, which did not reoccur after discharge from the hospital.

At the time of the accident, he was attending sixth grade at a regular school, played soccer, took swimming and karate lessons, and was independent in activities of daily living. He is an only child, lives with his mother, who is a high-school graduate; his father attended college for two years.

John was admitted to the SARAH Network by an interprofessional team 6 months after the accident. He presented with spastic tetraplegia and left-sided facial paralysis; he kept his mouth open most of the time. He was not attending school and was being seen at a public clinical rehabilitation facility, where treatment included daily sessions of physical therapy, occupational therapy, speech therapy, and water therapy in the pool. His family complained of fragmented assistance, lack of guidance, and failure to adequately attend to John's rehabilitation needs and social reinsertion.

A magnetic resonance imaging (MRI) scan showed an anterior lesion to the temporal lobe bilaterally, with impairment of the amygdala and hippocampus on the left; thalamic, parietal, and frontal lesions on the right; and parietal and frontal lesions on the left; and supretentorial ventricular dilation, ex-vacuum without the need of a ventriculo-peritoneal derivation valve.

12.6.2.2 Motor Evaluation

Upon admission to the rehabilitation program at SARAH, John presented with increased tonus in the four limbs, more pronounced on the right side. Babinski was present on the left. There was an extensor pattern of the lower limbs (feet in equinus and in right inversion) and flexor pattern of the upper limbs (elbow and wrists). When asked, John could flex and extend his right elbow and flex and extend his right knee, with no active movement of the lower left limb.

He had regular neck balance and no trunk control, gait, or voluntary grasping. He was totally dependent for activities of daily living and did not have a wheelchair. At home, John usually lay in bed or on a recliner-type seat, on which he was also fed and bathed. For longer distances, he was taken in the family car, and while at home he was carried around.

12.6.2.3 Neuropsychological Evaluation

During the period of admission, John underwent a qualitative assessment of his cognitive state. He responded to simple, contextual requests by smiling and directing his gaze.

After a consistent pattern of responses was established through conventionalization of signs, he was also submitted to Raven's Special Scale of the Colored Progressive Matrices. The data revealed a cognitive performance "definitively below average," with errors

---

* Not the patient's real name.

compatible with moderate intellectual deficits. John's answers were perseverant, albeit contextualized, also revealing difficulties with mental flexibility, planning, and abstraction.

12.6.2.4 Communication Strategy

Initially, John exhibited contextualized smiling and crying, sought visual contact and joint attention, and gave consistent responses to some of the questions he was asked by directing his gaze. He was able to vocalize some sounds but did not yet use them to effectively communicate. He had verbal comprehension of contextual events, but his capacity for verbal expression was compromised to the point of being unintelligible because of facial paralysis and severe dysarthria.

12.6.2.5 Evaluation of Visual, Auditive, and Perceptive Functions

John had visual deficits, characterized by limited field of vision and mild loss of visual acuity, with better performance on the left side. He was able to adjust the position of his head to improve his visual focus. He did not present any other sensorial impairments.

12.6.2.6 Neurorehabilitation Team Approach

AT tools were gradually introduced into John's neurorehabilitation process, during periods of inpatient treatment, according to his neurological progress and communication and social needs.

During his first inpatient stay at SARAH, the family was given a wheelchair, as per the rehabilitation team's indication, to attend to John's needs and functional level. The chair was customized with anatomical seat and backrest, enabling better inclination for his degree of neck and trunk control; the chair also had a headrest, seatbelts, and support for a table-board. This resource fostered better positioning and permitted greater stability during transport, playtime, and learning and eating activities; it also made it easier for the family to participate in these tasks. With better positioning in the wheelchair and the ability to actively move his upper limbs, John was able to get around more independently at home because he could manage the wheelchair back and forth for short distances over flat terrain using verbal commands.

With regards to communication, the team's initial goal was to re-establish a consistent pattern of affirmative and negative responses. Because he was able to say "e" for "yes" answers and a subtle movement of his head for "no," these were the conventionalized signs. His communication and cognitive progress were aided by the introduction of other AT devices: sound switches, boards with illustrations and, later, with letters, which were selected by using his communication signs or by having others do an oral sweep through the letters. The use of a sound switch was aimed primarily at greater control of his environment: John used it to call family members and became accustomed to it, later using it in computerized communication systems. The figure boards added to the possibilities of John's expression and speed in conversations. They were enlarged because of his vision impairment and allowed him to make an unlimited amount of words. To write, he would point at the letters with his right index finger. A special support was designed for adding the boards and reading materials onto the wheelchair, making it easier for John to engage in these activities. When he was discharged from this first inpatient stay, the family was guided through his return to school because he now possessed ways of communicating and getting around.

By the time he was admitted the second time for inpatient rehabilitation, John had already been reinserted back into sixth grade at the school he had been attending. The teachers asked for information and instruction about how to assess his learning process. At that time, the rehabilitation focus was primarily on strategies for cognitive and writing re-education. The SKM AT tool was added, with the switch John was already using, but without the sound device. He was able to write by scanning, turning on the switch with his right hand. A meeting was held with his teachers, at which modifications to the curriculum were suggested to help his learning process and facilitate his interaction with classmates, expand his communication, and master new content. Adaptations were also made to John's way of communicating by using the SKM and alphabet cards to write his answers or by pointing to the correct answer in multiple choice questions.

On John's third inpatient rehabilitation period, he was attending the same school and had passed to the seventh grade. He was using the communication board with the alphabet and months of the year on one side and days of the week and numbers on the reverse side. He had better neck and trunk balance and improved manual function. During this time, new boards were added, with ready words and phrases about the foods he ate, leisure activities and places, activities of daily life, names of friends, and feelings. These new boards aimed at speeding up and expanding his communication with other children. Improved manual function allowed John to use a conventional keyboard with larger letters that was placed on the same support as the boards on the left side within his field of vision. Figure 12.8 shows a rod affixed to his wheelchair to hold and better position the keyboard within his field of vision. Because using a mouse was not functional, a table-board with joystick and switch were made. Furthermore, the computer was reconfigured with new accessibility options: repeatedly pressed keyboard keys that froze up, short cuts, and extra-large letters on the screen. As his balance and manual function improved, John started training how to feed himself, with customization of eating paraphernalia, such as dishes that affixed to a table-board with raised edges to keep utensils from sliding off. A tubular bathing chair was also added, ensuring greater safety during bathtime and allowing John to more actively participate (he was able to soap up some parts of his body with his right hand).

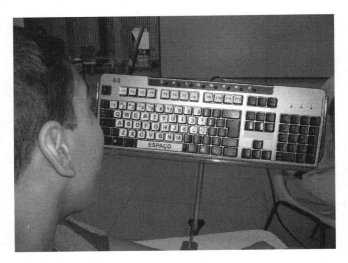

FIGURE 12.8
(See color insert.) Rod for holding a conventional keyboard for better positioning and viewing.

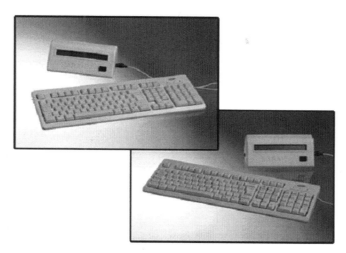

FIGURE 12.9
(See color insert.) Talker with keyboard.

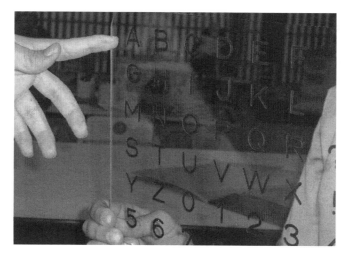

FIGURE 12.10
(See color insert.) Acrylic board for communication in the pool.

A fourth inpatient rehabilitation period included the introduction of a talker with keyboard (see Figure 12.9). A support was made for mounting the monitor to the table-board, which already had a rack for the keyboard.

Recording the ready phrases expanded John's means of communication in different settings and situations. This tool did not exclude the use of the word/letter boards. An acrylic board was made for John to use in the pool at school during swimtime with his classmates, such as the one in Figure 12.10. This transparent alphabet board also made his communication more similar to common exchanges, in which individuals speak face to face. Communication became more fluent and effective because the interlocutor was already able to read the words as John wrote them, rendering the exchanges more functional. Currently, John has used the talker in school on a daily basis and the communication board with family members. Table 12.2 details this process.

TABLE 12.2

Case 2: John

Bodily Functions	Activities and Participation	Environmental Factors	Assistive Technology
b117.2	d4103.4 (admission)	e1150 + 1 (admission)	– customized bathing chair
b164.2	d4103.3 (currently)	e1151 + 3 (currently)	– customized wheelchairs
b16700.1	d450.4 (admission	e1201 + 0	
b2100.1	and currently)	e1201 + 3	
b2101.2	d335.3 (admission)	e1251 + 0 (admission)	– sound switch
b230.0	d335.2 (currently)	e1251 + 3 (currently)	– verbalizations and "yes/no"
b320.4	d330.4 (admission	e1301 + 1 (admission)	signs
b7354. 4	and currently)	e1301 + 3 (currently)	– communication boards
b7300.2			– letter boards
			– keyboard with template and large adhesive letters
			– talker
	d440.4 (admission)	e1401 + 0 (admission)	– acrylic letter boards to use in
	d440.3 (currently)	e1401 + 3 (currently)	water
	d710.0	e355 + 2 (admission)	
		e355 + 4 (currently)	
		e410 + 4	
		e5852 + 4	
		e5850 + 2	

Bodily functions were classified according to data obtained in the initial evaluation; activities, participation, and environmental factors were classified according to performance at admission and today, in accordance with the rehabilitation process after the acquired injury.

12.7 Conclusions

These case studies show the importance of the functional application of AT tools in neurorehabilitation programs. Michael's case illustrates how assistive solutions enhance and foster the development of the child with brain injury. Notably, the use of technological resources should be customized to the child's cognitive and motor abilities, follow-up on his learning process, and attend to his setting and needs for social interaction. It is important to stress that the combined use of more and less technologically sophisticated devices can help expand the child's means of communicating, socializing, and acting more independently, with the freedom for self-expression and choice-making.

The case of John highlights how AT can contribute to helping the child return to activities of daily life, school, leisure, and community on the basis of his motor and neuropsychological potential. AT resources can be used in the neurorehabilitation of the child with TBI according to their recovery process and can be used temporarily or permanently, depending on the child's state. It is important to use AT tools adjusted to the child's different communication settings and needs, expanding their social interaction, as seen in Figure 12.11.

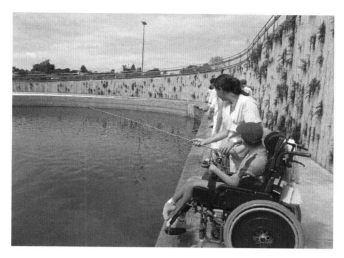

FIGURE 12.11
(See color insert.) AT resources that facilitate social interaction.

Summary of the Chapter

This chapter describes the role of the pediatric specialist in the neurorehabilitation process of the child that incorporates AT and its uses, applications, and indications. Two case studies, a child with CP and one with TBI, illustrate how AT impacted the children's development, recovery, and progress and how the pediatric specialist played an essential role in this process.

References

Bakeit, A. M. (1996). Effective teamwork in rehabilitation. *International Journal of Rehabilitation Research, 19*, 301–306.

Blackstone, S., Williams, M., and Wilkins, D. (2007). Key principles underlying AAC research. *Augmentative and Alternative Communication, 23*(3), 191–203. doi:10.1080/07434610701553684

Bottos, M., Feliciangeli, A., Sciuto, L., Gericke, C., and Vianello, A. (2001). Functional status of adults with cerebral palsy and implications for treatment of children. *Developmental Med Child Neurology, 43*(8), 516–528. doi:10.1017/S0012162201000950

Braga, L. W. (2000). Family participation in the rehabilitation of the child with traumatic brain injury. *Journal of Neupsychology Society, 6*, 388.

Braga, L. W. (2006). The context-sensitive family-based approach: Basic principles. In L. W. Braga, and A. Campos da Paz, Jr, (Eds.), *The Child with Traumatic Brain Injury or Cerebral Palsy: A Context-Sensitive, Family-Based Approach to Development* (pp. 1–16). Oxford, UK: Taylor & Francis.

Braga, L. W. (2009). Should we empower the family? *Developmental Neurorehabilitation, 12*(4), 179–180. doi:10.1080/17518420903102001

Braga, L. W., and Campos da Paz, Jr, A. (2006). *The Child with Traumatic Brain Injury or Cerebral Palsy: A Context-Sensitive, Family-Based Approach to Development.* Oxford, UK: Taylor & Francis.

Braga L. W., da Paz Júnior, A. C., and Ylvisaker, M. (2005). Direct clinician-delivered versus indirect family-supported rehabilitation of children with traumatic brain injury: a randomized controlled trial. *Brain Injury, 19*(10), 819–831. doi:10.1080/02699050500110165

Branson, D., and Demchak, M. (2009). The use of augmentative and alternative communication methods with infants and toddlers with disabilities: A research review. *Augmentative and Alternative Communication, 25*(4), 274–286. doi:10.3109/07434610903384529

Campos da Paz, Jr, A., Burnett, S. M., and Nomura, A. M. (1996). Cerebral palsy. In R. B. Duthie, *Mercers's Orthopedic Surgery.* London: Arnold.

Cattelani R, L. F. (1998). Traumatic brain injury in childhood: Intellectual, behavioural and social outcome into adulthood. *Brain Injury, 12*(4), 283–296. doi:10.1080/026990598122584

Copley, J., and Ziviani, J. (2007). Use of a team-based approach to assistive technology assessment and planning for children with multiple disabilities: A pilot study. *Assistive Technology, 19*(3), 109–125. doi:10.1080/10400435.2007.10131869

Fallon, K. A., Light, J., and Achenbach, A. (2003). The semantic organization patterns of young children: Implications for augmentative and alternative communication. *AAC Augmentative and Alternative Communication, 19*(2), 74–85. doi:10.1080/0743461031000112061

Fallon, K. A., Light, J. C., and Paige, T. K. (2001). Enhancing vocabulary selection for preschoolers who require augmentative and alternative communication (AAC). *American Journal Speech and Language Pathology, 10*(1), 81–94. doi:10.1044/1058–0360(2001/010)

Halper, A. S. (1993). Teams and teamwork: health care settings. *ASHA, 35*(6–7), 34–48.

Hinojosa, J., Sproat, C. T., Mankhetwit, S., and Anderson, J. (2002). Shifts in parent-therapist partnerships: Twelve years of change. *American Journal of Occupational Therapy, 56*(5), 556–563. doi:10.5014/ajot.56.5.556

Huang, I., Sugden, D., and Beveridge, S. (2009). Children's perceptions of their use of assistive devices in home and school settings. *Disability and Rehabilitation: Assistive Technology, 4*(2), 95–105. doi:10.1080/17483100802613701

Jahiel, R. I., and Scherer, M. J. (2010). Initial steps towards a theory and praxis of person-environment interaction in disability. *Disability and Rehabilitation, 32*(17), 1467–1474. doi:10.3109/09638280802590637

Jans, L. H., and Scherer, M. J. (2006). Assistive technology training: Diverse audiences and multidisciplinary content. *Disability and Rehabilitation: Assistive Technology, 1*(1–2), 69–77. doi:10.1080/09638280500167290

Kellegrew, D. (2000). Constructing daily routines: A qualitative examination of mothers with young children with disabilities. *American Journal Occupational Therapy, 54*(3), 252–259. doi:10.5014/ajot.54.3.252

Ketelaar, M, Vermeer, A., Hart, H., van Petegem-van Beek, E., and Helders, P. J. (2001). Effects of a functional therapy program on motor abilities of children with cerebral palsy. *Physical Therapy, 81*(9), 1534–1545.

King, J., Nelson, T., and Heye ML, Turturro, T. C., and Titus, M. N. D. (1998). Prescriptions, referrals, order writing, and the rehabilitation team function. In J. A. DeLisa, and Bruce M. Gans (Eds.), *Rehabilitation Medicine: Principles and Practice* (pp. 269–285). Philadelphia: Lippincott-Raven.

King, S., Teplicky, R., King, G., and Rosenbaum, P. (2004). Family-centered service for children with cerebral palsy and their families: A review of the literature. *Seminars in Pediatric Neurology, 11*(1), 78–86. doi:10.1016/j.spen.2004.01.009

Körner, M. (2010). Interprofessional teamwork in medical rehabilitation: A comparison of multidisciplinary and interdisciplinary team approach. *Clinical Rehabilitation, 24*(8), 745–754. doi:10.1177/0269215510367538

Leontiev, A. N. (1978). *O Desenvolvimento do Psiquismo.* Lisbon, Portugal: Livros Horizonte.

Lindsay, S., and Tsybina, I. (2011). Predictors of unmet needs for communication and mobility assistive devices among youth with a disability: The role of socio-cultural factors. *Disability and Rehabilitation: Assistive Technology, 6*(1), 10–21. doi:10.3109/17483107.2010.514972

McDougall, J., Wright, V., and Rosenbaum, P. (2010). The ICF model of functioning and disability: Incorporating quality of life and human development. *Developmental Neurorehabilitation, 13*(3), 204–211. doi:10.3109/17518421003620525

McDougall, J., Wright, V., Schmidt, J., Miller, L., and Lowry, K. (2011). Applying the ICF framework to study changes in quality-of-life for youth with chronic conditions. *Developmental Neurorehabilitation, 14*(1), 41–53. doi:10.3109/17518423.2010.521795

McNaughton, D., Rackensperger, T., Benedek-Wood, E., Krezman, C., Williams, B., and Light, J. (2008). "A child needs to be given a chance to succeed": Parents of individuals who use AAC describe the benefits and challenges of learning AAC technologies. *AAC Augmentative and Alternative Communication, 24*(1), 43–55. doi:10.1080/07434610701421007

Murchland, S., and Parkyn, H. (2010). Using assistive technology for schoolwork: The experience of children with physical disabilities. *Disability and Rehabilitation: Assistive Technology, 5*(6), 438–447. doi:10.3109/17483107.2010.481773

Murphy, J., Markova, I., Collins, S., and Moodie, E. (1996). AAC systems: Obstacles to effective use. *European Journal of Disorders of Communication, 31*(1), 31–44. doi:10.3109/13682829609033150

OPS/OMS. (2008). *Classificação Internacional de Funcionalidade, Incapacidade e Saúde*. São Paulo, Brazil: EDUSP.

Ostensjo S, C. E. (2003). Everyday functioning in young children with cerebral palsy: Functional skills, caregiver assistance, and modifications of the environment. *Developmental Medicine and Child Neurology, 45*(9), 603–612. Retrieved from http://www.ncbi.nlm.nih.gov/pubmed/12948327

Pennington, L., Goldbart, J., and Marshall, J. (2004). Speech and language therapy to improve the communication skills of children with cerebral palsy. *International Journal of Language & Communication Disorders, 39*(2), 151–170. doi:10.1080/13682820310001625598

Pueyo-Benito, R., and Vendrell-Gomez, P. (2002). [Neuropsychology of cerebral palsy]. *Revista de Neurología, 34*, 1080–1087.

Puyuelo, M. S. (2001). Problemas de linguagem na paralisia cerebral:diagnóstico e tratamento. In M. S. Puyuelo, P. Póo, C. Basil, and M. Le Métayer, (Eds.), *A Fonoaudiologia na Paralisia Cerebral: Diagnóstico e Tratamento* (pp. 17–80). São Paulo, Brazil: Santos Livraria Editora.

Raghavendra, P., Bornman, J., Grandlund, M., and Björck-Akesson, E. (2007). The World Health Organization's International Classification of Functioning, Disability and Health: Implications for clinical and research practice in the field of augmentative and alternative communication. *Augmentative and Alternative Communication, 23*(4), 349–361. doi:10.1080/07434610701650928

Ripat, J., and Woodgate, R. (2011). The intersection of culture, disability and assistive technology. *Disability and Rehabilitation: Assistive Technology, 6*(2), 87–96. doi:10.3109/17483107.2010.507859

Scherer, M. J. (1996). Outcomes of assistive technology use on quality of life. *Disability and Rehabilitation, 18*(9), 439–448. doi:10.3109/09638289609165907

Scherer, M. J. (2004). The matching person and technology model. In M. J. Scherer, (Ed.), *Connecting to Learn: Educational and Assistive Technology for People with Disabilities* (pp. 183–201). Washington, DC: American Psychological Association.

Scherer, M. J. (2005). Assessing the benefits of using assistive technologies and other supports for thinking, remembering and learning. *Disability and Rehabilitation, 27*(13), 731–739. doi:10.1080/09638280400014816

Scherer, M. J., and Craddock, G. M. (2002). Matching Person and Technology (MPT) assessment process. *Technology & Disability, 3*(14), 125–131. Retrieved from http://iospress.metapress.com/content/g0eft4mnlwly8y8g

Scherer, M. J., Craddock, G., and MacKeogh, T. (2011). The relationship of personal factors and subjective well-being to the use of assistive technology devices. *Disability and Rehabilitation, 33*(10), 811–817. doi:10.3109/09638288.2010.511418

Scherer, M. J., Sax, C. L., Vanbiervliet, A., Cushman, L. A., and Scherer, J. V. (2005). Predictors of assistive technology use: The importance of personal and psychosocial factors. *Disability and Rehabilitation, 27*(21), 1321–1331. doi:10.1080/09638280500164800

Skär, L. (2002). Disabled children's perceptions of technical aids, assistance and peers in play situations. *Scandinavian Journal of Caring Sciences, 16*(1), 27–33. doi: 10.1046/j.1471–6712.2002.00047.x

Stoner, J. B., Maureen, E., and Angell, R. L. (2010). Implementing augmentative and alternative communication in inclusive educational settings: A case study. *AAC Augmentative and Alternative Communication, 26*(2), 122–135. doi:10.3109/07434618.2010.481092

Strauss, D., Ojdana, K., Shavelle, R., and Rosenbloom, L. (2004). Decline in function and life expectancy of older persons with cerebral palsy. *Neurorehabilitation, 19,* 69–78. Retrieved from http://iospress.metapress.com/content/egevj8d1dyv9wpr7/

Vygostsky, L. V. (1984). *A Formação Social da Mente.* São Paulo, Brazil: Martins Fontes.

Vygotsky, L. V. (1991). *Pensamento e Linguagem.* São Paulo, Brazil: Martins Fontes.

Warzak, W. J., Allan, T. M., Ford, L. A., and Stefans, V. (1995). Common obstacles to the daily functioning of pediatric traumatically brain injured patients: Perceptions of caregivers and psychologists. *Child Health Care, 24*(2), 133–141. doi:10.1207/s15326888chc2402_5

Wilson, D. J., Mitchell, J. M., Kemp, B. J., Adkins, R. H., and Mann, W. (2009). Effects of assistive technology on functional decline in people aging with a disability. *Assistive Technology, 21*(4), 208–217. doi:10.1080/10400430903246068

Ylvisaker, M. (1998). *Traumatic Brain Injury Rehabilitation: Children and Adolescents.* Woburn, MA: Butterworth-Heinemann.

13

The Geriatrician

M. Pigliautile, L. Tiberio, P. Mecocci, and S. Federici

CONTENTS

13.1 Introduction

The word "geriatrics" was coined by Ignatz Leo Nascher (1863–1944), a Viennese man who worked as a physician in New York and who claimed that aging is not a disease but a period of life with its own physiology, requiring the need to treat geriatric medicine as a separate entity, as is done for pediatrics (Achenbaum 1995; Morley 2004). In the 1930s, Marjory Warren developed the principles of modern geriatric medicine in the United Kingdom by enhancing the environment, introducing active rehabilitation programs, and emphasizing the importance of the older person's motivation (Morley 2004).

Over time, geriatric medicine developed core values, a knowledge base, and clinical skills to improve the health, functioning, and well-being of older people and to afford appropriate palliative care, for which a marked expansion over the past three decades occurred to meet the growing needs for care of the aging population (American Geriatrics Society Core Writing Group of the Task Force on the Future of Geriatric Medicine 2005). In fact, the U.S. Census Bureau data (Kinsella and He 2009) reports an extraordinary demographic and epidemiological change that can be seen as a success story for public health policies and for socioeconomic development, consisting of an increase in the world's population aged 65 and over (from 7% in 2008 to 14% by 2040, with Japan in first position in the ranking countries with the oldest population followed by Italy and Germany), an increase in life expectancy, and a rise in the number of the oldest old (population aged 80 and above).

A geriatrician is consulted when an older person is frail and/or disabled (Fried 1994; Fried and Guralnik 1997; Fried et al. 2001, 2004, 2009), as Hazzard wrote,

> How often have I been asked over the past 30 years, "What is a geriatrician?" I cannot count the times and the ways that I have tried to answer this question. But clearly, even as the field has grown and matured, the public continues to have at best a vague idea of what a geriatrician is and does and why. […] I am a geriatrician. I specialize in the medical, psychological, and social care of old people. […] Perhaps my most typical patient is the old-fashioned picture of frailty, a man—or more often a woman—who lives on the razor's edge between independence and triggering a tragic cascade of diseases, disabilities, and complications that all too often prove irreversible. […] I am by definition an expert in subtlety and complexity. (2004, p. 161)

13.2 Analysis of the Older Patient: Diseases, Disability, and Frailty

Hazzard's words become clearer when considering the aging process. Aging is defined as an "accumulation of diverse deleterious changes in the cells and tissues with advancing age that increase the risk of disease and death" (Harman 2001, p. 2). Disease, disability, and frailty play an important role in the aging process.

13.2.1 Disease

Fried (2000) identified the 15 most prevalent conditions among people aged 65 years old or above in the United States: arthritis, hypertension, heart disease, hearing loss, influenza, injuries, orthopedic impairment, cataracts, chronic sinusitis, depression, malignant neoplasms, diabetes mellitus, visual impairment, urinary incontinence, and varicose veins.

Heron and colleagues (2009) found that heart disease, cancer, strokes, chronic lower respiratory tract disease, accidents (unintentional injuries), diabetes mellitus, and Alzheimer's disease were the seven leading causes of death in the United States in 2006.

Studies on comorbidity—the combination of additional diseases beyond an index disorder (Feinstein 1970)—and multimorbidity—the co-occurrence of diseases in the same person (Batstra et al. 2002)—have been conducted using different methods with the aim of identifying the relationship among disease clusters, health outcomes, and possible prevention programs (Guralnik 1996; de Groot et al. 2003; Marengoni et al. 2009). A recent study evaluated patterns of comorbidity and multimorbidity in an elderly population and found that chronic diseases were more likely to occur with comorbid conditions than alone (Marengoni et al. 2009). Hypertension and dementia were the most frequent diseases occurring with and without a comorbid disorder, whereas a few cases of heart failure and hip fracture occurred without any comorbidity. Heart failure and visual impairment were associated with the highest number of comorbid diseases and dementia with the lowest. Circulatory diseases were the most commonly co-occurring pairs of conditions. Co-occurring diseases clustered together beyond that which would be expected by chance and five major clusters were identified: Two of them were linked to vascular diseases, the others to dementia, diabetes mellitus, and malignancy.

Older age, female gender, and low socioeconomic status were found to be the main causes of multimorbidity, whereas disability and functional state decline, poor quality of life, and high health-care costs were the major consequences of multimorbidity (Marengoni et al. 2011). Considering epidemiological data on mental disorders in the older population, it is important to know that comorbid mental disorders are associated with functional status and quality of life, and that mental disorders increase the risk of death (Gijsen et al. 2001). In particular, dementia and depression are very common mental disorders in the elderly population. Approximately 24 million people have dementia in the world, with the number being projected to double every 20 years. Approximately 60% of dementia patients live in developing countries, and this proportion is predicted to increase to more than 70% by 2040 (Qiu et al. 2007). With respect to attendance rates due to the various forms of dementia, the main cause is Alzheimer's disease (50–80% of dementia cases), followed by Lewy body dementia (20%) and vascular dementia (5%; Corey-Bloom 2004). Considering the epidemiology of depression in the elderly, Alexopoulos (2005) reported 1–4% for major depression and 4–13% for minor depression. The incidence and prevalence of depression is double this in the oldest old, and the prevalence in medical settings is higher than in the community. Late-life depression is common in individuals with medical and psychosocial problems such as cognitive impairment, diseases, and social isolation. The care of depressed older people is complicated by a reciprocal interaction of depression with disability, medical illness, treatment adherence, and psychosocial factors (Alexopoulos et al. 2002). Depression is a predictor of disability in both sexes; in fact, it causes physical and social inactivity and the psychological aspects of depression even provoke a sense of disability (Tas et al. 2007).

13.2.2 Disability

Considering the interaction between disease and the environment, the concept of disability, in a biopsychosocial perspective, is an important aspect to consider in a society with an increasing number of old people. In a recent study (Landi et al. 2010), physical disability in aging was described as an effect of diseases plus physiological alterations connected to aging. In this view, social, economic, and behavioral factors and access to medical care modify the impact of the underlying causes. At the same time, disability is considered as an adverse health outcome and a risk factor for other adverse health outcomes. On the basis of several studies, the authors wrote that "disability, independent of its causes, may predict subsequent difficulty in instrumental and basic activities of daily living, and it has been associated with an increased risk of death, hospitalization, need for long term care, and higher health care expenditures" (Landi et al. 2010, p. 752).

During the last few decades, different scenarios have been proposed concerning the patterns of health trends in older people; these were resumed by Jagger (2000):

1. The compression of morbidity theory suggests that disease and disability will become compressed into a short period before death if changes in lifestyle delay the age –at onset and the progression of nonfatal disabling diseases (Fries 1980).

2. The opposite view, namely the expansion of morbidity theory, proposes that living longer implies living with a disabling disease such as Parkinson's disease, dementia, vision and hearing loss, and arthritis (Kramer 1980).

3. The third theory supports a dynamic equilibrium between an increase in the number of years lived with a disability and the number of years lived with a less severe disability (Manton 1982).

Many different studies have been dedicated to exploring the trends in mortality, morbidity, and disability. The U.S. Census Bureau (Kinsella and He 2009) reports that the prevalence of chronic conditions is increasing while disability is decreasing in developed countries, whereas the prevalence of disability is likely to increase in developing countries.

In the Rotterdam study, an analysis of the incidence of disability and its risk factors in multiple dimensions in community-dwelling women and men of older age, found that age, self-rated health, being overweight, depression, joint complaints, and medication use were predictors of disability for both men and women. Stroke, falling, and the presence of comorbidities predicted disability in men only, whereas having a partner, poor cognitive functioning, osteoarthritis, and morning stiffness predicted disability in women (Tas et al. 2007).

According to the compression morbidity theory, a recent study identified clinically distinct trajectories of disability in the last year of life and attempted to determine whether and how the distribution of these trajectories differed according to the condition leading to death (Gill et al. 2010). The results demonstrated that, for most of the decedents, the course of disability at the end of life did not follow a predictable pattern on the basis of the most common conditions leading to death: cancer, advanced dementia, organ failure, frailty, sudden death, and other conditions. Dementia was the condition with the least variation and was characterized by high levels of disability throughout the last year of life. For the other conditions, catastrophic disability was found a few months before death. The authors commented on evidence supporting the need to provide services at the end of life, especially for patients with dementia. In line with this, it was shown that dementia is the most important risk factor for the development of geriatric syndromes during hospitalization (Mecocci et al. 2005), suggesting that the hospital environment should be adapted to the needs of patients with cognitive problems.

Although it has been documented that disabilities and limitations have shown improvements over the last decade (Freedman et al. 2002), and that people are living longer than they did previously with less disability and fewer functional limitations (Christensen et al. 2009), older people (particularly of the oldest age) are often described as a "frail" group who are particularly vulnerable to diseases and functional disability and who are at a greater risk of losing the ability to manage their daily activities independently (Fried et al. 2001; Song et al. 2010).

13.2.3 Frailty

Frailty is defined as "a clinical state of increased vulnerability and decreased ability to maintain homeostasis that is age-related and centrally characterized by declines in functional reserve across multiple physiologic systems" (Fried et al. 2009, p. 634). A recent review identified different models of frailty coexisting in the literature where the "physical phenotype" and the "multidomain phenotype" that can be considered as extreme points on a continuum ranged from physical aspects to multiple aspects, respectively, including cognitive, functional, and social domains (Abellan van Kan et al. 2010). The main differences between the proposed models are due to the differences in considering physical, functional, cognitive, and social domains as components of the frailty model or as frailty outcomes. For example, disability is considered by many as a component of frailty and by others as an outcome; in fact, a survey of 62 geriatricians, focusing on the significance of the terms "frailty" and "disability," showed that 98% of the respondents considered frailty and disability to be two distinct entities with different prognoses and health-care implications (Fried et al. 2004). A different predictive capacity for clinical outcomes is associated with various models. The "physical phenotype" defines frailty as a biological syndrome of decreased physiological reserves resulting in a cumulative decline in all physiological systems and vulnerability to adverse outcomes and provides an operational definition by means of measurable items (exhaustion, weight loss, low energy expenditure, weak grip strength, and slow walking speed) that allow the classification of older people in "no frailty," "intermediate," and "frail" groups (Fried et al. 2001). This model supports the distinction among frailty, comorbidity, and disability. The physiological changes associated with aging can be considered as being the factors that contribute to frailty. Frailty can cause a risk of disability, but the fundamental concept is that although frailty, disability, and comorbidity are often associated, one is not synonymous with the other: Comorbidity represents an etiological factor of frailty and disability is an outcome of frailty (Fried et al. 2001, 2004). Disability can arise from a dysfunction in a single system or in many systems, but frailty always implies a multisystem dysfunction. Disability does not need to be associated with instability, whereas frailty always is (Rockwood et al. 2000). Frailty is a predictor of falls, hospitalization, disability, and death (Fried et al. 2001). The "multidomain phenotype" includes multidomain models resulting from regression models that consider cognitive, functional, and social aspects (Abellan van Kan et al. 2010). Frailty measures depending on the deficit identify frailty by means of comprehensive geriatric assessment. Rockwood and colleagues (1999) compiled a frailty index considering cognitive status, mood, motivation, communication, mobility balance, bowel and bladder functions, activities of daily living, nutrition, and social resources as well as several comorbidities. This index was highly predictive of death or institutionalization. More recently, a standard procedure for constructing a frailty index was proposed (Searle et al. 2008). On the basis of the idea that having more health deficits corresponds to a major probability of becoming fragile, the frailty index counts deficits in health (symptoms, signs, diseases, and disabilities or laboratory, radiographic, or electrocardiographic abnormalities). At the same time, in this theoretical framework, disability and dementia are components of the frailty index and are evaluated as poor clinical outcomes in the theoretical framework. The social domain receives particular attention because social isolation could have a strong impact on the development of dementia or disability (Abellan van Kan et al. 2010).

Now it appears clearer why Hazzard defines the geriatrician as an expert in subtlety and complexity. The explanation of these three main concepts highlights how complex this particular population is and the effective need of an expert physician. In fact, the care of older people differs from that of younger people for different reasons related to life expectancy, disease prevalence and comorbidity, social resources, goals of treatment, and preferences for care (Reuben et al. 2003).

13.3 Geriatric Assessment

The Geriatric Medicine Section of the European Union of Medical Specialists (UEMS) defines geriatric medicine as "a specialty of medicine concerned with physical, mental, functional and social conditions in acute, chronic, rehabilitative, preventive, and end of life care in older patients" with the aim to "optimise the functional status of the older person and improve the quality of life and autonomy" (2008, p. 1). Older patients are described as a group that requires a holistic approach and difficulties in the diagnostic process, response to treatment, and the need for social support are emphasized.

Straus and Tinetti (2009) identified five factors that distinguish clinical approaches toward elderly people from the traditional medicine proposed for young adult patients:

1. The difficulty in differentiating age-related physiological changes in organ systems from disease and the coexistence of chronic diseases;
2. The fact that distressing symptoms or impairments frequently depend on several factors (physical, psychological, social, environmental, etc.);
3. The difficulty for the physician in selecting and interpreting diagnostic tests that may be affected by age and comorbidity;
4. The variability observed in the importance that older patients assign to potential health outcomes; and
5. The involvement of caregivers who support the patients, provide information, and facilitate in terms of treatment, but who could also be a source of conflict when their goals do not coincide with those of the patient.

Unlike the traditional disease-oriented form of medical evaluation, the geriatric approach to the patient includes the assessment of cognitive, affective, functional, social, economic, environmental, and spiritual factors as well as a discussion about the patient's preferences regarding advance directives (Reuben and Rosen 2009), as illustrated in Figure 13.1.

In addition to medical history, a physical examination, and laboratory and ancillary tests, the geriatrician considers visual and hearing impairments, malnutrition/weight loss, urinary incontinence, balance and gait impairments, falling, and polypharmacy.

The assessment could be implemented by a single geriatrician or by a team of health professionals; in the latter case, the term "comprehensive geriatric assessment" (CGA) is used. This term was defined by a National Institute of Health (NIH) Consensus Development Conference in 1987 as a

> multidisciplinary evaluation in which the multiple problems of older persons are uncovered, described, and explained, if possible, and in which the resources and strengths of

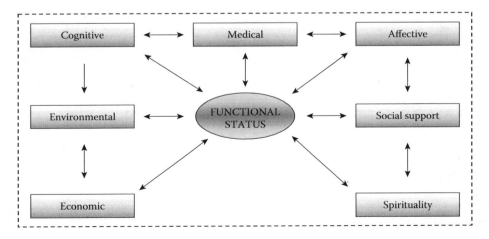

FIGURE 13.1
Interaction dimensions of the Geriatric Assessment. Modified from Reuben and Rosen (2009).

the person are catalogued, need for services assessed, and a coordinate care plan developed to focus interventions on the person's problems. (NIH Consensus Development Program, 1987).

and by Rubenstein as a "a multidimensional interdisciplinary diagnostic process intended to determine a frail elderly person's medical, psychosocial, and functional capabilities and problems in order to develop an overall plan for treatment and long-term follow-up" (Rubenstein 1995, p. 3). The goals of CGA have been summarized by Rubenstein (1995) as: enhancing diagnostic accuracy, optimizing medical treatment and living location, improving medical outcomes, improving function and quality of life, reducing unnecessary service usage, and arranging long-term care management.

A CGA can be performed in different health contexts, ranging from the hospital to the patient's home, and requires different programs, assessment instruments, and goals depending on the setting (Reuben and Rosen 2009).

Having identified impairments and disabilities through a comprehensive geriatric assessment, there are alternative ways of delivering care. One of these ways is rehabilitation, which represents a core element in the practice of medicine for older people.

In Section 13.4, a definition and an overview of geriatric rehabilitation are given that highlight the key relevant clinical diagnoses and rehabilitation interventions focusing on the role of assistive technology in the care process and everyday support of the frail and/ or disabled elderly.

13.4 Geriatric Rehabilitation

Rehabilitation is one of the basic elements of comprehensive geriatric care and it has been defined as "an active problem-solving and educational process, focused on disability and aiming to maximize the patient's participation in society and his or her well-being while reducing stress on the family" (Wade 1999, p. 176; see also Wade 1992). As described in previous sections, the elderly population is characterized by the presence of comorbidity, disability, and frailty, which requires appropriate geriatric rehabilitation services.

Geriatric rehabilitation has two main objectives: On the one hand, it limits the impact of disability and, on the other hand, it stimulates and strengthens residual abilities, encouraging and supporting motivation and needs through therapeutic interventions focused on the person and his or her living environment. The burden of a comorbid disease influences a patient's ability to tolerate a rehabilitative intervention. Therefore, an interdisciplinary approach should be adopted to achieve the best functional outcomes (Wells et al. 2003a).

Geriatric rehabilitation can be provided in a rehabilitation clinic, a subacute rehabilitation unit, a skilled nursing facility, or via home health assistance. The basic team consists of different subspecialty professionals, such as a physical therapist, who will assess a wide array of abilities, including strength, balance, transfer (rising from a chair), and walking. An occupational therapist evaluates self-care skills, activities of daily living, and the home environment. The occupational therapist can also provide training on how to use assistive technologies, incorporating meaningful activities to promote participation in everyday life. The occupational therapist assesses the patient's ability to perform his or her daily activities, whereas the physical therapist focuses on improving mobility. In addition, other professional members of the rehabilitation team are the speech therapist, nurse, social worker, dietician, psychologist, physiatrist, and pharmacist (Tsukuda 1990; Brown and Peel 2009). Rehabilitation treatment requires collaboration among team members, the patient, and his/her family. On the one hand, the patient should play an active part in the care and decision-making process, and, on the other, the family should ideally receive training on how to assist the older patient at home. This involvement influences not only rehabilitation outcomes but also the quality of life of the patient in all aspects: functional, physical, social, and emotional. A patient's satisfaction with care tends to be greater when there is such involvement (Toseland et al. 1996). This approach is in line with the biopsychosocial model, where the functioning of an older patient is not only seen in association with health condition but is also linked to personal and environmental factors. To prescribe an appropriate rehabilitation treatment, the health-care team should have a common understanding of health and functioning in a disability context. The International Classification of Functioning, Disability, and Health (ICF) model provides a helpful framework that illustrates why geriatric rehabilitation must be an interdisciplinary activity (WHO 2001).

Some common clinical problems in geriatric rehabilitation include hip fracture, stroke, and cognitive impairments, which have been discussed above (Wells et al. 2003b). The most serious risk factor for fracture is falling and frailty and, as a consequence, disability. Frequently, fractures occur at home, but they also occur just as frequently in hospital and in residential contexts. Appropriate preventive measures should be taken to protect the elderly who are at risk. Hip fractures require the most intense use of hospital resources and an intensive period of postoperative medical care and inpatient rehabilitation. The risk of stroke doubles every 10 years from the age of 55:72% of all strokes occur after the age of 65 (Feigin et al. 2003). Elderly patients suffering from a cerebrovascular accident have a clinical onset more severe than in younger patients, with a higher mortality rate by 30 days and a greater number of long-term admittances (Asplund et al. 1992).

Among the clinical factors that contribute toward the worst outcomes, two are very significant: the presence of a more severe initial clinical symptoms frame and reduced recovery capabilities (Nakayama et al. 1994).

The literature underlines the need for screening to identify patients who are most likely to benefit from geriatric rehabilitation. In this respect, CGA and the role of the geriatrician are very essential for two main reasons. Firstly, they offer a clear picture of the patient, the disease, and the possible health and social disadvantages that might result from the disability. Secondly, they decide upon the type of rehabilitation treatment to be used and the most appropriate intervention in terms of a technological aid.

An important goal of screening patients is in fact to identify comorbidities that may affect rehabilitation outcomes by evaluating functional impairment, medical complications, psychological functioning, and social support (Mosqueda 1993). Cognitive screening is also crucial in selecting patients for geriatric rehabilitation: Cognitive disorders are commonly and potentially critical regarding rehabilitation outcomes because they affect different aspects of treatment (e.g., difficulties related to understanding instructions or remembering information) (Ruchinskas and Curyto 2003). Cognitive impairments hinder the outcome of rehabilitation treatment (Patrick et al. 2001). Evidence from the literature shows that cognitive disorders are correlated with limited and poor results in functional and rehabilitation outcomes in elderly patients, particularly with regard to hip fractures (Colombo 2004). Cognitive disorders are considered as selection criteria for admission to a rehabilitation process. When a patient is suffering from a mild form of reduced cognition, there is good reason to be optimistic about rehabilitation outcomes. In addition, depression is a frequent complication after hip fracture or stroke that can negatively affect rehabilitation treatments. Furthermore, depression is a frequent complication after hip fracture or stroke; it may match with a cognitive impairment that is negatively affecting rehabilitation treatments. In general, depression is a very common disorder in the elderly and its effects on rehabilitation should be considered because persistent symptoms of depression are associated with a decline in cognitive and physical functioning (Wells et al. 2003b). In this respect, detailed neuropsychological screening is needed to detect cognitive impairment and depression and, consequently, to determine the course of further treatment (Ruchinskas and Curyto 2003).

Aside from medical conditions, several factors may influence the success of rehabilitation treatment (Brown and Peel 2009). When disability has been present for many years, the goals of treatment may be directed toward compensatory strategies or the treatment of deconditioning. Patients with low motivation require goals that are attainable and that can be reached in measurable steps to benefit from rehabilitation therapy. For patients nearing the end of rehabilitation, interventions should be focused on reducing the workload of the caregiver and the patient's discomfort. Critical circumstances, such as states of severe disability, malnutrition, the absence of a caregiver, financial limitations, and cultural beliefs, may limit the benefits from rehabilitation treatments, precluding the use of certain techniques and assistive solutions.

One of most commonly used interventions in geriatric rehabilitation, as well as in physical and cognitive exercise programs, includes the implementation of assistive solutions and the use of specific technological devices suitable for an individual's disability. The use of assistive technology enables the older person to interact more favorably with their life environment.

In Section 13.5, a definition of "assistive solution" and an overview of today's technologies for promoting independence and quality of life for elderly people with a disability will be given.

13.5 Assistive Solutions: A Challenge in Geriatric Rehabilitation

In recent years, awareness about the contribution that technological aids can make in supporting people with disabilities has increased, outlining the immense potential of assistive technology in helping elderly people with physical or cognitive limitations to perform activities of daily living. The International Standards Organization (ISO) 9999 (2007) defines technical aids as "any product, instrument, equipment or technical system used by a disabled person, especially produced or generally available, preventing, compensating, monitoring, relieving or neutralizing impairments, activity limitations and participation restrictions." The ICF adopts a more concise definition: "Any product, tool, equipment or technology adapted or designed specifically to improve the functioning of a disabled person" (WHO 2001, p. 164).

Technological development is one of the factors that pushed the WHO to reconsider the International Classification of Impairments, Disabilities, and Handicaps model on the basis of a linear causal relationship impairment → disability → handicap (WHO 1980, p. 11). According to the ICF, disability should not be seen as an attribute, but as a situation in which every individual could happen to find him/herself whenever there is a gap between individual capacity and environmental factors. To compensate for a disability, a technological device may not be sufficient. A merger is required between mainstream and assistive technologies with an assembly that is different from one person to another as the situation changes from one context to another. This merger can be designated as an assistive solution (AAATE 2003).

It is part of the ICF model of functioning and disability that environmental factors such as assistive technologies have the potential to reduce the impact of disability on a person's performance in all areas of daily living, and so increase the individual's autonomy and independence.

Within geriatric rehabilitation, assistive solutions may have the potential to enhance the outcomes of interventions through the systematic application of technological devices that meet the functional needs of people with cognitive and physical disabilities.

In this section, we will try to provide an overview of the areas where technological systems may offer support to the everyday life of the elderly and their caregivers. A recent field research study focused on the needs that the elderly and their caregivers expressed regarding the contribution of assistive technology to their everyday life and outlined four main areas of support: a need for the management of dementia symptoms, a need for social contacts to be maintained, a need for daily life activities, and a need for health monitoring and safety support (Lauriks et al. 2007).

The following section provides examples of commercially available and emerging assistive technologies for elderly people aimed at compensating for deficiencies such as memory and motor problems. A brief survey of socially assistive robotics systems is also given. Their main function is aimed at rehabilitation and at enhancing elderly health and psychological well-being.

13.5.1 Technological Devices for Elderly People With Cognitive Impairments

Assistive technologies to compensate for cognitive and neuropsychological disabilities take into account "cognitive prosthesis" or "cognitive orthosis" devices. Cognitive prostheses are computer-based systems that reduce the negative impact of disability on daily functional activities (Cole 1999). When these systems are used for rehabilitation purposes, it is necessary to design them with features that are highly customizable and easy to use. In general, cognitive aids include wearable devices, computer systems, personal digital assistants, and integrated sensory systems. They may improve the performance of elderly people with cognitive impairments and dementia through reminders or assistance in the execution of tasks (Gorman et al. 2003; Pollack et al. 2003; DeVaul 2004; Philipose et al. 2004; Mihailidis et al. 2008). Cognitive impairments are one of the reasons for medication nonadherence and treatment failure (Muir et al. 2001).

For example, cognitive prospective memory aids are context-aware technological aids that can help older people with cognitive disabilities to perform a programmed task (reminder systems) or they may provide a set of instructions related to the procedural guidance in activity execution (prompting systems). Reminder systems (e.g., electronic organizers, voice recorders, software for computers, communication devices, and personal digital assistants) are also very useful in case of difficulty in the management of medication therapy by older people. These devices can provide an alarm system, daily schedule planning, and the temporary or permanent storage of information to monitor medication use (McGarry Logue 2002).

The PEAT (Planning and Execution Assistant and Training) system is an example of automatic planning software that operates on a personal digital assistant or mobile phone. It provides personalized prompts to guide a person during the execution of a task (Levinson 1997). The ISAAC Cognitive Prosthetic Assistive Technology system is a hand-held cognitive prosthetic aid specifically designed for individuals who have a wide range of cognitive disabilities. It delivers individualized prompts and procedural information in a speech, audio, text, checklist, or graphic format. A case study involving two individuals with brain injury showed improved independence in activities of daily living and better communication with caregivers as a consequence of ISAAC (Gorman et al. 2003). Cognitive Orthosis for Assisting aCtivities in the Home (COACH) is a prototype system designed to support people with dementia in autonomously completing a hand-washing task. The COACH system provides prerecorded verbal prompts and uses a single video camera, neural networks, and plan recognition to automatically monitor the execution of the task. The results from a clinical trial with 10 elders with moderate to severe dementia showed significant improvements in the completion of hand-washing tasks without caregiver assistance after the use of the COACH system (Mihailidis et al. 2004).

Another problem associated with cognitive disability that accompanies the early stages of dementia, especially in the case of Alzheimer's dementia, is disorientation on not only the temporal level but also on the spatial level. Spatial-temporal disorientation is a threat to the safety of these patients and increases the apprehension and burden of caregivers. Global position system (GPS) technology provides some aids that include wrist watches with a GPS locator (GPS Locator Watch by Verify, and Digital Angel for Senior Wanderers). An integrated system using a wireless transceiver can detect the exact position of the older adult and allows caregivers to communicate and monitor the person from a distance (Parnes 2010). However, these technologies have not yet been widely validated and require further investigation, including long-term usage tests focused on identifying the key needs of both elderly people suffering dementia and their caregivers and on seeking ethical approval.

13.5.2 Technological Devices for Elderly People With Motor Disability

Daily activities also require the ability to move and interact with the environment as independently as possible. Osteoporosis, one of the most common bone diseases in the elderly population, and changes in visual and auditory perception can easily lead to a reduced personal mobility in old age. In this regard, there are several devices that claim to make life easier for seniors. Assistive technologies for older people with mobility limitations cover different products and intelligent systems, from bath lifts and rails, powered and autonomous wheelchairs, and smart walkers to upper/lower limb prosthetics.

The smart walker "Guido," the latest evolution of PAM-AID (Personal Adaptive Mobility Aid), was designed to facilitate the mobility of blind elderly people and focuses on power-assisted wall or corridor following (Lacey and Dawson-Howe 1998). The PAMM (Personal Aid for Mobility and Monitoring) device is aimed at supporting the navigation of elderly people who live independently or in senior assisted living facilities. It provides both guidance to destinations through preprogrammed maps, schedules, user commands, and sensed obstacles and continuous health monitoring (Yu et al. 2003). Wheelchair-mounted robotic arms (WMRAs) are devices with a manipulator arm on the wheelchair to provide assistance throughout the day (Alqasemi et al. 2005). Typical tasks of WRMAs include manipulating and moving objects, assistance with eating and drinking, and controlling communication devices and environment control units. Older adults can usually control the WRMA using a joystick, keypad, voice-command, or other input device.

The assistive robotic manipulator known as MANUS is a commercially available, WMRA that is able to assist older people with an upper-limb disability. Through a keypad and a joystick, the older person can drive MANUS manually, deciding the location and orientation to be achieved (Hok Kwee 1998; Driessen et al. 2001). Several studies have tested the effectiveness of an upper-limb robotic therapy that is based on the use of MANUS for improving motor outcomes among chronic stroke patients. The results showed positive benefits in trials with people who had moderate impairments, but also among severely impaired chronic stroke patients (Krebs et al. 2004).

13.5.3 Socially Assistive Robotics Systems

This section describes robotic devices for assisting elderly people. Assistive technologies that are based on robotic platforms may play an important role both in the rehabilitation domain and social assistance area. In the first case, the systems described in Section 13.5.2 offer support that is based on physical interaction (intelligent wheelchairs, artificial limbs, etc.). Socially assistive robots may be perceived as social entities that communicate with the user through social interaction. Social robots are divided into service robots (telepresence systems, reminding and monitoring) and companion robots. Some of these systems are available as trade products whereas others are still under development. Studies on socially assistive robots describe several devices for the maintenance of personal autonomy in terms of support for basic activities of daily living (eating, bathing, toileting, and dressing), the mobility of people (including shipping), and environmental and personal monitoring. Examples of these robots are "nursebot Pearl," which includes a system of reminders (e.g., medication, appointments in the program), telepresence (to allow the medical personnel and operators to interact remotely with a senior person who lives alone), and monitoring (for systematic supervising of the activity/health status of the person). Pearl is also a personal assistant and a social interaction system that facilitates contact with others (Pollack et al. 2003). The I-Cat robot is a robot cat that shows different facial expressions as an index of emotions. The studies on I-Cat focused on aspects of social interaction between older people and robots and on the effects of I-Cat behavior on its acceptance by elderly people (van Breemen et al. 2005). Through Care-O-Bot, older users can control lighting, heating, and air conditioning in their own homes and they can get in touch with a doctor or relatives. The Care-O-Bot robot is a mobile robotic home assistant designed to perform household tasks, media management, daytime management (e.g., time for medicine), the supervision of vital signs, and make emergency calls. It has the ability to guide a person around the house whilst avoiding obstacles and operates safely and reliably in different environments. The latest prototype, Care-O-Bot II, also has manipulator abilities that make it a more efficient assistant in the tasks of daily living (Graf et al. 2004). The Italian project RoboCare has developed an intelligent prototype system integrating robotic, sensory, and software agents to create innovative services for an elderly person at home. Its key feature is the ability to maintain continuity of behavior, such as ensuring the continuous monitoring of the state of an assisted elder and of his/ her domestic context, creating a context at the knowledge level around the actions that the assisted person performs, and providing contextualized interaction services aimed at proactive assistance for the assisted older adult (Cesta et al. 2003). Part of the research in RoboCare focused on an evaluation of elderly people's perception of assistive robots. The results showed how the acceptability of robotic devices in the home setting does not only depend on the practical benefits they can provide, but also on the complex relationships among cognitive, affective, and emotional components of people's images of a robot. The RP-7 In-Touch Health platform is a telepresence device that allows patients to be monitored remotely. Patients can see and hear their doctor in real time through a video-screen and speaker system. Patients prefer to see their doctor, even through a robot. Health-care professionals can make decisions based on vital signs transmitted in real time by visiting the patient remotely. The first results of a study conducted at the University of Maryland Hospital showed that most patients are comforted by the use of this robot because the platform enables them to maintain a more constant contact with health-care professionals (InTouch Health 2004).

13.6 Acceptance, Rejection, or Abandonment of an Assistive Technology

The acceptability and willingness by elderly people to use assistive solutions seem to be complex issues. A technological aid is a helpful support when used properly and designed appropriately on the basis of a user's characteristics and needs. Aging effects certainly have an influence on how willing older adults are to use existing technologies as well as how they learn to use new technologies. Personal factors such as age-related changes in perception, cognitive, and motor systems; anxiety; self-efficacy; and familiarity with technology represent strong predictors of technology adoption and its effective use (Czaja et al. 2006). McCreadie and Tinker (2005) suggested a complex model of acceptability in which the interaction between individual "felt need" for assistance and "product quality" play an important role. According to the authors, the synergy between individual needs and the personal life environment create the perception that a person needs help. In addition, if a technological device works properly, reliably, and safely, older people are more willing to accept and use it in everyday life. When a person accepts the technological aid only in terms of necessity and as a means of carrying out activities of daily life, acceptability is defined as reluctant. When the assistive solution is perceived as being part of one's own life, the acceptability is defined as grateful, and when a person considers the technological device as being a part of themselves, the acceptability is described as internal (Karmarkar et al. 2008). Another factor that influences the acceptability of assistive solutions is the perception of advantages or disadvantages of a device: If the perceived advantages outweigh the disadvantages, acceptability of the assistive solution increases. Cesta and colleagues (2011), in their study on the interaction of elderly people with an assistive technology domestic system, identified relevant issues about the acceptability of a robot by elderly users in the domestic environment. They found that elderly people recognize the practical advantages provided by an intelligent assistant, which can help the users in the management of everyday activities and age-related difficulties and makes them feel sure. According to the Technology Acceptance Model (TAM), perceived usefulness and perceived ease of use induce the user to acquire and use an assistive solution (Davis 1993). In addition, TAM indicates that the actual use of the system is predicted by the behavioral intention.

The acceptability of a specific support is probably influenced by the coping strategies elderly people commonly use to manage the weakening of their competences (Brandtstädter et al. 1990; Slangen-de Kort et al. 1998). Assimilative strategies involve an active modification of the environment to reach personal goals; conversely, accommodative strategies imply a personal adaptation to the environment. In this respect, it is clear that the acceptability of a technological support may depend on the extent to which it modifies the characteristics of older adult's home. In addition, another issue to be considered is the features of daily life for which the assistive solution is expected to be used. Environmental barriers (such as a two-story house) could limit the acceptability of an assistive solution, so it is important to assess physical environmental barriers in the home and in the outdoor environment (Iwarsson and Slaug 2001). Another factor affecting the acceptability of an assistive solution is the potential risk that using such a device will stigmatize the disabled person. Furthermore, the use of an assistive solution can indicate a change in personal competencies and this is associated with negative social judgments, affecting personal motivation and the adoption of a technological aid (Gitlin 1995).

Training in the use of a device is an important component for improving acceptability (Elliot 1991). One of the initial difficulties in the use of a device may be its installation, which might require skills and learning steps that are not always easy for an elderly person to learn, especially when there is the presence of cognitive deficits. Electronic systems, such as a reminder, may be difficult to manipulate and their interfaces could be too small and unclear to learn. Chiu and Man (2004) indicated that older adults who received training after discharge from the hospital showed a higher rate of satisfaction and usage of a device than older adults who did not receive training. A training program for the use of an assistive solution should provide client and family involvement in the selection of a device, follow-up care, and training in its use (Karmarkar et al. 2008).

Overall, the abandonment of an assistive device is often the result of an unsuccessful process of "matching person and technology" (Scherer 1998, 2002; Scherer and Craddock 2002). When providing an assistive solution, it is essential to conduct a careful evaluation of the potential user and to consider several steps before providing a technological aid. In this respect, the biopsychosocial model of the ICF can improve the selection of assistive solutions and help determine the best match of elderly user to a technological aid (Arthanat and Lenker 2004; Scherer 2005).

13.7 The Role of the Geriatrician in the Assistive Technology Assessment Process

When the user of a center for technical aid is an older person, the geriatrician should be involved in the assistive technology assessment (ATA) process as a professional consultant. Generally, an elderly person is admitted to a center for technical aid after a geriatric assessment. In an initial interview that is focused on gathering background information of the potential user, the geriatrician helps in reading and interpreting the data from the geriatric assessment.

In the multidisciplinary team, the geriatrician cooperates in deciding whether the data are sufficient for a "matching process" and, if necessary, he/she can assess the user or suggest instruments of assessment. To describe the user from an ICF perspective, the geriatrician relates the geriatric assessment dimensions to the ICF code, as illustrated in Table 13.1, because by adopting the ICF language the geriatrician is able to facilitate a dialogue with the other professional consultants of the multidisciplinary team.

When a description of the individual's level of functioning is obtained, the user's request is evaluated and the geriatrician informs about the hypothetical scenarios regarding the progression of a particular health condition and helps the team to identify factors that may influence the matching process in terms of acceptance and the risk of rejection or abandonment. When assessing the assistive solution proposed, the geriatrician intervenes in monitoring the health condition and in evaluating the efficacy of the device. If an environmental evaluation is necessary, the geriatrician should also be involved.

TABLE 13.1

Geriatric Assessment and ICF codes

GA	Components	Examples of tests and assessment techniques	ICF codes
Medical	Physical	Interview centre on clinical history, laboratory, imaging and other ancillary tests + Direct observations and functional testing + Hachinski Scale (Hachinski *et al.* 1975) Cumulative Illness Rating Scale (CIRS) (Parmelee *et al.* 1995)	BS and BF - all codes, depending on the health problems
	Visual impairment	Standard method: Snellen eye chart • Interviews and self-report: Activities of Daily Vision Scale • VF-14 ·, VFQ-25 • Cataract Symptom Scale •	BF: b210 - b229
	Hearing impairment	Interview · AudioScope 3 method • Whispered voice test • Hearing Handicap Inventory for the Elderly-Screening Version (HHIE-S) •	BF: b230 - b249
	Malnutrition/ weight loss	Initial visit: question about weight loss in the previous 6 months · Weighing patients at every office visit • Calculating body mass index • Nutritional Screening Initiative's 10-item checklist • Mini-Nutritional Assessment (MNA) •	BF: b510 - b539
	Urinary incontinence	Interview • Three incontinence questions (3IQ) •	BF: b620, b630, b639
	Balance and gait impairment and falling	Asking about falling in the last year • Asking about fear of falling • Timed up and go test • Gait speed over 10 m • Performance-Oriented Assessment of Mobility • Functional reach test •	BF: b235, b710 - b789
	Poly-pharmacy	Instructing the patient to bring in all current medications – both prescription and non-prescription medications – to each visit •	EF: e110
Cognitive	Global status	Mini Mental Status Examination (MMSE)*	BF:b114, b117, b140, b144, b167, b172, b176 AP:d130, d135, d160, d166, d170, d172, d310, d345, d440
		Addenbrooke's Cognitive Examination Revised (ACE-R) (Mioshi *et al.* 2006)	BF:b114, b117, b140, b144, b156, b167, b172, b176 AP:d130, d135, d160, d166, d170, d172, d310, d345, d440
	Attention	Digit Span *	BF:b140 AP:d135, d160

(Continued)

TABLE 13.1 (CONTINUED)

Geriatric Assessment and ICF codes

GA	Components	Examples of tests and assessment techniques	ICF codes
		Trial making test A and B (TMT) *	BF:b140 AP: d160, d220
		Stroop tests *	BF:b140 AP:d160, d220
		Corsi's Block-tapping test *	BF:b140 AP:d135, d160
	Memory	Benton Visual Retention Test (BVRT) *	BF:b144
		Auditory Verbal Learning Test (AVLT) *	BF:b144
		Babcock Story Recall Test (BSRT) *	BF:b144 AP:d325, d330
		Complex Figure Test (CFT): Recall administration *	BF:b144
	Concept formation and reasoning	Raven's Coloured Progressive Matrices (RCPM) *	BF:b164 AP:d163
		Proverbs and Similarities *	BF:b164 AP:d163, d310
		Wisconsin Card Sorting Test (WCST) *	BF:b164 AP: d220
	Construction	Coping Drawings *	BF:b176 AP:d130, d440
		Complex Figure Test (CFT): copy Administration *	BF:b164, b176 AP:d130, d440
		Clock face *	BF:b176 AP:d130, d440
	Language	Controlled Oral Word Association (COWA - sometimes labelled FAS) *	BF:b167 AP:d210
		Boston Naming Test (BNT) *	BF:167
		Category fluency *	BF:b167 AP:d210
		Token Test *	BF:b167 AP:d310
	Executive functions and motor performance	Tower of London *	BF:b164 AP:d163, d175, d210, d440
		Frontal Assessment Battery (FAB) *	BF:b164 AP:d163, d220
		Examination for Apraxia *	BF:b176 AP:d130, d440
Affective		Interview • Geriatric Depression Scale (GDS) (Yesavage 1983) • Patient Health Questionnaire-9 (PHQ-9) •	BF: b152
Functional		Activity Daily Living (ADL) (Katz *et al*. 1963)	BF:b176, b525, b620 AP:d410, d440, d450, d460, d465, d510, d520, d530, d540, d550, d560

TABLE 13.1 (CONTINUED)

Geriatric Assessment and ICF codes

GA	Components	Examples of tests and assessment techniques	ICF codes
Functional		Activity Daily Living (ADL) (Katz *et al.* 1963)	BF:b176, b525, b620 AP:d410, d440, d450, d460, d465, d510, d520, d530, d540, d550, d560
		Instrumental Activity Daily Living (IADL) (Lawton and Brody, 1969)	BF:b176 AP:d177, d230, d360, d440, d450, d460, d470, d475, d620, d630, d640 EF:e110, e165
Environmental		Interview about safety of the home environment • Interview about access to personal and medical services • Interview about driving function Checklist for patients and their families •.	AP: d475 EF: e115 - e125, e240, e310 - e340, e355, e360, e398, e465
Social Support		Interview about social history and quality of relationship • Interview about availability of assistance • Caregiver Burden Inventory (Novak and Guest 1989) Brief Symptom Inventory *	EF: e310, e320, e340, e355, e360, e410, e440
Economic		Interview about economic status and insurance •	AP: d870 EF: e165
Spirituality		Interview about religion or spirituality •	AP: d930 EF: e465
Advance Directives		Discussion about patients' goals and preferences •	All codes depending on the goals

The Geriatric assessment procedure is a multidimensional assessment that explores nine domains: medical, cognitive, affective, functional, environmental, social support, economic, spirituality and advance directives (first column). The domains comprehend several components reported in the second column. In the third column, an example of geriatric assessment techniques and test are presented. For a specific description of the assessment techniques and tests referring to the references if given, to Strauss and Tinetti (2009) for items with "+", to Reuben and Rosen (2009) for items with "•" and to Lezak, Howieson, and Loring (2004) for items with *.

The last column lists the ICF codes belonging to Body Structures (BS), Body Functions (BF), Activities and Participation (AP), Environmental Factors (EF) related to geriatric assessment.

Considering the state of the art, it seems important to reflect on two problems: on the one hand the scarce implementation of the ICF in geriatric medicine, and on the other the importance of training in assistive solutions by geriatricians. With respect to the first problem, it should be noted that the ICF offers a unique opportunity to describe and classify functioning, disability, and health in a common framework and in a common language, which would be very useful in a multidisciplinary team assessment. Moreover, although all member states of the World Health Organization (WHO) were invited to implement the ICF in the health sector (Stucki et al. 2005), different conceptualizations of disability coexist and several studies consider the transition from health to disability from the "the Disablement Process" perspective, proposed by Verbrugge and Jette (1994) and based on the model by Nagi (1964, 1965, 1991). Only in recent years has the concept of disability, in gerontology research, begun undergoing a profound transformation because of the adoption of the ICF language for the study of the late-life disability (Jette 2006, 2009; Freedman 2009; Guralnik and Ferrucci 2009). The refusal of the gerontological community to embrace the ICF language was due to two reasons (Freedman 2009). The first is the lack of accuracy in the crosswalk between the existing measures of functional limitation [activities of daily living (ADLs) and instrumental activities of daily living (IADLs)] and the ICF language. The second is that the ICF is not intended to be a dynamic model because it does not present a model of disability as a dynamic process. Jette (2006, 2009) invited the U.S. scientific community to adopt the ICF framework, putting into evidence the similarity and differences between the Nagi and ICF concepts and definitions, to use a common, international language in the rehabilitation field with the possibility of improving communication across national boundaries and disciplines, to facilitate interdisciplinary research, to ameliorate clinical care, and to dialogue with health policy and management. The National Health and Aging Trends Study (NHATS), a new resource for the scientific study of functioning in later life, appears promising in this direction because it was developed with both the ICF language and with a consideration of the Nagi roots. The NHATS is being conducted by the Johns Hopkins University Bloomberg School of Public Health with support from the National Institute on Aging and its scope is to foster research that will guide efforts to reduce disability, maximize health and independent functioning, and enhance quality of life at older ages. The NHATS supports studies of disability trends and trajectories in later life. One important objective is to work on developing, testing, and fielding a state-of-the-art disability instrument. Being part of the NHATS, Freedman (2009) puts into evidence the benefits that can be derived from the ICF language: the addition of the term "participation" to geriatrician vocabulary, the explicit and defined role for the environment, the availability of positive analogues for concepts that have traditionally been expressed in terms of loss in an advancement, and the distinction between capacity to perform and the actual performance of a range of activities. Recently, new assessment instrument tools for disability based on the ICF perspective were proposed as an alternative to the classic ADL and IADL (Rejeski et al. 2008).

Another important step to enhance the applicability of the ICF in clinical practice and research is the ICF Core Set Project created with the aim of selecting ICF domains that include "the least number of domains possible to be practical, but as many as required to be sufficiently comprehensive to cover the prototypical spectrum of limitations in functioning and health encountered in a specific condition" (Stucki et al. 2002, p. 936). The goal of the ICF Core Sets Project is to "serve as minimal standards for the assessment and reporting of functioning and health for clinical studies, clinical encounters and multi-professional comprehensive assessment" (Stucki et al. 2005, p. 350). A Core Set is developed by means of a consensus process that can be used as an assessment schema of individual problems and needs, prognoses, rehabilitation, and functioning in the acute and postacute condition for communication at a rehabilitation team conference (Grill and Stucki 2011).

Concerning the second problem of giving geriatricians a role in directing a patient to a center for technical aid, it is necessary to introduce training in assistive solutions for health professionals. At the same time, it is important to update and promote research on assistive solutions to diffuse the available knowledge about assistive solutions and to understand which factors determine the best match between an older user and technological aids.

In recent years, several studies have been dedicated to highlighting the ICF as a framework for the clinical assessment of people for assistive technology (Arthanat and Lenker 2004; Scherer, 2005). Referring to matching older users with technology, Scherer, Federici, and colleagues (2011) developed an ICF Core Set for Matching Older Adults with Dementia and Technology (MOADT) to provide a systematic coding scheme for health information systems and to establish a common language for describing the ATA. The MOADT represents a useful tool for better communication between the different centers for technical aid, institutes for geriatric rehabilitation, geriatric medical centers and institutes and people with dementia, their families, and caregivers. In the process of "matching older people and technology," it becomes essential that the geriatrician works with providers to identify appropriate technology for an older client.

To provide an example of the geriatrician as a professional consultant in a center for technical aid, a clinical case is described linking a geriatric assessment and the ICF perspective with an explanation of the factors that influence the matching process whilst considering a hypothetical scenario of the progression of a health condition.

13.8 Case Study and the ATA Process

Name: A.B.
Age: 73.3 years
Age at the beginning of disease: 70 years
Diagnosis: ICD-9-CM Diagnosis Code 331.0 Alzheimer's disease, I10 hypertension, M81.0 osteoporosis, F32.9 depression

Since the age of about 70, Mrs. A.B. began to notice memory problems (difficulties in naming, difficulties in finding personal effects, episodic memory deficits). As the months passed there was a slow worsening of her medical and functional conditions. Recently, she lost the ability to perform IADLs without assistance and she now frequently appears to be apathetic and depressed.

The anamnestic data show cataract surgery (at the age of 71), hypertension (at the age of 67), and osteoporosis (at the age of 62). At the age of 65, Mrs. A.B. presented depressive symptoms and underwent pharmacological treatment with citalopram. This treatment produced relevant benefits and was stopped after two years. One year ago, the same antidepressant drug was reintroduced. The family history shows a sibling who died from dementia (probably Alzheimer's disease) and a living sibling who has Parkinson's disease.

She is assessed every six months by a geriatric center to monitor the evolution of the disease and to maintain pharmacological treatment. Before the onset of the disease the patient spent time in housekeeping and in volunteering. In particular, she shopped for necessary items and worked for Caritas in the parochial center of the town. She was able to walk to services and the parochial center, and she was also a factory worker (she has eight years of education).

At the moment, Mrs. A.B. lives with her husband near the home of one of her two daughters. The town is very small and several services are within walking distance. Familiar people provide a valid form of support in allowing her to maintain her residual autonomy and to create situations for socialization and participation, but they are committed for the greater part of the day. If nobody is present, Mrs. A.B. spends her time watching television. If somebody indicates when they must be performed, she can carry out the ADLs by herself (dressing, toileting, transferring, continence, and feeding), except for having a bath because of her fear of falling. Regarding instrumental activities, she can dial a few well-known numbers and she can prepare food if her daughter suggests the procedure and quantity. She performs light daily tasks such as dishwashing and bed-making, but she has difficulty with laundry because she cannot choose the appropriate setting for the washing machine. She is not capable of dispensing her own medication because she has difficulty with recall. She undertakes limited travel in an automobile with the assistance of another person because she has problems with spatial orientation. Mrs. A.B. can also carry out simple activities such as paying in and withdrawing money from the bank. A familiar presence, stimulation, and activities seem to have a remissive effect on her depressive and apathetic symptoms. Mrs. A.B. sometimes seems anosognosic, but she refuses to have an external caregiver. In fact, for several weeks, a caregiver frequented the patient's home, but Mrs. A.B. presents delusions of jealousy.

- *Motor evaluation:* The present conditions of her motor condition are good. The patient is able to maintain a sitting position without support and to realize position transfers. Mrs. A.B. is able to maintain an erect position autonomously and she can walk without support. Pendular movements are present. The upper limbs present mobility and can be used for functional activities.

- *Neuropsychological test:* Mrs. A.B. is watchful, and she cooperates. She has difficulties in paying attention for longer periods; difficulties in shifting attention between different situations; and difficulties in planning actions, organizing her time, and in executing actions. She has spatial orientation impairment. Her episodic, semantic, and perspective memory are compromised. She can read and understand words, sentences, simple and complex orders, and short texts. She can produce short speeches, but her production is interrupted by frequent bouts of anomia. She can copy simple figures but she has difficulties with complex models. Her performance in concept formation and reasoning is within the normal limits.

- *Communication strategy:* She has the ability to communicate.

- *Evaluation of visual, perceptive, and motor functions:* She has no visual, perceptive, or motor impairments.

- *Aids and assistance:* At the moment, Mrs. A.B. has neither aids nor assistance.

- *Request:* Aids and assistance in monitoring health status, medication adherence, and support with the IADLs.

13.8.1 The Role of the Geriatrician in the ATA Process for the User A.B.

Mrs. A.B. is monitored by a geriatric center for the evolution of the disease and pharmacological treatment. In this case, the input data come from a CGA procedure, and the geriatrician at the center for technical aid has information regarding her medical, cognitive, affective, functional, environmental, social support, economic, spiritual, and advance directive domains.

Table 13.2 shows the correspondence between the dimensions of the geriatrician assessment and the ICF codes; Figure 13.2 illustrates the patient's profile from the point of view of the biopsychosocial model.

If the multidisciplinary team decides there are sufficient data for a matching process, then the selection of the proper technological aid is pursued. Because Alzheimer's disease is a progressive illness, an assistive solution requires monitoring adherence to pharmacological treatment by supporting the ADLs in a periodical follow-up.

TABLE 13.2

Geriatric Assessment of a Clinical Case

GA	Components	ICF codes	A.B.
Medical	Physical	BF:b280.0, b410.0, b415.0, b420.2, b430.0, b440.0, b510.0, b515.0, b525.0, b535.0, b540.0, b545.0, b555.0, b620.0, b710.0, b730.0, BS: s110.2, s710.0, s720.1, s730.0, s740.2, s750.0, s760.0	Hypertension Osteoporosis Alzheimer's disease
	Visual impairment	BF:b210.0, b215.0	No Visual Impairment Cataract Surgery in anamnestic data
	Hearing impairment	BF:b230.0	No hearing impairment
	Malnutrition/ weight loss	BF:b530.2	Weight loss in the last five months.
	Urinary incontinence	BF: b620.0	No urinary incontinence
Medical	Balance and gait impairment and falling	BF:b235.0, b710.2, b715.0, b730.0, b735.0, b740.0, b750.0, b755.0, b760.0, b765.0, b789.2	No balance or gait impairment. No falls.
	Poly-pharmacy	EF: e110	Current medication: ramipril (for hypertension), strontium ranelate (for osteoporosis), citalopram (for depression), rivastigmine (for dementia).
	Global status	BF:b114.2, b117.2, b140.2, b144.2, b156.0, b167.0, b172.1, b176.0 AP:d130.0, d135.0, d160.2, d166.0, d170.0, d172.1, d310.0, d345.0, d440.0	Cognitive deficit compatible with dementia
Cognitive	Attention	BF:b140.2 AP:d135.1, d160.2, d220.2	Deficits in short-term memory, in visual attention, in simple and alternate attention
	Memory	BF:b144.2 AP:d325.0,d330.0	Deficits in episodic and semantic memory.
	Concept formation and reasoning	BF:b164.0 AP:d163.1, d220.1, d310.0	Borderline performance
	Construction	BF:b176.2 AP: d130.0, d440.0	Difficulties in writing the numbers on a clock face and in copying complex figures
	Language	BF:b167.1 AP:d210.1, d310.0	Reduction in category fluency and anomia
	Executive functions and motor performance	BF:b164.2, b176.0 AP: d130.0, d163.2, d175.2, d220.1, d440.0	Difficulties in planning and set shifting
Affective		BF: b152.2	Depressive and apathetic symptoms.

(Continued)

TABLE 13.2 (CONTINUED)

Geriatric Assessment of a Clinical Case

GA	Components	ICF codes	A.B.
Functional		BF:b176.0, b525.0, b620.0 AP: d177.1, d230.1, d360.0, d410.0, d440.0, d450.0-d460.0, d475.9, d510.1, d520.0, d530.0, d540.0, d550.0, d560.0, d620.1, d630.1, d640.1 EF:e110.2, e165.0	Assistance with bathing for fear of falling; puts on clothes and dresses without any assistance, except for tying shoe laces. goes to toilet room, uses toilet, arranges clothes, and returns without any assistance (may use cane or walker for support and may use bedpan/urinal at night; moves in and out of bed and chair without assistance (may use cane or walker); controls bowel and bladder completely by herself; feeds herself without assistance; dials a few well-known numbers; shops independently for small purchases; prepares adequate meals if supplied with ingredients; performs light daily tasks such as dishwashing, bed making; launders small items; rinses stockings, etc.; travel limited to taxi or automobile with the assistance of another; is not capable of dispensing own medication; manages day-to-day purchases, but needs help with banking, major purchases, etc.
Environmental		AP: d475.9 EF: e110.0, e340+2, e355+1	Services within walking distance; Geriatric Assessment every six months; No car
Social Support		EF: e310+3, e320+2, e340+2, e355+1, e360+0, e410+3, e440+0	Familiar people are a valid support but they are committed for the greater part of the day; family and friends presence reduces depressive and apathetic symptoms.
Economic		AP: d870 EF: e165	No economic problems
Spirituality		AP: d930.2 EF: e465+3	Before the disease she had a rich social network linked to a parochial centre
Advance Directives		EF: e360+0	The patient refuses a non-familiar caregiver

The Geriatric assessment procedure, conducted using the instruments indicated in Table 13.1, explores nine domains: medical, cognitive, affective, functional, environmental, social support, economic, spiritual, and advance directives (first column). The domains include several components reported in the second column. The third column shows ICF codes for body structures (BS), body functions (BF), activities and participation (AP), and environmental factors (EF) related to A.B. geriatric assessment. In the fourth column, the condition of Mrs. A.B. is described.

The hypothetical future scenario configures a progressive worsening of cognitive deficit because of the progression of Alzheimer's disease. The possibility of her becoming lost when away from her home must be carefully considered because of her orientation deficits. At the same time, the possibility of walking to the parochial center or to the grocery store represents an opportunity for activity and participation to be maintained. Living in a small town represents an advantage in this sense. On the basis of the literature, Mrs. A.B. will lose her abilities in the ADLs, and difficulties with self-care and domestic life will manifest. If not stimulated by means of social and mental activities, Mrs. A.B. will suffer a worsening of apathetic and depressive symptoms with a reduction in participation. The assumptions of rivastigmine therapy include paying particular attention to the potential

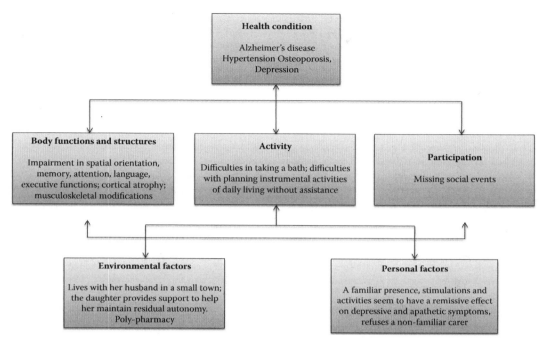

FIGURE 13.2
Patient's profile based on the Geriatric Assessment in a Centre for Technical Aids.

development of gastric symptoms and bradycardia. The presence of osteoporosis requires the prevention of falls and fractures with environmental devices. Because the patient developed delusions in response to an external caregiver, it is also important to instruct the family on the caregiver burden and to inform them about possible support groups, associations, and social services.

It should also be considered that although her difficulties with the IADLs are due to deficits in executive functions and prospective memory, if a suggestion is given with respect to plans of actions and their timing, the performance of Mrs. A.B. is good.

Considering all of these factors, assistive technological devices that could be assessed for Mrs. A.B. include

- Cognitive impairment devices such as reminder systems for medication adherence or a handheld cognitive prosthetic for guidance during the execution of daily tasks.
- A GPS locator system could be useful in compensating for spatio-temporal disorientation and for facilitating mobility of the patient, allowing the caregiver to have real-time information on the movements of the elderly lady.

13.9 Conclusions

This chapter illustrates the role of the geriatrician in relation to the main issues that characterize the aging of populations: disease, disability, and frailty. Although the idea of frailty is a clear concept, there are different definitions in the medical literature that emphasize different aspects. However, they are unanimous in considering frailty as a condition of multifactorial global functional decline that can easily lead to disability. This chapter follows the ICF definition of disability from the perspective of the biopsychosocial model outlines. This emphasizes that personal factors, environmental conditions, and the health of the individual merge to define the disability status.

The management of an elderly patient requires an approach that takes into account all of the factors that can affect health (illness, functional status, psychosocial situation, and environmental conditions). This procedure is called the comprehensive geriatric assessment (CGA) and is characterized by a multiprofessional team working with the objective of establishing priorities for the individualized plan of care. This chapter provides a detailed description of the procedure underlining the validity of this approach in the management of an elderly patient.

A care plan also provides rehabilitative treatments: in this chapter the clinical course of geriatric rehabilitation is described, emphasizing the importance of first performing a screening assessment of the patient, multidisciplinary interventions, and continuity of care. Assistive solutions can offer an important contribution to the practice of geriatric rehabilitation and continuity of care.

A description of state-of-the-art applications based on intelligent technologies is provided. Specifically, this chapter describes information and communications technology-based assistive living solutions for the elderly with cognitive and/or motor disabilities. Particular emphasis is given to the role that some individual factors have on technology acceptance by older users.

The role of the geriatrician is analyzed via a case study illustrating the Matching Person and Technology (MPT) assessment process. In a center for technical aid, the geriatrician could collaborate as a professional consultant to support a collaborative partnership between the service providers and the older user. A comprehensive geriatric assessment approach combined with an ICF model offer a unique opportunity to describe and classify functioning, disability, and health in a common framework with a universal language (Scherer et al. 2011; Stier-Jarmer et al. 2011). Furthermore, the MPT process also contributes to guiding the service provider in assistive technology decision-making and in the use of evidence-based outcome measures. Adoption of the ICF in geriatric medicine and geriatrician training in assistive solution is debated.

In conclusion, this chapter underlines the need to introduce training in assistive solutions for health professionals and to update and promote research in this area. Moreover, health workers need to be trained to spread the available knowledge about assistive solutions and to understand which factors best determine the match between an older user and technological aids. All of these factors need to take into account the ICF biopsychosocial framework (Arthanat and Lenker 2004; Scherer 2005; Scherer et al. 2011).

Summary of the Chapter

Heterogeneity in the health status of elderly patients requires a particular care approach, and geriatric medicine is the answer. To cope with, the geriatric assessment approach guides the geriatrician into considering the interaction between functional status and cognitive, medical, affective, environmental, social support, economic, and spirituality dimensions. Rehabilitation is the goal of the geriatric assessment, and the introduction of assistive solutions in geriatric rehabilitation makes possible a scenario in which the functioning of elderly people with physical or cognitive limitations is improved. This chapter provides an overview of the areas where technological systems may offer support to the everyday life of the elderly and their caregivers. The contribution of a geriatrician in a center for technical aid is described, linking the comprehensive geriatric assessment with the ICF model. The lack of implementation of the ICF and the requirement of training in assistive solutions for geriatricians and caregivers are discussed.

References

AAATE. (2003). AAATE position paper: A 2003 view on Technology and Disability Retrieved from http://www.aaate.net/

Abellan van Kan, G., Rolland, Y., Houles, M., Gillette-Guyonnet, S., Soto, M., and Vellas, B. (2010). The assessment of frailty in older adults. *Clinics in Geriatric Medicine, 26*(2), 275–286. doi:10.1016/j.cger.2010.02.002.

Achenbaum, W. A. (1995). *Crossing Frontiers: Gerontology Emerges as a Science.* New York: Cambridge University Press.

Alexopoulos, G. S. (2005). Depression in the elderly. *Lancet, 365*(9475), 1961–1970. doi:10.1016/S0140-6736(05)66665-2.

Alexopoulos, G. S., Buckwalter, K., Olin, J., Martinez, R., Wainscott, C., and Krishnan, K. R. R. (2002). Comorbidity of late life depression: An opportunity for research on mechanisms and treatment. *Biological Psychiatry, 52*(6), 543–558. doi:10.1016/S0006-3223(02)01468-3.

Alqasemi, R. M., McCaffrey, E. J., Edwards, K. D., and Dubey, R. V. (2005, Jun 28-Jul 1). *Analysis, Evaluation and development of Wheelchair-Mounted Robotic Arms.* Paper presented at the 9th International Conference on Rehabilitation Robotics: ICORR '05, Chicago. doi:10.1109/ICORR.2005.1501144.

American Geriatrics Society Core Writing Group of the Task Force on the Future of Geriatric Medicine. (2005). Caring for older Americans: The future of geriatric medicine. *Journal of American Geriatrics Society, 53*(Suppl 6), S245-S256. doi:10.1111/j.1532-5415.2005.53350.x.

Arthanat, S., and Lenker, J. A. (2004). *Evaluating the ICF as a Framework for Clinical Assessment of Persons for Assistive Technology Device Recommendation.* Paper presented at the 10th North American Collaborating Centre (NACC) Conference on ICF, Halifax, Nova Scotia. Retrieved from http://secure.cihi.ca/cihiweb/en/downloads/SajayArthanat_paper.pdf.

Asplund, K., Carlberg, B., and Sundström, G. (1992). Stroke in the elderly. *Cerebrovascular Diseases, 2*(3), 152-157. doi:10.1159/000109007.

Batstra, L., Bos, E. H., and Neeleman, J. (2002). Quantifying psychiatric comorbidity—Lessions from chronic disease epidemiology. *Social Psychiatry and Psychiatric Epidemiology, 37*(3), 105–111. doi:10.1007/s001270200001.

Brandtstädter, J., and Renner, G. (1990). Tenacious goal pursuit and flexible goal adjustment: Explication and age-related analysis of assimilative and accommodative strategies of coping. *Psychology and Aging, 5*(1), 58–67. doi:10.1037/0882-7974.5.1.58.

Brown, C. J., and Peel, C. (2009). Rehabilitation. In J. B. Halter, J. G. Ouslander, M. E. Tinetti, S. Studenski, K. P. High, and S. Asthana (Eds.), *Hazzard's Geriatric Medicine and Gerontology* (6th ed., pp. 343–358). New York: McGraw-Hill.

Cesta, A., Bahadori, S., Cortellessa, G., Grisetti, G., Giuliani, M., Locchi, L., et al. (2003, Jun 26–29). *The Robocare Project Cognitive Systems for the Care of the Elderly.* Paper presented at the International Conference on Aging, Disability and Independence: ICADI '03, Washington, DC.

Cesta, A., Cortellessa, G., Rasconi, R., Pecora, F., Scopelliti, M., and Tiberio, L. (2011). Monitoring elderly people with the Robocare Domestic Environment: Interaction synthesis and user evaluation. *Computational Intelligence, 27*(1), 60–82. doi:10.1111/j.1467-8640.2010.00372.x.

Chiu, C., W. Y., and Man, D. W. K. (2004). The effect of training older adults with stroke to use home-based assistive devices. *OTJR: Occupation, Participation and Health, 24*(3), 113–120.

Christensen, K., Doblhammer, G., Rau, R., and Vaupel, J. W. (2009). Ageing populations: The challenges ahead. *Lancet, 374*(9696), 1196–1208. doi:10.1016/S0140-6736(09)61460-4.

Cole, E. (1999). Cognitive prosthetics: An overview to a method of treatment. *NeuroRehabilitation, 12*(1), 39–51. Retrieved from http://iospress.metapress.com/content/fbkx9tj1l8q5tcga/

Colombo, M. (2004). Assistive technology: Mind the user! *Gerontechnology, 3*(1), 1–4. doi:10.4017/gt.2004.03.01.001.00.

Corey-Bloom, J. (2004). Alzheimer's disease. *Continuum, 10*(1), 29–57.

Czaja, S. J., Charness, N., Fisk, A. D., Hertzog, C., Nair, S. N., Rogers, W. A., et al. (2006). Factors predicting the use of technology: Findings from the Center for Research and Education on Aging and Technology Enhancement (CREATE). *Psychology and Aging, 21*(2), 333–352. doi:10.1037/0882-7974.21.2.333.

Davis, F. D. (1993). User acceptance of information technology: System characteristics, user perceptions and behavioral impacts. *International Journal of Man-Machine Studies, 38*(3), 475–487. doi:10.1006/imms.1993.1022.

de Groot, V., Beckerman, H., Lankhorst, G. J., and Bouter, L. M. (2003). How to measure comorbidity. A critical review of available methods. *Journal of Clinical Epidemiology, 56*(3), 221–229. doi:10.1016/S0895-4356(02)00585-1.

DeVaul, R. W. (2004). *The Memory Glasses: Wearable Computing for Just-In-Time Memory Support.* Doctoral Dissertation, Massachusetts Institute of Technology, Cambridge, MA. Retrieved from http://devaul.net/~rich/DeVaulDissertation.pdf.

Driessen, B., Evers, H., and van Woerden, J. (2001). MANUS—A wheelchair-mounted rehabilitation robot. *Proceedings of the Institution of Mechanical Engineers, Part H: Journal of Engineering in Medicine, 215*(3), 285–290. doi:10.1243/0954411011535876.

Elliot, R. (1991). *Assistive Technology for the Frail Elderly: An Introduction and Overview.* Philadelphia: University of Pennsylvania.

Feigin, V. L., Lawes, C. M., Bennett, D. A., and Anderson, C. S. (2003). Stroke epidemiology: A review of population-based studies of incidence, prevalence, and case-fatality in the late 20th century. *Lancet Neurology, 2*(1), 43–53. doi:10.1016/S1474-4422(03)00266-7.

Feinstein, A. R. (1970). The pre-therapeutic classification of co-morbidity in chronic disease. *Journal of Chronic Diseases, 23*(7), 455–468. doi:10.1016/0021-9681(70)90054-8.

Freedman, V. A. (2009). Adopting the ICF language for studying late-life disability: A field of dreams? *Journals of Gerontology. Series A, Biological Sciences and Medical Sciences, 64*(11), 1172–1174; discussion 1175–1176. doi:10.1093/gerona/glp095.

Freedman, V. A., Martin, L. G., and Schoeni, R. F. (2002). Recent trends in disability and functioning among older adults in the United States: A systematic review. *Journal of the American Medical Association, 288*(24), 3137–3146. doi:10.1001/jama.288.24.3137.

Fried, L. P. (1994). Frailty. In W. R. Hazzard, J. G. Ouslander, J. Blass, J. B. Halter and M. E. Tinetti (Eds.), *Principles of Geriatric Medicine and Gerontology* (3rd ed., pp. 1149–1155). New York: McGraw-Hill.

Fried, L. P. (2000). Epidemiology of aging. *Epidemiologic Reviews, 22*(1), 95–106.

Fried, L. P., Ferrucci, L., Darer, J., Williamson, J. D., and Anderson, G. (2004). Untangling the concepts of disability, frailty, and comorbidity: Implications for improved targeting and care. *Journals of Gerontology Series A: Biological Sciences and Medical Sciences, 59*(3), M255-M263. doi:10.1093/gerona/59.3.M255.

Fried, L. P., and Guralnik, J. M. (1997). Disability in older adults: Evidence regarding significance, etiology, and risk. *Journal of American Geriatrics Society, 45*(1), 92.

Fried, L. P., Tangen, C. M., Walston, J. D., Newman, A. B., Hirsch, C., Gottdiener, J., et al. (2001). Frailty in older adults: Evidence for a phenotype. *Journals of Gerontology, 56A*(3), M146-M156.

Fried, L. P., Walston, J. D., and Ferrucci, L. (2009). Frailty. In J. B. Halter, J. G. Ouslander, M. E. Tinetti, S. Studenski, K. P. High and S. Asthana (Eds.), *Hazzard's Geriatric Medicine and Gerontology* (6th ed., pp. 631–646). New York: McGraw-Hill.

Fries, J. F. (1980). Aging, natural death, and the compression of morbidity. *New England Journal of Medicine, 303*(3), 130–135. doi:10.1056/NEJM198007173030304.

Geriatric Medicine Section of UEMS. (2008). *Geriatric Medicine.* Retrieved from http://www.uems-geriatric medicine.org

Gijsen, R., Hoeymans, N., Schellevis, F. G., Ruwaard, D., Satariano, W. A., and van den Bos, G. A. M. (2001). Causes and consequences of comorbidity: A review. *Journal of Clinical Epidemiology, 54*(7), 661–674. doi:10.1016/s0895-4356(00)00363-2.

Gill, T. M., Gahbauer, E. A., Han, L., and Allore, H. G. (2010). Trajectories of disability in the last year of life. *New England Journal of Medicine, 362*(13), 1173–1180. doi:10.1056/NEJMoa0909087.

Gitlin, L. N. (1995). Why older people accept or reject assistive technology. *Generations, 19*(1), 41–46.

Gorman, P., Dayle, R., Hood, C.-A., and Rumrell, L. (2003). Effectiveness of the ISAAC cognitive prosthetic system for improving rehabilitation outcomes with neurofunctional impairment. *NeuroRehabilitation, 18*(1), 57–67. Retrieved from http://iospress.metapress.com/content/qb93q7w4qfh3r47y/

Graf, B., Hans, M., and Schraft, R. D. (2004). Care-O-Bot II—Development of a next generation robotic home assistant. *Autonomous Robots, 16*(2), 193–205. doi:10.1023/B:AURO.0000016865.35796.e9.

Grill, E., and Stucki, G. (2011). Criteria for validating comprehensive ICF Core Sets and developing brief ICF Core Set versions. *Journal of Rehabilitation Medicine, 43*(2), 87–91. doi:10.2340/16501977-0616.

Guralnik, J. M. (1996). Assessing the impact of comorbidity in the older population. *Annals of Epidemiology, 6*(5), 376–380. doi:10.1016/S1047-2797(96)00060-9.

Guralnik, J. M., and Ferrucci, L. (2009). The challenge of understanding the disablement process in older persons: Commentary responding to Jette AM. Toward a common language of disablement. *The Journals of Gerontology Series A: Biological Sciences and Medical Sciences, 64A*(11), 1169–1171. doi:10.1093/gerona/glp094.

Harman, D. (2001). Aging: Overview. *Annals of the New York Academy of Sciences, 286*(928), 1–21. doi:10.1111/j.1749-6632.2001.tb05631.x.

Hazzard, W. R. (2004). I am a geriatrician. *Journal of the American Geriatrics Society, 52*(1), 161. doi:10.1111/j.1532-5415.2004.52041.x.

Heron, M., Hoyert, D. L., Murphy, S. L., Xu, J., Kochanek, K. D., and Tejada-Vera, B. (2009). Deaths: Final data for 2006. *National Vital Statistic Report, 57*(14), 1–134.

Hok Kwee, H. (1998). Integrated control of MANUS manipulator and wheelchair enhanced by environmental eocking. *Robotica, 16*(5), 491–498. doi:10.1017/S0263574798000642.

International Standards Organization (ISO). (2007). *ISO 9999:2007 Assistive Products for Persons with Disability—Classification and Terminology.* Geneva, Switzerland: ISO.

InTouch Health. (2004). Advanced technology solutions for healthcare service providers Retrieved from http://www.intouch-health.com/index.html.

Iwarsson, S., and Slaug, B. (2001). *The Housing Enabler: An Instrument for Assessing and Analysing Accessibility Problems in Housing.* Staffanstorp, Sweden: Veten & Skapen & Slaug Data Management.

Jagger, C. (2000). Compression or expansion of morbidity: What does the future hold? *Age and Ageing, 29*(2), 93–94. doi:10.1093/ageing/29.2.93.

Jette, A. M. (2006). Toward a common language for function, disability, and health. *Physical Therapy, 86*(5), 726–734. Retrieved from http://www.physther.org/content/86/5/726.full.pdf + html.

Jette, A. M. (2009). Toward a common language of disablement. *Journals of Gerontology Series A: Biological Sciences and Medical Sciences, 64*(11), 1165–1168. doi:10.1093/gerona/glp093.

Karmarkar, A., Chavez, E., and Cooper, R. A. (2008). Technology for successful aging and disabilities. In A. Helal, M. Mokhtari and B. Abdulrazak (Eds.), *The Engineering Handbook of Smart Technology for Aging, Disability, and Independence* (pp. 27–48). Hoboken, NJ: John Wiley & Sons, Inc., doi:10.1002/9780470379424.ch1.

Kinsella, K., and He, W. (2009). *An Aging World: 2008. International Population Report*. Retrieved from http://www.census.gov/prod/2009pubs/p95-09-1.pdf.

Kramer, M. (1980). The rising pandemic of mental disorders and associated chronic diseases and disabilities. *Acta Psychiatrica Scandinavica, 62*(S285), 382–397. doi:10.1111/j.1600-0447.1980. tb07714.x.

Krebs, H., Ferraro, M., Buerger, S., Newbery, M., Makiyama, A., Sandmann, M., et al. (2004). Rehabilitation robotics: Pilot trial of a spatial extension for MIT-Manus. *Journal of NeuroEngineering and Rehabilitation, 1*(1), 5. doi:10.1186/1743-0003-1-5.

Lacey, G., and Dawson-Howe, K. M. (1998). The application of robotics to a mobility aid for the elderly blind. *Robotics and Autonomous Systems, 23*(4), 245–252. doi:10.1016/s0921-8890(98)00011-6.

Landi, F., Liperoti, R., Russo, A., Capoluongo, E., Barillaro, C., Pahor, M., et al. (2010). Disability, more than multimorbidity, was predictive of mortality among older persons aged 80 years and older. *Journal of Clinical Epidemiology, 63*(7), 752–759. doi:10.1016/j.jclinepi.2009.09.007.

Lauriks, S., Reinersmann, A., Van der Roest, H. G., Meiland, F. J., Davies, R. J., Moelaert, F., et al. (2007). Review of ICT-based services for identified unmet needs in people with dementia. *Ageing Research Reviews, 6*(3), 223–246. doi:10.1016/j.arr.2007.07.002.

Levinson, R. (1997). The Planning and Execution Assistant and Trainer (PEAT). *Journal of Head Trauma Rehabilitation, 12*(2), 85–91. doi:10.1097/00001199-199704000-00010.

Lezak, M. D., Howieson, D. B., Loring, D. W., Hannay, H. J., and Fischer, J. S. (2004). *Neuropsychological assessment* (4th ed.). New York: Oxford University Press.

Manton, K. G. (1982). Changing concepts of morbidity and mortality in the elderly population. *Milbank Memorial Fund Quarterly. Health and Society, 60*(2), 183–244. doi:10.2307/3349767.

Marengoni, A., Angleman, S., Melis, R., Mangialasche, F., Karp, A., Garmen, A., et al. (2011). Aging with multimorbidity: A systematic review of the literature. *Ageing Research Reviews*. doi:10.1016/j.arr.2011.03.003.

Marengoni, A., Rizzuto, D., Wang, H. X., Winblad, B., and Fratiglioni, L. (2009). Patterns of chronic multimorbidity in the elderly population. *Journal of American Geriatrics Society, 57*(2), 225–230. doi:10.1111/j.1532-5415.2008.02109.x.

McCreadie, C., and Tinker, A. (2005). The acceptability of assistive technology to older people. *Ageing and Society, 25*(1), 91–110. doi:10.1017/S0144686X0400248X.

McGarry Logue, R. (2002). Self-medication and the elderly: How technology can help. *American Journal of Nursing, 102*(7), 51–55.

Mecocci, P., von Strauss, E., Cherubini, A., Ercolani, S., Mariani, E., Senin, U., et al. (2005). Cognitive impairment is the major risk factor for development of geriatric syndromes during hospitalization: Results from the GIFA study. *Dementia and Geriatric Cognitive Disorders, 20*(4), 262–269. doi:10.1159/000087440.

Mihailidis, A., Barbenel, J. C., and Fernie, G. (2004). The efficacy of an intelligent cognitive orthosis to facilitate handwashing by persons with moderate to severe dementia. *Neuropsychological Rehabilitation, 14*(1–2), 135–171. doi:10.1080/09602010343000156.

Mihailidis, A., Boger, J., Craig, T., and Hoey, J. (2008). The COACH prompting system to assist older adults with dementia through handwashing: An efficacy study. *BMC Geriatrics, 8*(1), 28. doi:10.1186/1471-2318-8-28.

Morley, J. E. (2004). A brief history of geriatrics. *Journals of Gerontology. Series A, Biological Sciences and Medical Sciences, 59*(11), 1132–1152. doi:10.1093/gerona/59.11.1132.

Mosqueda, L. A. (1993). Assessment of rehabilitation potential. *Clinics in Geriatric Medicine, 9*(4), 689–703.

Muir, A. J., Sanders, L. L., Wilkinson, W. E., and Schmader, K. (2001). Reducing medication regimen complexity: A controlled trial. *Journal of General Internal Medicine, 16*(2), 77–82. doi:10.1046/j.1525-1497.2001.016002077.x.

Nagi, S. Z. (1964). A study in the evaluation of disability and rehabilitation potential: Concepts, methods, and procedures. *American Journal of Public Health and the Nation's Health, 54*(9), 1568–1579. doi:10.2105/ajph.54.9.1568.

Nagi, S. Z. (1965). Some conceptual issues in disability and rehabilitation. In M. B. Sussman (Ed.), *Sociology and Rehabilitation* (pp. 100–113). Washington, DC: American Sociological Association.

Nagi, S. Z. (1991). Disability concepts revisited: Implications for prevention. In A. M. Pope and A. R. Tarlov (Eds.), *Disability in America: Toward a National Agenda for Prevention* (pp. 309–327). Washington, DC: National Academy Press.

Nakayama, H., Jorgensen, H. S., Raaschou, H. O., and Olsen, T. S. (1994). The influence of age on stroke outcome. The Copenhagen Stroke Study. *Stroke, 25*(4), 808–813. doi:10.1161/01.STR.25.4.808.

NIH Consensus Development Program. (1987). *Geriatric Assessment Methods for Clinical Decision Making. NIH Consens Statement.* (6/13). Retrieved from http://consensus.nih.gov/1987/1987 GeriatricAssessment065html.htm.

Parnes, R. B. (2010). *GPS Technology and Alzheimer's Disease: Novel Use for an Existing Technology.* Retrieved from http://www.thirdage.com/

Patrick, L., Knoefel, F., Gaskowski, P., and Rexroth, D. (2001). Medical comorbidity and rehabilitation efficiency in geriatric inpatients. *Journal of American Geriatrics Society, 49*(11), 1471–1477. doi:10.1046/j.1532-5415.2001.4911239.x.

Philipose, M., Fishkin, K. P., Perkowitz, M., Patterson, D. J., Fox, D., Kautz, H., et al. (2004). Inferring activities from interactions with objects. *Pervasive Computing, IEEE, 3*(4), 50–57. doi:10.1109/MPRV.2004.7.

Pollack, M. E., Brown, L., Colbry, D., McCarthy, C. E., Orosz, C., Peintner, B., et al. (2003). Autominder: An intelligent cognitive orthotic system for people with memory impairment. *Robotics and Autonomous Systems, 44*(3–4), 273–282. doi:10.1016/S0921-8890(03)00077-0.

Qiu, C., De Ronchi, D., and Fratiglioni, L. (2007). The epidemiology of the dementias: An update. *Current Opinion in Psychiatry, 20*(4), 380–385. doi:10.1097/YCO.0b013e32816ebc7b.

Rejeski, W. J., Ip, E. H., Marsh, A. P., Miller, M. E., and Farmer, D. F. (2008). Measuring disability in older adults: The International Classification System of Functioning, Disability and Health (ICF) framework. *Geriatrics and Gerontology International, 8*(1), 48–54. doi:10.1111/j.1447-0594.2008.00446.x.

Reuben, D. B., and Rosen, S. (2009). Principles of geriatric assessment. In J. B. Halter, J. G. Ouslander, M. E. Tinetti, S. Studenski, K. P. High and S. Asthana (Eds.), *Hazzard's Geriatric Medicine and Gerontology* (6th ed., pp. 141–152). New York: McGraw-Hill.

Reuben, D. B., Shekelle, P. G., and Wenger, N. S. (2003). Quality of care for older persons at the dawn of the third millennium. *Journal of American Geriatrics Society, 51*(Suppl 7), S346–S350. doi:10.1046/j.1365-2389.2003.51346.x.

Rockwood, K., Hogan, D. B., and MacKnight, C. (2000). Conceptualisation and measurement of frailty in elderly people. *Drugs and Aging, 17*(4), 295–302. doi:10.2165/00002512-200017040-00005.

Rockwood, K., Stadnyk, K., MacKnight, C., McDowell, I., Hebert, R., and Hogan, D. B. (1999). A brief clinical instrument to classify frailty in elderly people. *Lancet, 353*(9148), 205–206. doi:10.1016/S0140-6736(98)04402-X.

Rubenstein, L. Z. (1995). An overview of comprehensive geriatric assessment: Rationale, history, programs models, basic components. In L. Z. Rubenstein, D. Wieland and R. Bernabei (Eds.), *Geriatric Assessment Technology: The State of the Art* (pp. 1–9). New York: Oxford University Press.

Ruchinskas, R. A., and Curyto, K. J. (2003). Cognitive screening in geriatric rehabilitation. *Rehabilitation Psychology, 48*(1), 14–22. doi:10.1037/0090-5550.48.1.14.

Scherer, M. J. (Ed.). (1998). *Matching Person & Technology. A Series of Assessments for Evaluating Predispositions to and Outcomes of Technology Use in Rehabilitation, Education, the Workplace & Other Settings.* Webster, NY: The Institute for Matching Person & Technology, Inc.

Scherer, M. J. (2002). Introduction. In M. J. Scherer (Ed.), *Assistive Technology: Matching Device and Consumer for Successful Rehabilitation* (pp. 3–13). Washington, DC: American Psychological Association.

Scherer, M. J. (2005). *Cross-Walking the ICF to a Measure of Assistive Technology Predisposition and Use*. Paper presented at the 11th World Health Organization (WHO) North American Collaborating Centre (NACC) Conference on the International Classification of Functioning, Disability and Health (ICF), Rochester, MN.

Scherer, M. J., and Craddock, G. (2002). Matching Person & Technology (MPT) assessment process. *Technology & Disability, 3*(14), 125–131. Retrieved from http://iospress.metapress.com/content/g0eft4mnlwly8y8g.

Scherer, M. J., Federici, S., Tiberio, L., Pigliautile, M., Corradi, F., and Meloni, F. (2011). ICF Core set for Matching Older Adults with Dementia and Technology. *Ageing International, 36*. doi:10.1007/s12126-010-9093-9.

Searle, S. D., Mitnitski, A., Gahbauer, E. A., Gill, T. M., and Rockwood, K. (2008). A standard procedure for creating a frailty index. *BMC Geriatrics, 8*(24), 1–10. doi:10.1186/1471-2318-8-24

Slangen-de Kort, Y. A. W., Midden, C. J. H., and van Wagenberg, A. F. (1998). Predictors of the adaptive problem-solving of older persons in their homes. *Journal of Environmental Psychology, 18*(2), 187–197. doi:10.1006/jevp.1998.0083.

Song, X., Mitnitski, A., and Rockwood, K. (2010). Prevalence and 10-year outcomes of frailty in older adults in relation to deficit accumulation. *Journal of American Geriatrics Society, 58*(4), 681–687. doi:10.1111/j.1532-5415.2010.02764.x.

Stier-Jarmer, M., Grill, E., Muller, M., Strobl, R., Quittan, M., and Stucki, G. (2011). Validation of the comprehensive ICF Core Set for patients in geriatric post-acute rehabilitation facilities. *Journal of Rehabilitation Medicine, 43*(2), 102–112. doi:10.2340/16501977-0617.

Straus, S. E., and Tinetti, M. E. (2009). Evaluation, management, and decision making with the older patient. In J. B. Halter, J. G. Ouslander, M. E. Tinetti, S. Studenski, K. P. High and S. Asthana (Eds.), *Hazzard's Geriatric Medicine and Gerontology* (6th ed., pp. 133–140). New York: McGraw-Hill.

Stucki, G., Ewert, T., and Cieza, A. (2002). Value and application of the ICF in rehabilitation medicine. *Disability and Rehabilitation, 24*(17), 932–938. doi:10.1080/09638280210148594.

Stucki, G., Üstün, T. B., and Melvin, J. (2005). Applying the ICF for the acute hospital and early post-acute rehabilitation facilities. *Disability and Rehabilitation, 27*(7/8), 349–352. doi:10.1080/09638280400013941.

Tas, U., Verhagen, A. P., Bierma-Zeinstra, S. M., Hofman, A., Odding, E., Pols, H. A., et al. (2007). Incidence and risk factors of disability in the elderly: The Rotterdam Study. *Preventive Medicine, 44*(3), 272–278. doi:10.1016/j.ypmed.2006.11.007.

Toseland, R. W., O'Donnell, J. C., Engelhardt, J. B., Hendler, S. A., Richie, J. T., and Jue, D. (1996). Outpatient geriatric evaluation and management. Results of a randomized trial. *Medical Care, 34*(6), 624–640. doi:10.1097/00005650-199606000-00011.

Tsukuda, R. A. (1990). Interdisciplinary collaboration: Teamwork in geriatrics. In C. K. Cassel, D. E. Riesenberg, L. B. Sorensen and J. R. Walsh (Eds.), *Geriatric Medicine* (2nd ed., pp. 668–675). New York: Springer-Verlag.

van Breemen, A., Yan, X., and Meerbeek, B. (2005, Jul 25–29). *iCat: An Animated User-Interface Robot with Personality*. Paper presented at the 4th International Joint Conference on Autonomous Agents and Multiagent Systems: AAMAS '05, Utrecht, The Netherlands. doi:10.1145/1082473.1082823.

Verbrugge, L. M., and Jette, A. M. (1994). The disablement process. *Social Science and Medicine, 38*(1), 1–14. doi:10.1016/0277-9536(94)90294-1.

Wade, D. T. (1992). Stroke: Rehabilitation and long-term care. *The Lancet, 339*(8796), 791–793. doi:10.1016/0140-6736(92)91906-o.

Wade, D. T. (1999). Rehabilitation therapy after stroke. *Lancet, 354*(9174), 176–177. doi:10.1016/S0140-6736(99)90064-8.

Wells, J. L., Seabrook, J. A., Stolee, P., Borrie, M. J., and Knoefel, F. (2003a). State of the art in geriatric rehabilitation. Part I: Review of frailty and comprehensive geriatric. *Archives of Physical Medicine and Rehabilitation, 84*(6), 890–897. doi:10.1016/S0003-9993(02)04929-8.

Wells, J. L., Seabrook, J. A., Stolee, P., Borrie, M. J., and Knoefel, F. (2003b). State of the art in geriatric rehabilitation. Part II: clinical challenges. *Archives of Physical Medicine and Rehabilitation, 84*(6), 898–903. doi:10.1016/S0003-9993(02)04930-4.

World Health Organization (WHO). (1980). *ICIDH: International Classification of Impairments, Disabilities, and Handicaps. A Manual Of Classification Relating to the Consequences of Disease.* Geneva, Switzerland: WHO.

World Health Organization (WHO). (2001). *ICF: International Classification of Functioning, Disability, and Health.* Geneva, Switzerland: WHO.

Yu, H., Spenko, M., and Dubowsky, S. (2003). An adaptive shared control system for an intelligent mobility aid for the elderly. *Autonomous Robots, 15*(1), 53–66. doi:10.1023/a:1024488717009.

14

Role of Speech–Language Pathologists in Assitive Technology Assessments

K. Hill and V. Corsi

CONTENTS

14.1 Description of the Professional Profile

A speech–language pathologist (SLP) is a professional trained to evaluate and treat people who have communication and swallowing disorders. A person must have the required academic training and clinical experience to be certified or licensed as an SLP. The SLP is then able to diagnose and treat disorders across the life span pertaining to speech, language, voice, or swallowing. The specific course requirements and extent of clinical training vary internationally across curricula and awarded degrees. In some countries, professionals may practice as speech therapists with a 2- or 4-year degree. However, the more accepted standard for delivering clinical SLP services requires completion of a Master's degree. In North America, SLPs become independent practitioners after earning a Master's degree in communication science and disorders, completing a clinical fellowship year, and receiving a Certificate of Clinical Competence from the American Speech–Language-Hearing Association (ASHA). An advanced degree may be earned through a clinical doctorate program with an emphasis on medical speech–language and swallowing disorders. The PhD is the terminal degree for the profession.

ASHA standards have typically been applied with some modification worldwide. The standards vetted by ASHA will be used in this paper to describe the professional role and responsibilities of the SLP in practicing on the AT assessment team. The standards reflect an optimal model to strive for internationally in developing curricula, clinical/educational certificate and credentialing programs, and clinical services that hold the interest of the individual with a disability paramount. ASHA members are committed to ensuring that all people with communication disorders receive services to optimize communication (ASHA 2004a). Many individuals being treated by SLPs for communication disorders have disabilities that require the use of assistive technology (AT).

The *Scope of Practice in Speech–Language Pathology* (ASHA 2007) includes a framework for clinical practice and the professional roles and activities of SLPs employed in a variety of clinical/educational settings (see Figure 14.1). The ASHA documents identified within the framework support the expectation and provision of the highest-quality, evidence-based services from SLPs. The profession has identified and described the role of SLPs in providing AT services in various preferred practice patterns, position statements, guidelines, and knowledge and skills documents. Regardless of the extent of training, a certified SLP may perform clinical, educational, and advocacy services across the *Scope of Practice* with the expectation of adherence to the *Code of Ethics* (ASHA 2010) and specific principles therein.

The principle that SLPs shall provide all services competently may seem obvious. Also, apparent may be principles that address client confidentially and nondiscriminatory conduct. Additionally, clinicians are expected to engage in only those aspects of service consistent with their level of education, training, and experience (Principle of Ethics Rule

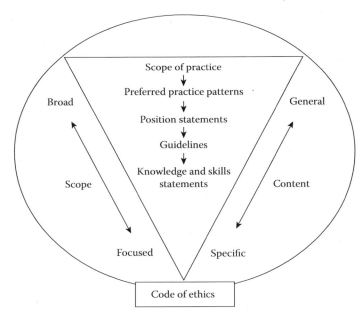

FIGURE 14.1
Conceptual framework of ASHA practice documents. (American Speech–Language-Hearing Association (ASHA). *Scope of Practice in Speech–Language Pathology* [Scope of Practice], 2007. Retrieved from http://www.asha.org/policy)

II-b). Therefore, as professionals SLPs are expected to refer when appropriate to ensure that clients are being provided with high-quality service. Another rule indicates that life-long learning is required to maintain and enhance professional competence. Gaining knowledge and skills related to the highest quality of professional care in AT training and experience may become challenging. Continuing education and specialty certification are methods to document life-long learning. When in doubt about the ability to maximize an individual's potential, to err on the side of holding paramount the welfare of the persons served professionally is advised (Principle of Ethics I).

14.1.1 Assistive Technology Teams and the SLP

Collaborative teaming has been a widely acknowledged and accepted approach to con-ducting AT assessments (Swengel and Marquette 1997; Cook and Hussey 2002). The concepts of multidisciplinary, interdisciplinary, and transdisciplinary teams imply that several related clinical, rehabilitational, and educational service personnel are included on AT teams. AT team members, in addition to the SLP, may include families, therapists, edu-cators, counselors, psychologists, rehabilitation specialists, engineers, vendors, and manu-facturers as well as the individual central to the team (Hill et al. 1998). Consequently, AT teams have many overlapping and shared roles and responsibilities, making coordination and responsibility of services challenging (Lieber et al. 1997).

Establishing a collaborative team culture is essential to developing effective AT teams (Bodine and Melonis 2005). A principle to establishing effective team management and col-laboration is that the knowledge and skills of various team members are honored, yet the responsibility in assessing and implementing the AT plan is shared (Haines and Robertson 2005). Whether the team follows a multidisciplinary, interdisciplinary, or transdisciplinary model, each member is aware of each others' role and responsibilities. Therefore, identi-fying the role of the SLP along with the roles of the other members on the team becomes essential to optimizing the performance and outcomes for an individual using AT.

SLPs bring specific knowledge and skills about the oral and written communication and listening and reading skills of the individual under consideration. Although these domains overlap with the knowledge and skills of other AT team members, the com-petence or expertise of addressing these cognitive-linguistic domains and functional communication of an individual is critical to the Matching Persons and Technology (MPT) process (Hill and Scherer 2008). Consequently, successful collaborative teaming is dependent on team members having regular opportunities to share their expertise, identify common goals, build plans of support, and determine responsibilities (Hunt et al. 2004).

The expected roles of SLPs working with individuals who rely on augmentative and alternative communication (AAC) apply to the responsibilities of SLPs on AT teams (ASHA 2004b):

- Conduct a comprehensive assessment of the individual who requires AT;
- Provide assessment and documentation of AT methods, components, and strate-gies evaluated and selected;
- Evaluate the effectiveness and usefulness of the chosen AT;
- Develop and implement intervention plans;
- Advocate for increased responsiveness and funding needs; and
- Coordinate and collaborate AT services that optimize performance and outcomes;

The SLP may be asked to assume the role of case manager or team leader because the domains of communication are frequently areas of concern for many AT cases (ASHA 2004b). The life experience of individuals who are AT speakers and/or writers is affected by their achieved communication competence. Consequently, the SLP is in the position of discussing how communication influences all other aspects of daily living and life skills. The SLP is the professional who frequently works with the various other professionals, delivers services to the individual and/or family, and expresses the expectation to optimize communication to promote or maintain the highest quality of life.

14.1.2 Evidence-Based Practice and SLPs

Authority-based approaches to making AT decisions have historically placed teams in the position of relying on "expert opinions" and hierarchical approaches to matching persons with technology (Hill and Romich 2007). Historically, teams subscribed to an established "authority" rather than feeling bombarded by the full range of options and endless list of features and components in selecting an AT intervention. However, today SLPs apply the principles of evidence-based practice (EBP) to their decision-making with the incorporation of data collection and outcomes measurement in guiding the provision of services (ASHA 2001).

Dollaghan (2007) states that the goal of EBP is to reduce uncertainty about clinical decisions. Uncertainty is reduced by having a fully informed patient, identifying his or her preferences, and using the best evidence. Best evidence has been identified and described by several authors (Sackett et al. 2000; Dollaghan 2007; Law and MacDermid 2008) to include (1) external or research evidence, (2) internal or clinical evidence, and (3) personal evidence. The ability and experience to fully inform individuals and families and appraise and integrate these three critical types of evidence requires competence in the following domains (ASHA 2002a):

- Knowledge and skill in using systematic observation;
- Knowledge and skill in identifying and measuring outcomes;
- Skill in preparing, monitoring, documenting, and analyzing goals, objectives, procedures, and progress; and
- Knowledge of performance ratings for technology interventions.

The experienced SLP supports the AT team in applying EBP to the assessment and intervention processes. Figure 14.2 (Hill and Romich 2003) serves as a system model for AT service delivery that starts and ends with the interests of the individual with a disability and their family. The process starts with characterizing the individual. Characterizing the individual is a crucial process that identifies, classifies, and prioritizes the areas and problems associated with a disability and an individual's level of functioning. Given the compiled profile, the team may need to gather additional assessment data. The SLP may realize that additional evaluation of the individual's receptive and expressive language, written language skills, and literacy abilities will be needed to proceed through the EBP steps. If individuals are using any AT currently for oral and written communication, then baseline performance data will also need to be collected by the SLP.

All too frequently, adding procedures to collect diagnostic clinical and educational data is overlooked or considered too time-consuming by AT teams. However, without a complete picture of the individual's capabilities the entire EBP process is threatened.

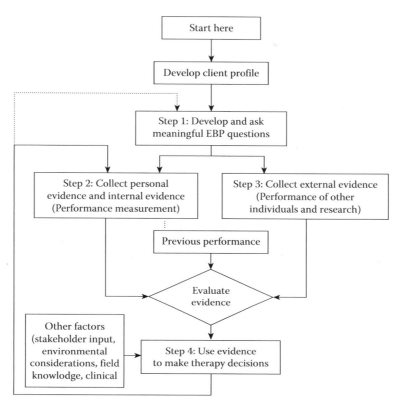

FIGURE 14.2
Four-step model for EBP. (Hill, K. and Romich, B., *AAC Evidence-Based Clinical Practice: A Model for Sucess.* AAC Institute Press. Pittsburgh, PA, 2003.)

In reality, the feature match process is extended by avoiding full characterization of the individual (e.g., complete clinical and personal evidence). AT teams starting at the level of matching the person with technology often find themselves in a "trial-and-error" process, repeating trials and/or needing more time for additional AT trials. The wide range of speech, language, and communication abilities and behavioral characteristics common among children and adults diagnosed with autism spectrum disorder (ASD) demands that SLPs collect and interpret quantitative clinical data regarding these domains at the start of considering AT interventions. No two adults referred for an AT evaluation with a diagnosis of aphasia present with the same residual abilities related to an oral-motor speech or oral and written language disorder. AT teams cannot assume that the individual's current rehabilitation and educational records contain the diagnostic data needed to proceed through the EBP and MPT processes. The SLP is a team member whose role may be to review the records and suggest what additional testing, interviewing, and observations are needed to improve the assessment outcome.

The data gathered from all team members that characterize the individual supports the team in formulating well-built, value-based questions. These meaningful questions lead to locating the best external evidence or to identifying strategies to gather more authentic clinical/educational and personal evidence (Hill 2006). The SLP may suggest posing two types of questions: background and foreground (Sackett et al. 2000). The team may start by asking background questions if their experience is limited and/or if information is missing related to a particular disorder or condition. For example, the AT team may ask background questions seeking additional evidence on the characteristics of fragile X syndrome or the side effects of baclofen. However, a foreground question is formulated to search for research evidence to guide decisions.

The acronym PICO used by Sackett et al. (2000) provides a structure that includes identifying the type of *patient* or *problem*, a broadly defined *intervention*, a *comparison* intervention, and an *outcome*. Experience with EBP is needed to distinguish the elements of a PICO question and determine the level of detail regarding the intervention, comparison, and outcome components of the question. Consider the following PICO questions supporting the goal to reduce the uncertainty of a decision about an AT solution:

- For a college student with cerebral palsy (P), will word prediction (I) or orthographic word selection (C) result in the greatest increase in selection rate (bits per second) and average communication rate (words per minute) (O) for generating writing assignments for college classes and personal correspondence?

- For an adult with severe Broca's aphasia (P), would computer-based AT using a visual scene user interface for word retrieval (I) or a grid-type interface with core and activity rows (C) lead to the greater increases in accurate word order and utterance length (O) for conversations with family?

- For a child with autism (P), what approach would result in greater gains in accurate word recognition and word fluency (O) during oral reading tasks: computer-based AT software based on a four-block model (I) or traditional instruction with no technology support (C)?

In each of the above examples, the knowledge and skills of the SLP can be tapped into pinpoint the elements and extent of detail of the question. If the client is a child with ASD (as above), is that enough detail for the question? Detailed client information regarding emergent or elementary literacy skills may be added. Perhaps the (P) could indicate that the child was at the "phonology-metaphonology" transition of language acquisition? The SLP may have knowledge and skills about specific interventions and recommendations about comparison strategies that include posing the alternative as "no treatment." Finally, the SLP can recommend outcome elements that match the intervention, are measurable, and are considered critical to optimizing communication.

Once the best or most meaningful question is formulated, the search continues to locate and appraise the external evidence. McKibbon et el. (1995) emphasize that the best research-derived evidence is valid, important, and applicable. Research evidence is appraised based on levels of evidence. SLPs are trained to identify not only the strength of the evidence, but to also use the acronym POEM to evaluate if the evidence is patient-oriented evidence that matters (Dollaghan 2007). However, SLPs realize that POEM on treatment effectiveness for individuals with significant disabilities frequently is limited. Therefore, at times, perhaps a single case study may be the best evidence to support an AT decision.

EBP does not rely on external evidence alone. The clinical and personal evidence gathered by the SLP are the two other EBP components required to guide decision-making. Additional clinical and personal evidence (e.g., quantitative and qualitative data) may be needed as the AT team evaluates all of the evidence. At this point, a functional analysis and psycho-socio-environmental evaluations that address the specific context of use are conducted. Note how the EBP model (Figure 14.2) depicts a continuous loop in collecting and evaluating the evidence. In the end, teams place the individual's benefits first when applying EBP, pose specific questions of direct practical importance, objectively and efficiently evaluate the current best evidence, and take appropriate action guided by evidence (Gibbs 2003).

14.1.3 AT Assessments and the SLP

Applying the systematic steps of the EBP model becomes even more critical when no standardized battery of tests compose the AT evaluation. Minimal research exists to support a specific AT evaluation model (Hill and Scherer 2008). In addition, no current, standardized, evidence-based AT procedures exist to determine if an individual would benefit from AT. However, evidence is available to identify procedures for conducting reliable, valid, and dynamic or authentic assessments that can be recommended to collect data to identify an individual's abilities, needs, and expectations. These data are then used for the feature match process.

A primary role for the SLP as a team member assessing an individual for AT is to collect, analyze, and interpret evidence (data) related to speech, language, oral and written communication, swallowing abilities, needs, and expectations. The unique knowledge that SLPs bring to the AT evaluation is their ability to assess the subsystems of language— phonology, morphology, syntax, semantics, and pragmatics—as they relate to spoken and written language (ASHA 2001). Consequently, the SLP answers questions that the team has about an individual's basic language knowledge at the level of sounds, words, sentences, and interactive conversation regardless of whether the communication disorder is developmental in nature or acquired.

For the pediatric population with disabilities and associated communication disorders, the SLP contributes evidence related to how the child is progressing through the transitions of speech and language acquisition. Three major transitions take place during the first 5 years of life (Paul 1997): (1) pragmatics to semantics, (2) semantics to syntax, and (3) phonology to metaphonology. Following a developmental model provides evidence to guide SLPs and the AT team in determining the capabilities of the child and the cognitive-linguistic requirements of an AT intervention (Hill 2009). In addition, these transitions provide benchmarks for when, what, and how to collect data to monitor the effectiveness of AT interventions and when to modify or revise AT decisions.

For the adult population with disabilities and associated communication disorders, the SLP contributes evidence related to the type, severity, and prognosis of the disorder. Adults with acquired communication disorders who may benefit from AT must be evaluated to determine a course of AT treatment to support regaining skills (e.g., aphasia or traumatic brain injury). In other cases, the individual may be evaluated to determine an AT solution to maintain function across the course of the underlying disease complex (e.g., amyotrophic lateral sclerosis or Huntington's chorea). In either case, the SLP contributes evidence by administering clinically, linguistically, and culturally appropriate approaches to assess the current cognitive-linguistic abilities. This information then serves as baseline data.

A clear distinction exists among the type of assessments conducted to identify speech, language, and overall oral and written communication capacities. A thorough and comprehensive evaluation of cognitive-linguistic skills is paramount to beginning the feature-match process. For both the pediatric and adult populations who may benefit from AT, identifying the shared and distinctive targets assessed by the SLP and other educational or rehabilitation professionals highlights the importance in collecting thorough evidence. Table 14.1 illustrates the overlapping domains of language and literacy assessed by SLPs

TABLE 14.1

Illustration of the Overlapping Domains of Language and Literacy Assessed by SLPs and Educational AT Team Members

Language	Overlapping	Literacy
Speaking and Listening	*Literate Language*	*Reading and Writing*
• Form and content for social and personal uses	• Academic and metalinguistic uses	• Letter knowledge
• Phonemic awareness	• Abstract and figurative content	• Word reading
• Lexical retrieval	• Decontexualized and formal forms	• Spelling
• Auditory memory	• Print concepts	• Punctuation
• Articulation	• Formal oral contexts	• Reading fluency
• Fluency	• Print contexts	• Reading comprehension
• Voice		• Writing composition

Source: Adapted from Ukrainetz, T. A., and Fresquez, E. F. (2003). "What isn't language?" A qualitative study of the role of the school Speech–Language pathologist. *Language, Speech, and Hearing Services in Schools, 34,* 284–298.

and teachers (Ukrainetz and Fresquez 2003). Such detailed reporting of specific parameters of language and literacy provide clear targets/markers for matching the operational requirements for various AT intervention. Similar language and literacy abilities and/or executive functioning skills can be identified to show the distinctive and shared targets that are evaluated by SLPs and rehabilitation professionals working with adult populations. These results are used for matching the AT requirements and features.

The SLP is responsible for assessing the relationship that the domains of communication competence (i.e., linguistic, social, strategic, and operational) (Light 1989; Kovach 2009) may have on the individual's ability to benefit from various AT interventions. These domains have been identified as important to the feature match process and for monitoring outcomes. The linguistic and social domains require evaluating data on the various subsystems of language identified earlier in this section. The strategic and operational domains involve an individual's use of AT features and require evaluating data on executive functions and the cognitive, sensory, and perceptual domains.

Finally, as part of the AT assessment battery, SLPs will include procedures that are applicable to everyday life. The use of ecological inventories and daily journals may help to identify variables or barriers to successful implementation of AT interventions (Beukelman and Mirenda 2005). Conducting a task analysis to identify the operational requirements of AT under consideration or a discrepancy analysis to identify the performance of peers on similar tasks may provide insight for feature matching. Interviewing is conducted to identify the client's or family's values, expectations, beliefs, and goals. However, AT assessments limited to ecological inventories, interviews, and observations in activities of daily living will fail to gather the evidence needed to be most effective in the feature match process.

14.1.4 Matching Persons With Technology and SLPs

The MPT model is best applied at the point of selection and trial of the AT interventions and then used to determine the outcomes of the process of matching the person and the AT device/system (Scherer 2002, 2004; Scherer and Craddock 2002). As noted above, external, clinical, and personal evidence is collected and vetted to arrive at the process of identifying or matching the features and components of an AT device/system for

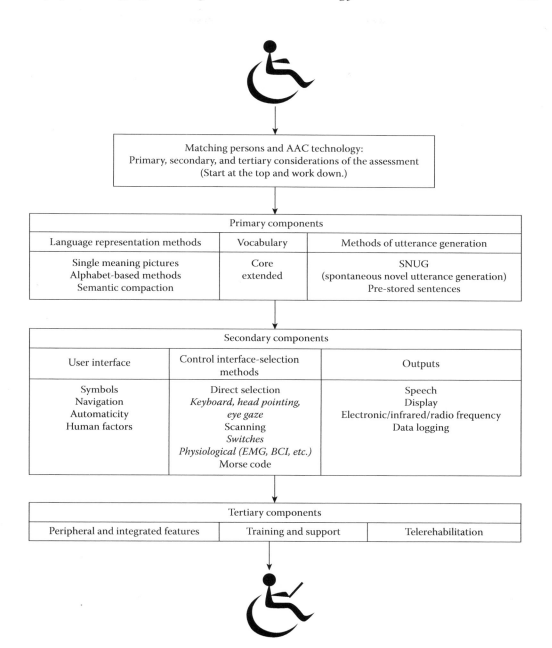

FIGURE 14.3
Diagram representing the primary, secondary, and tertiary components to consider during an AT assessment. (Hill, K. and Scherer, M., *Proceedings of the Twenty-Third Annual Conference "Technology and Persons with Disabilities,"* California State University, Northridge, CA, 2008.)

demonstration and trial (Figure 14.3). The features of AAC systems have been identified as primary, secondary, and tertiary components (Romich et al. 2005; Cooper et al. 2009). This approach places more value on features that enhance communication performance and productivity than typical feature listings or coding categories used for funding (Hill et al. 2007). A similar performance-based approach may be taken for AT pertaining to oral

TABLE 14.2

Case Example of Performance Data Comparing Original and Selected AAC Systems at the End of the First Month of Training

Performance Data and Outcomes Measurement	Original AAC System	New AAC System
Frequency of LRMs:		
Spelling	97%	6%
Word prediction	2%	3%
Single-meaning pictures	1%	1%
Semantic compaction	Not supported by system	90%
Mean length of utterance in Words (MLU-w)	2.8	5.5
Average communication rate: direct keyboard	1.0 wpm	6.5 wpm
Peak communication rate: direct keyboard	Not able to calculate	21 wpm
Average communication rate: optical head pointing	N/A	5.3 wpm
Peak communication rate: optical head pointing	N/A	17.4 wpm

N/A, not applicable; wpm, words per minute.

and written communication because features that enhance the speakers' or writers' performance and ultimately well-being have higher value (Hill and Scherer 2008).

The primary, secondary, and tertiary AT components used for oral and written communication are identified in Table 14.2. Primary components focus on the language parameters of the AT system. These language-based components are compared to the assessment data contributed by the SLP and relate to how the speaker or writer generates spoken or written messages. Because many AT systems include stored vocabulary and messages, how the speaker or writer accesses the two vocabulary categories of core (high frequency) words and extended (specific to a topic or activity) words affects performance. In addition, features for spontaneous, novel utterance generation (SNUG) or access to preprogrammed utterances/messages influence spoken and written productions and should be identified as available or not.

Secondary components relate to the user and control interfaces and output options. The primary components influence the user interface, or what the speaker or writer sees, and how the individual accesses AT. If the speaker/writer requires letter-by-letter spelling, then the user interface may be a standard keyboard. However, if the speaker/writer requires word prediction as a feature, then a touch-screen monitor may be included as the user interface. Sensory, perceptual, and motor skills will influence the interfaces and selection methods. Therefore, the evidence from the SLP regarding cognitive-linguistic abilities and executive functioning skills will influence the use and arrangement of symbols/lexemes, navigational features of the user interface, and other related human factor principles. These capacities assessed by the SLP may also provide insight into the selection of AT system outputs.

Tertiary components relate to additional supports that influence short- and long-term effectiveness of the selected AT. Again, the SLP can provide insights into the use of peripherals and integration of an AT system with other devices. For example, many AAC speakers want mobile access to phones and are interested in integrating an AAC system with phone access. Individuals using computers to support written communication desire integrating environmental controls with the computer for more independent control of other electronic devices in the home. The SLP may also recommend specific trainings and supports for the individual, family, and team. Several manufacturers provide initial in-home installation and training on AT and offer Internet-based trainings that do not require travel to another location. Finally, more SLPs are offering telerehabilitation services to support training and intervention for clients using AT.

The MPT process is client-centered and requires that the individual, including family or significant others, participate in the selection of AT options. The SLP may have the role of explaining the full range of AT solutions along the continuum of no technology to high-performance technology. In addition, the SLP may explain and demonstrate the various AT components related to speech and oral and written language and communication. This instructional and demonstration time ensures that the client and family are fully informed of all of the options and are actively involved in the selection of the AT interventions considered for trial.

Individuals and/or family members may enter the MPT process with preconceived notions about the type of AT they want. By providing an overview of the range of AT options and descriptions of AT in terms of primary, secondary, and tertiary components, the person and family gain an appreciation of the complex nature of the MPT process (Hill and Scherer 2008). Although off-the-shelf products may be a final solution, the selected AT more frequently includes features that provide more flexibility and customization for the person's unique capabilities than products not designed for specific populations with disabilities. With limited knowledge, an individual may have high satisfaction with an AT solution, but once they are fully informed about the performance differences that exist among the available solutions their initial satisfaction vanishes. Consequently, the external, internal, and personal evidence gathered by the SLP is used to support the details for the feature match.

14.1.5 Evaluation of the Effectiveness and Usefulness of the AT

The trial portion of the MPT process requires collecting quantitative and qualitative data to evaluate the effectiveness and usefulness of the AT intervention. It is typical in the United States for third-party payers to require that the AT team provide documentation for at least three trials on similar solutions before making a selection. Although three trials may be documented, the AT team must have reviewed the range of solutions and a detailed comparison among the possible AT options. Because no research evidence exists regarding the length required for an AT trial, the professional opinion of the AT team along with the choice of the individual and family makes the decision about the trial lengths.

Baseline data on any current AT that were collected at the start of the assessment can be compared with data collected during the AT trials. Automated performance monitoring provides quantitative data that are based on units of measurement to use at the trial stage (Hill and Romich 2001). The built-in data logging feature of several AT systems, integrated software, or external tools offer effective and efficient methods for monitoring gains in performance or for comparing AT solutions under consideration. The SLP's role includes identifying the most reliable and valid measures to monitor performance and recommending the methods to collect oral and written language samples.

The collection and analysis of language samples is the most authentic procedure for identifying communication competence (Light and Binger 1998; Paul 2007; Hill 2009). The parameters used to measure communication competence are the same across cohorts and the life span. The parameters used to determine the severity of a communication disorder are also valid for AT speakers and writers. The SLP selects those measurements that will provide the most reliable and valid data for decision-making and monitoring progress. Typical data related to the subsystems of language (semantics, morphology, and syntax) include the measures of vocabulary, syntactic diversity, and the length and complexity of utterances.

Various language sampling contexts may be recommended to collect the most representative example of an individual's language functioning (Dollaghan et al. 1990). Various factors have been found to affect the quality of the language, such as the visual and auditory prompts of the tasks (Shadden 1998) or asking for a description rather than a narrative (Duchan 1991). McNeil et al. (2002) have validated a story retell procedure for adults. Hill (2001) compared an interview and picture description task for AAC speakers and found both contexts to be reliable and valid to report communication performance. Obviously, the most representative sampling would come from the AT speakers' or writers' communication during activities of daily living. Without using automated data logging, capturing these data would be impossible.

Language activity monitoring (LAM) refers to a principle and set of tools that places primary value on the use of language samples in making decisions about AT solutions for spoken and written communication. LAM principles focus on the importance of collecting and analyzing the parameters of communication used across contexts, environments, and the life span. LAM tools record a log file to document the use of an AAC/AT system. The LAM log file starts with a header and includes a privacy statement, the device sending the information, the current software version, and the date (Hill 2004). The data format has been standardized for analysis programs to accept the data from different sources. In addition, the standard format ensures that the log file can be (1) readily uploaded or saved on a computer, (2) readily interpretable by AT teams, (3) easily visually inspected to identify possible treatment targets, and (4) suitable for standard language analysis. Figure 14.4 represents the process when LAM is a built-in feature of an AAC system. KeyLAM (AAC Institute 2009) software allows the computer to record a log file when other AAC systems are used or when the AT writer is using a computer.

The time stamp element of LAM and other performance measurement tools provide quantitative data that other observational and video or audio recording tools and software cannot provide. The Performance Report Tool (PeRT) (AAC Institute 2001; Romich et al. 2003) allows SLPs to create a transcript from LAM data. It also automatically generates a two-page report that contains 17 summary measures, some with graphic representation and various appendices related to vocabulary and utterance use. Compass software (Koester et al. 2003; Koester Performance Research 2007) measures AT writer's skills in various kinds of computer interactions to help AT teams evaluate computer access. The various

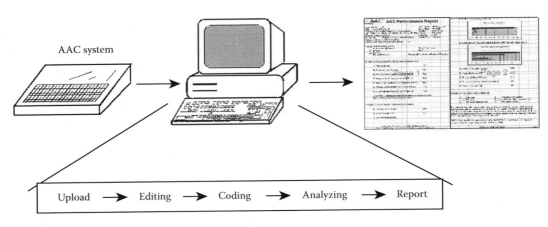

FIGURE 14.4
Diagram representing the LAM process uploading a log file to generate a performance report. (Hill, K., *Topics in Language Disorders: Language and Augmented Communication*, 24, 18–30, 2004.)

skills assessed include keyboard and mouse use, navigation through menus, and switch use. The SLP can provide insights into determining which sampling tasks would be most representative for reporting data for AT decision-making.

14.1.6 Development and Implementation of AT Intervention Plans

The AT assessment and MPT processes are not concluded without the development of an intervention plan. Now, the International Classification of Functioning, Disability, and Health (ICF) (WHO 1992) has elevated therapy and technology to more strongly match the desired activity and participation of the AT user (Cooper 2007). When surveyed, individuals with disabilities and family members expressed a clear sense of maximizing potential and independence as an important outcome (Pain et al. 1998). Therefore, the focus of intervention is not on the recommended AT, but is client-centered and aimed at optimizing the client's performance and outcomes using the chosen AT.

For individuals with communication disorders, therapy or treatment will include goals and objectives to support gains in speech and the subsystems of language. These would be the identical evidence-based treatments if AT had not been recommended. Evidence-based intervention methods are used with children for language acquisition goals. Evidence-based strategies are used in therapy to support regaining language for adults with aphasia. In addition, AT may frequently support targeting deficits in speech–language comprehension and/or expression by the use of voice output, written modes of communications, and other educational and clinical software features.

14.1.7 The SLP's Role in Advocacy

The National Joint Committee (NJC) for the Communication Needs of Persons with Severe Disabilities has proposed that all people, regardless of the severity of their disabilities, have a basic right to use communication as a means of affecting how they live. Indeed, consideration of AT should not be based on exclusionary criteria in determining eligibility for AT supports and services (Kangas and Lloyd 1988; NJC 2002). Rather, the ICF acknowledges the rights and dignity of individuals with disabilities and encourages AT teams to look at how an individual falls on a continuum of participation in daily activities and environments (Huer et al. 2006; Huer and Hill 2007). Therefore, SLPs advocate for a zero exclusion policy when institutional or administrative policies may be in place that first determines individuals' eligibility.

14.1.8 Specific Learning Disabilities

In relation to the above, with regard to the role and function of the SLP within a team for the evaluation and treatment of language pathologies mediated by AT, and considering in particular written communication disorders, it is useful to give a brief examination of some aspects linked to what are defined as specific learning disabilities (SLDs) (dyslexia, dysorthography, dysgraphia, and dyscalculia). These disorders are of enormous clinical relevance, affecting approximately 5% of the population (Prasher and Kapadia 2006; Lagae 2008), and an ineffective and superficial management has had, and may continue to have, a considerable social impact (e.g., Zabel and Nigro 1999).

SLDs are developmental disorders affecting children—male and female, intelligent and healthy and thus unharmed from a neurological and sensory point of view—who have had normal sociocultural and scholastic opportunities and despite this are unable to learn, or rather to manage with sufficient confidence, the process of reading (in this case, dyslexia), writing (dysorthography and dysgraphia when the quality of the written line is affected), and mathematical calculation (dyscalculia). These disorders may present in isolation or in association with each other and do not depend in any way, from an etiological point of view, on relational or psychological problems in general. However, in some cases they may unfortunately become the cause of psychological difficulties rather than fully developed psychopathologies of, for example, an anxious or depressive nature (Rourke and Fuerst 1991; Daniel et al. 2006; Morgan and Fuchs 2007).

In this respect, the role of an SLP would appear very important both in contributing to assessment and, above all, in rehabilitation. This is true even if the SLDs are only in part linked to language, or rather to linguistic functions inasmuch as the processes of reading, writing, and calculation involve other areas and cognitive processes such as visuoperceptive and visuospatial skills, visuomotor integration, attention, executive functions, and short- and long-term memory. In other words, reading, referring to the Representional Redescription (RR) model proposed by A. Karmiloff Smith (1992, p. 17), is a process that "modularizes," that is, it tends to become highly automatic, and for such modularization to occur, according to Moskovitch and Umiltà (1990) and, contrary to the hypothesis of Fodor (1983), it would be necessary to turn to other processes enabling the assembly of submodules (see Moscovitch and Umiltà, 1990, p. 12). In fact, reading, according to Moscovitch and Umiltà's model, would be included among the third type of module, that is, those that are assembled on a voluntary basis, departing from the second type of module, in this case, language and visuoperceptive functions, which on the contrary would be assembled without voluntary intervention (indeed, one refers to the acquisition of language, rather than learning) (Moscovitch and Umiltà 1990, pp. 16–18). This "assemblage" occurs thanks to the attentional resources dedicated by the supervisory attentional system, as hypothesized by Shallice (1988).

To conclude, from this perspective first-type modules (the assemblage of which generates second-type modules) would be those of Fodor, not assembled and with functional specificity. For example, the perception of colors, acoustic frequencies, visual and acoustic localization, depth, and faces would be first-type modules. From this approach there emerges a model for reading of the following type (Figure 14.5).

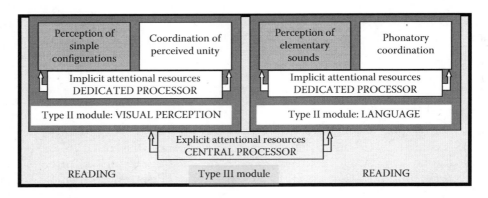

FIGURE 14.5

Illustration of reading as a third-type module formed by different possible second-type modules, visuoperception and language, which in turn are formed by simpler first-type modules such as perception of simple configurations and perception of elementary sounds at the top of the diagram. (Moscovitch, and Umiltà, C. *Modular Deficits in Alzheimer-Type Dementia*, Cambridge, MA: MIT Press, 1990.)

As Figure 14.5 shows, it is difficult to find one reading disorder with the same underlying problems as another. In fact, with reference to reading as a third-type module, it can be seen from the diagram that the malfunction, which results ultimately in a reading disorder, may concern any one of the modules or submodules concerned (in generally different ways): the attentional resources and executive functions (central processor), language (language) or any of its components (e.g., perception of elementary sounds), visuoperceptual aspects (e.g., coordination of perceived unities), and visuospatial attention. In other words, the malfunctioning of one or more of the processes indicated above will be manifested according to different profiles, thus demonstrating the notable heterogeneity of reading disorders.

From the model we are able to say that a reading disorder may depend upon the hypodevelopment of or damage to one or more of the several subcomponents (the central processor, dedicated processor, and several first- or second-type modules in various percentages). In reality, the situation is even more complex if one considers the complete functional architecture of reading: I refer to the two-way model (e.g. Shallice 1988). The graphic/phonological system of conversion alone, according to Moscovitch and Umiltà (1990), would already constitute a third-type module.*

With reference to dyslexia, given the neuropsychological complexity of the process, the moment of assessment is extremely delicate. The etiology of the disorder, although still not yet perfectly known (Esgate et al. 2005), in the light of the most recent theories, is multifactorial (Manis et al. 1996; Segalowitz and Rapin 2002; Esgate et al. 2005) and it would therefore be necessary in the assessment to define a profile of neuropsychological function that could (as previously illustrated) vary considerably from case to case.

In the case of a child diagnosed with dyslexia, the disorder could be based on linguistic difficulties (for example, phonological or metaphonological) or visuoperceptual (for example, visual search, visuospatial attention with consequent crowding effect), or both of the above, thus considerably aggravating the clinical picture. There could also be (again according to the model previously set forth) difficulties at the level of attentional resources and executive functions necessary for the assemblage of the submodules (for example, working memory, inhibition and control of irrelevant stimuli, and planning).

From this perspective it is possible to identify an effective treatment, specific and targeted, making use of all that AT can offer nowadays. In England (HMSO 1995) and in the United States (US 2004), a SLD such as dyslexia is considered a true disability: "A disability can arise from a wide range of impairments which can be: developmental, such as autistic spectrum disorders (ASD), dyslexia and dyspraxia, learning difficulties" (HMSO 1995 A6) and is therefore considered as falling within the purview of the general law on disability:

> The term "child with a disability" means a child with—mental retardation, hearing impairments (including deafness), speech or language impairments, visual impairments (including blindness), serious emotional disturbance (hereinafter referred to as "emotional disturbance"), orthopedic impairments, autism, traumatic brain injury, other health impairments, or specific learning disabilities (US 2004, Sec. 620).

On the contrary, in Italy, from a legal point of view a SLD is not considered a disability, and so a specific law was passed (No. 170) in October 2010 with the aim of protecting the

---

* In Italy, this research is being performed by Professor F. Benso (University of Genova), whose publications on the subject are currently available only in Italian: Benso, F. (2010). *Sistema Attentivo-Esecutivo e Lettura. Un Approccio Neuropsicologico alla Dislessia.* Torino, IT: Il Leone Verde; Idem (2004). *Neuropsicologia Dell'Attenzione. Teoria e Trattamenti nei Disturbi dell'Apprendimento.* Pisa, Italy: Edizioni del Cerro.

right to learn and study in individuals with SLDs (Repubblica Italiana 2010). This law provides indications regarding the type of path that should be taken in each individual case to be organized within the school system. This approach, defined as a Personalized Didactic Plan, is to be drawn up by the school via the Class Council with the collaboration of the specialists who have made the diagnosis and assumed responsibility for rehabilitation.

It is therefore a "right" for students of any order and level (also in universities) to have access to compensatory tools and dispensatory strategies. With regard to the former (compensatory tools), AT can be of great benefit, using tools ranging from a simple calculator to a computer equipped with textbooks in digital format; an example of a dispensatory strategy would be a reduced workload, to be set with close attention to quality rather than quantity, or, with regard to foreign languages (in Italy, for example, English) it would be legitimate to focus upon oral rather than written aspects when setting didactic objectives. At the same time, it is a "duty" for schools and teachers to know these tools and to permit and promote their use, enabling children and young people to understand how these techniques and tools represent an opportunity to favor the emergence of their potential and intelligence, which otherwise risk remaining unexpressed, giving rise to considerable frustration, rather than instruments for labeling them as incapable, which unfortunately often occurs. The risk that children and young people perceive the suggested tools as an advantage or as assistance granted because "in any case they aren't able" is closely linked to the still limited knowledge of SLDs in many countries (including Italy) and the fact that, culturally, these difficulties do not yet form a part of our habits and culture. In other words, a child with dyscalculia "needs" a calculator or a Pythagorean table just as a short- or long-sighted child "needs" glasses. However, although a teacher would never dream of requiring a child to fulfill a task without glasses, should he or she need them, calculators or conceptual maps are frequently taken away from children with a SLD because of an absurd and incomprehensible sense of "justice" with regard to the others (who, not having a SLD, do not have any need for compensatory tools to practice their skills).

Here it should be emphasized that the use of tools provided by AT should always be studied and organized by the school with the assistance of the specialists concerned, who will be able to provide the most specific indications on a case-by-case basis that are linked to the diagnosis and particular neuropsychological profile of each child/young person and, using the appropriate tests, identify the most suitable enabling (exercise-based) and compensatory tools. This agreement between the specialists and the school must naturally be shared and accepted by the family.

The diagnostic criteria are those established by international classifications:

- *DSM IV* (APA 2000): Learning Disorders/Academic Skills Disorders [315] are diagnosed when
  - The results obtained by the subject in individually administered standardized tests on reading, mathematics, or written expression are significantly lower than to be expected on the basis of age, education, and level of intelligence;
  - Learning problems interfere in a significant manner with school results and with everyday activities requiring reading, mathematical, and written abilities.
- *ICD-10*—Diagnostic characteristics (WHO 1992): Specific developmental disorders relating to scholastic abilities F81
  - These are "disorders in which the normal patterns of skill acquisition are disturbed from the early stages of development. This is not simply a consequence

of a lack of opportunity to learn, it is not solely a result of mental retardation, and it is not due to any form of acquired brain trauma or disease." These disorders, on the contrary, derive from anomalies in cognitive processes linked to a greater extent to some form of biological dysfunction. As with the majority of other developmental disorders, these conditions are markedly more common in males.

In Italy, as in other countries, a Consensus Conference was organized (last updated in April 2011; see the Dislexya Italian Association's website [http://www.aiditalia.org/]) to establish further shared guidelines regarding diagnostic criteria (completed with the necessary neuropsychological investigations) and the professionals involved in multidisciplinary teams responsible for evaluation, providing indications for management. With regard to the latter, there are two principal routes that may, depending on the case in hand, be alternative or parallel. These are

1. A strictly rehabilitational route, which will aim to
   - Recover the deficit (the neurocognitive deficit underlying the disorder). For example, in line with the points previously illustrated, it would be useful in the diagnostic process to clarify the level at which the "breaking point" is located, whether this may be linguistic, visuoperceptual, or linked to attentional resources, and to take this as the basis for rehabilitation using the appropriate tools;

   and/or

   - Work directly on the task in itself (for instance, reading). An approach to rehabilitation centered on the task of reading, taking into consideration the context and type of orthography in which it is located (more or less transparent), again in this case should be specific and targeted and should work on single aspects in accordance with the two-way model of reading (Coltheart 1987; Shallice 1988; Zorzi 2005) such as visual analysis, grapheme-phoneme conversion, metaphonological analysis, and phonemic synthesis, with regard to sublexical reading (phonological decoding), and the construction of an orthographic lexicon with (for example) tachistoscopic presentation of words with growing complexity of the phonotactic structure, by lexical reading. For each of the aspects listed, numerous types of specific rehabilitational software are available (see, for example, Abledata.com [http://www.abledata.com], or EASTIN [http://www.eastin.info]).

   The aim of this approach to rehabilitation is not the complete remission of the symptoms, which would be unrealistic, but the achievement of a level of mastery of the process sufficient to enable compatibility with autonomous study. On the other hand, even in relation to writing in general, it is possible to reach a level of control of the process permitting effective written communication, clear from a morphosyntactic point of view, even if orthographical errors are likely to be present. The likelihood of attaining these objectives is greater the earlier the moment of diagnosis and the more targeted and specific the approach to rehabilitation. In some cases, rehabilitation as described above may not reach the set objectives on account of numerous variables (aside from delayed diagnosis and intervention, i.e., at over 9 years of age), including the severity of the disorder. This severity depends on the level to which the affected individual function is compromised and how many functions are involved in determining the symptom (for example, difficulty of reading). The path of rehabilitation is considered to be concluded when

- Reasonable objectives have been reached;
- The advanced age of the subject means that the effectiveness of the intervention can no longer be guaranteed; and
- In some cases, further improvements cannot be achieved.

2. A compensatory path aims, instead, to guarantee to the individual, despite the continuation of the difficulty (for instance, nonautomatic reading, which is therefore not functional for study purposes), access to information, with the possibility of undertaking a regular path of study, thus providing access to the consequent professional opportunities.

From this perspective, AT managed by a specialist team (as presented earlier in the chapter) is of fundamental importance.

The introduction of speech synthesis,* which is, along with the use of texts in digital format, now provided for by current regulations, enables the acquisition of information through listening, circumventing the problem of reading.

It should be emphasized that the use of vocal synthesis for studying does not undermine reading skills; if anything, it helps improve them. By personalizing the speed of the reader and highlighting the text, which can be followed while it is read by the vocal synthesizer, it enables indirect training in the process of reading.

Vocal synthesis is a program that enables the computer to read a text that must obviously, therefore, be inserted in digital form; a voice, with an intonation ever closer to natural patterns, enables the user to decodify and listen as necessary, thus avoiding the obstacle of nonautomatic reading.

The objective of vocal synthesis is to provide a reader able to decode in the place of the user who may experience difficulty in doing so, rather like a mother or teacher who, aware of the tiredness reading may provoke and the resulting limited comprehension, decides to read aloud. The child is thereby finally able to listen and maintain sufficient attentional resources, which are generally lost in the tiring process of nonautomatic reading, to understand the meaning of the text. Compared with a person such as a mother or teacher who reads the text for the child or the young person, vocal synthesis has the advantage of rendering the subject autonomous. Thanks to this tool, a child with reading difficulties does not need to be accompanied by others and, using a computer, may autonomously access information.

The problem that often confronts young people starting to use vocal synthesis is that there may still be difficulties of comprehension that cannot be recovered through the use of the tool. This is certainly not due to problems related to intelligence (see diagnostic criteria for inclusion/exclusion) but rather, in general, to the impoverishment of metacognitive resources. In other words, these children or young people, distracted by the difficulties of decodification imposed by dyslexia, make enormous efforts to learn the process of reading itself and therefore only with difficulty do they activate the resources necessary to ask themselves, "What purpose does this process serve? Why read?" These resources are

---

* Speech synthesis is a technique for the artificial reproduction of the human voice. A system used for this purpose is described as a vocal synthesizer and can be achieved by means of software or hardware. Systems of vocal synthesis are also known as text-to-speech (TTS) systems because of the possibility that they provide conversion of text to spoken word. There are also systems able to convert phonetic symbols into speech (Wikipedia.org).

metacognitive skills such as searching for key words, identifying the principal character in a story, distinguishing what is salient from what is not and relating it to prior knowledge, etc. In these cases, before young people experience another failure, it is necessary to help them with interventions of a psychopedagogic nature to enable the recovery of these so-called metacognitive resources and to work on study methods in general, using compensatory tools that will finally enable the student to have the "energy" necessary to acquire an effective method.

In line with the provisions of the model of the ATA process in a center for technical aid, the specialist team should decide which of the two paths should be taken by a child diagnosed with a SLD. Bearing in mind the age of the subject, the extent of the disorder, and the possibility of intervening directly in the deficit, the team decides if it is appropriate to take an approach aimed at rehabilitation or to undertake a compensatory route. In general, a child between 6 and 9 years of age, and therefore at a stage in which the developmental window of the functions in question is still open and sensitive to further development, and who has not previously undertaken a course of rehabilitation will take the route of specific, targeted rehabilitation with the aid of relevant software. On the other hand, an older child or one who has already undertaken the specific rehabilitation path will take the compensatory route, with the aim of guaranteeing the most general learning processes covered in school, using the appropriate compensatory tools. In this case, the principal objective is that of guaranteeing access to information that may be filtered or lost in the case of nonautomatized reading and writing. This will enable the subject to deal with data and to manipulate them, enabling, in accordance with Karmiloff's RR model (1992), a behavioral mastery with possible representational redescription. This procedure, when well managed, enables the regular development of potentialities that, if not activated and trained, might not emerge, thus not favoring overall cognitive development.

In a help center, at the moment of planning a path using compensatory tools, tests are proposed using software and/or specific tools in direct contact with the child or young person to identify those most suitable for the specific situation, whereas enabling software (rehabilitational) is advised on the basis of the problems that emerge in the context of clinical evaluation and at the center for technical aid. Project planning is performed, where possible, in agreement with the health-care professionals following the progress of the child or young person and always with the teachers and family involved. A follow-up is periodically performed (normally every six months to one year) to decide, by means of a new evaluation, whether to continue with the use of enabling tools or to concentrate instead on compensatory ones. The team that decides upon the use of AT is always available for consultation by teachers, families, and health-care professionals should variations to the initial project become necessary.

Along with the identification of the appropriate tools to use, there is guaranteed training in their use for the child or young person, teachers, the family, and health-care professionals, if present. At the end of the AT evaluation, indications regarding the most appropriate personalization of the software and tools are given.

In conclusion, having a SLD means having a disorder only in a society such as the one in which we currently live, which (fortunately for all) requires literacy; in fact, children with SLDs begin to demonstrate their "disorder" only when they enter school and have to gauge their abilities in terms of the acquisition of reading, writing, and mathematical skills. In many cases, this disorder can be practically "annulled" through the introduction of adequate techniques for teaching reading and writing by using the appropriate tools chosen on a case-by-case basis. The possibility of enabling many children and young people with SLDs to learn, study serenely, and to prepare themselves for satisfactory integration in the adult world, making the most of their own real potential, would seem closely linked to a cultural change (perhaps only just begun) that, through a knowledge of the way in which these disorders function and the consequent use of the appropriate tools, will render study more fulfilling for most young people.

14.2 Case Evaluation in a Multidisciplinary Team or as a Professional Consultant

The following is a case study documented by Hill (2006) that exemplifies following the EBP steps and uses performance and outcomes measurement to monitor gains toward achieving short- and long-term goals of intervention. A multidisciplinary team approach was involved in the assessment process. As a client-centered principle, the client managed the team that consisted of the SLP clinical supervisor, graduate students in SLP training, an AT consultant, a rehabilitation engineer, a rehabilitation counselor, a university advisor, and a parent. The goals and objectives of intervention reflect the ICF model. The client self-identified the need to re-evaluate his use of AT because he was failing his first semester at the university. His goal was to receive a four-year degree, become gainfully employed, and live independently.

14.2.1 Characterizing the Client

The case involves a 22-year-old college student with cerebral palsy. He was referred to the AT center of a university by the university's office for students with disabilities. The referral indicated the need to identify strategies to improve communication and academic performance. The student had a high school diploma and an associate degree in accounting from another college. He transferred at the start of the semester into a four-year degree program. High school and college transcripts, medical records, and other educational testing records were reviewed. Standardized screening indicated no hearing or visual acuity problems. Spoken and written language samples confirmed linguistic and communication competence. Other standardized instruments indicated that auditory comprehension and vocabulary skills were within normal adult ranges. Performance data on current use of an AAC system and computer were collected and reviewed. Interviewing was used to collect personal evidence about the client's values and needs for spoken and written communication and participation in other daily living activities. The ICF was used to support the activities and level of participation expected by the client. His expressed values were consistent with the desire to be a "faster, more efficient" communicator with comments that he did not appreciate having his messages "guessed" by other people. He valued being able to use his own words rather than having pre-stored messages. In addition, he valued that all of his AT could be integrated and upgraded to work as efficiently and effectively as possible.

14.2.2 Step 1: Asking Meaningful EBP Questions

The team discussed the PICO format of asking questions to seek the evidence that mattered for this client. The patient was an adult with cerebral palsy enrolled in college; his current AT was used as the intervention; the comparison was an alternative language representation method; and the outcome was increased communication rate and communication fluency. However, the following three questions summarize value-based questions that were asked by all team members:

1. Is the client's communication rate as fast as others of similar profile?
2. Is the client's use of alphabet-based approaches the most effective language representation method possible?
3. Is the client's use of a touch-screen, page-based display the most effective technology solution?

14.2.3 Step 2: Collecting Clinical and Personal Evidence

Traditional methods of observation and LAM tools were used for this process (Hill and Romich 2001). The PeRT software was used to analyze language samples and generate a performance report. Although traditional methods of observation allowed for the collection of the multimodal aspects of communication, only LAM tools provided the accuracy needed to monitor change or make comparisons among interventions. In addition, the measurement of communication and selection rate requires a time stamp for calculating standardized units of measure (Romich and Hill 1999).

On the basis of the formulated EBP questions, the following performance measures were critical to obtain: (1) average and peak communication rate, (2) communication rate of language representation methods, (3) selection rate, (4) mean length of utterance, and (5) frequency of complete utterances.

14.2.4 Step 3: Locating and Reviewing Research Evidence

The electronic search for evidence resulted in eight studies that were used to provide external evidence to guide decisions. These studies were summarized by the SLPs and shared with the team. An electronic database managed by the author was mined to find performance data of individuals with similar profiles (Hill et al. 2000). The results provided information on the performance achieved by others using AT systems under consideration. In addition, the client joined an online discussion group to seek user input on satisfaction with various AAC/AT options. He shared responses to his queries from the discussion group with the team as well as content on related topics that he felt pertained to his situation.

14.2.5 Step 4: Using the Evidence

This step involved using the external, clinical, and personal evidence for the MPT process. The primary, secondary, and tertiary features were discussed and demonstrated to the client with trials. The client requested the following three trial periods before making a decision about AAC and/or AT: (1) his current AAC device with modifications and current computer arrangement, (2) an upgraded touch-screen AAC system to emulate with the computer, and (3) a hybrid AAC system to emulate with the computer.

The primary components became the major features for the client to select. Identifying the various language representation methods (LRMs) used to generate communication for spoken or written language would influence performance. Becoming aware of how core and extended vocabulary could be stored and retrieved was a feature that he had not previously considered. Because the client preferred not to use pre-stored messages, but wanted SNUG to be his primary means of communicating, customizing a bank of preprogrammed sentences was not considered.

The secondary components offered a wide range of options to consider and manipulate. The SLPs on the team and the AT consultant were more involved in discussing, demonstrating, and comparing the various language software with pre-stored vocabulary configurations, different numbers of display locations, symbol types, color display options, sizes of touch screens, etc. In addition, given the client's significantly reduced selection rate on his current systems, the team suggested evaluating alternative access methods as a means to increase communication rate. The client indicated that he wanted the option to switch between direct keyboard selection and optical head pointing, depending on his physical status during the day. Other features that were considered desirable by the client included infrared control for computer access and environmental control and data logging. In comparing the various AAC systems under consideration, the client found value in the following secondary features: core and activity row configuration to access vocabulary, icon prediction, icon tutor, and easy access to display status and tool box customization.

The central tertiary component important to the client was being able to use the AAC system with a computer. Setting up the peripherals in the dorm was needed for this to happen. In addition, mounting solutions and fabrication of other peripherals were needed and performed by the rehabilitation engineer. The client also took into consideration services offered by the manufacturer.

Step 4 involved a clinical summary at the end of three months. The summary was written to describe the result of the assessment and trial process and culminated in submitting a funding request for a new AAC system and updates to computer access. Training and intervention on the new communication technology included a 1-hour therapy session once a week for three months. The built-in LAM feature provided an efficient method for monitoring progress by both the client and the SLPs and prompted discussion about treatment outcomes. Within three months of treatment, the client had learned his new language application program and was selecting words using semantic compaction 90% of the time. His average communication rate was 6.7 words per minute and peak communication of 21 words per minute with direct keyboard selection. For this case, the use of semantic compaction was 16 times faster than spelling. By the end of the academic year, performance and outcomes data indicated significant gains, that overall spoken and written communication were more effective and efficient, and that user satisfaction was high.

Table 14.2 compares the client's performance on his original system with his performance on his new system at the end of the first month. Using PeRT allowed for precise and accurate reporting of performance measures during the assessment and intervention processes. The performance reports provided an ongoing, reliable record of progress for treatment outcomes. In addition to improvements in his communication performance in various social environments, his communication in classes was also considered to be improving. With an improvement in his grades, withdrawal was no longer considered necessary. Two years later, the client graduated from the university with a four-year degree. He has met his long-term goals by being gainfully-employed and living independently.

14.3 Conclusions

Our case adheres to the precepts of a client-driven process to reach an AT solution that allows the individual to reach their highest potential within the ICF framework. The client's request, which is based on his concern over his school performance, triggered the referral and assessment processes. The client invited specific members to the team, taking into consideration how the components of the ICF model related to him: his body functions and structure, personal, and environmental factors. The SLP became the team coordinator and manager because the primary area of concern related to the significant discrepancy in his spoken and written communication with his college peers.

The final AT solution was identified by applying the principles of EBP. This included becoming familiar with resources and services to support the long-term effectiveness of the AT solutions. In our client's case, after he was shown video clips of individuals speaking with high-performance voice output systems, he shared that he had never met another AAC speaker. The team conducting his previous evaluation had never performed an assessment for an AAC system and computer access, and he had not been made aware of environmental controls. His original team had made decisions on the basis of "ease of use at first encounter, rather than long-term effectiveness." His first AT team found an immediate solution, but it was not the most effective, efficient, or satisfying AT solution. During separate conversations with the client and his family, we came to realize that they had no idea that individuals with severe communication and physical disabilities were communicating so effectively and fast using an AAC system.

At the first assessment session, the client was introduced to various Internet resources through the AAC Institute web site (http://www.aacinstitute.org). He was encouraged to post questions about the AT assessment process to members of a discussion group to be a better advocate for himself. Internet resources can provide access to information that is current and useful when sources are carefully and prudently evaluated.

Today the SLP on AT teams is expected to conscientiously and judiciously use the best evidence or data to support decisions that fit into the ICF framework. SLPs practicing the principles in this chapter "place the client's benefits first when applying evidence of direct practical importance to planning" (Gibbs 2003). Our case is an example that individuals who are AAC speakers believe that the fundamental, desired outcome of independent spoken and written communication can be achieved with appropriate technology and appropriate long-term, often intensive intervention strategies (Creech 1995; Hill et al. 2007). Our client's quality of life was dramatically enhanced by striving for a solution that resulted in the most effective, independent communication as well as integrating other AT solutions together. AT teams that are client-driven and include the family and significant others can feel secure that the client's benefits are placed first when evidence is used judiciously and conscientiously within an organized framework.

Summary of the Chapter

The chapter highlights the knowledge and skills the that the SLP contributes to the AT team. The SLP is one member of a collaborative, dedicated group of people who work together to reach the best solution for a client. The SLP provides unique clinical measures related to an individual's speech, language, oral and written communication, listening, reading, and swallowing capabilities. In addition, the SLP contributes performance measures and functional analysis of speaking and writing skills to support AT solutions. The use of LAM resources and tools provide evidence to quantify client achievement of specified goals with respect to effectiveness, efficiency, and satisfaction in desired activities and environments. Personal well-being and life experience are directly related to an individual's ability to communicate as effectively as possible.

Acknowledgments

Katya Hill contributed to the entire study except for Section 14.1.8, which was reviewed by Corsi Valerio.

References

AAC Institute. (2001). *Performance Report Tool* (PeRT) [computer software]. Pittsburgh, PA: AAC Institute.

AAC Institute. (2009). *KeyLAM* [computer software]. Pittsburgh, PA: AAC Institute.

American Speech–Language-Hearing Association (ASHA). (2001). *Roles and Responsibilities of Speech–Language Pathologists with Respect to Reading and Writing in Children and Adolescents* [Guidelines]. Retrieved from http://www.asha.org/policy

American Speech–Language-Hearing Association (ASHA). (2002a). *Augmentative and Alternative Communication: Knowledge and Skills for Service Delivery* [Knowledge and Skills]. Retrieved from http://www.asha.org/policy

American Speech–Language-Hearing Association (ASHA). (2002b). *Knowledge and Skills Needed by Speech–Language Pathologists with Respect to Reading and Writing in Children and Adolescents* [Knowledge and Skills]. Retrieved from http://www.asha.org/policy

American Speech–Language-Hearing Association (ASHA). (2004a). *Preferred Practice Patterns for the Profession of Speech–Language Pathology* [Preferred Practice Patterns]. Retrieved from http://www.asha.org/policy

American Speech–Language-Hearing Association (ASHA). (2004b). *Roles and Responsibilities of Speech–Language Pathologists with Respect to Augmentative and Alternative Communication: Technical Report* [Technical Report]. Retrieved from http://www.asha.org/policy

American Speech–Language-Hearing Association (ASHA). (2007). *Scope of Practice in Speech–Language Pathology* [Scope of Practice]. Retrieved from http://www.asha.org/policy

American Speech–Language-Hearing Association (ASHA). (2010). *Code of Ethics* [Ethics]. Retrieved from http://www.asha.org/policy

American Psychiatric Association (APA). (2000). *Diagnostic and Statistical Manual of Mental Disorders: DSM-IV-TR*. Arlington, VA: APA.

Beukelman, D., and Mirenda, P. (2005). *Augmentative and Alternative Communication: Management of Severe Communication Disorders in Children and Adults* (3rd ed.). Baltimore: Paul H. Brookes Publishing Co.

Bodine, C., and Melonis, M. (2005). Teaming and assistive technology in educational settings. In D. Edyburn, K. Higgins, and R. Boone, (Eds.), *Handbook of Special Education* (pp. 209–227). Whitefish Bay, WI: Knowledge by Design, Inc.

Coltheart, M. (1987). *Attention and Performance XII: The Psychology of Reading*. London: Psychology Press.

Cook, A. M., and Hussey, S. M. (2002). *Assistive Technologies: Principles and Practice* (2nd ed.). St. Louis, MO: Mosby.

Cooper, R. A. (2007). Introduction. In R. R. Cooper, H. Ohnabe, and D. A. Hobson, (Eds.), *An Introduction to Rehabilitation Engineering* (pp. 1–18). New York: Taylor & Francis Group.

Cooper, R. A., Roberts, B. R., Hill, K., Karg, P. Karmarkar, A., Lane, A. K., et al. (2009). Seating, assistive technology, and equipment. In J. Stein, R. L. Harvey, R. F. Macko, C. J. Winstein, and R. D. Zorowitz, (Eds.), *Stroke Recovery and Rehabilitation* (pp. 543–568). New York: Demos Medical Publishing.

Cooper, R. A., Ohnabe, H., and Hobson, A. D. (2007). *An Introduction to Rehabilitation Engineering.* Boca Raton, FL: CRC Press.

Creech, R. (1995). Outcomes: Choosing our directions—Our freedom is the field's reason for being. In *Proceedings of the Third Annual Pittsburgh Employment Conference.* Pittsburgh, PA: SHOUT Press, 3, pp. 9–12.

Daniel, S. S., Walsh, A. K., Goldston, D. B., Arnold, E. M., Reboussin, B. A., and Wood, F. B. (2006). Suicide, school dropout, and reading problems among adolescents. *Journal of Learning Disabilities, 39*(6), 507–514. doi:10.1177/00222194060390060301

Dollaghan, C. A. (2007). *The Handbook for Evidence-Based Practice in Communication Disorders.* Baltimore, MD: Paul H. Brookes Publishing Co.

Dollaghan, C. A., Campbell T. F., and Tomlin, R. (1990). Video narration as a language sampling context. *Journal of Speech and Hearing Disorders, 55,* 582–590.

Duchan, J. (1991). Everyday events: Their role in language assessment and intervention. In T. Gallaher, (Ed.), *Pragmatics of Language: Clinical Practice Issues* (pp. 43–98). San Diego: Singular.

Esgate, A., Groome, D., and Baker, K. (2005). *An Introduction to Applied Cognitive Psychology.* London: Psychology Press.

Fodor, J. A. (1983). *The Modularity of Mind.* Cambridge, MA: MIT Press.

Gibbs, L. B. (2003). *Evidence-Based Practice for Helping Professions: A Practical Guide with Integrated Multimedia.* Pacific Grove, CA: Thompson Brookes/Cole.

Haines, L., and Robertson, G. (2005). Teamwork needs technology. In D. Edybum, K. Higgins, and R. Boone, (Eds.), *Handbook of Special Education Technology Research and Practice* (pp. 455–480). Whitefish Bay, WI: Knowledge by Design.

Hill, K. (2001). *The Development of a Model for Automated Performance Measurement and the Establishment of Performance Indices for Augmented Communicators under Two Sampling Conditions.* Dissertation Abstracts International, *62*(05), 2293 (UMI No. 3103368).

Hill, K. (2004). AAC evidence-based practice and language activity monitoring. *Topics in Language Disorders: Language and Augmented Communication, 24,* 18–30.

Hill, K. (2006). A case study model for augmentative and alternative communication. *Assistive Technology Outcomes and Benefits, 3*(1).

Hill, K. (2009). Data collection and monitoring AAC intervention in the schools. *ASHA Perspectives on Augmentative and Alternative Communication 18,* 58–64. doi:10.1044/aac18.2.58

Hill, K. J., Baker, B., and Romich, B.A. (2007). Augmentative and alternative communication technology. In R. A. Cooper, H. Ohnabe, and D. A. Hobson, (Eds.), *An Introduction to Rehabilitation Engineering* (pp. 355–384). Boca Raton, FL: Taylor & Francis.

Hill, K., Dollaghan, C., and Nyberg, E. (2000). *AAC Language Sample Library for Intervention, Outcomes Measurement, and Research.* Presented at the Annual American Speech–Language-Hearing (ASHA) Annual Convention. Washington DC. November 16–19.

Hill, K., Glennen, S., and Lytton, R. (1998). The Role of Manufacturers' Consultants in Delivering AAC Services. In *Proceedings of the 8th ISAAC Biennial Conference.* Dublin, Ireland.

Hill, K., and Romich, B. (2001). A language activity monitor for supporting AAC evidence-based clinical practice. *Assistive Technology, 13,* 12–22.

Hill, K. and Romich, B. (2003). *AAC Evidence-Based Clinical Practice: A Model for Success.* Pittsburgh, PA: AAC Institute Press.

Hill, K., and Romich, B. (2007). *AAC Evidence-Based Practice: Four Steps to Optimized Communication.* Pittsburgh, PA: AAC Institute Press.

Hill, K., Romich, B. and Hurd, R. (2007). *Family and Consumer Perceptions of AAC Evidence-Based Practice.* Poster at the 8th Annual Conference of the ASHA Division on AAC. Atlanta, GA.

Hill, K., and Scherer, M. (2008). Matching Persons & Technology: Data-Driven AAC Assessment. *Proceedings of the Twenty-Third Annual Conference "Technology and Persons with Disabilities,"* California State University, Northridge, CA.

HMSO. (1995). *Disability Discrimination Act*. Retrieved from http://www.legislation.hmso.gov.uk/

Huer, M. D., and Hill, K. (2007). *AAC and the Rights and dignity of Persons with Disabilities*. Workshop at the 2007 RESNA Annual Conference. Phoenix, AZ. June 15–19.

Huer, M., Hill, K., and Loncke, F. (2006). International Policy Trends and AAC. In *Proceedings of the ISAAC Biennial 2006 Conference*. Dusseldorf, Germany. July 29–August 5, 2006.

Hunt, P., Soto, G., Maier, J., Liboiron, N., and Bae, S. (2004). Collaborative teaming to support preschoolers with severe disabilities who are placed in general education early childhood programs. *Topics in Early Childhood Special Education, 24*(3), 123–142.

Kangas, K., and Lloyd, L. (1988). Early cognitive skills as prerequisites to augmentative and alternative communication use: What are we waiting for? *Augmentative and Alternative Communication, 4*, 211–221.

Karmiloff-Smith, A. (1992). *Beyond Modularity: A Developmental Perspective on Cognitive Science*. Cambridge, MA: MIT Press.

Koester, H. H., LoPresti, E., Ashlock, G., McMillan, W., Moore, P., and Simpson, R. (2003). Compass: Software for Computer Skills Assessment. In *Proceedings of CSUN 2003 International Conference on Technology and Persons with Disabilities*, Los Angeles, CA. March 2003.

Koester Performance Research. (2007). COMPASS [computer software]. Ann Arbor, MI: Koester Performance Research.

Kovach, T. M. (2009). *Augmentative and Alternative Communication Profile: A Continuum of Learning*. East Moline, IL: LinguiSystems.

Lagae, L. (2008). Learning disabilities: definitions, epidemiology, diagnosis, and intervention strategies. *Pediatric Clinics of North America, 55*(6), 1259–1268. doi:10.1016/j.pcl.2008.08.001

Law, M. L., and MacDermid, J. (2008). *Evidence-Based Rehabilitation*. Thorofare, NJ: SLACK Inc.

Lieber, J., Beckman, P. J., Hanson, M. J., Janko, S., Marquart, J. M., Horn, E., et al. (1997). The impact of changing roles on the relationships between professionals in inclusive programs for young children. *Early Education and Development, 8*, 67–82.

Light, J. (1989). Toward a definition of communicative competence for individuals using augmentative and alternative communication systems. *Augmentative and Alternative Communication, 5*, 137–144.

Light, J., and Binger, C. (1998). *Building Communicative Competence with Individuals Who Use Augmentative and Alternative Communication*. Baltimore, MD: Paul H. Brookes Publishing Co.

Manis, F. R., Seidenberg, M. S., Doi, L. M., McBride-Chang, C., and Petersen, A. (1996). On the bases of two subtypes of development dyslexia. *Cognition, 58*(2), 157–195. doi:10.1016/0010-0277(95)00679-6.

McKibbon, K. A., Wilczynski, N., Hayward, R. S., Walker-Dilks, C., and Haynes, R. B. (1995). *The Medical Literature As a Resource for Evidence Based Care. Working Paper from the Health Information Research Unit*, McMaster University, Ontario, Canada.

McNeil, M. R., Doyle, P. J., Park, G. H., Fossett, T. R. D., Brodsky, M. B. (2002). Increasing the sensitivity of the Story Retell Procedure for the discrimination of normal elderly subjects from persons with aphasia. *Aphasiology, 16*(8), 815–822.

Morgan, P. L., and Fuchs, D. (2007). Is there a bidirectional relationship between children's reading skills and reading motivation? *Exceptional Children, 73*(2), 165–183.

Moscovitch, M., and Umiltà, C. (1990). Modularity and neuropsychology: Modules and central processes in attention and memory. In M. F. Schwartz, (Ed.), *Modular Deficits in Alzheimer-Type Dementia* (pp. 1–59). Cambridge, MA: MIT Press.

National Joint Committee for the Communicative Needs of Persons with Severe Disabilities (NJC). (2002). Access to communication services and supports: Concerns regarding the application of restrictive "eligibility." *Communication Disorders Quarterly, 23*(2), 145–153.

Ninni, K. M., Brownstein, L. (1999). Patient outcome as a selection criterion in determining treatment mode. *Perfusion, 14*(3), 213–218.

Pain, K., Dunn, M., Anderson, G., Darrah, J., and Kratochvil, M. (1998). Quality of life: What does it mean in rehabilitation? *Journal of Rehabilitation, 64*(2), 5–11.

Paul, R. (1997). Facilitating transitions in language development for children using AAC. *Augmentative and Alternative Communication, 13*, 141–148.

Paul, R. (2007). *Language Disorders from Infancy through Adolescence* (3rd ed.). St. Louis, MO: Mosby Elsevier.

Prasher, V. P., and Kapadia, H. M. (2006). Epidemiology of learning disability and comorbid conditions. *Psychiatry, 5*(9), 302–305. doi:10.1053/j.mppsy.2006.06.010

Repubblica Italiana. (2010). Legge 170/10: Nuove norme in materia di disturbi specifici di apprendimento in ambito scolastico (10G0192). *Gazzetta Ufficiale della Repubblica Italiana—Serie Generale, 244,* 1–3.

Romich, B., and Hill, K. (1999). A language activity monitor for AAC and writing systems: Clinical intervention, outcomes measurements, and research. In *Proceedings for the RESNA '99 Annual Conference.* Long Beach, CA. pp 19–21.

Romich, B., Hill, K., Seagull, A., Ahmad, N., Strecker, J., and Gotla, K. (2003). AAC Performance Report Tool. In *Proceedings of the RESNA 2001 Annual Conference* [CD-ROM]. Atlanta, GA: RESNA Press.

Romich, B., Vanderheiden, G., and Hill, K. (2005). Augmentative communication. In J. D. Bronzino, (Ed.), *The Biomedical Engineering Handbook,* (3rd ed). Boca Raton, FL: CRC Press.

Rourke, B. P., and Fuerst, D. R. (1991). *Learning Disabilities and Psychosocial Functioning: A Neuropsychological Perspective.* New York: Guilford Press.

Sackett, D. L, Strauss, S. E., Richardson, W. S., Rosenberg, W., and Haynes, R. B. (2000). Evidence-based medicine: How to practice and teach EBM. Edinburgh, Scotland: Churchill Livingstone.

Sackett, D. L., Rosenberg, W. McGray, J. M., Haynes, R. B., and Richardson, W. S. (1996). Evidence-based medicine: What it is and what it isn't. *British Medical Journal, 321,* 71–72.

Scherer, M. J. (Ed.). (2002). *Assistive Technology: Matching Device and Consumer for Successful Rehabilitation.* Washington, DC: APA Books.

Scherer, M. J. (2004). The Matching Person and Technology Model. In Scherer, M.J. (Ed.), *Connecting to Learn: Educational and Assistive Technology for People with Disabilities* (pp. 183–201). Washington, DC: APA.

Scherer, M. J., and Craddock, G. M. (2002). Matching Person and Technology (MPT) assessment process. *Technology & Disability, 3*(14), 125–131.

Segalowitz, S. J., and Rapin, I. (2002). *Handbook of Neuropsychology: Child Neuropsychology* (Vol. 8 Pt. 1). Amsterdam, The Netherlands: Elsevier Health Sciences.

Shadden, B. B., Burnette, R. B., Eikenberry, B. R., and DiBrezzo, R. (1991). All discourse tasks are not created equal. *Clinical Aphasiology, 20,* 327–341.

Shallice, T. (1988). *From Neuropsychology to Mental Structure.* Cambridge, UK: Cambridge University Press.

Swengel, K., and Marquette, J. (1997). Service delivery in AAC. In S. L. Glennon, and D. Decoste, (Eds.), *Handbook of Augmentative and Alternative Communication* (pp. 21–57). San Diego: Singular Publishing Group.

Ukrainetz, T. A., and Fresquez, E. F. (2003). "What isn't language?" A qualitative study of the role of the school Speech–Language pathologist. *Language, Speech, and Hearing Services in Schools, 34,* 284–298.

U.S. Government (US). (2004). *Individuals with Disabilities Education Act.* Public Law 108–446, December 3, 2004.

World Health Organization (WHO). (1992). *ICD-10: International Statistical Classification of Diseases and Related Health Problems, 10th Revision* (Vol. 1–3). Geneva, Switzerland: WHO.

Zabel, R. H., and Nigro, F. A. (1999). Juvenile offenders with behavioral disorders, learning disabilities, and no disabilities: Self-reports of personal, family, and school characteristics. *Behavioral Disorders, 25*(1), 22–40.

Zorzi, M. (2005). Computational models of reading. In G. Houghton, (Ed.), *Connectionist Models in Cognitive Psychology* (pp. 403–444). London: Psychology Press.

Section III

Assistive Technology Devices and Services

S. Federici and M. J. Scherer

Introduction

Today much information about assistive technologies (ATs) can be obtained from many databases and web sites on the World Wide Web (WWW).* However, we can make a clear distinction between databases and web sites: AT web sites mostly aim to present a catalogue of technologies for a specific kind of disability, such as the American Printing House for the Blind (http://www.aph.org/), or for other specific groups of disabilities, such as the Cambium Learning Technology Company web site (http://www.intellitools.com/). Databases are more focused on the diffusion of technical information about equipment by collecting a very extensive list of ATs.

The two largest and most complete databases of devices are[†]

- AbleData.com (http://www.abledata.com): Supported by the National Institute on Disability and Rehabilitation Research in 1996, this database currently provides information on approximately 40,000 products classified into 20 areas. It also offers information on noncommercial prototypes, customized and one-of-a-kind products, and do-it-yourself designs.
- The European Assistive Technology Information Network (EASTIN, http://www.eastin.info): In 2003, some of the best-known expert information providers in Europe joined together to create a comprehensive information service on AT, which currently offers information on 66,269 products.

---

* A complete list of AT databases and web sites can be found at http://www.a4access.org/atia.htm.
† The number of products on http://www.abledata.com and http://www.eastin.info was retrieved in May 2011.

The impressive number of products offered by those databases is evidence of the growth in AT devices that has occurred. In fact, when we consider the increase in products presented by the AbleData database from 1996 to 2011, we see that the number of products has doubled (Halverson and Belknap 1996). This rapid increase in the amount of online information about AT products underscores the need and desire for technologies that meet the diverse needs of people with disabilities in all facets of their lives: from products for medical treatment to supports for school, work, and self-care to equipment for housekeeping, recreation, and sexual activity.

Company investments in the improvement of AT have led to the development of new products as well as product upgrading and updating. Simultaneously, literature appears on product usability, use versus discard, and on the optimal matching of user and technology. By aiming to analyze both the interaction between the user and the technology in the assistive technology assessment (ATA) process and the development of new ATs, Section III is focused on the idea that it is impossible to represent the most recent ATs without losing the race with the advancement of technology, in which something that is new today becomes outdated in a week. To avoid the possibility of discussing outdated technology, the five chapters making up Section III (Chapters 15–19) are focused on new landscapes in AT development and research by presenting technologies that are not now available on web sites and databases (such as brain–computer interface technologies) while emphasizing new concepts and methods for improving the next generation of ATs.

Presentation of the Chapters of Section III

The chapters in Section III are organized in conceptual order from the most theoretical—the role of user experience evaluation in the ATA process—to the most concrete—adapted physical activity and equipment for sport activities. (Table III. 1).

Chapter 15, "Systemic User Experience," presents a theoretical framework of the role of user experience (Section 15.1) in the ATA process using an integrated approach of evaluation in the rehabilitation system. The user experience (UX) holistic perspective and definition are presented along with the concepts of usability and accessibility (Sections 15.2.1 and 15.2.2). The authors introduce a new conceptual perspective that is based on the

TABLE III.1

Chapters of Section III

Chapter	Topic
15	Systemic User Experience (Borsci, Kurosu, Mele, and Federici)
16	Web Solutions for Rehabilitation and Daily Life (Liotta, Di Giacomo, Magni, and Corradi)
17	Brain–Computer Interfaces: The New Landscape in Assistive Technology (Pasqualotto, Federici, Olivetti Belardinelli, and Birbaumer)
18	New Rehabilitation Possibilities for Persons with Multiple Disabilities through the Use of Microswitch Technology (Lancioni, Singh, O'Reilly, O'Sigafoos, Oliva, and Basili)
19	Methods and Technologies for Leisure, Recreation and an Accessible Sport (Capio, Mascolo, and Sit)

UX framework and integrated model of interaction evaluation (Section 15.3.1). The authors endorse the assumption that UX evaluation concerns not only the user's experience with an assigned technology but also the user's experience of the action of the center for technical aid (i.e., ATA process functioning), proposing an ATA process under the lens of UX evaluation to assess both the relation between the AT and the users and that between the users and the center for technical aid (Section 15.4.1). Finally, the authors present different examples concerning the application of the UX framework to the design process of systems for rehabilitation (Sections 15.4.2 and 15.4.2.1).

All of the other chapters in Section III, by aiming to present new landscapes and visionary AT projects, are explicitly or implicitly linked to the integrated model presented in Chapter 15.

In Chapter 16, "Web Solutions for Rehabilitation and Daily Life," Liotta, Di Giacomo, Magni, and Corradi focus on the relationship between users and new ATs. The authors present two studies that share a user-centered design (UCD) perspective (Norman and Draper 1986) to reduce the digital device neutralizing barriers due to both the physical and the virtual environment. The authors' theoretical background endorses the perspective provided by the World Health Organization (WHO) that considers "the use of information, communication, and related technologies for rehabilitation as an emerging resource that can enhance the capacity and accessibility of rehabilitation measures by providing interventions remotely" (WHO and World Bank 2011, p. 118).

Chapter 16 describes new Web technologies by making two assumptions about the WWW:

1. The WWW is a means of accessing and using information—AT, to allow users to achieve their goal (i.e., accessing and using information), has to reduce the digital divide by increasing the accessibility and usability of websites and search engines.

2. The WWW is a means of providing a service—AT, to allow users to obtain a service (i.e., rehabilitation), uses the Internet to provide a remote/online service.

The first AT presented, called WhatsOnWeb, is a clustering web search engine (Section 16.2) that makes use of both the information visualization approach (Sections 16.2.3 and 16.2.3.1) and the sonification of the graphical elements of the interface (see Chapter 15, Section 4.2 and Chapter 16, Section 16.2.3.2) to improve the effectiveness and efficiency of Web searching for blind users. The WhatsOnWeb evaluation results (Sections 16.2.3.3, 16.2.3.3.1, and 16.2.3.3.2) are presented to analyze the properties and features of this technology as an assistive device.

The second AT discussed is called Nu!Reha Desk, a telemedicine tool for rehabilitation (Sections 16.3.1 and 16.3.2) created to supply personalized exercises for execution at home by users in a distant but monitored manner. The system has been designed as a main application for extending the "traditional approach" of the neurological rehabilitation service (Sections 16.3.3 and 16.3.4). The Nu!Reha evaluation results are presented to discuss the role of AT in providing distance data to practitioners to optimize users' access to a rehabilitation program (Sections 16.3.5 and 16.3.5.1).

Chapter 17, "Brain–Computer Interfaces: The New Landscape in Assistive Technology," discusses brain–computer interfaces (BCIs) for restoring communication and movement in patients with severe and multiple disabilities (Section 17.1). It presents the history of BCIs and brain activity measures (Sections 17.2.1–17.2.4 and 17.3). The authors endorse the idea that BCIs are information and communication technologies that support the daily life activities of people with disabilities (Section 17.7). In this sense, BCI technologies are ATs that aim not to compensate for a deficit but to promote the user's social participation.

Chapter 17 presents BCI applications for different rehabilitation goals, such as (1) the use of BCIs as communication tools for individuals with neurodegenerative and motor diseases, for example, Guillain Barré syndrome, amyotrophic lateral sclerosis, locked-in syndrome, and so on (Sections 17.4.1 and 17.4.2); (2) the use of BCIs for motor restoration in patients with stroke or traumatic brain or spinal cord injury (Sections 17.5.1 and 17.5.2); and (3) the use of BCIs for treatment of behavioral disorders such as epilepsy and attention deficit hyperactivity disorder (Sections 17.6.1 and 17.6.2).

Chapter 18, "New Rehabilitation Opportunities for Persons with Multiple Disabilities through the Use of Microswitch Technology," discusses the role of microswitch technologies and voice output communication aids (VOCAs) to help persons with profound and multiple disabilities to learn to control relevant stimuli in their environment and achieve social contact through simple responses. The chapter presents different studies on the application of microswitch technology to (1) monitor small (nontypical) responses of people with minimal motor behavior (Section 18.2); (2) allow the person direct access to different types of stimulation by using a combination of two or more microswitches (Section 18.2.1); and (3) allow the person direct access to stimulation as well as the possibility of calling for social attention and interaction by the use of microswitches combined with VOCAs (Section 18.3). The results obtained by the experimental applications led the authors to suggest the possibility of using combinations of ATs as microswitches and VOCAs in rehabilitation programs that aim to increase people's adaptive responses to the environment and to allow direct social contact between the person and caregivers (Sections 18.4 through 18.4.2).

Section III ends with Chapter 19, "Methods and Technologies for Leisure, Recreation and an Accessible Sport." The authors of this chapter, aiming to promote programs of adapted physical activity (APA), discuss the methods and technologies that facilitate accessible sport via self-efficacy theories for enabling sports participation for all (Sections 19.1.1–19.2.2). The relation between sports and disability is analyzed from historical, biomedical, and sociopsychological points of view (Sections 19.3–19.3.3), and, at the same time, the authors underline the essential role of technical improvement of the ATs (e.g., mobility devices, wheelchairs, and prostheses) not only to promote sports and social participation activities but also to extend the "sports for all" idea in both developed and developing countries (Sections 19.4–19.4.3).

This chapter gives readers the opportunity to think about AT from a historical point of view, overcoming the medical approach of technical-fix (Roulstone 1998), whereas the authors clearly underline the role of the equipment not only as a means of "access" or for "rehabilitation" but also as a right for the promotion of leisure, recreation, and physical activities.

All of Section III's authors, like those of other sections of this book, agree with the book's editors' set of concepts as stated in the Introduction to Section I. Moreover, the authors directly or indirectly address the following concept definitions:

- Accessibility—Three Definitions:
  1. Accessibility as the means to opportunities and possibilities: "The art of ensuring that, to as large an extent as possible, facilities are available to people whether or not they have impairments of one sort or another" (Berners-Lee and Fischetti 1999).

2. Accessibility as access to information and communication technology: The Web Accessibility Initiative (WAI) defines accessibility as allowing people with disabilities to "perceive, understand, navigate and interact with the web" (2006).

3. Accessibility as access to a usable interface: ISO 9241-171 defines accessibility as the "usability of a product, service, environment, or facility by people with the widest range of capabilities" (ISO 2008).

- Sonification: This is a process of "transformation of data relations into perceived relations in an acoustic signal for the purposes of facilitating communication or interpretation" (Kramer et al. 1997, p. 3).

- Usability: This is the extent to which a product can be used by specified users to achieve specified goals with effectiveness, efficiency, and satisfaction in a specified context of use (ISO 1998).

    - *Effectiveness* is the accuracy and completeness with which users achieve specified goals;

    - *Efficiency* is the resources expended in relation to the accuracy and completeness with which users achieve goals; and

    - *Satisfaction* is the freedom from discomfort and positive attitudes toward the use of the product when users achieve goals.

In medicine and rehabilitation, a further distinction is made between efficacy and effectiveness as follows (Haynes 1999; Marley 2000):

- *Efficacy* refers to the accuracy and completeness with which users achieve specific goals under controlled or ideal conditions (e.g., within a clinic or rehabilitation setting).

- *Effectiveness* refers to the accuracy and completeness with which users achieve specific goals under real-world conditions.

- **Universal Design or Design for All (UD):** In the context of human–computer interaction, this implies a proactive approach toward products and environments that can be accessible and usable by the broadest possible end-user population, without the need for additional adaptations or specialized (re-)design. This approach refers to "the conscious effort to consider and take account of the widest possible range of end user requirements throughout the development life-cycle of products or services" (Akoumianakis and Stephanidis 2001).

- **User-Centered Design (UCD):** This term was first originated in Donald Norman's research laboratory at the University of California in the 1980s (Norman and Draper 1986). UCD is a design process characterized by a cycle of tests and re-tests of the technology. In the first series of tests run to optimize the interface, experts analyze how subjects are likely to use the prototype of the interface; in this first step, experts try to simulate the behavior of a common user following the guidelines of a user's model. Then, in the second series of tests, users are involved in a prototype analysis to further identify interface problems and to allow a redesign of the information architecture. Following the results of these two different cycles of tests (one performed by experts and one by users), the UCD model is able to take into account the needs and abilities of people and, therefore, is also able to optimize the interface according to these same needs and abilities, rather than forcing users to adapt themselves to an interface that is strictly dependent on the developer's model.

Section III is designed according to two main conceptual frameworks: the first is the integrated model of interaction evaluation and the second is the ATA process. The first framework allows us to propose the user experience evaluation as the core of the assignation process for achieving the rehabilitation priority indicated by the WHO, which is "to ensure access to appropriate, timely, affordable, and high-quality rehabilitation interventions" (WHO & World Bank 2011, p. 121) to provide ATs that are "suited to the environment" and "suitable for the user" by also granting "an adequate follow-up to ensure safe and efficient use" (WHO & World Bank 2011, p. 118). In fact, the UX evaluation is applied for measuring (and improving) both the user's interaction with the AT and the assessment of the whole ATA process as perceived by the users.

Following the integrated model of interaction evaluation (see Chapter 15), the accessibility and usability of a system are not understood as characteristics regarding two separate interacting entities but rather as one intrasystemic relation in which both object and subject are just moments in a multiphase process of empirical observation. All of Section III's chapters are focused on the idea that the interaction between user and environment through the AT is an intrasystemic relation that can be evaluated by the integrated model to assess the quality of the match or determine whether the environment has to be changed to improve the intrasystemic relation between user and AT (Federici and Borsci 2010). During an assignation, the process of a center for technical aid itself may be considered as a system interface by which a user can reach a goal. In this sense, we might evaluate the user experience in the ATA process on two levels: (1) the UX evaluation of the ATA process itself, i.e., the degree of accessibility and usability in the relationship between the users and the center for technical aid; and (2) the UX evaluation of the assistive solutions provided by the AT process, i.e., the matching of users with technical solutions.

Following the second framework regarding the ATA process, each chapter of Section III is organized to discuss technologies and models related to one or more steps of the process as follows:

- Chapter 15 is related to the following steps: (1) access of the user to the center for technical aid, i.e., the contact and accessibility of the center; (2) the user's checking of a solution, i.e., the user's evaluation; (3) the collection of data from users; (4) the multidisciplinary team meeting analysis of the case; and (5) the multidisciplinary team evaluation.

- Chapter 16 is related to the following steps: (1) the user's checking of a solution; (2) the user's living solution, i.e., the user's/client's adoption of the solution; (3) the collection of data from users; (4) the multidisciplinary team meeting analysis of the case; and (5) the multidisciplinary team evaluation.

- Chapters 17 and 18 are related to the following steps: (1) the user's living solution; (2) the multidisciplinary team meeting analysis of the case; and (3) the multidisciplinary team evaluation.

- Chapter 19 is related to the step of the user's living solution.

Taken as a whole, the chapters in Section III form a pathway to the optimal match of person and technology, the ultimate quality of which is determined from the end-user at various times post-AT acquisition.

References

Akoumianakis, D., and Stephanidis, C. (2001). *Universal Design in HCI: A Critical Review of Current Research and Practice*. Paper presented at the ACM Conference on Human Factors in Computing Systems: Universal Design: Towards Universal Access in the Information Society: CHI 2001, Seattle, WA. Retrieved from http://www.ics.forth.gr/hci/files/ch12001/akoumianakis.pdf

Berners-Lee, T., and Fischetti, M. (1999). *Weaving the Web: The Original Design and Ultimate Destiny of the World Wide Web by 1st Inventor*. London: Orion Business.

Federici, S., and Borsci, S. (2010). Usability evaluation: Models, methods, and applications. In J. Stone and M. Blouin (Eds.), *International Encyclopedia of Rehabilitation*. Buffalo, NY: Center for International Rehabilitation Research Information and Exchange (CIRRIE). Retrieved from http://cirrie.buffalo.edu/encyclopedia/article.php?id=277&language=en

Halverson, L., and Belknap, K. A. (1996). *Informed Consumer's Guide to Assistive Technology for People with Spinal Cord Injuries*. Retrieved from http://www.abledata.com/abledata_docs/icg-spin.htm

Haynes, B. (1999). Can it work? Does it work? Is it worth it? *British Medical Journal, 319*(7211), 652–653

International Standards Organization (ISO). (1998). *ISO 9241–11: Ergonomic Requirements for Office Work with Visual Display Terminals*. Geneva, Switzerland: ISO.

International Standards Organization (ISO). (2008). *ISO 9241–171: Ergonomics of Human-System Interaction—Part 171: Guidance on Software Accessibility*. Geneva, Switzerland: ISO.

Kramer, G., Walker, B., Bonebright, T., Cook, P., Flowers, J., Miner, N., et al. (1997). *Sonification Report: Status of the Field and Research Agenda*. Retrieved from http://sonify.psych.gatech.edu/publications/pdfs/1999-NSF-Report.pdf

Marley, J. E. (2000). Efficacy, effectiveness, efficiency. *Australian Prescriber, 23*(6), 114–115.

Norman, D. A., and Draper, S. W. (1986). *User-Centered System Design: New Perspectives on Human-Computer Interaction*. London: Lawrence Erlbaum Associates.

Roulstone, A. (1998). Researching a disabling society: The case of employment and new technology. In T. Shakespeare (Ed.), *The Disability Reader: Social Science Perspectives* (pp. 110–128). London: Cassell.

Web Accessibility Initiative (WAI). (2006). Introduction to Web Accessibility. Retrieved from http://www.w3.org/WAI/intro/accessibility.php

World Health Organization (WHO), and World Bank. (2011). *World Report on Disability*. Geneva, Switzerland: WHO.

15

Systemic User Experience

S. Borsci, M. Kurosu, M. L. Mele, and S. Federici

CONTENTS

15.1 Introduction

The term User eXperience (UX), proposed in the 1990s by Donald A. Norman and colleagues (1995) is focused on pleasure, value, and on performance during a human-system interaction. In the design process of the interaction, the usability of the system is a necessary but not sufficient condition for obtaining (designing or evaluating) a good level of UX; indeed, although usability is a dimension of the interaction, UX is a holistic perspective on how a user feels about using a system. There are various definitions regarding UX, including the one provided by Norman in explaining the UX term as "all aspects of the user's interactions with the product: how it is perceived, learned and used. It includes ease of use and, most important of all, the needs that the product fulfils" (1998, p. 47), and the definition provided by Garrett, "how the product behaves and is used in the real world" (2003, p. 17). Recently, the International Organization for Standardization (ISO) 9241-210 (1999) defined it as "a person's perceptions and responses that result from the use or anticipated use of a product, system or service." The ISO also states that

> User experience is a consequence of the presentation, functionality, system performance, interactive behaviour, and assistive capabilities of an interactive system, both hardware and software [...]. It is also a consequence of the user's prior experiences, attitudes, skills, habits and personality (ISO 1999).

Because of this, a total of 30 usability professionals and other people joined together in a workshop that was held in Dagstuhl, Germany, in 2010, and Virpi Roto and other editors summarized the discussion in the "User Experience White Paper" (Roto et al. 2011).

The UX is a complex concept that includes and extends the usability dimensions, without completely overcoming it. Many authors underline the areas in which UX goes beyond usability (Hassenzahl and Tractinsky 2006; Law et al. 2007). Those areas are well summarized by Petrie and Bevan as follows:

- *UX is more holistic than usability*: As previously discussed, usability focuses on performance of and satisfaction with users' tasks and their achievement in defined contexts of use; UX takes a more holistic view, aiming for a balance between task-oriented aspects and other nontask-oriented aspects (often called hedonic aspects) of eSystem use and possession, such as beauty, challenge, stimulation, and self-expression.

- *UX is more focused on subjective perception of the system than usability*: Usability has emphasized objective measures of its components, such as percentage of tasks achieved for effectiveness and task completion times and error rates for efficiency; UX is more concerned with users' subjective reactions to eSystems, their perceptions of the eSystems themselves, and their interaction with them.

- *UX is more focused on positive aspects of the system than usability*: Usability has often focused on the removal of barriers or problems in eSystems as the methodology for improving them; UX is more concerned with the positive aspects of eSystem use and how to maximize them, whether those positive aspects be joy, happiness, or engagement (Petrie and Bevan 2009).

Although the accessibility and the usability refer to the quality of the device and system in access and in use that can be described objectively, the concept of UX relates to such subjective aspects as an expected experience and perception and memory on the part of the user. In other words, quality traits such as usability and reliability can be regarded as independent variables whereas the UX is a dependent variable that will be influenced by the quality traits of devices and systems to be used. This means that consideration of the quality traits alone will not necessarily lead to a good UX. We should consider something more to achieve a better UX. This stance of putting an emphasis on the resulting UX is better than just focusing on the quality traits.

Experience was one of the key concepts in the area of marketing, especially in its relation to the formation of expectation. Establishing a good expectation on the part of consumers is one of the goals of marketing activity. But the marketing approach is less concerned about how people use the device or system, on which aspect user engineering has been focused.

Thus, Kurosu and Ando (2008) and also Kurosu (2010) combined these two concepts of experience and proposed a four-phase model of UX that was based on the idea that people will change their stance from the consumer to the user before and after the purchase of the system, as shown in Figure 15.1. In the first phase, people as consumers shape their expectancy both in subjective ways (e.g., simple desire) and in objective ways (e.g., foreseeable usage) for the device and system on the basis of various pieces of information obtained through such ephemera as advertisements and TV commercials, as well as other such media (e.g., web sites, journal articles, and information from friends). What the marketing approach has been emphasizing is this phase of UX. Thereafter, people obtain an

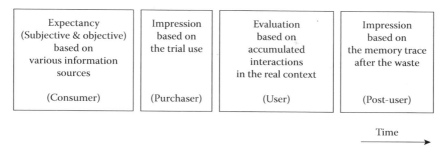

Expectancy (Subjective & objective) based on various information sources	Impression based on the trial use	Evaluation based on accumulated interactions in the real context	Impression based on the memory trace after the waste
(Consumer)	(Purchaser)	(User)	(Post-user)

Time →

FIGURE 15.1
The four phases of user experience.

impression of the device and system on the basis of a trial use if they are interested in it and motivated toward purchasing it. Usability testing as a summative evaluation is measuring what corresponds to this phase. Usability testing is one type of the interactive experience, but it does not represent the total UX because the length of the test only lasts for approximately 2 h on average and is too short to be regarded as UX.

After the purchase, people become the user and start interacting with the system in a real context. The repetitive interactions in the real environment will be stored in the memory of the user one by one, thus forming an evaluation of the system. Because this part of UX as the evaluation is a cumulative experience stored in memory, its level goes up or down depending on the quality of interaction at any time. Regarding adequate length of the evaluation, ISO 9241-210 (2010) claims that 6–12 months is necessary, and the Users Award Program in Sweden conducts an evaluation of information technology (IT) systems 9 months after installation.

Especially with regard to the third phase of UX, stakeholders who design the device and system have to assess both the quality of the system architecture (accessibility) and the quality of the system in use (usability) under the lens of user experience to evaluate the interaction.

After wasting the device and the system, there still remains a trace of impression in the memory. This information will serve as a basis for searching a new device or system as a consumer in the next cyclical stage. Thus, these four phases will form a spiral structure.

The UX perspective strongly emphasizes the point that it is not possible to obtain a realistic evaluation by analyzing only the functionality of the system, especially in an experimental setting, by using specific tools that enable evaluation of the device and system with a certain degree of objectivity (i.e., automatic evaluation and expert evaluation). In this sense, the UX accomplishes the User Centered Design (UCD) or the Human Centered Design (HCD) philosophy, by shifting the focus from an old perspective of design and evaluation focused only on the engineering aspects of the system to the new perspective that enables the consideration of users' experience with the system in the real environment.

It is not sufficient just to consider the object (device and system) and the subject (user) as two polarities for the interaction. The weakness of this dichotomy model is the insufficiency in taking into account the intrasystemic relation between system and user as an emergent independent reality not reducible to components (system and user) (Federici et al. 2005; Federici and Borsci 2010). In this sense, a member of the design team who tries to evaluate the interaction has to be an evaluator of the intrasystemic relation between system and user by taking into account the perspective both of the object and the subject (see Figure 15.2).

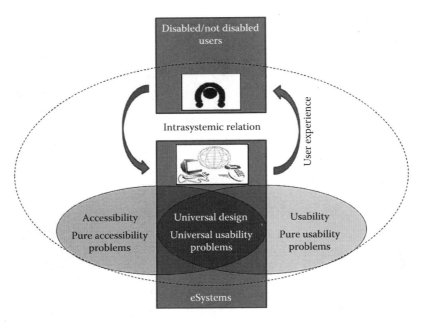

FIGURE 15.2
(See color insert.) The intrasystemic relation between users and eSystems. UX is represented as the user perspective in the intrasystemic relation of action and feedback with the eSystem (Federici et al. 2005; Federici and Borsci 2010). The universal design properties that make up the eSystem are obtained by the intersection of the accessibility and the usability of the eSystem. By following Petrie and Kheir (2007), the universal usability problems represent interaction problems of usability and accessibility that are found by all kinds of users in a bad intrasystemic relation because of a bad UX (universal design problems). When the problems affect mostly disabled people's interaction, we may use the term "pure accessibility problems," when the problems do not pertain to disabled users' interaction, we may use the term "pure usability problems." However, between these two extremes there are many different degrees of interaction problems that affect the UX of disabled and nondisabled users.

15.2 From Accessibility and Usability of Systems to the Users' Experience of Systems

15.2.1 The Relationship Between Accessibility and Usability

In the field of HCI, there have been various definitions of the concept of usability. But today, there is a shared definition originally provided by ISO 9241-11 (1998). This standard defines usability as "the extent to which a system, product or service can be used by specified users to achieve specified goals with effectiveness, efficiency and satisfaction in a specified context of use." On the other hand, with regard to the accessibility concept, there is no unique and complete definition that is able to describe the dimensions under evaluation. For example, according to ISO 9241-20 (2009), the definition of accessibility is "the usability of a product, service, environment or facility by people with the widest range of capabilities." In this definition, the relationship between usability and accessibility is not in parallel but is inclusive.

In fact, the concept of accessibility is linked to the rights of "access" to a wide "range of services, information, cultural exchanges, identity reaffirmations and social transactions […] seen as a basic right of citizens in many advanced society contexts" (Roulstone

2010, p. 9). In this sense, "Web accessibility" means that "people with disabilities can use the Web [...] more specifically [they] can perceive, understand, navigate, and interact with the Web" (WAI 2006). Di Blas and colleagues state that "W3C guidelines only guarantee 'technical readability,' i.e., the very fact that screen readers can work; they do not ensure at all the fact that the Website is 'accessible' by blind users, in the sense that blind users can effectively access it." (2004, p. 1).

These authors underline that the most important aim of the World Wide Web Consortium (W3C) is to ensure an effective user experience, or "usable accessibility" (Di Blas et al. 2004).

However, it is interesting that accessibility has a less comprehensive definition whereas it has a more defined and shared method of assessment than usability. Indeed, accessibility focuses on the objective analysis of the system through the conformance to international guidelines, whereas the usability evaluation does not have a unified and shared methodology. The usability evaluation focuses on the users' achievement of the goal regarding effectiveness and efficiency and on their satisfaction, and it results in a more subjective, and so less reducible, characteristic for assessment. This difference in evaluation between accessibility and usability turns in an impressive set of reliable and valid evaluation methods for usability.

Despite the differences among the evaluation objectives, the concept of accessibility and usability are inter-related because they are two ways to detect interaction problems from different angles. As Petrie and Kheir emphasized, accessibility and usability problems can be seen as two overlapping sets, which would include three categories as follows (see Figure 15.2):

> [i] Problems that only affect disabled people; these can be termed "pure accessibility" problems; [ii] Problems that only affect non-disabled people; these can be termed "pure usability" problems; [iii] Problems that affect both disabled and non-disabled people; these can be termed "universal usability" problems. Accessibility problems were not a complete sub-set of usability problems. (2007, p. 398; please see also Shneirderman 2003; Horton 2007; Lazar 2007).

In this sense, accessibility problems are not the subset of usability problems, nor are usability problems the subset of accessibility problems.

15.2.2 An Overview of the Usability Standards

Organizations in charge of international standardization include the International Organization for Standardization (ISO), the International Electrotechnical Commission (IEC), and the Comité Européen de Normalisation (CEN). In addition to these, there are local organizations such as Japanese Industrial Standards (JIS), Deutsches Institut für Normung (DIN), British Standards Institute (BSI), and American National Standards Institute (ANSI). They have issued many standards and documents in terms of usability and accessibility, sometimes in conjunction with each other. Usually, international standards are established first, and some of them will be translated as local standards. But sometimes local standards become international standards, as in the case of JIS X8341-1 (2006) and ISO 9241-20 (2009).

Regarding usability, many standards and documents were published by the Technical Committee (TC) on the ergonomics of ISO (see http://www.iso.org). In the ISO/TC159, there are four Subcommittees (SC), i.e., SC1, SC2, SC3, and SC4, in which SC4 is in charge of the "Ergonomics of Human-System Interaction." In SC4, there are 11 Working Groups (WG), in which WG6 is in charge of "Human-Centered Design Processes for Interactive Systems."

This WG6 of the TC159 published some of the most important standards on usability, such as

- *ISO 9241-11 (1998):* This standard provided practitioners with the concept definition of usability and three subconcepts: effectiveness, efficiency, and satisfaction. Today, this is regarded as the world standard in terms of the definition of usability.

- *ISO 9241-171 (2008):* This standard is also important for its definition of the HCD and UX. The description of how it can be achieved is also an important part of this standard. The four-stage model of HCD, including (1) understanding and specifying the context of use, (2) specifying the user requirements, (3) producing design solutions, and (4) evaluating the designs against requirements, is a world-famous scheme today.

- *ISO/TR 18529 (2000):* This document is a first attempt to expand the scope of HCD from just the design that ISO 9241-171 described to the whole life cycle and specified set of methods that should be adopted in each activity.

- *ISO/TR 16982 (2002):* This document presents sets of methods that should be adopted in each stage of the HCD process as described in ISO 9241-210; however, there is still argument regarding the validity of the description.

- *ISO/PAS 18152 (2003):* This document, known as ISO/TR 16982 (2002), is an extension of the HCD concept and of the approach to the life cycle. This standard proposed a human-systems (HS) model for the assessment of the maturity of an organization in performing the processes that make a system usable, healthy, and safe. This process is composed of four human-systems components: HS.1, life-cycle involvement; HS.2, human factors integration; HS.3, usability engineering (the same as that described in ISO 9241-210); and HS.4, human resources.

The standards described above are focused on good design process. Another series of standards aims to introduce the concept of "ease of operation": ISO 20282-1 (2006a), ISO/TS 20282-2 (2006b), ISO/PAS 20282-3 (2007a), and ISO/PAS 20282-4 (2007b). These standards refer to the usability of everyday products in which the ease of operation is defined as the functionality of the product and correct operation of the user interface is strictly linked to usability. However, there is still an international debate on the adequate position of these standards.

Another set of standards on usability came from the committee JTC 1 on information technology, and in particular from the group SC 7 on software and systems engineering.

- *ISO/IEC 25062 (2006c):* This standard defines the document format for usability testing as an evaluation method. The point here is that ISO 9241-11 (1998) provided the key concepts, especially on the definition of usability concept, and ISO 9241-171 (2008) showed the process on how to conduct the HCD. Following on from ISO 9241-171 (2008), other usability standards and documents appeared such as ISO/TR 18529 (2000), ISO/PAS 18152 (2003), ISO/TR 16982 (2002), the ISO 20282 (2006a) series, and ISO/IEC 25062 (2006c). Now, some of them are going to be reorganized as the ISO 9241-200 series including 210, 220, and 230 (2010). Part 200 is planned so as to redefine related concepts.

This brief overview underlines how the concept of usability is extended and related to many dimensions of HCI. In particular, in analyzing the usability-related standards there is an evident interrelation with the concept of accessibility expressed in some national and international definitions of accessibility, such as Section 508 of the U.S. Rehabilitation Act of 1973 (e.g., see the web site for understanding and implementing the requirements of Section 508, http://www.section508.gov), the JIS X8341 series in Japan, and the definitions of WAI, which found in the usability standards an application. The relation between accessibility and usability is clearly expressed in ISO/IEC Guide 71 (2001), which expresses the standard that takes into account the needs of older persons and persons with disabilities in the interaction, in ISO 9241-20 (2009), which described the accessibility guidelines for information/communication technology equipment and services, and in ISO 9241-171 (2008), which proposes guidance on software accessibility.

The relationship between usability and accessibility is particularly evident in the ISO/IEC Guide 71 (2001), in which it is recognized that accessibility and usability are important for both products and services because "some people with very extensive and complex disabilities may have requirements for access to the product." This guide

> Describes a process by which the needs of older persons and persons with disabilities may be considered in the development of standards; provides tables to enable standards developers to relate the relevant clauses of a standard to the factors which should be considered to ensure that all abilities are addressed; offers descriptions of body functions or human abilities and the practical implications of impairment; offers a list of sources that standards developers can use to investigate more detailed and specific guidance materials. (ISO 2001).

As we have seen in this section, the inter-relation between accessibility and usability concepts is clearly marked by both the standards and the UX theoretical approach. Although this relation is evident, practitioners are accustomed to doing a split in the evaluation process of products in two uncorrelated steps: the evaluation of accessibility and the evaluation of usability. In these two steps, the accessibility represents the evaluation of the objective access to the interaction, as the measure of the way the architecture accomplishes the standards (i.e., objectivity), and the usability represents the evaluation of the subjective use of the interaction (i.e., subjectivity). This strong division between objective and subjective aspects of interaction is a limitation of the UX studies that can be recomposed only by an integrated model of interaction evaluation (Federici and Borsci 2010).

15.3 Evaluation of Systems

15.3.1 A Conceptual Framework: An Integrated Model of Interaction Evaluation

The relation between accessibility and usability, as we claim, is often reduced superficially to that of objectivity and subjectivity (Federici et al. 2005; Federici and Borsci 2010). However, this simplification does not catch all of the aspects involved in the interaction between technology and user (Annett 2002; Kirakowski 2002). As Federici and Borsci claim,

> Accessibility refers to the interface code that allows a user to access and achieve the information (e.g., a user can read a text alternative description of a figure by a screen reader), usability pertains to the subjective perception (satisfaction) of the interface structure's efficiency and effectiveness (e.g., a user is satisfied because they can immediately

achieve the information they are looking for). However, when the relationship between accessibility and usability is defined in this bi-polar way, accessibility might be established as the objective end of the user interaction, while usability could be correlated to the subjective aspects, as determined by users' inherent individual differences. From this perspective, a technological product is reduced to a neutral entity that functions independently from its user in a neutral environment. As a result, a machine could be perfectly accessible but not usable. Consequently, usability does not pertain at all to the technological aspects of a machine functioning, but to the cognitive and functional aspects of the individual differences. (2010, p. 2).

Therefore, as Federici and colleagues (2005) state, when objective and subjective elements are referred to accessibility and usability in a user-computer interaction, they cannot be considered as separate entities, but as two different moments both included in the continuum of empirical observation. Each entity is not considered separately from its observer during the interpretative/reconstructive process because the entity is known by the subject only as an observed and perceived object (Figure 15.3).

From this viewpoint, accessibility and usability are not understood as characteristics regarding two separate interacting entities but rather as one intrasystemic relation in which both object and subject are just moments in a multiphase process of empirical observation. This prevents the existence of userless technological products, thereby guaranteeing that the accessibility of a machine always refers only to the possible entrance and exit of a signal needed to fulfill the task for which it was designed, and that it is in constant relation either to its designer or to its user. In this sense, a machine should not be accessible and yet unusable at the same time.

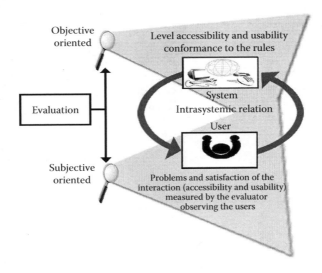

FIGURE 15.3
(See color insert.) The possible evaluation perspectives during the evaluation of the intrasystemic dialogue between user and system: the objective-oriented and the subjective-oriented perspectives. The interaction evaluation has to take into account not only the properties of a single dimension (the accessibility or the usability), but also the relations that bind the objective part of the interaction to the subjective one (and vice versa). In this context, accessibility and usability are considered as necessary steps for the evaluation of the intrasystemic relation between interface and user.

For Federici and Borsci (2010), according to the integrated model, accessibility and usability do not refer to the objective and subjective factors of the user/technology relationship, but rather to a bidirectional way of observing the interaction. Actually, this represents two outlooks from which the one and only observed reality of the user/technology system is drawn. Accessibility of an environment is therefore defined based on how it allows the user to initiate and terminate the operation that completes the machine's task (functioning construct), whereas its usability is based on the user's perception of the user/technology interaction (user performance). The functioning construct of a system is the basis for standard rules (e.g., Web Content Accessibility Guidelines) against which accessibility levels are controlled and assessed. The user performance in relation to the functioning construct of a machine allows us to deduce scales (e.g., efficiency, satisfaction, cognitive load, and helpfulness) of usability scores.

The object of the evaluation cannot be merely reduced to the artifact or to the user: what is to be evaluated is the functionality of the intrasystemic dialogue between the user (i.e., the subjective dimension of the interaction) and interface (i.e., the objective dimension of the interaction). The accessibility and the usability estimations, then, need to be understood as the measurements of the possibility for the user to achieve their goals navigating the given interface. The evaluation of the intrasystemic relation between user and technology includes object-oriented methods as well as subject-oriented ones; still, the overall evaluation cannot be obtained by the simple addition of the results coming from the two different methods but by an evaluation process able to consider and integrate both the accessibility and usability dimensions. An integrated model of usability evaluation is compatible with a universal model of disability whereby ability/disability are viewed within a continuum. Using ability/disability to refer to an individual functioning in a real context can only have a theoretical interest because nobody has a complete absence of disability or complete absence of ability (Zola 1989; Bickenbach et al. 1999; WHO 2001). Therefore, ability/disability are referred to by the activities performed by an individual, originating from the environment and valued by a predetermined functioning construct. These activities can change the topology of an environment, and the construct with respect to the process and measure expected of its functioning.

The model proposed by Federici and Borsci (2010) is based on the UX framework and on the idea that UX problems are originated by a distance between the models used to reason about the system, to anticipate its behaviour and to explain why it reacts as it does (Craik 1943) by the designer of the technological product and by the user of the product. Mental models, considered according to Norman's (1983) definition of "system causality conveyance," are those collections of knowledge and skills that lead the subject in the interaction (user) or in the creation (designer) of an interface. From the point of view of the evaluation process, we need to consider that

- *The developer's cognitive processes* involved in the design of the system are mostly connected to problem-solving strategies, to the representation of knowledge, and to expertise in complex task environments. Although these processes have been analyzed deeply, the difficulties due to the "simulation" process have never been properly studied in depth. When designing an interface, the developers simulate how a user would perform to achieve their goals; therefore, the designer develops the functions of the system according to their idea of a potential user and of a hypothetical interaction. Furthermore, there are many stakeholders involved in the development process, including the planner, the designer, the advertising people, the salesperson in the retail market, etc., who may not have the same image regarding the system. In this way, the designer is forced to integrate their design skills with their ability to simulate the user's behavior. The application of standard models offered by several international guidelines on accessibility and usability, indeed, although it is able to represent the typical user's behavior to a certain extent, is not enough to grant the success of a product. Therefore, to deliver a satisfactory product, the designer needs to possess to a certain extent the ability to "simulate" the possible user's behavior. However, the ability to "simulate" someone else's behavior consists of one of the hardest and most complex cognitive processes that a human being can perform (Meltzoff and Decety 2003; Decety and Jackson 2004).

- *The user's cognitive process:* The user's interaction with the system is quite different from the designer's process. First of all, it is a fact that, by interacting with the interface, the user applies the same cognitive processes used by the designer in the creation of the interface (i.e., problem-solving, representation of knowledge and expertise). Thanks to these shared processes, the user is able to "operate" in the interface (i.e., the interface is understandable and usable). However, whereas the designer applies these shared cognitive processes during their simulation of a hypothetical user's behavior (i.e., in the design of the information architecture), the actual user does not need any simulation of the designer's intention: Their cognitive processes are used only to perform actions in the interface and they do not need to forget about their mental model. Therefore, the actions performed by the user in the interface are not based on an "imagined" or "simulated" developer; the actions are experienced directly.

The distance separating the designer and the user in the interaction mostly depends on the different ways of applying their mental model: the designer's simulation of the interaction and the user's interaction with the system. The distance between designer and user can be reduced by the actors' competences to adapt the mental model to the action required (i.e., simulate and interact). The more competent a designer is in simulating the hypothetical user, the smaller the distance separating their mental model from that of the actual user; the more competent a user is in the system functioning, the smaller the distance from the conceptual model of the interface (and therefore from the designer's model).

Both the user and the designer are part of the object we need to measure (the interaction). Therefore, we cannot use as standards of measurement either the expectations on how the system should work (i.e., the designer's perspective) or the experience and the satisfaction perceived by the users in the interaction with the system (i.e., the user's perspective). In fact, both of these perspectives are only a part of what we need to measure. In this sense, we need to find an external unit of measurement able to generalize the relation between the two. This standard unit we want to introduce can be observed only by introducing an external model (i.e., evaluator's model) able to estimate the distance between the two actors involved in the intrasystemic interaction. This model should be created on the base of the available guidelines—e.g., Web Content Accessibility Guidelines 2.0, Heuristic list, and design principle etc.—and usability evaluation methods (UEMs) for subjective- and objective-oriented observation. An evaluator's model so created will be able to introduce a new conventional unit of measurement, the reliability of which will be granted by the agreement of the international scientific community. Moreover, this new unit of measurement should also respect the principles of economy (i.e., efficiency and efficacy), meaning that it should be able to lessen the costs for the identification of problems in an interaction evaluation.

In this sense, the interaction problems are considered as the units of the distance between the two mental models (Figure 15.4). The evaluator's mental model, just like the other two,

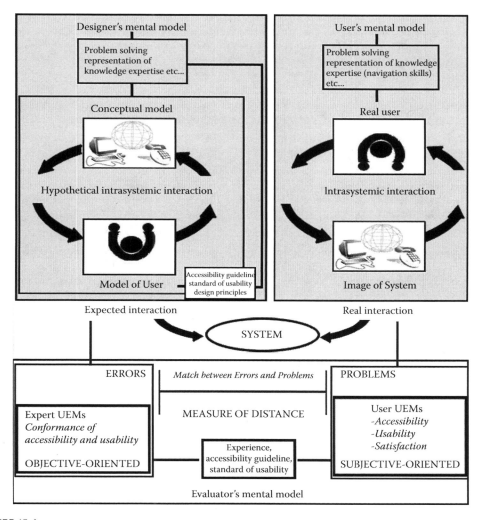

FIGURE 15.4
The role of the evaluator's mental model from the perspective of the UX evaluation: The designer's mental model is embodied in the system by the conceptual model. The developer designs the system in relation to his or her experience, representation of knowledge, etc. The designer, taking into account standards and guidelines, images an expected interaction according to the user model. The real user applies their mental model in the interaction with the image of the system, including the manual and other information sources such as the Internet. The user in the "real interaction" experiences problems whereas the designed system contains the errors. The evaluator mental model is involved in the evaluation using the UEM to observe the object and the subject and measure the distance between the designer's and the user's mental models.

is composed of the evaluator's expertise and knowledge. Still, two other components influence the evaluation process:

1. The international accessibility and design guidelines that determine the standards the evaluator has to take into account when evaluating the interface properties (accessibility and usability).
2. The techniques actually applied by the evaluator for evaluating accessibility, usability, and satisfaction. The use of a specific technique forces the evaluator to adapt his or her mental model to the perspective endorsed by the technique. In other words, because the specific techniques used for the evaluation influence the mental model adopted by the evaluator, the evaluation outcome largely depends on the applied techniques.

At the end of the evaluation process, the evaluator should have obtained the level of accessibility; the level of usability; the degree of satisfaction; and, as indirect estimation, the measure of the distance between the designer's and the user's mental model as the distance between the technology functions—the conceptual model created by the designer's mental model—and the function of technology that is really perceived by users. The evaluators obtain the measure of the interaction distance matching the errors of the object, analyzed by expert analysis (objective-oriented) with the problems observed by the users' evaluation (subjective-oriented). This match shows the distance between the interaction imagined by the designer for a hypothetical user and the interaction perceived by the real user.

15.4 Example of the UX Concept Application in Design Systems for Rehabilitation

15.4.1 UX in the Assistive Technology Assessment Process

By using the integrated approach in the rehabilitation system, we might consider that the UX evaluation does not concern only the users' experience with an assigned technology, but also the users' experience of the whole assistive technology assessment (ATA) process functioning (i.e., action of the center for technical aid), that can be considered as the degree of accessibility and usability of the service.

In fact, the assignation process of a center for technical aids may be considered as a system interface itself by which a user can reach a goal. In this sense, we can evaluate the UX experience of the ATA process on two levels (see Figure 15.5):

1. The first level concerns the UX evaluation of the ATA process (i.e., degree of accessibility and usability in the relationship between the users and the center for technical aids). This level of evaluation is linked to managerial solutions that are able to grant access to and use of the service. Even if this level is far from the classic use of the UX evaluations, concerning the economical and managerial dimensions, it is necessary for guaranteeing the correct evaluation of the assistive technology (AT) (second level). Indeed, the design of a good ATA process is the best way to obtain a satisfied match between user and technology.

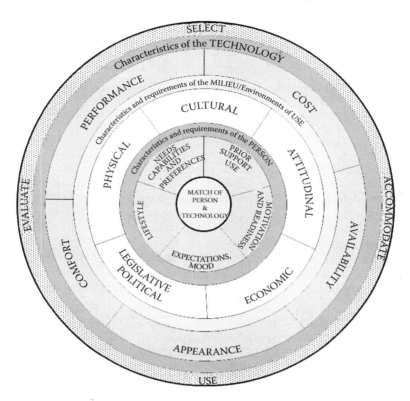

FIGURE 15.5
The Matching Person and Technology model, as shown in this diagram, with AT as the example, occurs within and requires assessment of the context of environmental and personal factors.

To do that, the ATA process has to be evaluated by those dimensions, described by Scherer and DiCowden (2008), of well-being that involve person, milieu, and technology.

Accessibility at this level is determined by the possibility and the satisfaction of the contacts, measured by the following dimensions: the costs perceived by the users in terms of use and access to the service for obtaining the goal, the possibility to reach the service (availability), the ease of contact (comfort), the expectation of the users (appearance), and the users' perceived (or known) performance of the service. The efficiency in the ATA process is guaranteed by the collection of data and by the center for technical aid's staff (multidisciplinary team). The efficiency, defined as the "Resources expended in relation to the accuracy and completeness with which users achieve goals" (ISO 1998), is measured by the costs in terms of time and workload perceived by users to obtain the AT. In this step the efficiency of the process, defined as "Accuracy and completeness with which users achieve specified goals" (ISO 1998), is strictly related to the efficacy in ideal conditions. In fact, before the users' UX evaluation of the AT and the use of the AT in a daily life condition, it is impossible to measure the real effectiveness of the process and the satisfaction of the user.

2. The second level is the UX evaluation of the assistive solutions (i.e., the matching of users with technical solutions). This step is the core of the matching process, when the user is involved in the trial of the AT and in the evaluation of the UX. After the match, it is possible to measure the effectiveness in the real world of the AT and the satisfaction of the user both with the AT and the ATA process by a survey and questionnaires (Figure 15.6).

The UX evaluation is one of the most important steps for achieving the rehabilitation priority indicated by the World Health Organization that is "to ensure access to appropriate, timely, affordable, and high-quality rehabilitation interventions" (WHO 2011, p. 121) to provide ATs that are "suited to the environment" and "suitable for the user" by also granting an "adequate follow-up to ensure safe and efficient use" (WHO & the World Bank 2011, p. 118). In fact, the UX evaluation is applied for measuring both the interaction with the AT and the assessment of the whole ATA process as perceived by the users to evaluate and improve them.

Another kind of application of the UX framework is the design of the product. In the next sections we will describe the sonification concept to create a particular kind of

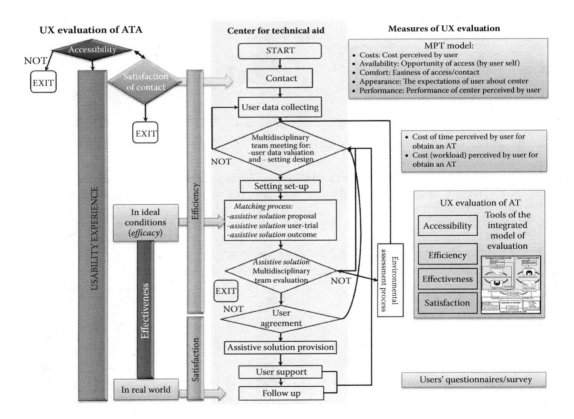

FIGURE 15.6
(See color insert.) The dimensions and the measures of the UX evaluation of the model's functioning of the ATA process of a center for technical aid. In this schema, the UX evaluation of the AT, with its dimensions, is part of the efficiency and efficacy evaluation of the relationship between the user and the center for technical aid.

technology for blind users to exemplify how the UX and cognitive concepts can be used to create innovation and open up possibilities for disabled people.

15.4.2 Sonification of the System

The way the representation of space is processed has long been discussed in the literature. Many authors analyzed whether spatial representation is directly guided by visual experience or is indeed related to some other different sensory ways that allow equivalent spatial representations. Although some authors pointed out that visual experience is of the utmost importance for the processing of spatial cues (Thinus-Blanc and Gaunet 1997), there is a broad consensus that the spatial representation of information is independent from the way the sensory inputs are displayed. In particular, some studies highlighted that blind subjects show better performance in processing spatial auditory inputs than sighted people (Zimmer 2001; Avraamides et al. 2004; Mast et al. 2007). Moreover, as Bryant (1992, 1997) pointed out, blind people show a motion ability functionally equivalent to the visually guided method in sighted people in performing spatial exploration tasks guided only by natural acoustic cues. Starting from these suggestions, an amodal system of spatial representation has been proposed by explaining the involvement of the auditory, haptic, and kinesthetic information in the spatial mapping processing of people with visual disabilities (Millar 1994). These findings seem to be in contrast with other studies stating both that spatial understanding is directly related to visual experience and that less efficient spatial capabilities are due to a lack of visual experience (Ungar et al. 1997).

Starting from these findings, in the last 30 years many research studies in different fields have been involved in studying different ways to transmit spatial information through nonvisual sensory channels, paying special attention to sonification methods as an alternative to visual and haptic traditional methods. This alternative approach to conveying spatial information should be especially useful in complex scenarios in which visual overload or several distractors and incomplete signals due to visual noise could occur. By conveying information about the spatial location of its source (Brunetti et al. 2005, 2008), the nature of sound seems to be able to communicate the complexity of either static or dynamic data representations by keeping their inner relations unchanged. As defined by Kramer and colleagues, sonification is "the transformation of data relations into perceived relations in an acoustic signal for the purposes of facilitating communication or interpretation" (1997, p. 3). Since the 1980s, a growing number of works—especially in computer science and related fields—have focused on the implementation of different ways of conveying spatial information through nonvisual sensory channels to improve the nonvisual access to spatial information. For example, in the late 1980s some researchers designed and tested different systems based on sounds representing spatial cues, highlighting that human-computer interaction could be improved by means of nonverbal acoustic signals on graphic interfaces (Sumikawa et al. 1985; Gaver, 1986; Blattner et al. 1989). Moreover, in the 1990s Barfield and colleagues (1991) and Brewster (1997, 1998) designed nonspeech interfaces that were based on the use of earcones, that is to say musical patterns providing navigational cues into hierarchical menus. By analyzing the recognition performances occurring after the interaction session of blind users with the interface, the authors verified the efficacy of the nonverbal acoustic items. Blind subjects showed a high rate of accuracy in recognition tasks, highlighting that the proposed system seems to be able to be used in spatial orientation tasks (Barfield et al. 1991; Brewster 1997). To maintain the correspondence between visual and acoustic spatial positions of items, a broad number of researchers proposed loudspeaker-based systems. For example, Lakatos (1993) proposed a system based on speakers transmitting complex auditory-spatial signals to analyze the pattern recognition performance of sighted users; moreover, Golledge and colleagues (1991) and Shinn-Cunningham and colleagues (1996) designed a system that simulates realistic sound sources from different locations by using loudspeakers.

The application of sonification techniques to the design process seems to be useful in creating mobility aids, i.e., electronic travel aids (ETAs) able to "detect the environment within a certain range or distance, process reflected information, and furnish the user with certain information in an intelligible and useful manner" (Farmer and Smith 1998 p. 238). Sonar techniques are the most used blind mobility aids and allow users to perceive the spatial information of the environment by means of a source that transduces an ultrasound signal into an auditory or haptic feedback (Kay 1964). As defined by Farmer and Smith (1998), it is possible to distinguish four categories of ETAs:

1. Devices with a single output for object preview, for example, devices emitting audiotactile feedback indicating the obstacles encountered in the user's path—e.g., the *Mowat Sensor* (Morrissette et al. 1981) or the *Sonicguide* (Kay 1974);

2. Devices with a multiple output for object preview, for example, the Laser Cane proposed by Benjamin, a walking cane receiving and transmitting spatial signals to help blind people to explore and move within an urban environment (1973, 1974);

3. Devices providing both object preview and environmental information, for example, the Kay's Advanced Spatial Perception Aid Technology—KASPA (2000), an ultrasonic device (needing approximately a month of training) designed to allow users to avoid obstacles during their mobility in the surrounding environment (Kay 2001);

4. Devices using artificial intelligence as a component, for example, the Sonic Pathfinder, a sonification tool designed by Heyes (1984) to help blind people to avoid obstacles by translating the objects found in front of the users into musical notes conveyed by five input/output loudspeaker devices.

Unless all mentioned studies are focused on sensory substitution for blind people, a critical issue emerges: None of the proposed systems and models have been evaluated by assessing the accessibility and the usability of the corresponding sonification devices, showing a lack of an effective user-centered approach in the design process. This question could be explained by noting that most of the above-mentioned studies have been carried out by conducting the design process through an objective perspective. In fact, users have been involved only after the prototype was developed, excluding in this way the subjective perspective, which is fundamental to analyzing the components of the interaction between user and the sonification interface.

One of the first studies that attempted to build a sonification system by following a user-centered approach was proposed in the 1990s by Meijer (1992), who carried out an experimental analysis of the system in an everyday life context. In his work, Meijer introduced the *vOICe* system, a software created to "allow blind people literally to see through sounds" by a continuous horizontal scan of the real-life environment, which is recorded by a head-mounted camera analyzing and translating the surrounding scene into a sine wave acoustic signal. To detect the neural activation in sighted and blind subjects during the object recognition tasks, the *vOICe* system has been recently analyzed by using fMRI (Amedi et al. 2007). Following this technique, the authors found that the spatial navigation by means of *vOICe* is related to the activation of lateral-occipital tactile visual areas—generally used to encode visual spatial information—in response to auditory stimuli (Merabet et al. 2008). More recently, Zhao of the Human Computer Interaction Laboratory at the University of Maryland proposed a new sonification technique able to transmit georeferenced data by means of haptic and auditory signals (Zhao et al. 2004, 2005) and implemented a new system called *iSonic*, a sonification tool that allows people with visual disabilities to explore georeferenced maps by means of haptic and auditory information combined by following exploration techniques. The *iSonic* usability was tested on people who had been totally blind for a long time (Zhao et al. 2008), blindfolded, and congenitally and acquired blind users (Olivetti Belardinelli et al. 2007). Starting from these usability studies, the authors suggested that during the spatial orientation, totally or partially blind subjects show their preferences for a body-centered strategy that was based on corporal reference points, rather than for an allocentric strategy, often adopted in mental rotation and scanning tasks (Olivetti Belardinelli et al. 2009; Delogu et al. 2010).

15.4.2.1 Application of a UX Framework for Designing a Sonified Visual Web Search Engine

In 2009, the Department of Computer Engineering (DIEI) of the University of Perugia and the Interuniversity Centre for Research on Cognitive Processing in Natural and Artificial Systems (ECONA) implemented a sonificated system on *WhatsOnWeb* (Di Giacomo 2007), an accessible visual web search clustering engine that transmits the indexed information related to the requested query in one single page by using graph-drawing methods on semantically clustered data. In this way, *WhatsOnWeb* is able to overcome the efficiency limitation of the top-down representation (the Search Engine Report Pages—SERPs) adopted by the commonly used search engines (Federici et al. 2008, 2010b). The sonificated version of *WhatsOnWeb* has been tested on blind and sighted users by using the Partial Concurrent Thinking Aloud technique (Federici et al. 2010a, 2010c), an evaluation protocol that overcomes the limits encountered during the evaluation with blind subjects using the concurrent and the retrospective verbal protocols. In this usability study, blind subjects showed a better motion ability than sighted people in performing spatial exploration guided only by auditory cues (Mele et al. 2009; Rugo et al. 2009). Allowing the users with disabilities an easier mapping of the elements in the interface, the application of the sonification to the web interface significantly improves the access and the use of the systems (Mele et al. 2010).

From an overall review of the above-mentioned studies, it appears that the sonification approach seems to be an effective way to transmit spatial information (e.g., graphic or environmental data). As highlighted by many studies, people with visual disabilities show spatial capabilities equivalent to sighted users in performing both spatial orientation tasks and spatial recall tasks. Starting from these evidences, many authors support the "amodal hypothesis" by explaining the involvement of an amodal system in spatial mapping processing of the auditory, haptic, and kinesthetic information of blind people. However, almost all of the systems mentioned in the previous section have not been developed under the user-centered design approach by taking into account end-users' needs. Most of the proposed sonification tools require long training sessions to be efficiently used and may lead to a cognitive overload.

The role of both user-centered design and the integrated model of interaction evaluation is today a main point for developing ATs that are mediators that are able to allow users to overcome their (virtual or physical) environment barriers. In this section, we discussed the sonification concept for design by a UX framework of a technology—*WhatsOnWeb*—which is a communication technology that users can interact with through several alternative input devices (e.g., brain computer interaction). In Chapter 16, we will analyze the design and evaluation of *WhatsOnWeb* and telemedicine tools (Nu!Rhea Desk) that are not only described as the means by which users can obtain their goals (i.e., as an AT) but also as eAssistive Solutions (eAS) that are able to increase the user's well-being in a specific context of use.

15.5 Conclusions

By presenting a complete review of usability standards and a deep analysis of the difference between usability and the UX concept, this work discusses the UX framework in the field of rehabilitation. The chapter is divided into four parts:

1. The first section illustrates the different approaches and fields of application behind User eXperience, that is to say, a holistic perspective on how a user feels about using a system or, following the ISO (1999) definition, "a consequence of the presentation, functionality, system performance, interactive behaviour, and assistive capabilities of an interactive system, both hardware and software."

2. In the second section, we describe both the usability and accessibility theoretical constructs and their relation with the UX perspective, by analyzing the differences among the evaluation objectives, the concept of accessibility, and the concept of usability under the UX theoretical approach. A brief overview of international standards on usability is shown here.

3. The third section introduces an integrated model of interaction evaluation, a new conceptual perspective that is based on the UX framework that focuses on the intrasystemic dialogue between user and system within the interaction environment. Following this new approach, the accessibility and usability evaluation processes become a bidirectional way of observing the person-technology interaction rather than merely objective/subjective factors.

4. Finally, in the fourth section we present different examples concerning the application of the UX framework to the design process of systems for rehabilitation. First, the analysis within the ATA process is shown. Moreover, an overview of the state of the art concerning sonification methods is illustrated. Finally, we introduce a visual sonificated web search clustering engine called *WhatsOnWeb*, a new communication technology developed by following a user-centered design process.

The evaluation of the interaction between users and eSystems is analyzed by an integrated model of interaction in which the relation between the designers' and the users' mental models are evaluated by the evaluator's mental model from both the objective and the subjective points of view. The new perspective endorsed by the chapters is that the UX concepts can be used not only to set up an evaluation of the users' interaction with AT, but also to organize and evaluate the ATA process, and to design (or redesign) new technologies able to overcome the barriers usually experienced by disabled users. In particular, the redesign of a sonificated web search engine is presented as an example of the growing need of the UX approach in the AT design.

Summary of the Chapter

This chapter discusses the relation and the role of the constructs of accessibility and usability under the user experience theoretical approach. An integrated model of interaction evaluation, a new evaluation perspective based on the user experience, is presented as a framework not only to set up an evaluation of the users' interaction with assistive technology, but also to organize and evaluate the Assistive Technology Assessment process.

References

Amedi, A., Stern, W. M., Camprodon, J. A., Bermpohl, F., Merabet, L., Rotman, S., et al. (2007). Shape conveyed by visual-to-auditory sensory substitution activates the lateral occipital complex. *Nature Neuroscience, 10*(6), 687–689. doi:10.1038/nn1912

Annett, J. (2002). Subjective rating scales in ergonomics: A reply. *Ergonomics, 45*(14), 1042–1046. doi:10.1080/00140130210166762

Avraamides, M. N., Loomis, J. M., Klatzky, R. L., and Golledge, R. G. (2004). Functional equivalence of spatial representations derived from vision and language: Evidence from allocentric judgments. *Journal of Experimental Psychology: Learning, Memory, and Cognition, 30*(4), 801–814. doi:10.1037/0278-7393.30.4.804

Barfield, W., Rosenberg, C., and Levasseur, G. (1991). The use of icons, earcons, and commands in the design of an online hierarchical menu. *IEEE Transactions on Professional Communication, 34*(2), 8. doi:10.1109/47.87619

Benjamin, J. M. J. (1973). *The New C-5 Laser Cane for the Blind*. Paper presented at the Proceedings of the 1973 Carnahan Conference on Electronic Prosthetics, New York.

Benjamin, J. M. J. (1974). The laser cane. *Bulletin of Prosthetics Research, 11*(2), 443–450.

Bickenbach, J. E., Chatterji, S., Badley, E. M., and Üstün, T. B. (1999). Models of disablement, universalism and the international classification of impairments, disabilities and handicaps. *Social Science and Medicine, 48*(9), 1173–1187. doi:10.1016/S0277-9536(98)00441-9

Blattner, M. M., Sumikawa, D. A., and Greenberg, R. M. (1989). Earcons and icons: Their structure and common design principles. *Human-Computer Interaction, 4*(1), 11–44. doi:10.1207/s15327051hci0401_1

Brewster, S. A. (1997). Using non-speech sound to overcome information overload. *Displays, 17*(3–4), 179–189. doi:10.1016/S0141-9382(96)01034-7

Brewster, S. A. (1998). Using nonspeech sounds to provide navigation cues. *ACM Transactions on Computer-Human Interaction (TOCHI), 5*(3), 224–259. doi:10.1145/292834.292839

Brunetti, M., Belardinelli, P., Caulo, M., Del Gratta, C., Della Penna, S., Ferretti, A., et al. (2005). Human brain activation during passive listening to sounds from different locations: An fMRI and MEG study. *Human Brain Mapping, 26*(4), 251–261. doi:10.1002/hbm.20164

Brunetti, M., Della Penna, S., Ferretti, A., Del Gratta, C., Cianflone, F., Belardinelli, P., et al. (2008). A frontoparietal network for spatial attention reorienting in the auditory domain: A human fMRI/MEG study of functional and temporal dynamics. *Cerebral Cortex, 18*(5), 1139–1147. doi:10.1093/cercor/bhm145

Bryant, D. J. (1992). A spatial representation system in humans. *Psycoloquy, 3*(16). Retrieved from http://www.cogsci.ecs.soton.ac.uk/cgi/psyc/psummary?3.16

Bryant, D. J. (1997). Representing space in language and perception. *Mind and Language, 12*(3–4), 239–264. doi:10.1111/j.1468-0017.1997.tb00073.x

Craik, K. (1943). *The Nature of Exploration*. Cambridge, UK: Cambridge University Press.

Decety, J., and Jackson, P. L. (2004). The functional architecture of human empathy. *Behavioral and Cognitive Neuroscience Reviews, 3*(2), 71–100. doi:10.1177/1534582304267187

Delogu, F., Palmiero, M., Federici, S., Zhao, H., Plaisant, C., and Olivetti Belardinelli, M. (2010). Non-visual exploration of geographic maps: Does sonification help? *Disability and Rehabilitation: Assistive Technology, 5*(3), 164–174. doi:10.3109/17483100903100277

Di Blas, N., Paolini, P., and Speroni, M. (2004). "Usable Accessibility" to the Web for blind Users. Paper presented at the 8th ERCIM Workshop: User Interfaces for All, Vienna, Austria. Retrieved from http://citeseerx.ist.psu.edu/viewdoc/summary?doi = 10.1.1.110.8239. doi:10.1.1.110.8239

Di Giacomo, E., Didimo, W., Grilli, L., and Liotta, G. (2007). Graph visualization techniques for web clustering engines. *IEEE Transactions on Visualization and Computer Graphics, 13*(2), 294–304. doi:10.1109/TVCG.2007.40

Farmer, L. W., and Smith, D. L. (1998). Adaptive technology. In B. B. Blasch, W. R. Wiener, and R. Welsh (Eds.), *Foundations of Orientation and Mobility* (2nd ed., pp. 231–259). New York: American Foundation for the Blind Press.

Federici, S., and Borsci, S. (2010). Usability evaluation: Models, methods, and applications. In J. Stone and M. Blouin (Eds.), *International Encyclopedia of Rehabilitation* (pp. 1–17). Buffalo, NY: Center for International Rehabilitation Research Information and Exchange (CIRRIE). Retrieved from http://cirrie.buffalo.edu/encyclopedia/article.php?id = 277&language = en

Federici, S., Borsci, S., and Mele, M. L. (2010a). Usability evaluation with screen reader users: A video presentation of the PCTA's experimental setting and rules. *Cognitive Processing, 11*(3), 285–288. doi:10.1007/s10339-010-0365-9

Federici, S., Borsci, S., Mele, M. L., and Stamerra, G. (2008). Global Rank: Tra popolarità e qualità dei siti Web. [Global Rank: Between popularity and quality of web sites]. *Psicotech, 6*(1), 7–23. doi:10.1400/113633

Federici, S., Borsci, S., Mele, M. L., and Stamerra, G. (2010b). Web popularity: An illusory perception of a qualitative order in information. *Universal Access in the Information Society, 9*(4), 375–386. doi:10.1007/s10209-009-0179-7

Federici, S., Borsci, S., and Stamerra, G. (2010c). Web usability evaluation with screen reader users: Implementation of the Partial Concurrent Thinking Aloud technique. *Cognitive Processing, 11*(3), 263–272. doi:10.1007/s10339-009-0347-y

Federici, S., Micangeli, A., Ruspantini, I., Borgianni, S., Corradi, F., Pasqualotto, E., et al. (2005). Checking an integrated model of web accessibility and usability evaluation for disabled people. *Disability and Rehabilitation, 27*(13), 781–790. doi:10.1080/09638280400014766

Garrett, J. J. (2003). *The Elements of User Experience: User-Centered Design for the Web*. New York: New Riders Press.

Gaver, W. W. (1986). Auditory icons: Using sound in computer interfaces. *Human-Computer Interaction, 2*(2), 167. doi:10.1207/s15327051hci0202_3

Golledge, R. G., Loomis, J. M., Klatzky, R. L., Flury, A., and Yang, X. L. (1991). Designing a personal guidance system to aid navigation without sight: progress on the GIS component. *International Journal of Geographical Information Systems, 5*(4), 373–395. doi:10.1080/02693799108927864

GSA's IT Accessibility and Workforce (ITAW). (2010). Resources for understanding and implementing Section 508. Retrieved from http://www.section508.gov

Hassenzahl, M., and Tractinsky, N. (2006). User experience—A research agenda. *Behaviour & Information Technology, 25*(2), 91–97. doi:10.1080/01449290500330331

Heyes, A. D. (1984). Sonic Pathfinder: A programmable guidance aid for the blind. *Electronics & Wireless World, 90*(1579), 26–29 and 62.

Horton, S. (2005). *Access by Design: A Guide to Universal Usability for Web Designers*. New York: New Riders Press.

International Standards Organization (ISO). (1998). *ISO 9241-11: Ergonomic Requirements for Office Work with Visual Display Terminals*. Geneva, Switzerland: ISO.

International Standards Organization (ISO). (1999). *ISO 13407: Human-Centred Design Processes for Interactive Systems*. Geneva, Switzerland: ISO.

International Standards Organization (ISO). (2000). *ISO/TR 18529: Ergonomics–Ergonomics of Human-System Interaction—Human-Centred Lifecycle Process Descriptions*. Geneva, Switzerland: ISO.

International Standards Organization (ISO). (2001). *ISO/IEC Guide 71: Guidelines for Standards Developers to Address the Needs of Older Persons and Persons with Disabilities*. Geneva, Switzerland: ISO.

International Standards Organization (ISO). (2002). *ISO/TR 16982: Ergonomics of Human-System Interaction–Usability Methods Supporting Human-Centred Design*. Geneva, Switzerland: ISO.

International Standards Organization (ISO). (2003). *ISO/PAS 18152: Ergonomics of Human-System Interaction – Specification for the Process Assessment of Human-System Issues*. Geneva, Switzerland: ISO.

International Standards Organization (ISO). (2006a). *ISO 20282-1: Ease of Operation of Everyday Products–Part 1: Design Requirements for Context of Use and User Characteristics*. Geneva, Switzerland: ISO.

International Standards Organization (ISO). (2006b). *ISO 20282-2: Ease of Operation of Everyday Products–Part 2: Test Method for Walk-Up-and-Use Products*. Geneva, Switzerland: ISO.

International Standards Organization (ISO). (2006c). *ISO/IEC 25062: Software Engineering–Software Product Quality Requirements and Evaluation (SQuaRE)—Common Industry Format (CIF) for Usability Test Reports*. Geneva, Switerland: ISO.

International Standards Organization (ISO). (2007a). *ISO/PAS 20282-3: Ease of Operation of Everyday Products–Part 3: Test Methods for Consumer Products*. Geneva, Switzerland: ISO.

International Standards Organization (ISO). (2007b). *ISO/PAS 20282-4: Ease of Operation of Everyday Products–Part 4: Test Method for the Installation of Consumer Products*. Geneva, Switzerland: ISO.

International Standards Organization (ISO). (2008). *ISO 9241-171: Ergonomics of Human-System Interaction–Part 171: Guidance on Software Accessibility*. Geneva, Switzerland: ISO.

International Standards Organization (ISO). (2009). *ISO 9241-20: Ergonomics of Human-System Interaction—Part 20: Accessibility Guidelines for Information/Communication Technology (ICT) Equipment and Services*. Geneva, Switzerland: ISO.

International Standards Organization (ISO). (2010). *ISO 9241-210: Ergonomics of Human-System Interaction—Part 210: Human-Centred Design for Interactive Systems*. Geneva, Switzerland: ISO.

Japanese Standards Association (JSA). (2006). *JIS X 8341-5*. Tokyo: JSA.

Kay, L. (1964). An ultrasonic sensing probe as a mobility aid for the blind. *Ultrasonics, 2*(2), 53–59. doi:10.1016/0041-624X(64)90382-8

Kay, L. (1974). A sonar aid to enhance spatial perception of the blind: Engineering design and evaluation. *Radio and Electronic Engineer, 44*(11), 605–627. doi:10.1049/ree.1974.0148

Kay, L. (2000). Auditory perception of objects by blind persons, using a bioacoustic high resolution sonar. *Journal of the Acoustical Society of America, 107*(6), 3266–3275.

Kay, L. (2001). Bioacoustic spatial perception by humans: A controlled laboratory measurement of spatial resolution without distal cues. *The Journal of the Acoustical Society of America, 109*(2), 803–808. doi:10.1121/1.1336138

Kirakowski, J. (2002). Is ergonomics empirical? *Ergonomics, 45*(14–15), 995–997. doi:10.1080/00140130210166889

Kramer, G., Walker, B., Bonebright, T., Cook, P., Flowers, J., Miner, N., et al. (1997). Sonification report: Status of the field and research agenda. Retrieved from http://sonify.psych.gatech.edu/publications/pdfs/1999-NSF-Report.pdf

Kurosu, M. (2010). *Concept Structure of UX (User Experience) and Its Measurement*. Paper presented at the APCHI & Ergofuture 2010: Joint International Conference of APCHI (Asia Pacific Computer Human Interaction) 2010 and Ergofuture 2010, Bali, Indonesia. Retrieved from http://iea.cc/upload/Ergofuture%202010%20Brochure.pdf

Kurosu, M., and Ando, M. (2008). *The Psychology of Non-Selection and Waste: A Tentative Approach for Constructing the User Behavior Theory Based on the Artifact Development Analysis.* Paper presented at the 74th Annual Convention of Japanese Psychological Association, Osaka University, Japan. Retrieved from http://www.wdc-jp.biz/jpa/conf2010/

Lakatos, S. (1993). Recognition of complex auditory-spatial patterns. *Perception, 22*(3), 363–374.

Law, E. L.-C., Vermeeren, A. P. O. S., Hassenzahl, M., and Blythe, M. (2007, September 3–7). *Towards a UX Manifesto.* Paper presented at the Proceedings of the 21st British HCI Group Annual Conference on People and Computers: HCI '07, University of Lancaster, UK.

Lazar, J. (Ed.). (2007). *Universal Usability: Designing Computer Interfaces for Diverse User Populations.* West Sussex, UK: Wiley and Sons.

Mast, F., Jäncke, L., Loomis, J. M., Klatzky, R. L., Avraamides, M., Lippa, Y., et al. (2007). *Functional Equivalence of Spatial Images Produced by Perception and Spatial Language.* Berlin: Springer. doi:10.1007/978-0-387-71978-8_3

Meijer, P. B. L. (1992). An experimental system for auditory image representations. *Biomedical Engineering, IEEE Transactions on, 39*(2), 112–121. doi:10.1109/10.121642

Mele, M. L., Borsci, S., Rugo, A., Federici, S., Liotta, G., Trotta, F., et al. (2009). An accessible web searching: An on-going research project. In P. L. Emiliani, L. Burzagli, A. Como, F. Gabbanini and A.-L. Salminen (Eds.), *Assistive Technology from Adapted Equipment to Inclusive Environments: AAATE '09* (Vol. 25, p. 854). Florence, Italy: IOS Press. doi:10.3233/978-1-60750-042-1-854

Mele, M. L., Federici, S., Borsci, S., and Liotta, G. (2010). Beyond a visuocentric way of a visual web search clustering engine: The sonification of *WhatsOnWeb.* In K. Miesenberger, J. Klaus, W. Zagler and A. Karshmer (Eds.), *Computers Helping People with Special Needs* (Vol. 1, pp. 351–357). Berlin: Springer. doi:10.1007/978-3-642-14097-6_56

Meltzoff, A. N., and Decety, J. (2003). What imitation tells us about social cognition: A rapprochement between developmental psychology and cognitive neuroscience. *Philosophical Transactions of the Royal Society of London. Series B, Biological Sciences, 358*(1431), 491–500. doi:10.1098/rstb.2002.1261

Merabet, L., Pogge, D., Stern, W. M., Bhatt, E., Hemond, C., Maguire, S., et al. (2008). *Activation of Visual Cortex Using Crossmodal Retinotopic Mapping.* Paper presented at the 14th Annual Meeting of the Organization for Human Brain Mapping (OHBM): HBM '08, Melbourne, Australia. Retrieved from http://www.seeingwithsound.com/hbm2008.html

Millar, S. (1994). *Understanding and Representing Space: Theory and Evidence from Studies with Blind and Sighted Children.* New York: Oxford University Press.

Morrissette, D. L., Goodrich, G. L., and Hennessey, J. J. (1981). A follow-up study of the Mowat Sensor's applications, frequency of use, and maintenance reliability. *Journal of Visual Impairment and Blindness, 75*(6), 244–247.

Norman, D. A. (1983). Some observations on mental models. In D. Gentner and A. L. Steven (Eds.), *Mental Models* (pp. 7–14). Hillsdale, NJ: Lawrence Earlbaum Associates.

Norman, D. A. (1998). *The Invisible Computer: Why Good Products Can Fail, the Personal Computer is So Complex, and Information Appliances are the Solution.* Cambridge, MA: MIT Press.

Norman, D. A., Miller, J., and Henderson, A. (1995, May 7–11). *What You See, Some of What's in the Future, and How We Go about Doing It: HI at Apple Computer.* Paper presented at the Conference Companion on Human Factors in Computing Systems: CHI '95, Denver, CO. doi:10.1145/223355.223477

Olivetti Belardinelli, M., Federici, S., Delogu, F., and Palmiero, M. (2009). Sonification of spatial information: Audio-tactile exploration strategies by normal and blind subjects. In C. Stephanidis (Ed.), *Universal Access in HCI, Part II, HCII 2009, LNCS 5615* (pp. 557–563). Berlin: Springer-Verlag. doi:10.1007/978-3-642-02710-9_62

Olivetti Belardinelli, M., Santangelo, V., Botta, F., and Federici, S. (2007). Are vertical meridian effects due to audio-visual interference? A new confirmation with deaf subjects. *Disability and Rehabilitation, 29*(10), 797–804. doi:10.1080/09638280600919780

Petrie, H., and Bevan, N. (2009). The evaluation of accessibility, usability, and user experience. In C. Stephanidis (Ed.), *The Universal Access Handbook* (pp. 299–314). Boca Raton, FL: CRC Press.

Petrie, H., and Kheir, O. (2007). *The Relationship between Accessibility and Usability of Websites.* Paper presented at the Proceedings of the SIGCHI conference on Human Factors in Computing Systems, San Jose, CA. Retrieved from http://doi.acm.org/10.1145/1240624.1240688. doi:10.1145/1240624.1240688

Roto, V., Law, E., Vermeeren, A., and Hoonhout, J. (2011). *User Experience White Paper. Result from Dagstuhl Seminar on Demarcating User Experience, September 15–18, 2010.* Retrieved from http://www.allaboutux.org/files/UX-WhitePaper.pdf

Roulstone, A. (2010). Access and accessibility. In J. Stone and M. Blouin (Eds.), *International Encyclopedia of Rehabilitation* (pp. 1–12). Buffalo, NY: Center for International Rehabilitation Research Information and Exchange (CIRRIE). Retrieved from http://cirrie.buffalo.edu/encyclopedia/article.php?id = 153&language = en

Rugo, A., Mele, M. L., Liotta, G., Trotta, F., Di Giacomo, E., Borsci, S., et al. (2009). A visual sonificated web search clustering engine. *Cognitive Processing, 10*(Suppl 2), 286–289. doi:10.1007/s10339-009-0317-4

Scherer, M. J., and DiCowden, M. A. (2008). Organizing future research and intervention efforts on the impact and effects of gender differences on disability and rehabilitation: The usefulness of the International Classification of Functioning, Disability and Health (ICF). *Disability and Rehabilitation, 30*(3), 161–165. doi:10.1080/09638280701532292

Shinn-Cunningham, B. G., Zurek, P. M., Stutman, E. R., and Berkovitz, R. (1996). *Perception of Azimuth for Sources Simulated Using Two Loudspeakers in Natural Listening Environments.* Paper presented at the 19th Association for Research in Otolaryngology Midwinter Meeting, St. Petersburg Beach, FL.

Shneiderman, B. (2003). *Leonardo's Laptop: Human Needs and the New Computing Technologies.* Cambridge, MA: MIT Press.

Sumikawa, K. A., Blattner, M. M., Joy, K. I., and Greenberg, R. M. (1985). *Guidelines for the Syntactic Design of Audio Cues in Computer Interfaces.* (UCRL-93464).

Thinus-Blanc, C., and Gaunet, F. (1997). Representation of space in blind persons: Vision as a spatial sense? *Psychological Bulletin, 121*(1), 20–42. doi:10.1037/0033-2909.121.1.20

Ungar, S., Blades, M., and Spencer, C. (1997). Strategies for knowledge acquisition from cartographic maps by blind and visually impaired adults. *Cartographic Journal, 34*(2), 93–110.

Web Accessibility Initiative (WAI). (2006). Introduction to Web Accessibility. Retrieved from http://www.w3.org/WAI/intro/accessibility.php

World Health Organization (WHO). (2001). *ICF: International Classification of Functioning, Disability, and Health.* Geneva, Switzerland: WHO.

World Health Organization (WHO), and World Bank. (2011). *World Report on Disability.* Geneva, Switzerland: WHO.

Zhao, H., Plaisant, C., and Shneiderman, B. (2005). *"I Hear the Pattern": Interactive Sonification of Geographical Data Patterns.* Paper presented at the CHI '05 extended abstracts on Human factors in computing systems, Portland, OR. Retrieved from http://portal.acm.org/citation.cfm?doid = 1056808.1057052

Zhao, H., Plaisant, C., Shneiderman, B., and Duraiswami, R. (2004, July 6–9). *Sonification of Geo-Referenced Data for Auditory Information Seeking: Design Principle and Pilot Study.* Paper presented at the 10th Meeting of the International Conference on Auditory Display: ICAD '04, Sydney, Australia. doi:10.1.1.140.8467-1

Zhao, H., Plaisant, C., Shneiderman, B., and Lazar, J. (2008). Data sonification for users with visual Impairment. *ACM Transactions on Computer-Human Interaction, 15*(1), 1–28. doi:10.1145/1352782.1352786

Zimmer, H. D. (2001). The interface between language and visuo-spatial representations. In M. Denis, R. Logie, C. Cornoldo, M. de Vega and J. EngelKamp (Eds.), *Imagery, Language and Visuo-Spatial Thinking* (pp. 109–136). London: Psychology Press.

Zola, I. K. (1989). Toward the necessary universalizing of a disability policy. *Milbank Quarterly, 67*(Suppl 2 Pt. 2), 401–428. doi:10.2307/3350151

16

Web Solutions for Rehabilitation and Daily Life

G. Liotta, E. Di Giacomo, R. Magni, and F. Corradi

CONTENTS

16.1 Introduction

This chapter presents two studies: the first one discusses the design and the evaluation process of a tool for extending the possibility for disabled users to search and access the information on the Internet; the second discusses the development of a telemedicine tool for rehabilitation. Both the tools are created by a User Centered Design perspective (Norman, 1983) with a test–retest process:

- The first tool, called WhatsOnWeb, is a sonified clustering web search engine that makes use of visualization techniques to improve the effectiveness and efficiency of web searching. The whole information is presented to the user simultaneously in an interactive and sonified visual map, simplifying the user's ability to access and find information. This technology is very important in a world in which more than two Exabytes of new information are created every year (Lyman and Varian, 2003).

- The second tool, under the trademark Nu!Reha*, is a digital desk with a software platform created for the implementation of telerehabilitation services in European countries. The Nu!Reha Desk can supply personalized exercises to be executed at home by users in a distant, monitored manner. The main technical feature is constituted by an asynchronous link between the home system (portable unit) and the professional installation, which allows off-line data monitoring and configuration of the exercise.

16.2 The Simplification of the World Wide Web for Disabled Users: The WhatsOnWeb Search Engine

16.2.1 Introduction

Computers have become an essential and increasingly pervasive tool in everyday life, in both the professional and the personal entertainment spheres. Unfortunately, disabled people, face serious difficulties in using traditional input or output devices such as keyboards, mice, or screens because such devices require precise abilities to accomplish even the simplest tasks. Think for example of the use of the hands for the mouse or the use of the eyes for reading the screen.

In this section, we describe emerging human–computer interaction paradigms that are based on sophisticated diagrammatic interfaces that aim to overcome some of the limitations of the existing approaches to make computer applications accessible for impaired people. We concentrate on the simple but rather common task of searching the Web. Although the general theory behind the described approach is unique, we distinguish between diagrammatic interfaces for the visually impaired and motion-impaired people. This distinction depends on the fact that visually impaired people have major problems with traditional output devices whereas motion-impaired people cannot easily use input devices. In the rest of this introduction, we shortly recall the state of the art about the most commonly used devices and technologies; we also highlight their main shortcomings.

The assistive technologies proposed in the literature for visually impaired people have to translate the information to be conveyed to the user into forms that can be received by the user with senses distinct from the view, such as touch or hearing. The success of Braille-based interfaces (Roberts et al. 2000) have been limited in the past both because of the low levels of Braille literacy (some estimates are 20%) and the high cost of refreshable Braille displays (Zhao et al. 2008) The most popular technologies for blind people are those based on screen readers (Slatin and Rush 2003) because they have low costs, short training time, and do not require additional hardware. A screen reader is a software program that provides synthesized speech, representing what appears on the screen and alternative text provided by the application. Although the solutions based on screen readers are very effective in many situations, they present also some limitations. Firstly, a screen reader can easily translate textual informations into speech, but it may be difficult to convey graphical information (pictures, charts, or diagrams). Secondly, the time necessary to read the screen content can be very long and therefore the interaction between the user and the computer applications can be slowed down. For example, consider the task of searching a web page

---

* Nu!Reha is a trademark of Pragma Engineering srl.

with a standard search engine (e.g., Google). In response to the user's query, the engine returns a long list of results. Before the user can select the result he/she is interested in, he/she has to wait a relatively long time to hear the reading of each result.

At the same time, to overcome the barriers in the interaction between motion-impaired users and computers, several alternative input devices have been studied including, e.g., brain–computer interaction (BCI) (Chin et al. 2006), eye movement detection (Fejtová et al. 2006), tongue control (Struijk 2006), and speech/sound interaction (Manaris et al. 2002; Sporka et al. 2006). These devices allow the end-user to interact with the computer by performing a sequence of commands in which each command corresponds to selecting one from a very limited number of options. Conceptually, this is equivalent to having a keyboard with very few keys, possibly a single button. In other words, these input devices can be modeled as systems with a reduced number of statuses (only two for the single-button case). Even if these alternative devices partially overcome the barriers in interaction for the end-users, the overall interaction becomes slow and convoluted because the number of commands required to complete a single task increases with the loss of expressiveness of the input device. For example, searching a document in the Web with an interface operated by BCI technologies requires translating each keyboard and mouse command into a sequence of binary choices imposed by the two control statuses of a typical BCI.

16.2.2 The Interaction Model

Different approaches have been proposed in the literature to overcome the digital divide for motion-impaired people. We classify existing approaches with respect to the hierarchical model of Figure 16.1. This figure describes the interaction between a user and a computer as a traversal of a stack of four different layers: the task layer, the operation layer, the command layer, and the action layer.

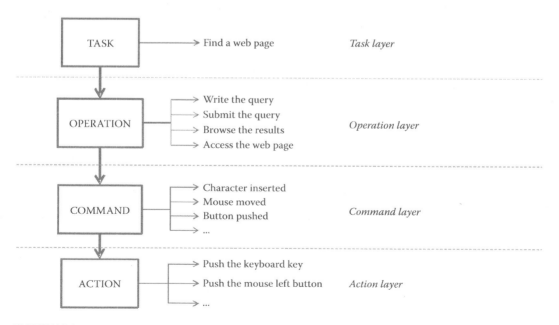

FIGURE 16.1
A hierarchical model for human-computer interaction.

When a user interacts with a computer, his/her goal is to perform some tasks that are specified in the task layer. For example, the user may want to search a file in the file system, or send an e-mail, or search a page in the Web. The choice of a task triggers activities at the lower levels of the hierarchy.

At the operation layer, the user has to execute a number of operations. For example, if the task selected by the user is that of searching the Web, the user's operation consists of writing the query, submitting the query, browsing the results, and eventually accessing those web pages he/she is looking for.

Each operation then translates into a set of commands at the command layer. A command corresponds to an event detected by the program, e.g., the insertion of a character, a click of the mouse, or the selection of an icon on the screen.

The user sends commands to the computer by performing a suitable number of actions at the action layer. An action is performed by interacting with the input device and it corresponds to simple acts such as pressing a key on the keyboard to write a character or executing a "double click" by pressing twice the left button of the mouse.

Notice that, for able-bodied people, there is typically a one-to-one correspondence between the actions and the commands, i.e., each action executed results in a command sent to the computer. This is not necessarily true for disabled people who use alternative input devices. For example, typing a single character (the command) using a binary switch can require operating the switch (the action) several times.

We now use the model of interaction described above to classify existing approaches that have been proposed in the literature to overcome the digital divide for motion-impaired people. Depending on the layer of the stack to which these approaches refer, we distinguish between action layer approaches and command layer approaches.

Action layer approaches focus on the design and realization of alternative input devices that allow disabled people to interact with standard software applications. In terms of the interaction model of Figure 16.1, these approaches allow motion-impaired people to perform the same set of commands as the able-bodied ones by means of a different set of actions. For example, an impaired user might move the mouse cursor by means of the voice or by moving the eyes. Depending on the user's disability and on the actions he/she can perform, different devices have been considered in this context. Examples include speech/sound-based interfaces (Manaris et al. 2002; Sporka et al. 2006), eye movement detection (Fejtová et al. 2006), EMG interfaces (Chin et al. 2006), and a light-spot operated mouse (Itoh 2006).

The advantage of action layer approaches is that they do not require the software to be modified, and therefore the impaired people can potentially use any computer application. Unfortunately, there are some drawbacks to take into account within these approaches. One disadvantage is that a long training period is required to reach a good level of usability. Also, obtaining an alternative input device that can completely replace a keyboard and mouse can be a difficult result to achieve, especially for individuals with particularly severe disabilities. Therefore the execution of the commands remains a major bottleneck for an efficient interaction.

Command layer approaches address the above-mentioned problem by using alternative input devices, the effectiveness of which is enhanced by means of software adaptation layers. These software layers act as a bridge between the standard applications and the input devices. An example of this approach is the use of scanners (Ntoa et al. 2004). Scanners highlight software controls (e.g., software buttons or menu items) in a predefined order. The user may choose one of the highlighted controls by using an input device with just two statuses, such as a BCI or a single button. Another example is the use of force-feedback gravity wells, i.e., attractive basins that pull the cursor to the center of an on-screen target (Hwang et al. 2003). These techniques are designed to help users who have tremor, spasm, and co-ordination difficulties to perform "point and click" tasks more quickly and accurately.

Referring to Figure 16.1, command layer approaches allow the user to execute the same operations as in the standard interaction, but they require him/her to perform a different set of commands. As an example, consider the operation of sending a query to a search engine. With standard input devices, the following commands must be executed: "Move the mouse to the search button" and "Press the button." The same operation performed with a scanner consists of the scanner highlighting the search button and the user executing a single command, namely "Activate the highlighted button."

The major drawback of command layer approaches is that although the actions to be performed by the user on the input devices are in general reduced or simplified, the time needed to execute a single command typically increases. For example, pressing a button using a scanner requires significantly more time than pressing the same button with a mouse because of the time needed to scan the whole set of command options. Also, to offer a seamless integration between the adaptation layer and any application software, the latter should adhere to precise software design rules that in most cases have not been taken into account in the design of the application software.

16.2.3 The Information Visualization Approach

The information visualization approach (IVA) aims to overcome the main disadvantages of the action layer approaches and command layer approaches that have been described in the previous section. The main characteristic of this approach is to act at the operation layer of the hierarchical model of Figure 16.1. The idea is to change the set of operations associated with the execution of a task in such a way that the total number of corresponding commands is reduced. Reducing the number of commands aims at compensating for the loss of efficiency that a motion-impaired person must pay in executing them because of the limited number of statuses available in his/her alternative input device.

To achieve this goal, enhanced information visualization technologies can be used. Visual representations, obtained by using geometric primitives and transformation, colors, and other visual objects, translate data into a visible form that highlights important features that would be otherwise hardly identifiable or even hidden. It follows that, when compared with different possible representations of the information space associated with a task, visual representations are more efficient in conveying information. This is due to two main reasons. On one hand, visual representations take advantage of the human eye's broad bandwidth connection into the brain to allow users to see, explore, and understand large amounts of information at once. On the other hand, the use of visual objects makes the acquisition of information more intuitive and immediate, and therefore the cognitive elaboration is reduced.

Thus, IVA makes the end-user interact with a computer in which data are presented in a nontraditional way by means of sophisticated diagrammatic interfaces. All non-IVA interaction paradigms aim at reducing the discomfort of motion-impaired individuals within the classical iconic representation of the data offered by traditional operating systems. They do not try to compensate the reduced expressiveness of the input devices by enlarging the amount of information that can be visually processed by the end-user in the same time frame.

For example, consider the task of searching a page on the Web. A possible set of operations is as follows: write the query, submit the query, scan the list of results, and access the web page. One of the efficiency bottlenecks for the motion impaired would be scanning the list of results, which can be very long. IVA changes this critical operation. Traditionally, search engine results are presented as a list of pages that are sequentially scanned. An alternative presentation could be the following: pages are grouped into different categories, in which each category contains pages that are semantically coherent; furthermore, possible relations between different categories are explicitly showed. In this scenario, the number of commands associated with the browsing can be significantly reduced because the information space to be searched by the end-user looking for a page is naturally narrowed by selecting categories or subcategories and by discarding large quantities of uninteresting pages with a single command. A snapshot of a possible diagrammatic interface for this specific operation is given in Figure 16.2, which represents the output of a visual web search engine called WhatsOnWeb (Di Giacomo et al. 2007).

16.2.3.1 The Application Information Visualization Approach: The Web Accessibility for Disabled Users

We propose a new interaction paradigm between computers and disabled users. The objective is both to make the impaired people capable of using a computer in a more efficient way and to take advantage of this gained efficiency in an aid assessment process that exploits the Web to easily convey information of any kind to impaired people. The leading idea is that the use of sophisticated information visualization technologies can significantly affect the cognitive efficiency of a user that browses the Web, even if this user is blind (Di Giacomo et al. 2010). Information visualization conveys abstract information in intuitive ways. Visual representations and interaction techniques take advantage of the human eye's broad bandwidth pathway into the mind to allow users to see, explore, and understand large amounts of information at once. Furthermore, it has been shown that spatial representation can be independent by the sensorial way in which it is perceived (Avraamides et al. 2004), leading to the hypothesis of an amodal spatial representation (Bryant 1992). The screen readers are an effective solution for several software applications adapted by blind people. However, because the quantity of nontextual conveyed

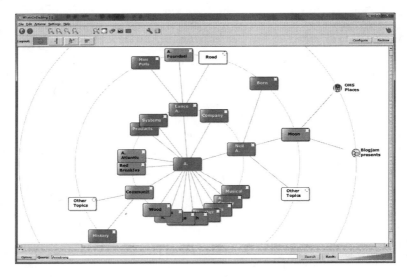

FIGURE 16.2
(See color insert.) Example of diagrammatic interface that reduces the search commands to be executed when accessing a page on the Web.

information through the Web is constantly increasing, screen readers show clear limits. Also, even in those cases in which the output is typically text, such as for the output of a web search engine, the interaction between a blind person and a computer can become slow and convoluted because of the many lines of text that a screen reader may need to read before leading the user to the wanted information. Also in this case, it would be very useful to adopt techniques such as those described in the previous section that convey a great amount of information in an intuitive and concise manner. For example, the use of a visual map of semantic categories could significantly reduce the amount of time needed to explore the results space and to find the desired information.

The adoption of solutions on the basis of the information visualization may seem impossible for blind people because of their disability. However, many studies agree that the spatial representation of information is independent from the way in which the sensory inputs are displayed; in particular, some authors pointed out that blind subjects have a better performance in processing spatial auditory inputs than sighted people (de Vega et al. 2001; Avraamides et al. 2004). Indeed, it has been highlighted that blind people show a motion ability in performing spatial exploration tasks guided by only natural acoustic cues, functionally equivalent to the visually guided way for sighted people (Bryant 1992). Even more, the nature of sound seems to be able to communicate the complexity of visual representations of data (Kramer 1994). Therefore, one can use information visualization approaches similar to those described in the previous section coupled with sonification techniques. Sonification is the way to "represent data relations into perceived relations in an acoustic signal for the purposes of facilitating communication and interpretation" (Kramer et al. 1997).

16.2.3.2 A Sonification Example

As a case study, we report recent experimental research about the sonification of WhatsOnWeb (Rugo et al. 2009; Mele et al. 2010). In most of the sonificated (see Chapter 15) systems, priority is usually given to the mapping of the sound attribution to data, but not to the interactivity with the user. To overcome this limit and to guarantee that the sonification represents both the interaction design and information, Zhao and colleagues (2008) provided the Action by Design Component (ADC) framework, a sonification model designed to permit an active and dynamic navigation into the interaction environment. For this reason, the ACD framework was chosen as a theoretical background for the sonification of WhatsOnWeb, in which the indexed data are organized by semantic correlations resulting in abstract information.

The sonification of WhatsOnWeb is combined with visual events describing global and particular browsing information. Although the global information is visualized after "search" action, the temporization technique provides an increase in the intensity of each category. From the first to the last ranking organization result is guaranteed to the user through an overall overview of information that allows the first mental representation of the framework that users are going to browse. The complexity of the tone of each node is related with the complexity of its paraverbal information. For example, while browsing a category, a harmonic chord will be executed, suggesting the semantic links with the other peaks. A low-latency (less than 100 ms) of short sounds have been used to grant a kind of active interaction in which sound information processing and keeping does not implicate a short-term memory overload (Atkinson and Shiffrin 1971). Moreover, WhatsOnWeb browsing is granted by the auditory reiterable feedback, which provides spatial information to facilitate user orientation. Indeed, WhatsOnWeb provides the user with a persistent signal that indicates his/her current position in the interface, as it happens in visual navigation. Spatial cues are uttered by a stereo-audio overview, which simulates the position of selected nodes within a Cartesian coordinate plane; the information identification and memorization is strengthened by a verbal feedback voiced by an integrated synthesizer.

Three different sonification models have been tested for WhatsOnWeb. The sound's volume, pitch, tone, blinking, and grid reference are used to transmit visual features in a univocal way. In the first model, called the VolumeSonification model, the Euclidean distance coding for a node compared to a significant reference is rendered through the sound volume level, whereas the panning is used to strengthen the node detection on the abscissas axis as absolute information. The second model, called the BlinkAndPitchSonification model, conveys spatial relations through an independent mapping of the two axes of the Cartesian plane (x,y), respectively, with the frequency of the sound blinking together with panning and with the note pitch. Finally, to optimize the graphic representation in terms of sound, the PanAndPitchSonification model has been created solely considering the panning for the x-axis and the pitch for the y-axis.

16.2.3.3 A Usability Evaluation

In this section, we describe an experimental analysis of the re-engineered and sonificated WhatsOnWeb (Mele et al. 2010). This analysis evaluated the usability of the different visual layouts: TreeMap, Layered Radial, and Spiral TreeMap.

16.2.3.3.1 Experimental Procedures

Phase 1: The first phase investigated the usability of the sonificated WhatsOnWeb by an expert evaluation. Three experts with more than 5 years of experience in the usability evaluation assessed the software by the Nielsen's heuristic list (Nielsen 1994). A user scenario was performed to test each of the implemented layouts. In particular, the experts' tasks were to test the usability and the layout differences among the three models of sonification: PanAndPitch, PitchAndVolume, and BlinkAndPitch. The heuristic evaluation identified a small set of usability issues with a medium and high level of severity, suggesting that it was necessary to redesign the layout. Finally, all of the evaluators suggested unification of two of the sonification models—PanAndPitch and BlinkAndPitch—proposing a new model called PanAndPitchBlinking. The PanAndPitchBlinking model conveys spatiality through the two axes of the Cartesian plane (x,y) by using the panning technique (x-axis) and the note pitch (y-axis) and it uses the blink effect to represent the rank order of each vertex.

Phase 2: After the usability issues reported by the experts were fixed, a usability test was performed with two groups of participants: four totally blind users and four sighted users (mean age 28 years, equally distributed by sex). This phase of evaluation aimed at investigating both the quality of users' interaction with the visual and sonificated WhatsOnWeb and the users' satisfaction. To achieve these evaluation goals, we used the Partial Concurrent Thinking Aloud (PCTA) (Mele et al. 2009) and the System Usability Scale (SUS) (Brooke 1996) questionnaires. Each user tested WhatsOnWeb after a clear and essential description of the task and a preliminary exploration (lasting 3 min) of the layout. The experimental task, provided by a scenario, consisted of an exhaustive search of the meaning of the word "Armstrong" by using the WhatsOnWeb search engine. The keyboard navigation was performed by using either three typologies of layout—Radial, Layered, and Spiral TreeMap—or the PanAndPitch Blinking sonification. At the end of the evaluation session, all of the subjects were interviewed about their layout preferences and finally they were asked to complete the SUS survey.

16.2.3.3.2 Experimental Results

Problems identified during the PCTA protocols were collected and matched with the heuristic analysis of the first evaluation phase. All of the subjects found 19 problems: 9 of which were related to visual performance and 11 to auditory performance. The one-way analysis of variance (ANOVA), performed by SPSS 18 on task completion times for each layout, shows no significant differences ($p > 0.05$) between the two groups and between the kind of layout—layered layout (sighted M = 50.25", blind M = 132.5"), Spiral TreeMap layout (sighted M = 263.25", blind M = 236")—whereas considerable difference was found on the Radial layout ($F(1,6) = 13,690; p < 0.05$). The analysis of the SUS score shows no significant differences ($p > 0.01$) between the two participants' groups. Therefore, because these results highlight similar levels of efficacy, efficiency, and satisfaction between the two groups for both information presentation modalities, the sonificated modality and the visual modality performances seem to be homogeneous.

16.3 The Telemedicine: The Nu!Reha Desk

16.3.1 Introduction to Telemedicine

During last 15 years, intensive development of technological applications in the fields of medicine and rehabilitation has been observed, with the main reason being technological development [mainly in information and communication technologies (ICT)] itself, which is "horizontally" influencing all of the frameworks of our lives, but also the increasing demand of innovative services. Many definitions have been applied to identify these services on the basis of the specific application (i.e., telecardiology) and the specific technology used (Internet based, mobile carrier based), but the most usable and comprehensive term is still "medicine at a distance." This definition introduces two fundamental concepts telemedicine is a specific realization in the framework of "traditional" medicine, and the ability to influence people's well-being, health. and therapy at a distance. Another important aspect is the chance to apply the concept of distance interaction to management and the "social" activities linked to medical services, such as the need for a second opinion, teleconsulting, the safety monitoring of disabled and elderly people, and medical education (online courses, blended learning) (Mair et al. 2000; Wootton 2001). In this sense "telemedicine" is a large framework encompassing a number of different activities, both front- and back-office, in the medical and paramedical sectors, which are largely affecting organizational profiles and educational activities (curricular and continuous medical education).

The diffusion of telemedicine is not clearly confined into geographical boundaries: Many examples are found in developed countries as well as in emerging economies and underdeveloped countries. The applications of telemedicine are clearly chosen on the basis of needs and cost/benefit balances with different results, i.e., the application of remote services in the case of war scenarios or adverse natural occurrences (Llewellyn 1995). In some cases, some applications are recognized as part of a well-known intervention protocol (Pettersen et al. 1999; Salvador et al. 2005).

The variety of applications is increasing because they belong to different areas of medicine. The first applications reported just focused on teleradiology, telepathology, and telecardiology because they manage easy-to-transmit data even with a low bandwidth connection.

Since its primordial application, the two main drivers of telemedicine were, firstly, the chance to reach underserved users to provide sanitary services, as in the case of rural areas or people living in adverse climatic conditions, and, second, the chance to exploit ICT to propose innovative solutions for the organization of sanitary services in terms of efficacy and efficiency. Nowadays, several studies demonstrate the chance to reach large populations of users, even in large areas, as well as the chance to manage information efficiently among different professional profiles (Balch and Tichenor 1997; Balch et al. 2006). Recently, an increasing number of projects have proposed the direct involvement of "informed" users in the exploitation of telemedicine services, going on to redefine the relationships between agents of the sanitary services.

Literature reviews, carried out analyzing pilot telemedicine experiences, demonstrated that only a small amount of them were producing actual benefits with respect to traditional approaches. However, it is important to note that most of these studies were developed without updated technologies and in some cases without the availability of traditional alternatives (Strode et al. 1999; Whitten et al. 2002). What is emerging is the need to carry out telemedicine applications, including "cost-effectiveness" evaluations (in comparison with traditional services), as an integral part of service design and analysis.

An important issue involving users and professionals is the problem related to the treatment and management of privacy data. From a technical point of view, three main key points are to be highlighted: confidentiality (granting access only to authorized agents), integrity (no modification of user data), and availability (related to rights to access data). At present, some tentative designs of shared standards have been considered to reach interoperability among systems and applications, saving the need to design and exploit autonomously designed telemedicine services.

16.3.2 Telerehabilitation

In the general framework of telemedicine applications, more recently telerehabilitation has been developed: hence, a number of practical applications are already available supported by the technological achievements of the last decade (1999–2010). These applications are designed for distance rehabilitation by means of ICT as the media to transmit therapy data (Lathan et al. 1999). The main driver for these applications compared with traditional systems was the chance to supply rehabilitation to users living in rural areas (Torsney 2003): Remote access is allowing the users to access sanitary services (Hauber et al. 2002).

Another benefit of telerehabilitation is the prolonging of the rehabilitative time at home, considering that, in some cases, intensive rehabilitation can ensure an effective recovery from the impairment. The chance to extend the rehabilitative activities can also be useful in the chronic phase, when the "lowering" of the function can also be caused by the "not-used" condition (Taub et al. 2000). Telerehabilitation has a large number of applications with different complexities (from a simple telephone teleconsultation to distance operated rehab exercise monitoring).

16.3.3 The Nu!Reha Platform

The platform represents the final realization resulting from an intense experimental period in which concept design has been explored (Scattareggia et al. 2004; Zampolini et al. 2007; Huijgen et al. 2008). The main idea is to supply personalized exercises for execution at home by users in a distant, monitored manner. The system has been designed to be a main application of part of the neurological rehabilitation service as an extension of the "traditional approach." The main technical feature includes an asynchronous link between the home system (portable unit) and the professional installation, which allows offline data monitoring and configuration of the exercises.

16.3.4 Proposed Approach

The experimental paradigm of the Nu!Reha Desk has been the use of the technological features with the facilitation of motor recovery. In fact, according to the most recent studies, motor action is facilitated by a significant contextual environment. On the basis of these observations in rehabilitation, a therapy based on the task has been developed (Smith et al. 1999; Michelle et al. 2007).

Taking into account this organization of motor control, a virtual reality approach seems to be inapplicable in rehabilitation activity; therefore, the system is based on the use of a purposely conceived "activity desk" for the execution of occupational therapy tasks and exercises, allowing different grasping actions and interactions with sensorized objects. The device is composed of a base unit and a list of components that have different functionalities and scopes of utilization depending on their connection to the base unit.

- *The base unit:* The desk supporting the core structure of the system (both hardware and software). It is intended as the basic module of the whole system: All other modules or subsystems are to be connected to this unit.
- *Control pad:* It allows the control of the system interface by the caregiver assisting the patient during the exercises.
- *Shelf:* A shelf-like tool useful for the execution of vertical-displacement-based exercises; it is equipped with an array of infrared proximity sensors allowing the detection of the presence of a sensorized object (an object covered by reflective labels).
- *Keyboard module:* Module for the execution of exercises consisting of inputting a sequence of numbers with a telephone/POS-like keyboard.
- *Radio frequency tool:* A plastic cylinder containing an internal transceiver that allows for its horizontal localization.
- *Video cameras and supports:* A couple of webcams with articulated stands supplied for the video recording of the exercises performed by the patient.
- *Accessories:* A list of accessories is supplied to keep the system usage simple and feasible; accessories include a sensorized pen, plastic jars and cups, a book-like reproduction, and foam cubes.

By means of accessories and sensors, a number of different exercises can be configured directly by the therapist allowing a full customizable environment in which to perform different grasp/grip actions and upper limb movements. Writing and pregraphism exercises and vertical and horizontal object displacements can be performed and monitored by the system.

The system (PU) is based on a sensorized LCD surface placed in front of the patient and acting as an interface and working area for the execution of exercises. A single board computer placed inside of the table supports the execution of all tasks and acquisitions requested by each exercise. A WiFi interface allows the connection to external LAN or ADSL connections for data uploading and configuration retrieval from an external server.

A typical exercise includes the utilization of one or more sensorized accessories for the execution of contextual activities as provided by occupational therapy. For example, an exercise typology could include interaction with the sensorized pen (similar in weight and dimension to a normal pen) on the plastic surface of the screen. It understands a "writing" exercise (based on the writing performance) and/or a "pregraphism" exercise (based on trajectories) as shown in Figure 16.3.

Another exercise typology utilizes a plastic jar inside of the radio frequency tool. It is localized on the sensorized area, allowing the monitoring of horizontal displacement through the positions suggested by the exercise, as shown in Figure 16.4.

16.3.5 Clinical Evaluation

The Nu!Reha Desk is commercially available as a tool for the implementation of "telerehabilitation services" in European Union countries. Several studies on clinical efficacy are running at present, and the Nu!Reha Desk has been applied to users with different impairments and rehabilitative objectives.

The clinical evaluation reported refers to the feasibility study performed during the execution of the "Hellodoc" project. The project, supported by the eTen initiative, was undertaken in the period 2005–2007 by a European consortium coordinated by the ISS-Istituto Superiore di Sanità, which is the technical body of the Italian Health Ministry. During the

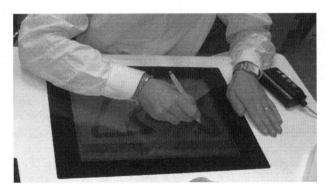

FIGURE 16.3
(See color insert.) Nu!Reha Desk example of writing or "pre-graphism" exercise.

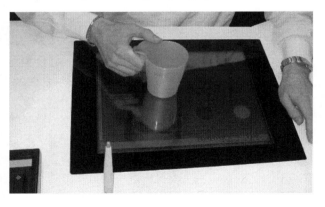

FIGURE 16.4
(See color insert.) Nu!Reha Desk example of physical contextual activities exercise.

execution of the clinical trials (Hermens et al. 2007), prototype portable units were used with the same functionality as the Nu!Reha platform (not engineered, certified and aesthetically refined). The users in the trial were recruited from groups of multiple sclerosis (MS), traumatic brain injury (TBI), and stroke patients (because the system was originally conceived for neurological rehabilitation). The inclusion criteria were

1. Age over 18 years;
2. Established diagnosis of MS, stroke, or TBI;
3. Taking more than 25 s to perform the nine-hole peg test;
4. Ability to move at least one peg in 180 s during the nine-hole peg test;
5. Sufficient autonomous functioning;
6. Internet connection or telephone line and reachable Internet provider;
7. Stable clinical status; and
8. Living at home.

The third and the fourth criteria include only users whose arm abilities were in the mid-range between severe impairment and little impairment because these criteria make use of a recognized clinical evaluation tool, which consists of a nine-hole matrix in which pegs of specific dimensions should be inserted. The exclusion criteria were

1. Disturbed upper limb function not related to MS, TBI, or stroke;
2. Serious cognitive and/or behavioral problems;
3. Serious emotional problems;
4. Major visual problems;
5. Communication problems;
6. Medical complications; and
7. Other problems possibly contraindicating autonomous exercise at home.

The scheme of clinical trials was based on the ABA application of the telerehabilitation tool for the intervention group, comparing the results from the control group. The duration chosen for the application of rehabilitation at home was four weeks, which was considered sufficient to reveal the effects of the proposed activities. Figure 16.5 is the flow chart of the experimental design.

T0 is the first assessment, after the application of the inclusion criteria, after which users were randomly assigned to the intervention or control group. At T1, a second assessment was provided (after a period of 1 month), whereas at T2 an assessment after 1 month of telerehabilitation activity (intervention group) was performed.

16.3.5.1 Results and Discussion

The experimental trial included 47 men and 34 women with an average age of 48 years. They were distributed among the three impairment causes (16 stroke, 30 TBI, and 35 MS). At the end of the trial it was shown that the intensity of treatment (control group with usual care versus intervention group with telerehabilitation) was nearly the same (9 h/month versus 9.5 h/month). It is outside of the scope of this chapter to investigate and describe specific assessment tools utilized or to go into a detailed analysis of the assessment results

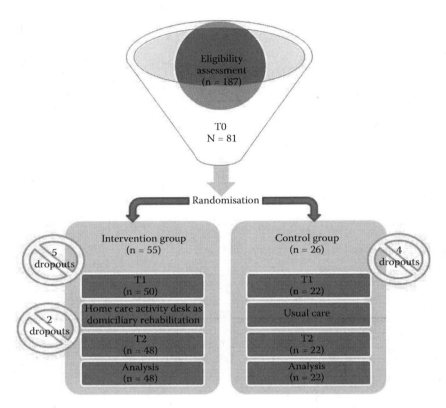

FIGURE 16.5
(See color insert.) Flow chart of the experimental design for the clinical evaluation of the Nu!Reha Desk.

obtained because this is available in the literature. Considering all of the impairment causes, a significantly small difference has been revealed in assessing both groups during the intervention period: There are always different results in the confidence intervals for the chosen measurement tools.

In general, the results for the included set of patients demonstrate the equivalence between the telerehabilitation and usual care groups, in which patients who more often showed improvement with respect to usual care were those who will use the telerehabilitation system more frequently.

During the clinical trials, a first assessment of user satisfaction was also performed based on direct questions for therapists and patients making use of telerehabilitation systems [those with Visual Analogue Scale (VAS) scores below 30 were considered to be dissatisfied, those with scores between 31 and 69 as satisfied, and those with scores 70 and over were considered fully satisfied]. The results were encouraging with regard to user acceptance on both sides: Only the aesthetical aspects were considered to be unsatisfactory (prototype versions of Nu!Reha Desk) as well as the difficulty of some tasks related to the activity to be executed (patients).

16.3.6 Future Evolutions

The promising scenario about teletherapy applied to rehabilitation is the involvement of the whole community of potential users (patients and families, health-care suppliers, health-care payers). Each party is clearly more sensible to different aspects understood by the use of this type of solution: Availability and ease of use to increase the intensity and duration of treatments, new opportunities to optimize recovery and patient follow-up, and a general reduction in the costs of treatment sessions. All of these expectations will pass through a kind of "cultural" evolution in understanding and conception, i.e., passing from the present "new tool application" to a "service-centered" adoption concept, which means the parallel growth of

- *Technological solutions:* Reliable, replicable, easy to use, low-cost, integrated, and interoperable.
- *Clinical consensus:* Convergence about solutions, validation criteria, adoption, and service shaping.
- *Education:* Mostly of the personnel involved in health-care supplier applications as an integral part of their curricular or CME (Continuous Medical Education) provisions.
- *Reimbursement policy:* Regional/national rules to recognize the cost of teletreatments as they will be covered by private or public allowances.
- *User acceptance:* As a routine service, therapy at home (even in the absence of a rehab professional) should involve the final beneficiary with a careful assessment of needs and preferences.

Leaving the so-called "pilot phase", all of these aspects will be taken into account because they could support the next evolution/adoption of innovative technological solutions.

These processes are placed inside of the more general frame of "personalized medicine," which will be the growing trend for the future dealing with genomics, pharmacogenomics, predictive models, cultural and ethical issues, etc.

16.4 Conclusions

The two studies presented in this chapter discussed the design of two kinds of technology: one to simplify the use of web technology in daily life (WhatsOnWeb) and one to improve the telemedicine tool applied in the rehabilitation processes (Nu!Reha Desk). These technologies, by the use of the user-centered design perspective, aim to open up new possibilities of well-being for disabled users by widening user access and management of information (WhatsOnWeb) or to access a rehabilitation process despite the physical barriers (Nu!Reha Desk). These two studies implicitly underline the important role played by the user-centered design process for the improvement of users' daily lives and well-being, showing the new kind of technological solutions that, on the one hand, allow users to work in the physical environment by the mediation of the virtual one (Nu!Reha), and on the other (WhatsOnWeb) to simplify the interaction of the users with the virtual systems. The two studies show that the most important way forward for the evolution of interaction technologies is strictly focused on the design of the relationship between the users and the technology to overcome the barriers due to both the physical and the virtual environment.

Summary of the Chapter

This chapter presents two studies: the first one discusses the design and the evaluation process of a tool for extending the possibility for disabled users to search and access the information on the Internet (WhatsOnWeb); the second discusses the development of a telemedicine tool for rehabilitation (Nu!Reha). WhatsOnWeb can widen the ability of web users to search and access information through a semantic and spatial organization of information. This tool, by its sonification algorithm, becomes an important tool for visually impaired users because it allows this kind of user to explore the spatial organization of the retrieved information without performance differences to those of nonimpaired users. Also, the use of the user-centered perspective allows the designer to set up the WhatsOnWeb technology for brain–computer interface use with locked-in subjects to spread the semantic web possibility of searching in the World Wide Web. The second technology, the Nu!Reha Desk, is a telemedicine system that can include in the rehabilitation process disabled users without easy access to practitioners. The analysis of the user experience of this technology, and in particular the ease of learning perceived by the users, is the core for the implementation of this tool to optimize access to the rehabilitation process.

References

Atkinson, R. C., and Shiffrin, R. M. (1971). The control of short-term memory. *Scientific American,* 225(2), 82–90.

Avraamides, M. N., Loomis, J. M., Klatzky, R. L., and Golledge, R. G. (2004). Functional equivalence of spatial representations derived from vision and language: Evidence from allocentric judgments. *Journal of Experimental Psychology: Learning, Memory, and Cognition,* 30(4), 801–814.

Balch, D., Rosenthal, D., and Taylor, C. (2006). *The 2005 "Last Chance Bravo" Bioterrorism Exercise: A Report on the Efficacy of Communications Technologies and Telemedicine for Disaster Response.* Paper presented at the SAIS 2006 Proceedings. Paper 9. http://aisel.aisnet.org/sais2006/9

Balch, D. C., and Tichenor, J. M. (1997). Telemedicine expanding the scope of health care information. *Journal of the American Medical Informatics Association:JAMIA,* 4(1), 1–5.

Brooke, J. (1996). SUS: A quick and dirty usability scale. In P. W. Jordan, B. Thomas, B. A. Weerdmeester and A. L. McClelland (Eds.), *Usability Evaluation in Industry.* Boca Raton, FL: CRC Press.

Bryant, D. J. (1992). A spatial representation system in humans. *Psycoloquy,* 3(16).

Chin, C., Barreto, A., and Alonso, M. (2006). Electromyogram-based cursor control system for users with motor disabilities. In K. Miesenberger, J. Klaus, W. Zagler and A. Karshmer (Eds.), *Computers Helping People with Special Needs* (Vol. 4061, pp. 905–912). Berlin/Heidelberg: Springer.

de Vega, M., Cocude, M., Denis, M., Rodrigo, M. J., and Zimmer, H. D. (2001). The interface between language and visuo-spatial representations. In M. Denis, R. H. Logie, C. Cornoldi, M. de Vega and J. Engelkamp (Eds.), *Imagery, Language and Visuo-Spatial Thinking.* Hove, UK: Psychology Press.

Di Giacomo, E., Didimo, W., Grilli, L., and Liotta, G. (2007). Graph visualization techniques for web clustering engines. *IEEE Transactions on Visualization and Computer Graphics,* 13(2), 294–304. doi: 10.1109/PACIFICVIS.2008.4475473

Di Giacomo, E., Liotta, G., and Federici, S. (2010). *Information Visualization Techniques for Motion Impaired People.* Paper presented at the 3rd International Conference on Health Informatics (HEALTHINF 2010). http://www.scitepress.org/DigitalLibrary/User/ViewPaper.aspx. doi: 10.5220/0002758403610366

Fejtová, M., Fejt, J., and Štěpánková, O. (2006). Eye as an actuator. In K. Miesenberger, J. Klaus, W. Zagler and A. Karshmer (Eds.), *Computers Helping People with Special Needs* (Vol. 4061, pp. 954–961), Berlin/Heidelberg: Springer.

Hauber, R. P., Vesmarovich, S., and Dufour, L. (2002). The use of computers and the Internet as a source of health information for people with disabilities. *Rehabilation Nursing, 27*(4), 142–145.

Hermens, H., Huijgen, B., Giacomozzi, C., Ilsbroukx, S., Macellari, V., Prats, E., et al. (2007). Clinical assessment of the HELLODOC tele-rehabilitation service. *Annali dell'Istituto Superire di Sanita, 44*(2), 154–163.

Hersh, W. R., Hickam, D. H., Severance, S. M., Dana, T. L., Pyle Krages, K., and Helfand, M. (2006). Diagnosis, access and outcomes: Update of a systematic review of telemedicine services. *Journal of Telemedicine and Telecare, 12*(Suppl 2), 3–31. doi: 10.1258/135763306778393117

Huijgen, B. C., Vollenbroek-Hutten, M. M., Zampolini, M., Opisso, E., Bernabeu, M., Van Nieuwenhoven, J., et al. (2008). Feasibility of a home-based telerehabilitation system compared to usual care: Arm/hand function in patients with stroke, traumatic brain injury and multiple sclerosis. *Journal of Telemedicine and Telecare, 14*(5), 249–256. doi: 10.1258/jtt.2008.080104

Hwang, F., Keates, S., Langdon, P., and Clarkson, P. J. (2003). *Multiple Haptic Targets for Motion-Impaired Computer Users*. Paper presented at the Proceedings of the SIGCHI Conference on Human Factors in Computing Systems, Ft. Lauderdale, FL.

Itoh, K. (2006). Light spot operated mouse emulator for cervical spinal-cord injured PC users. In K. Miesenberger, J. Klaus, W. Zagler and A. Karshmer (Eds.), *Computers Helping People with Special Needs* (Vol. 4061, pp. 973–980–980), Berlin/Heidelberg: Springer.

Kramer, G. (1994). *Auditory Display: Sonification, Audification, and Auditory Interfaces*. Reading, MA: Addison Wesley.

Kramer, G., Walker, B., Bonebright, T., Cook, P., Flowers, J., Miner, N., and Neuhoff, J. (1997). *Sonification Report: Status of the Field and Research Agenda*, International Community for Auditory Display. Retrieved from http://sonify.psych.gatech.edu/publications/pdfs/1999-nsf-report.pdf

Lathan, C. E., Kinsella, A., Rosen, M. J., Winters, J., and Trepagnier, C. (1999). Aspects of human factors engineering in home telemedicine and telerehabilitation systems. *Telemedicine Journal, 5*(2), 169–175. doi: 10.1089/107830299312131

Llewellyn, C. (1995). The role of telemedicine in disaster medicine. *Journal of Medical Systems, 19*(1), 29–34. doi: 10.1007/bf02257188

Lyman, P., and Varian, H. R. (2003). *How Much Information 2003*. Berkeley, CA: University of California at Berkeley, School of Information Management and Systems.

Mair, F., Whitten, P., May, C., and Doolittle, G. C. (2000). Patients' perceptions of a telemedicine specialty clinic. *Journal of Telemedicine and Telecare, 6*(1), 36–40. doi: 10.1258/1357633001933925

Manaris, B., McGivers, M., and Lagoudakis, M. (2002). A listening keyboard for users with motor impairments—A usability study. *International Journal of Speech Technology, 5*(4), 371–388. doi: 10.1.1.13.8194

Mele, M. L., Borsci, S., Rugo, A., Federici, S., Liotta, G., Trotta, F., and Di Giacomo, E. (2009). *An Accessible Web Searching: An On-Going Research Project* (Assistive Technology Research Series ed. Vol. 25). Amsterdam: IOS press. doi: 10.3233/978-1-60750-042-1-854.

Mele, M. L., Federici, S., Borsci, S., and Liotta, G. (2010). *Beyond A Visuocentric Way of a Visual Web Search Clustering Engine: The Sonification of WhatsOnWeb*. Paper presented at the Proceedings of the 12th International Conference on Computers Helping People with Special Needs: Part I, Vienna, Austria. doi: 10.1007/978-3-642-14097-6_56.

Michelle, J. J., Kimberly, J. W., John, A., Dominic, N., Elaine, S., Judith, K., et al. (2007). Task-oriented and purposeful robot-assisted therapy. In S. S. Kommu (Ed.), *Rehabilitation Robotics*. Vienna, Austria: InTech.

Nielsen, J. (1994). *Enhancing the Explanatory Power of Usability Heuristics*. Paper presented at the Proceedings of the SIGCHI Conference on Human Factors in Computing Systems: Celebrating Interdependence, Boston, MA.

Norman, D. A. (1983). Some observations on mental models. In D. Gentner and A. Steven (Eds.), *Mental Models* (pp. 7–14). Hillsdale, NJ: Lawrence Erlbaum Associates.

Ntoa, S., Savidis, A., and Stephanidis, C. (2004). FastScanner: An accessibility tool for motor impaired users. In K. Miesenberger, J. Klaus, W. Zagler, and D. Burger (Eds.), *Computers Helping People with Special Needs* (Vol. 3118, pp. 626–626). Berlin/Heidelberg: Springer.

Pettersen, S., Uldal, S. B., Baardsgard, A., Amundsen, M., Myrvang, R., Nordvag, D., and Stenmarkl, H. (1999). The North Norwegian Health Net. *Journal of Telemedicine and Telecare*, 5(Suppl 1), 34–36. doi: 10.1258/1357633991932469

Roberts, J., Slattery, O., and Kardos, D. (2000). 49.2: Rotating-wheel Braille display for continuous refreshable Braille. *SID Symposium Digest of Technical Papers*, 31(1), 1130–1133. doi: 10.1889/1.1832864

Roulstone, A. (2010). Access and accessibility. In J. H. Stone and M. Blouin (Eds.), *International Encyclopedia of Rehabilitation*.

Rugo, A., Mele, M., Liotta, G., Trotta, F., Di Giacomo, E., Borsci, S., and Federici, S. (2009). A visual sonificated web search clustering engine. *Cognitive Processing*, 10(0), 286–289. doi: 10.1007/s10339–009–0317–4.

Salvador, C. H., Carrasco, M. P., de Mingo, M. A. G., Carrero, A. M., Montes, J. M., Martin, L. S., Monteagudo, J. L. (2005). Airmed-cardio: A GSM and Internet services-based system for out-of-hospital follow-up of cardiac patients. *Information Technology in Biomedicine, IEEE Transactions on* 9(1), 73. doi:10.1109/TITB.2004.840067

Scattareggia, M. S., Nowe, A., Zaia, A., Cucinotta, A., Magni, R., Magnino, F., et al. (2004). H-Cad: A new approach for home rehabilitation. *International Journal Of Rehabilitation Research* 27(Suppl 1), 110–111.

Slatin, J., and Rush, S. (2003). *Maximum Accessibility*. Reading, MA: Addison-Wesley.

Smith, G. V., Silver, K. H. C., Goldberg, A. P., and Macko, R. F. (1999). "Task-oriented" exercise improves hamstring strength and spastic reflexes in chronic stroke patients. *Stroke*, 30(10), 2112–2118.

Sporka, J., Kurniawan, H., and Slavík, P. (2006). Acoustic control of mouse pointer. *Universal Access in the Information Society*, 4(3), 237–245. doi: 10.1007/s10209–005–0010-z

Strode, S. W., Gustke, S., and Allen, A. (1999). Technical and clinical progress in telemedicine. *JAMA: The Journal of the American Medical Association*, 281(12), 1066–1068. doi: 10.1001/jama.281.12.1066

Struijk, L. (2006). A tongue based control for disabled people. In K. Miesenberger, J. Klaus, W. Zagler and A. Karshmer (Eds.), *Computers Helping People with Special Needs* (Vol. 4061, pp. 913–918). Berlin/Heidelberg: Springer.

Taub, E., Uswatte, G., van der Lee, J. H., Lankhorst, G. J., Bouter, L. M., and Wagenaar, R. C. (2000). Constraint-induced movement therapy and massed practice. *Stroke*, 31(4), 983–991.

Torsney, K. (2003). Advantages and disadvantages of telerehabilitation for persons with neurological disabilities. *Neurorehabilitation*, 18(2), 183–185.

Whitten, P. S., Mair, F. S., Haycox, A., May, C. R., Williams, T. L., and Hellmich, S. (2002). Systematic review of cost effectiveness studies of telemedicine interventions. *BMJ*, 324(7351), 1434–1437. doi: 10.1136/bmj.324.7351.1434

Wootton, R. (2001). Telemedicine. *BMJ*, 323(7312), 557–560. doi: 10.1136/bmj.323.7312.557

Zampolini, M., Baratta, S., Schifini, F., Spitali, C., Todeschini, E., Bernabeu, M., et al. (2007). *Upper Limb Telerehabilitation with Home Care and Activity Desk (HCAD) system*. Paper presented at Virtual Rehabilitation 2007, Venice, Italy.

Zhao, H., Plaisant, C., Shneiderman, B., and Lazar, J. (2008). Data sonification for users with visual impairment: A case study with georeferenced data. *ACM Transactions on Computer-Human Interaction*, 15(1), 1–28. doi: 10.1145/1352782.1352786

17

Brain–Computer Interfaces: The New Landscape in Assistive Technology

E. Pasqualotto, S. Federici, M. Olivetti Belardinelli, and N. Birbaumer

CONTENTS

17.1 What Is a Brain–Computer Interface?

A brain–computer interface (BCI) provides a direct connection between the brain and an external device, such as a computer or any other system capable of receiving a signal. In June 1999, the First International Meeting on Brain–Computer Interface Technology took place at the Rensselaerville Institute (Albany, NY). The aims of this first meeting, which 50 researchers from 22 different research groups attended, were to review the state of the art of BCI research and to define a shared set of procedures, methods, and definitions. During this meeting, it was established that "a brain–computer interface is a communication system that does not depend on the brain's normal output pathways of peripheral nerves and muscles" (Wolpaw et al. 2000). In a BCI, neuromuscular activity is not necessary for the production of the activity that is needed to convey the message (Pasqualotto et al. 2011a).

A BCI may be an assistive technology (AT) that allows communication in people that are paralyzed or have severe motor deficits. Most ATs usually require control by using muscles. For this reason, people with disabilities leading to progressive motor degeneration, such as amyotrophic lateral sclerosis (ALS), brainstem stroke, or severe cerebral palsy, lack any communication device. In recent years, thanks to refined technologies, different systems that enable a connection between the brain and a machine (e.g., a computer) have been developed.

A BCI uses the electrical, magnetic, and metabolic activity generated by neurons to give an input to an AT. This usually happens by measuring brain activity with brain imaging techniques. Different electrophysiological recordings are possible: invasive and noninvasive (Lebedev and Nicolelis 2006). The invasive method uses electrocorticography (ECoG), which is characterized by intracranial recordings of electrical activity, or direct activity of single neurons or neural assemblies. The noninvasive methods use electroencephalography (EEG), magnetoencephalography (MEG), functional magnetic resonance imaging (fMRI), and near-infrared spectroscopy (NIRS) to allow control over a personal computer or peripheral device. This kind of method is mostly used to enable paralyzed patients to develop a communication channel with the outside world (Wolpaw et al. 2002). BCI research usually focuses on EEG because of the portability and the low cost of this technique. To focus on patients, we will mainly present EEG-based BCI, providing some information on BCIs that are based on other techniques.

A century has passed since the discovery of the EEG (Swartz and Goldensohn 1998), and more than 30 years have gone by from the attempt to create an interface that is able to establish a direct connection between the brain and machines. Over the past 20 years, BCIs have seen a remarkable increase involving several research groups all over the world.

BCI systems consist of two separate functional blocks: a transducer, which translates the person's brain activity into usable control signals, and the peripheral device (Mason et al. 2005). The transducer is made of different parts (see Figure 17.1). Generally, there are sensors that record brain activity, which usually has a very small amplitude and needs to be amplified. To be usable, this signal needs to be cleaned from artifacts. Finally, often by using complex mathematical algorithms, the specific feature of the brain activity that will be used as an input can be extracted and translated. The assistive device component uses these control signals to perform a desired activity or function.

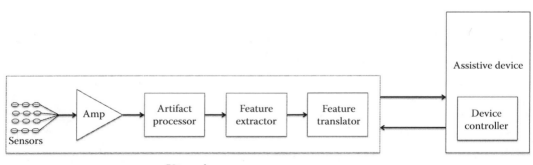

FIGURE 17.1
(See color insert.) Generally, the sensors record brain activity, which needs to be amplified. Then, the signal must be cleaned from artifacts. Finally, the feature of the brain activity that will be used as an input can be extracted and translated by an algorithm. The assistive device component uses these control signals to perform a desired activity or function.

17.2 Measuring Brain Activity

17.2.1 EEG

Electroencephalography (EEG) is a measure of the electrical activity of the brain. It is usually measured using multiple disk-shaped silver-silver chloride electrodes (Ag-AgCl electrodes) of dimensions in the range of 2–12 mm on the scalp. It usually requires the use of a conductive paste to reduce skin impedance, although dry electrodes that do not require a paste are in development (Popescu et al. 2007). The EEG recorded on the scalp reflects the sum of synchronous electrical activity of millions of pyramidal cells.

Neurons are excitable by voltage changes across their membranes. Because of the attenuation of the neuronal signal, it is only possible to record signals coming from the dendrites; therefore, EEG has a good temporal resolution but a poor spatial resolution. Although it is possible to record signals on the order of milliseconds, the spatial resolution is poor (around 1 cm) compared with other techniques (see Table 17.1).

17.2.2 MEG

Magnetoencephalography (MEG) is a measure of changes to the magnetic fields. This means that although maintaining the temporal resolution of the EEG (they measure the same signal), the spatial resolution is better. MEG is considered as a compromise because it offers the same temporal resolution of the EEG, but a spatial resolution closer to other techniques, such as fMRI.

The advantages of MEG are counterbalanced by its costs. Apart from the costs of the machine itself, MEG requires a magnetically shielded room to shield from all magnetic fields coming from outside of the head and to record only the magnetic fields of the brain. These magnetic fields are on the order of few femtotesla (10^{-15} T). Not only can the Earth's magnetic field interfere with MEG, but so can any electric source nearby that produces detectable fields. The brain's magnetic fields are sensed by superconducting quantum interference devices (SQUIDs) positioned in the helmet of the MEG.

17.2.3 fMRI

Functional magnetic resonance imaging (fMRI) uses a very strong magnet located inside of a horizontal tube, where a person can be positioned, to generate a stable magnetic field

TABLE 17.1

Comparison of Different Techniques to Measure Brain Activity

	Temporal Resolution	Spatial Resolution	Portability	Cost
EEG	~1 ms	~1 cm	High	Low
MEG	~1 ms	~1 mm	Not portable	Very high
fMRI	4–5 s	<1 mm	Not portable	High
NIRS	4–5 s	<3 cm	Low	Moderate

EEG and MEG have better temporal resolution, although MRI has the best spatial resolution. EEG is a quite portable technique, and NIRS might be considered as acceptably portable, whereas MEG and fMRI cannot be moved.

that is able to align hydrogen atoms. When the atomic nuclei are in a magnetic field, the protons inside tend to line up in the same direction. If these protons are hit by radio waves, their alignment is altered, inducing the protons to spin. In the process of returning to their original orientation, the protons resound with a short radio signal that is sent to a receiver, which processes the signals. fMRI is accurate within a millimeter, but it has the great disadvantage of being able to record a scan only every second, therefore presenting a low temporal resolution.

17.2.4 fNIRS

Functional near-infrared spectroscopy (fNIRS) uses the oxygen metabolism to measure brain activity. Whereas the fMRI measures the concentration of oxyhemoglobin and deoxyhemoglobin using their magnetic properties, NIRS measures the absorption of the near-infrared region of the electromagnetic spectrum in tissues.

The function of NIRS is easily explained with an example that almost everyone has experienced as a child. By placing a flashlight against a finger extremity, the light is still visible, although it has travelled through several centimeters of tissues. By using high peak laser diodes, light penetrates the scalp. The light passes through the superficial tissues of the head to the brain, and then from the brain to optodes (optical electrodes) that detect the light reflection or absorption. On this path, hemoglobin absorbs part of the light in different ways depending on whether it is oxygenated or deoxygenated. In this way, it is possible to have a measure of the concentration of blood and thus of brain activity. The NIRS systems have several advantages compared to other techniques: they are relatively portable and have an acceptable spatial resolution, although the temporal resolution is limited as in fMRI.

17.3 History of BCIs

In 1929, the German neuropsychiatrist Hans Berger (1873–1941), professor of psychiatry and director of the Jena Psychiatric University Clinic, published in *Zeitschrift für die Gesamte Neurologie und Psychiatrie* the paper "Über das Elektrenkephalogramm des Menschen" (Berger 1929), the first of 14 reports on the electroencephalogram. This system was supposedly able to measure potential differences of the brain from the scalp. Berger, who discovered the alpha rhythm, was the first to record an encephalogram. The new method did not gain immediate success until confirmation arrived from other scientists such as Adrian, Lennox, Gibbs, and Jasper (Wiedemann 1994). Over the following years, the technique became popular and several EEG laboratories were created for both clinical and research purposes.

At the time Hans Berger invented the EEG, he could not imagine that 40 years later, electroencephalography would be used to control machines exploiting brain impulses (Vidal 1973). Since the early years of the 1970s, the idea of using operant conditioning of neural events to control an external device became appealing. The goal was ambitious and the technology was advanced enough to adapt EEG systems for this purpose.

In 1968, Joseph Kamiya showed in a crucial paper that the alpha rhythm in humans could be subjected to operant conditioning. He showed that people learn to discriminate the presence and the absence of the alpha rhythm.* Moreover, using feedback, they could be trained to change the alpha rhythm's frequency. This paper deeply influenced the EEG field and it is considered the beginning of the neurofeedback area, which influenced the idea of using this control of brain waves to gain control of an external device.

The Advanced Research Projects Agency (ARPA, now renamed the Defense Advanced Research Projects Agency, or DARPA) and other government agencies funded several research projects,[†] and by the early 1970s they became interested in developing technologies "that would permit a more immersed and intimate interaction between humans and computers and would include so-called bionic applications" (Vidal 1999). Two projects are worth mentioning from these years: the first directed by Dr. George Lawrence, and the second directed by Dr. Jacques Vidal.

The first project was an internal project of ARPA. Dr. Lawrence's focus was on autoregulation and cognitive biofeedback, aiming to develop new techniques that would enhance human performance. Their focus was mainly on military applications because their aim was to enhance the performance of military personnel engaged in tasks demanding high mental loads (Wolpaw et al. 2000). This research did not produce valuable results, although it produced some interesting insights on biofeedback. After this project, the focus was shifted to a different approach.

At the University of California–Los Angeles (UCLA), an important project funded by the National Science Foundation (NSF), and then by ARPA, gained attention. In this research project, the term "brain–computer interface" was used for the first time in a scientific article (Vidal 1973). Dr. Vidal, Director of the Brain–Computer Interface Laboratory at UCLA, was the head of this project. One of the most interesting outcomes of this project was to show the possibility of using single-trial visual evoked potentials (VEPs) as a communication channel (Vidal 1977). Vidal used computer-generated visual stimulation and sophisticated signal processing to allow a subject to control a cursor positioned in a maze on a display. It was possible to control the cursor by a sequence of turns in four different directions.

According to Wolpaw and colleagues (2000), Vidal highlighted the significance of discriminating between the EEG activity and the electromyographic (EMG) activity coming from the scalp or facial muscles. For this reason, one of the aims of the First International Meeting on BCI was to define BCIs to exclude the muscular activity.

Over the next two decades, BCI grew as a research field, taking advantage of a better understanding of brain processes and functions and of the new personal computer era that brought cheap and powerful machines. Few of the current BCI applications are actually dedicated to restore communication and movement in patients with severe and multiple disabilities (Lebedev and Nicolelis 2006; Birbaumer et al. 2008; Daly and Wolpaw 2008).

Several BCI software programs were developed to serve as a general platform for different applications. These tools were generally open-source, easy to set up, and could also be modified and adapted to new research paradigms. BCI2000 (Schalk et al. 2004; Mellinger and Schalk 2007), BioSig (Schlögl et al. 2007), and Open-VIBE (Arrouet et al. 2005) are examples of computer platforms that can be used to record, analyze, and translate the EEG signal into a BCI application.

---

* The alpha rhythm, discovered by Hans Berger, is an oscillation in the frequency range of 8–12 Hz. It originates in the occipital lobe and it is usually associated with a wakeful relaxed state with closed eye
† ARPA funded the project ARPANET, which later became what we now know as the Internet.

17.4 Communication

17.4.1 Potential Users

BCIs are intended to be used by those disabled individuals for whom other common ATs are ineffective because of their dependency on voluntary muscular control. Neurodegenerative and motor diseases, such as Guillain Barré syndrome, ALS, brainstem stroke, and traumatic or metabolic brain disease, may lead to severe or complete motor paralysis, making communication hard or impossible (Kübler and Birbaumer 2008). In 1966, Plum and Posner (1966) tried to define the locked-in syndrome (LIS), a condition of quadriplegia and anarthria leading to a state of complete paralysis without impairing cognition. In this state, the classical LIS condition, patients have residual eye movements that may be used for communication (Feldman 1971). Subsequently, Bauer and colleagues (1979) added to this classical definition two more stages. Incomplete LIS is a state in which some residual movements, such as the control of a finger or of some facial muscles, are still preserved and may therefore be used for communication. Total LIS or complete LIS (CLIS) is a state in which all eye movements are compromised and a condition of total immobility persists.

As Birbaumer and colleagues state, "These locked-in patients ultimately become unable to express themselves and to communicate even their most basic wishes or desires, as they can no longer control their muscles to activate communication devices" (Birbaumer et al. 1999).

Because of the inability of these patients to communicate, their condition may be misdiagnosed as a vegetative state or coma instead of LIS (Gallo and Fontanarosa 1989). There are reports claiming that it may take several years before LIS patients are recognized as being conscious (Laureys et al. 2005), although it has been shown that it is possible to obtain minimal consciousness behavioral signs with simple contingent conditioning (Lancioni et al. 2008). LIS patients in a medically stable condition with appropriate medical care could have a normal life expectancy of several decades (Doble et al. 2003).

Although in classical and incomplete LIS some residual movements are preserved and used as communication channels, for example using eye tracking systems (Calvo et al. 2008) or mechanical switches (Lancioni et al. 2008; 2009, 2010), only a BCI could potentially be used in all types of LIS (see Table 17.2). Moreover, other devices are often too difficult to use compared with BCIs.

In the future, people with less severe disabilities may also benefit from this technology. At present, several problems still need to be resolved. No study has so far proven the

TABLE 17.2

A Comparison of Some Technologies

	Eye Tracker	Etran	Switch	Joystick	BCI
Incomplete LIS	X	X	X	X	X
LIS	X	X	X	X	X
CLIS					X

Although all technologies such as the eye tracker, the Etran table, mechanical switch, or joysticks can be used in incomplete and classical LIS, only the BCI may be used during the entire progression of the disease.

long-term reliability of BCIs, and although there are studies that demonstrated the influence of mood and motivation on BCI performance (Nijboer et al. 2010), we do not know whether the use of such a technology may or may not improve the quality of life. Several studies have shown that ALS patients with adequate care and basic communication systems have a reasonable quality of life (Simmons et al. 2000; Robbins et al. 2001; Lulé et al. 2009; Matuz et al. 2010).

17.4.2 Development

The first published "mental prostheses" was the P300 Speller developed by Farwell and Donchin (1988). This system, which is still used in many applications, records the P300 event-related potential. This potential is a positive deflection of the EEG 300-ms post-stimulus, and it is elicited by focusing the attention on a series of stimuli events, with some rare or unexpected stimuli. The P300 Speller uses this procedure, which is called the "oddball paradigm," intensifying random rows and columns of a matrix containing the letters of the alphabet and other commands (see Figure 17.2). When the patient wishes to communicate, he/she focuses attention on a letter of the matrix. In this way, the content becomes relevant and rare (in a 6 × 6 matrix, 12 intensifications occur but only 2 identify a single cell, 1 for the row and 1 for the column), thus eliciting a P300 potential.

Several applications based on the P300 Speller were built for communication and entertainment, and it is currently one of the most used BCIs. Studies on the P300 Speller for communication (Donchin et al. 2000) and on its use to control Internet browsers and e-mails (Karim et al. 2006; Bensch et al. 2007; Mugler et al. 2008, 2010), painting applications (Münbinger et al. 2010), and real and virtual environments (Bayliss 2003; Cincotti et al. 2009), were published.

Using a different technique, Birbaumer and colleagues were the first to provide an experimental verification of the use of a BCI to communicate with ALS LIS patients

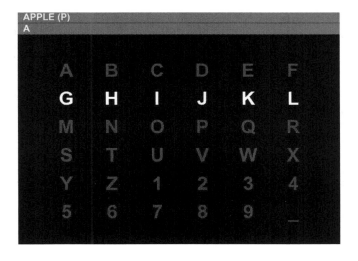

FIGURE 17.2
(See color insert.) The P300 signal is elicited by focusing attention on a series of stimuli events, which comprise rare, unexpected or relevant stimuli. In order to create this effect, the P300 Speller randomly intensifies rows and columns of the matrix containing the letters of the alphabet and other commands. When the patient wishes to communicate something, he/she focuses attention on a cell of the matrix while the rows and columns are intensifying.

(Birbaumer et al. 1999). Whereas the P300 Speller used a "natural" phenomenon of brain activity, Birbaumer and colleagues used a technique closer to neurofeedback, the conditioning of slow cortical potentials (SCPs). Many studies previously demonstrated that people have been able to voluntarily self-regulate brain activity through feedback and reward with neurofeedback. Expectations were high, and hasty statements about its clinical success that were based on single case studies were made, discrediting the field early on. In 1969, Miller claimed operant control of autonomic and central functions in curarized rats, proving that voluntary operant regulation of bodily functions was possible and thus excluding the mediation of the motor system through curarization (Miller 1969). Despite the initial excitement, the results of this experiment were impossible to replicate (Dworkin and Miller 1986). As Birbaumer, Ramos Murguialday, Weber, and Montoya have claimed (2009), the overstatements made about biofeedback and the Miller (1969) and Dworkin and Miller (1986) incident halted public funding of large, controlled clinical studies, although some indications of biofeedback's efficiency were available. Only some years later has it been shown that consistent SCP self-regulation may affect the number of ictal events in some patients with drug-resistant epilepsy (Rockstroh et al. 1993; Kotchoubey et al. 2001). The same positive effect has also been reported using biofeedback of skin conductance responses (GSR) (Nagai et al. 2004), confirming previous reports of the decrease in negative SCPs at the cortical level during GSR control and thus increasing seizure thresholds (Birbaumer et al. 1990; Rockstroh et al. 1993; Kotchoubey et al. 2001).

SCPs usually last from 300 ms to several seconds. Polarization variations originate from depolarization of the apical dendritic tree, in the upper cortical layer, provoked by a series of synchronous activations mainly resulting from thalamo-cortical afferents. This system regulates the excitation (with negative potentials) and the inhibition (with positive potentials) of cortical circuits.

In those studies that used training and visual feedback of positive SCPs in focal epilepsies, some patients achieved virtually 100% accuracy in the control of SCPs after extensive training over 30–50 sessions. This important result paved the way for the use of SCPs on ALS patients as a means of communication (Birbaumer et al. 1999).

In a typical experiment, patients are presented with two target goals at the top and at the bottom of the screen. Continuous feedback is given using a cursor that moves based on SCP amplitude. To learn how to regulate SCP amplitude, patients are told that negative and positive SCP amplitudes are elicited by moving the cursor toward the top rectangle and the bottom rectangle, respectively (Kübler et al. 2001; Kübler and Birbaumer, 2008). To reinforce the association between brain control and cursor during the training phase, a smiling face appears in the center of the screen when the association is correct. When patients achieve good control in the training phase (approximately 75% of trials in which targets were reached correctly), they are provided with the Language Support Program (LSP) (Birbaumer et al. 2000; Neumann et al. 2003). The same goals on the top and bottom part of the screen are used to present a dichotomous version of letters. At each step, the user can either accept or block the target letter. To select a letter, patients usually move the cursor downward, producing cortical positivity. Selection speed is not high: On several occasions, subjects had to be trained for months to be able to control SCPs (Kübler et al. 2001; Kübler and Birbaumer, 2008).

To improve the subject's performance, it is necessary to have algorithms that classify the different components of the EEG as accurately as possible. Therefore, the study and implementation of different mathematical algorithms for EEG classification was necessary for both offline and online use (Hinterberger et al. 2003; Dornhege et al. 2007). For this purpose, a virtual international competition is held regularly to validate signal processing and classification methods for BCIs, and the results are published in peer-reviewed journals. Many researchers have taken up this challenge (Sajda et al. 2003; Blankertz et al. 2004, 2006).

A key point in using BCIs with LIS patients is their usefulness as a cognitive rehabilitation device. At the present moment, CLIS patients are not able to communicate with BCI devices (Kübler and Birbaumer 2008). In 2007, one study reported 17 CLIS patients trained with a NIRS-based BCI (Naito et al. 2007). Questions requiring simple "yes" and "no" answers were presented to the patients. The "yes" answer was associated with an increase in the blood oxygenation of the patients, whereas the "no" answer was associated with a decrease. Seven patients achieved 70% correctness, although the study suffered from a lack of quantification and definition of the clinical criteria used for the CLIS patients (Birbaumer et al. 2009).

It has been frequently proposed that LIS patients lack communication because of the progression of the disease (Sellers and Donchin 2006). Birbaumer (2006) and Kübler and Birbaumer (2008) explained that in long-term paralyzed patients, intentional thoughts are rarely followed by rewarding or punishing stimuli, causing a decrease of causal contingency perception between the thought and its consequences, which progressively extinguishes in the complete locked-in state. Extensive use of a BCI beginning before the locked-in state may potentially help in providing the rewarding stimuli necessary for causal attribution, supposedly preventing a complete lack of communication.

17.5 Motor Restoration

17.5.1 Potential Users

Severe injuries of the motor system, such as a stroke or traumatic brain or spinal cord injury, may lead to paralysis or semiparalysis of the limbs. Depending on the severity and location of the injury, these diseases can cause breathing difficulties, numbness, and sensory changes as well as severe weakness or paralysis of the limbs. When injuries occur at the chest level of the spinal cord, there can be a condition called paraplegia, impairing motor and/or sensory functions of the lower limbs. When the injury occurs at the neck level of the spinal cord, impairment can occur at the upper and lower limbs, and injuries at the trunk level can cause breathing problems. This condition is known as tetraplegia or quadriplegia.

It has been reported that in 2005, in the United States, approximately 250,000 persons were surviving a spinal cord injury (Wyndaele and Wyndaele 2006). It has also been estimated that the annual incidence in the United States of spinal cord injuries is approximately 11,000 new cases each year, not considering people who do not survive the accident. Stroke is also a major concern for public health. Approximately 750,000 strokes occur each year in the United States (Carandang et al. 2006). In the United Kingdom, approximately 50% of stroke survivors are left dependent on other people for everyday activities (Rothwell et al. 2004), whereas in Germany one-third of the patients that survive the first year present with hemiplegia (Millán et al. 2010). Nearly one-third of stroke patients are not able to use the paralyzed limb one year after the injury (Lai et al. 2002), and no effective treatment is available (Birbaumer et al. 2008; Buch et al. 2008), causing a considerable negative impact on the patients, their families, and the society.

17.5.2 BCI in Movement Restoration

BCIs could be used to activate devices for assisting movements. In addition to using brain signals to control wheelchairs (Rebsamen et al. 2007; Galán et al. 2008; Iturrate et al. 2009; Millán et al. 2010), a challenge is to use them to control devices that could assist the movements of the limbs.

Functional reorganization of the motor cortex plays either an adaptive or a maladaptive role in modifying the intact cortical tissue (Nudo et al. 2001). Since the first successful attempt to train a tetraplegic patient to control a device applied to hand muscles using the mu rhythm (Pfurtscheller et al. 2000), BCIs have been considered possible rehabilitation devices (Dobkin 2007). The use of BCIs in motor retraining was extended to other techniques using invasive methods with implanted electrodes in tetraplegic patients (Hochberg et al. 2006) or noninvasive MEG-modulated mu rhythms to control a hand orthosis (Birbaumer 2006; Buch et al. 2008).

By recording the brain activity, it is possible to detect cortical activity originating from the sensorimotor areas; this activity varies between 8 and 12 Hz and is present if subjects are not engaged in processing motor information or in producing or imagining movement. Sensorimotor rhythm (SMR) is produced during inactivity and is caused by thalamo-cortical circuits. Such rhythms have different terms (Wolpaw et al. 2003). By using event-related synchronization (ERS) (mu-increase) and desynchronization (ERD) (mu-decrease), Pfurtscheller and colleagues trained a patient to operate a hand orthosis by imagination of specific motor commands. Afterward, they convincingly demonstrated the potential usefulness of SMR-BCIs for motor restoration of hand grasp functions (Pfurtscheller et al. 2003a, 2003b). Using the beta oscillations generated by patients while imagining foot movement, Pfurtscheller and colleagues were able to analyze and classify the EEG with a BCI and to use the output signal to control a functional electrical stimulation (FES) device. A FES device is a system that uses electrical stimulation to stimulate peripheral nerves controlling specific muscles, or groups of them, to activate lost bodily functions such as grasping, walking and standing, and bowel and bladder management. Generally, FES systems for grasping are limited by the fact that only the patients who maintain voluntary control of the shoulder and elbow are able to use these devices (Millán et al. 2010). Thus, showing the feasibility of the combination of a BCI and an FES device, Pfurtscheller's work gave an important impulse to the BCI community (Pfurtscheller et al. 2003a, 2003b). In this study, a tetraplegic patient after a long training period was able to trigger the FES device by imagining foot movements. Stimulating the forearm nerves, the FES device activated the required movements to grasp with the paralyzed hand a cylinder placed in front of the patient.

The use of an MEG-BCI was exploited, showing as proof of concept successful BCI control of grasping functions in healthy subjects (Mellinger et al. 2007) and in stroke patients (Buch et al. 2008). The system used the activity of three of the 275 MEG sensors to control the orthosis; the patient opened the hand by increasing the mu rhythm, and by decreasing the mu rhythm the patient closed the hand. Patients with chronic hand plegia resulting from stroke participated in 13–22 training sessions to gain control of the orthosis. At the end of the training, they were able to control the opening and closing functions of an orthosis attached to the plegic hand, but no one showed clinical improvements in the completely paralyzed hands without the prosthetic device. An important effect of the training was the refocusing of MEG activity, which provided the first evidence that training with a BCI may result in cortical reorganization (Birbaumer et al. 2009). As a further evidence of brain reorganization after BCI training, Caria and colleagues (2011) found increased lateralization toward the ipsilesional sensorimotor regions in a patient with severe hand paresis after using a MEG- and EEG-based BCI in combination with physiotherapy.

17.6 BCI and Behavioral Disorders

17.6.1 Epilepsy and ADHD

Researchers have used neurofeedback training with various EEG measures to treat patients with pharmacologically intractable or insufficiently tractable diseases, such as intractable epilepsy and attention deficit hyperactivity disorder (ADHD). Epilepsy is a severe neurological disorder that is characterized by seizures, caused by an excessive and synchronous activity of the central nervous system (CNS). This abnormal activity causes symptoms that vary depending on the type of epilepsy and can affect patients in different ways. A seizure can last from few seconds to minutes, sometimes with loss of consciousness and/or loss of muscular control, with tonic, clonic, and myoclonic muscle spasms, or a mixture of these. The World Health Organization (WHO) estimates that epilepsy affects at least 50 million people worldwide (Dua et al. 2006). Epilepsy can be treated pharmacologically, but some people do not respond to any medications.

Other potential users of BCIs are ADHD patients. ADHD is a neurodevelopmental disorder, with inattention, hyperactivity, and impulsivity (Zwi et al. 2000). The term ADHD and the disorder is a controversial issue. The extent to which symptoms are considered pathological varies and should be assessed in the context of the child's developmental level. A prevalent theory links this disorder to abnormal development in the dopaminergic and noradrenergic cortico-subcortical networks, which are important for executive functions and the regulation of attention. Approximately 3–5% of children are affected by ADHD, and they are usually treated with stimulants that decrease impulsivity and hyperactivity and increase attention. Nevertheless, there is a strong demand for nonpharmacological treatments because of several concerns about the use of stimulant medication during development (Strehl et al. 2006).

17.6.2 Neurofeedback in Epilepsy and ADHD

The first clinical application was the use of slow cortical potential (SCP) regulation to control untreatable epileptic seizures (Kotchoubey et al. 2001). As previously mentioned (see Section 17.4.1), several studies have shown that learning to control SCPs affects the number of ictal events in patients with drug-resistant epilepsy (mostly with secondarily generalized seizures) (Rockstroh et al. 1993; Kotchoubey et al. 2001). A more recent study, which included the self-regulation of SCPs in a behavioral self-management program, confirmed that more than half of the patients involved had significant reductions in the number of seizures (Strehl et al. 2005).

By using similar procedures, BCIs have shown good success in the treatment of children with ADHD (Strehl et al. 2006; Fuchs et al. 2003). In these studies, although with small samples, it was shown that it is possible to improve attention and vigilance (for a complete review on the effects of different treatments on ADHD, refer to Toplak et al. 2008). Thus, the mitigation of ADHD symptoms obtained with SCP self-regulation is comparable to the improvements obtained with medication without any negative side effects (Birbaumer and Cohen 2007).

These groundbreaking studies highlighted the possibility of modifying cognitive functions, paving the road for new applications of BCI technology. One of the most recent directions concerning clinical applications is the use of a BOLD regulation-based BCI to treat emotional disorders such as psychopathy and schizophrenia (Birbaumer et al. 2005, 2008). Several studies have shown that it is possible to control emotion-related brain activity using real-time fMRI (rt-fMRI) (Weiskopf et al. 2003, 2004a, 2004b; Phan et al. 2004; Caria et al. 2007). In a typical experiment, subjects try to increase and decrease the BOLD response from a region of interest. The BOLD response is usually displayed on a screen giving feedback to the subjects with a delay of approximately 1–3 s. By using this protocol, several studies have already explored the feasibility of self-regulation of different brain regions. The regulation of the BOLD response from premotor and motor areas can lead to changes in the motor response speed, whereas from parahippocampal areas it can lead to changes in explicit memory performance (Weiskopf et al. 2004b, 2007). The regulation of the anterior cingulate region leads to decrease of pain (deCharms et al. 2005). Finally, regulation of the anterior insula can lead to changes in negative emotional responses (Caria et al. 2007; Lee et al. 2011) as face perception (Ruiz et al. 2011).

The feasibility of a NIRS-BCI was exploited by measuring oxygenated and deoxygenated hemoglobin changes during left- and right-hand motor imagery in five healthy subjects (Sitaram et al. 2007). By using a Hidden Markov Model (HMM) algorithm, Sitaram and colleagues successfully classified the imagery of the two hands with an accuracy of 89%.

17.7 Assistive Technologies and BCI

BCIs represent one of the most pioneering fields in AT. Therefore, it is necessary to consider the complexity of the assignment process of ATs. As recently pointed out, BCIs might be seen as an AT in the area of information and communication technologies (AT ICT) (Millán et al. 2010): "AT ICT products are understood to be devices for helping a person to receive, send, produce and/or process information in different forms" (ISO 2007). According to this definition, BCIs should be considered as ATs that support daily life activities. It is important to match person and technology to avoid dissatisfaction and abandonment (Louise-Bender Pape et al. 2002). It is widely accepted that personal factors can serve as significant barriers and facilitators to the use of AT (Scherer et al. 2011). The predisposition to the use of technology could depend on personal and psychosocial characteristics, such as users' personality, quality of life, abilities, and beliefs (Scherer et al. 2005). ATs are not considered as deficit compensation systems, but they involve personal well-being and social participation. Only considering the use in a real environment could it be possible to meet the needs of its intended users and to entail the consideration of a broad range of functional and nonfunctional attributes (Stephanidis et al. 1998). The notion of quality integrates the traditional concept of usability (Abran et al. 2003) and includes aspects that are not easily measurable on the basis of performance criteria.

The proper BCI should be assessed based on the individual needs and specifics of the health conditions of the patient (Nijboer et al. 2010). Although it was shown that ALS patients can use SCPs (Birbaumer et al. 1999), P300 (Sellers and Donchin 2006), and SMRs (Kübler et al. 2005), it has still not been demonstrated that completely locked-in patients could use these technologies (Kübler and Birbaumer 2008). However, Birbaumer and colleagues successfully tested a new procedure with CLIS successfully (personal communication).

Although there is a well-established tradition in BCI research, there are only few studies on the usability of BCIs (Pasqualotto et al. 2009, 2011b, 2011c) and a general lack of assessment studies (Pasqualotto et al. 2011a). However, considering BCIs for communication as an example, we can identify some limitations.

Only few studies have involved LIS patients in the long-term use of BCIs, and none of them proved long-term efficacy. Although this technology is supposed to be usable for a long time, studies with LIS patients generally only lasted a few hours. The effects of EEG changes on long-term use of a BCI have not been assessed yet.

Another two problematic points that could affect the patients' evaluation of the technology (and therefore affect the probability of abandonment) are the usability and aesthetics of BCIs. At present, aesthetics could be seen as a secondary problem in the use of this technology. However, it is important to note that traditional EEG is not appealing to patients because of the electrodes and the cables; conductive paste that tends to dry up in a few hours, thus needing replacement; and caps required for electrode placement. The possible use of dry EEG electrodes and wireless technology (Popescu et al. 2007; Gargiulo et al. 2010; Grozea et al. 2011) will probably improve the usability and therefore the acceptance of BCIs.

Moreover, it is still necessary to improve the software to simplify operations. Although several open-source platforms exist, handling communication still requires an external operator. An alternative technical solution could be the hybrid BCI designed by Pfurtscheller and colleagues (2010). A BCI usually relies on a single brain signal. A hybrid BCI could consist instead of two or more different signals (such as EEG and GSR) and use one of them as a "brain switch" or as a "selector" to detect a brain state that functions as a command.

To assess, it is necessary to identify the right tools for this process, and most of the classical psychological questionnaires and physiological measures cannot be applied to paralyzed persons (Birbaumer 2006). Parallel to the development of the BCI technology, tools for evaluation should become available for those who will perform the assessment process to match the technology with the users.

17.8 Conclusions

Beginning in the 1970s, the idea of communicating directly through brain activity shifted from science fiction to actual applications. The increase of studies, funding, and papers during the 1990s lead a large BCI community, documented in the First International Meeting on Brain–Computer Interface Technology in 1999, to establish a shared definition: A BCI is a psychophysiological system that does not depend on the brain's normal output pathways of peripheral nerves and muscles.

Two different methods of electrophysiological recordings are normally used: invasive and noninvasive. The invasive electrocorticography, which is characterized by intracranial recordings of electrical activity with macroscopic electrodes or microelectrodes, records directly from single neurons. The noninvasive method uses electroencephalography, magnetoencephalography, functional magnetic resonance imaging, and near-infrared spectroscopy to allow for control of a personal computer or a peripheral device. BCI research usually focuses on EEG because of the portability and the affordable costs. However, NIRS in particular seems to be promising.

Most of the current BCI applications are dedicated to the restoration of communication and movement in patients with severe and multiple disabilities. As a means of communication, BCIs have been developed for severely paralyzed patients. Neurodegenerative and motor diseases may lead to severe or complete paralysis, making communication difficult or impossible. ATs are ineffective with these patients because of their requirement for voluntary muscular control. By using different components of EEG activity, several applications have been developed. The P300 Speller is probably one of the most used applications, not only for communication, but also for the control of Internet browsers and e-mail clients, painting applications, and real and virtual environments. However, CLIS patients cannot use it because of compromised vision and/or cognition. By using SCPs it has been shown that ALS LIS patients could use BCIs. Intentional thoughts are rarely followed by rewarding stimuli in long-term paralyzed patients, resulting in a lack of causal contingency perception between the thought and its consequences, which may result in the extinction of goal-directed thinking in the CLIS. Thus, extensive use of a BCI before the CLIS may assist in providing the rewarding stimuli necessary for causal attribution.

Stroke and traumatic brain or spinal cord injury may lead to paralysis or semiparalysis of the limbs. BCIs may activate devices for assistive movements. Pfurtscheller showed that a tetraplegic patient could control a device applied to hand muscles using the mu rhythm. An MEG-BCI was used to control grasping functions in stroke patients. This study also showed that training with a BCI may result in cortical reorganization.

Finally, BCIs could be used to treat patients with diseases that are pharmacologically intractable or insufficiently tractable, such as some types of epilepsy and ADHD. In fact, it has been shown that there is a positive effect on attention and vigilance in ADHD patients. Moreover, the mitigation of symptoms obtained with SCP self-regulation is comparable to the improvements obtained with medication. Another clinical application is the use of a BOLD regulation-based BCI to treat emotional disorders, such as psychopathy and schizophrenia. The self-regulation of specific brain areas can lead to changes in motor response speed, explicit memory performance, and downregulation of pain and in emotional responses such as face perception.

Although BCIs represent one of the most pioneering fields in AT, it is necessary to work on an assessment process to avoid dissatisfaction and abandonment. Personal factors can serve as significant barriers and facilitators to the use of AT; therefore, only when considering the real use is it possible to meet the needs of its intended users.

The proper BCI, and the specific brain signals that should be used, need to be assessed considering the individual needs and health conditions of the patient. There have been only a few studies on the usability of BCIs, and assessment studies are generally lacking. It is necessary to identify the right tools for the assignment and evaluation process because most classical psychological questionnaires and physiological measures cannot be applied to the life of a paralyzed person.

Summary of the Chapter

In this chapter, we analyzed what a BCI is and how it could be considered as an AT. First, we underlined the definition of AT: A BCI is a communication system that does not depend on the brain's normal output pathways of peripheral nerves and muscles. We then explained the basis of the different techniques for measuring brain activity, highlighting for each the pros and cons. We then described the historical excursus from the 1970s to the most recent advances and applications. Furthermore, we described the practical uses of BCIs, which are communication, motor restoration, and clinical treatment of diseases that are not pharmacologically tractable. Finally, we analyzed the perspective of a center for technical aid and the requirements to assess the assignment and evaluation process to match BCIs and patients.

References

Abran, A., Khelifi, A., Suryn, W., and Seffah, A. (2003). Usability meanings and interpretations in ISO standards. *Software Quality Journal, 11*(4), 325–338.

Arrouet, C., Congedo, M., Marvie, J. E., Lamarche, F., Lécuyer, A., and Arnaldi, B. (2005). Open-Vibe: A 3D platform for real-time neuroscience. *Journal of Neurotherapy, 9*(1), 3–25.

Bauer, G., Gerstenbrand, F., and Rumpl, E. (1979). Varieties of the locked-in syndrome. *Journal of Neurology, 221*, 77–91.

Bayliss, J. D. (2003). Use of the evoked potential P3 component for control in a virtual apartment. *IEEE Transactions on Neural Systems and Rehabilitation Engineering, 11*(2), 113–116. doi:10.1109/TNSRE.2003.814438

Bensch, M., Karim, A. A., Mellinger, J., Hinterberger, T., Tangermann, M., Bogdan, M., et al. (2007). Nessi: An EEG-controlled web browser for severely paralyzed patients. *Computational Intelligence and Neuroscience, 2007*, 71863. doi:10.1155/2007/71863

Berger, H. (1929). Uber das elektrenkephalogramm des menschen. *Zeitschrift Für Die Gesamte Neurologie Und Psychiatrie, 87*, 527–570.

Birbaumer, N. (2006). Breaking the silence: Brain–computer interfaces (BCI) for communication and motor control. *Psychophysiology, 43*(6), 517–532. doi:10.1111/j.1469–8986.2006.00456.x

Birbaumer, N., and Cohen, L. G. (2007). Brain–computer interfaces: Communication and restoration of movement in paralysis. *The Journal of Physiology, 579*(Pt 3), 621–636. doi:10.1113/jphysiol.2006.125633

Birbaumer, N., Elbert, T., Canavan, A. G., and Rockstroh, B. (1990). Slow potentials of the cerebral cortex and behavior. *Physiological Reviews, 70*(1), 1–41.

Birbaumer, N., Ghanayim, N., Hinterberger, T., Iversen, I., Kotchoubey, B., Kübler, A., et al. (1999). A spelling device for the paralysed. *Nature, 398*(6725), 297–298.

Birbaumer, N., Kübler, A., Ghanayim, N., Hinterberger, T., Perelmouter, J., Kaiser, J., et al. (2000). The thought translation device (TTD) for completely paralyzed patients. *IEEE Transactions on Rehabilitation Engineering, 8*(2), 190–193.

Birbaumer, N., Murguialday, A. R., and Cohen, L. (2008). Brain–computer interface in paralysis. *Current Opinion in Neurology, 21*(6), 634–638. doi:10.1097/WCO.0b013e328315ee2d

Birbaumer, N., Ramos Murguialday, A., Weber, C., and Montoya, P. (2009). Neurofeedback and brain–computer interface clinical applications. *International Review of Neurobiology, 86*, 107–117. doi:10.1016/S0074–7742(09)86008-X

Birbaumer, N., Veit, R., Lotze, M., Erb, M., Hermann, C., Grodd, W., and Flor, H. (2005). Deficient fear conditioning in psychopathy: A functional magnetic resonance imaging study. *Archives of General Psychiatry, 62*(7), 799–805. doi:10.1001/archpsyc.62.7.799

Blankertz, B., Müller, K. R., Curio, G., Vaughan, T. M., Schalk, G., Wolpaw, J. R., et al. (2004). The BCI competition 2003: Progress and perspectives in detection and discrimination of EEG single trials. *IEEE Transactions on Biomedical Engineering, 51*(6), 1044–1051. doi:10.1109/TBME.2004.826692

Blankertz, B., Müller, K. R., Krusienski, D. J., Schalk, G., Wolpaw, J. R., Schlögl, A., et al. (2006). The BCI competition. III: Validating alternative approaches to actual BCI problems. *IEEE Transactions on Neural Systems and Rehabilitation Engineering, 14*(2), 153–159. doi:10.1109/TNSRE.2006.875642

Buch, E., Weber, C., Cohen, L. G., Braun, C., Dimyan, M. A., Ard, T., et al. (2008). Think to move: A neuromagnetic brain–computer interface (BCI) system for chronic stroke. *Stroke: A Journal of Cerebral Circulation, 39*(3), 910–917. doi:10.1161/STROKEAHA.107.505313

Calvo, A., Chiò, A., Castellina, E., Corno, F., Farinetti, L., Ghiglione, P., et al. (2008). Eye tracking impact on quality-of-life of ALS patients. In *Lecture Notes in Computer Science: Computers helping people with special needs.* (Vol. 5105 pp. 70–77). Heidelberg, Germany: Springer. doi:10.1007/978–3-540–70540–6_9

Carandang, R., Seshadri, S., Beiser, A., Kelly-Hayes, M., Kase, C. S., Kannel, W. B., and Wolf, P. A. (2006). Trends in incidence, lifetime risk, severity, and 30-day mortality of stroke over the past 50 years. *JAMA: The Journal of the American Medical Association, 296*(24), 2939–2946. doi:10.1001/jama.296.24.2939

Caria, A., Veit, R., Sitaram, R., Lotze, M., Weiskopf, N., Grodd, W., and Birbaumer, N. (2007). Regulation of anterior insular cortex activity using real-time fMRI. *Neuroimage, 35*(3), 1238–1246. doi:10.1016/j.neuroimage.2007.01.018

Caria, A., Weber, C., Brötz, D., Ramos, A., Ticini, L. F., Gharabaghi, A., et al. (2011). Chronic stroke recovery after combined BCI training and physiotherapy: A case report. *Psychophysiology, 48*(4), 578–582. doi:10.1111/j.1469–8986.2010.01117.x

Cincotti, F., Quitadamo, L., Aloise, F., Bianchi, L., Babiloni, F., and Mattia, D. (2009). Interacting with the environment through non-invasive brain–computer interfaces. *Universal Access in Human-Computer Interaction. Intelligent and Ubiquitous Interaction Environments,* 483–492.

Daly, J. J., and Wolpaw, J. R. (2008). Brain–Computer interfaces in neurological rehabilitation. *IEEE Transactions on Neural Systems and Rehabilitation Engineering, 7*(11), 1032–1043. doi:10.1016/S1474–4422(08)70223–0

deCharms, R. C., Maeda, F., Glover, G. H., Ludlow, D., Pauly, J. M., Soneji, D., et al. (2005). Control over brain activation and pain learned by using real-time functional MRI. *Proceedings of the National Academy of Sciences of the United States of America, 102*(51), 18626–18631. doi:10.1073/pnas.0505210102

Dobkin, B. H. (2007). Brain–computer interface technology as a tool to augment plasticity and outcomes for neurological rehabilitation. *The Journal of Physiology, 579*(Pt 3), 637–642. doi:10.1113/jphysiol.2006.123067

Doble, J. E., Haig, A. J., Anderson, C., and Katz, R. (2003). Impairment, activity, participation, life satisfaction, and survival in persons with locked-in syndrome for over a decade: Follow-up on a previously reported cohort. *The Journal of Head Trauma Rehabilitation, 18*(5), 435.

Donchin, E., Spencer, K. M., and Wijesinghe, R. (2000). The mental prosthesis: Assessing the speed of a p300-based brain–computer interface. *IEEE Transactions on Rehabilitation Engineering, 8*(2), 174–179.

Dornhege, G., Millán, J. d. R., Hinterberger, T., McFarland, D. J., and Müler, K. R. (2007). *Toward Brain–Computer Interfacing.* Cambridge MA: MIT Press

Dua, T., de Boer, H. M., Prilipko, L. L., and Saxena, S. (2006). Epilepsy care in the world: Results of an ILAE/IBE/WHO global campaign against epilepsy survey. *Epilepsia, 47*(7), 1225–1231. doi:10.1111/j.1528–1167.2006.00595.x

Dworkin, B. R., and Miller, N. E. (1986). Failure to replicate visceral learning in the acute curarized rat preparation. *Behavioral Neuroscience, 100*(3), 299–314.

Farwell, L. A., and Donchin, E. (1988). Talking off the top of your head: Toward a mental prosthesis utilizing event-related brain potentials. *Electroencephalography and Clinical Neurophysiology, 70*(6), 510–523.

Feldman, M. H. (1971). Physiological observations in a chronic case of "locked-in" syndrome. *Neurology, 21*(5), 459–478.

Fuchs, T., Birbaumer, N., Lutzenberger, W., Gruzelier, J. H., and Kaiser, J. (2003). Neurofeedback training for attention-deficit/ hyperactivity disorder in children: A comparison with methylphenidate. *Applied Psychophysiology and Biofeedback, 28*, 1–12.

Galán, F., Nuttin, M., Lew, E., Ferrez, P. W., Vanacker, G., Philips, J., et al. (2008). A brain-actuated wheelchair: Asynchronous and non-invasive brain–computer interfaces for continuous control of robots. *Clinical Neurophysiology, 119*(9), 2159–2169. doi:10.1016/j.clinph.2008.06.001

Gallo, U. E., and Fontanarosa, P. B. (1989). Locked-in syndrome: Report of a case. *The American Journal of Emergency Medicine, 7*(6), 581–583.

Gargiulo, G., Bifulco, P., Cesarelli, M., Jin, C., McEwan, A., and van Schaik, A. (2010). Wearable dry sensors with bluetooth connection for use in remote patient monitoring systems. *Studies in Health Technology and Informatics, 161*, 57–65.

Grozea, C., Voinescu, C. D., and Fazli, S. (2011). Bristle-Sensors—Low-cost flexible passive dry EEG electrodes for neurofeedback and BCI applications. *Journal of Neural Engineering, 8*(2), 025008. doi:10.1088/1741–2560/8/2/025008

Hinterberger, T., Kübler, A., Kaiser, J., Neumann, N., and Birbaumer, N. (2003). A brain–computer interface (BCI) for the locked-in: Comparison of different EEG classifications for the thought translation device. *Clinical Neurophysiology, 114*(3), 416–425.

Hochberg, L. R., Serruya, M. D., Friehs, G. M., Mukand, J. A., Saleh, M., Caplan, A. H., et al. (2006). Neuronal ensemble control of prosthetic devices by a human with tetraplegia. *Nature, 442*(7099), 164–171. doi:10.1038/nature04970

International Standard Organization (ISO). (2007). *ISO 9999:2007 Assistive Products for Persons with Disability. Classification and Terminology.* Geneva, Switzerland: ISO.

Iturrate, I., Antelis, J., Kübler, A., and Minguez, J. (2009). Non-invasive brain-actuated wheelchair based on a P300 neurophysiological protocol and automated navigation. *IEEE Transactions on Robotics, 25*(3), 614–627.

Kamiya, J. (1968). Conscious control of brain waves. *Psychology Today, 1*(11), 56–60.

Karim, A. A., Hinterberger, T., Richter, J., Mellinger, J., Neumann, N., Flor, H., et al. (2006). Neural internet: Web surfing with brain potentials for the completely paralyzed. *Neurorehabilitation and Neural Repair, 20*(4), 508–515. doi:10.1177/1545968306290661

Kotchoubey, B., Strehl, U., Uhlmann, C., Holzapfel, S., König, M., Fröscher, W., et al. (2001). Modification of slow cortical potentials in patients with refractory epilepsy: A controlled outcome study. *Epilepsia, 42*(3), 406–416.

Kübler, A., and Birbaumer, N. (2008). Brain–computer interfaces and communication in paralysis: Extinction of goal directed thinking in completely paralysed patients? *Clinical Neurophysiology, 119*(11), 2658–2666. doi:10.1016/j.clinph.2008.06.019

Kübler, A., Neumann, N., Kaiser, J., Kotchoubey, B., Hinterberger, T., and Birbaumer, N. (2001). Brain–computer communication: Self-regulation of slow cortical potentials for verbal communication. *Archives of Physical Medicine and Rehabilitation, 82*(11), 1533–1539.

Kübler, A., Nijboer, F., Mellinger, J., Vaughan, T. M., Pawelzik, H., Schalk, G., et al. (2005). Patients with ALS can use sensorimotor rhythms to operate a brain–computer interface. *Neurology, 64*(10), 1775–1777. doi:10.1212/01.WNL.0000158616.43002.6D

Lai, S. M., Studenski, S., Duncan, P. W., and Perera, S. (2002). Persisting consequences of stroke measured by the stroke impact scale. *Stroke: A Journal of Cerebral Circulation, 33*(7), 1840–1844.

Lancioni, G. E., O'Reilly, M. F., Singh, N. N., Sigafoos, J., Oliva, D., Antonucci, M., et al. (2008). Microswitch-Based programs for persons with multiple disabilities: An overview of some recent developments. *Perceptual and Motor Skills, 106*(2), 355–370.

Lancioni, G. E., Saponaro, F., Singh, N. N., O'Reilly, M. F., Sigafoos, J., and Oliva, D. (2010). A microswitch to enable a woman with acquired brain injury and profound multiple disabilities to access environmental stimulation with lip movements. *Perceptual and Motor Skills, 110*(2), 488–492.

Laureys, S., Pellas, F., Van Eeckhout, P., Ghorbel, S., Schnakers, C., Perrin, F., et al. (2005). The locked-in syndrome: What is it like to be conscious but paralyzed and voiceless? *Progress in Brain Research, 150*, 495–511. doi:10.1016/S0079–6123(05)50034–7

Lebedev, M. A., and Nicolelis, M. A. (2006). Brain-Machine interfaces: Past, present and future. *Trends in Neurosciences, 29*(9), 536–546. doi:10.1016/j.tins.2006.07.004

Lee, S., Ruiz, S., Caria, A., Veit, R., Birbaumer, N., and Sitaram, R. (2011). Detection of cerebral reorganization induced by real-time fMRI feedback training of insula activation: A multivariate investigation. *Neurorehabilitation and Neural Repair, 25*(3), 259–267. doi:10.1177/1545968310385128

Louise-Bender Pape, T., Kim, J., and Weiner, B. (2002). The shaping of individual meanings assigned to assistive technology: A review of personal factors. *Disability and Rehabilitation, 24*(1–3), 5–20.

Lulé, D., Zickler, C., Häcker, S., Bruno, M. A., Demertzi, A., Pellas, F., et al. (2009). Life can be worth living in locked-in syndrome. *Progress in Brain Research, 177,* 339–351. doi:10.1016/S0079-6123(09)17723-3

Mason, S. G., Jackson, M. M., and Birch, G. E. (2005). A general framework for characterizing studies of brain interface technology. *Annals of Biomedical Engineering, 33*(11), 1653–1670. doi:10.1007/s10439-005-7706-3

Matuz, T., Birbaumer, N., Hautzinger, M., and Kübler, A. (2010). Coping with amyotrophic lateral sclerosis: An integrative view. *Journal of Neurology, Neurosurgery & Psychiatry, 81*(8), 893–898. doi:10.1136/jnnp.2009.201285

Mellinger, J., and Schalk, G. (2007). BCI2000: A general-purpose software platform for BCI research. In G. Dornhege, J. d. R. Millán, T. Hinterberger, D. J. McFarland, and K. R. Müller (Eds.), *Toward Brain–Computer Interfacing.* Cambridge MA: MIT Press.

Mellinger, J., Schalk, G., Braun, C., Preissl, H., Rosenstiel, W., Birbaumer, N., and Kübler, A. (2007). An meg-based brain–computer interface (BCI). *Neuroimage, 36*(3), 581–593 doi:10.1016/j.neuroimage.2007.03.019

Millán, J. d. R., Rupp, R., Müller-Putz, G. R., Murray-Smith, R., Giugliemma, C., Tangermann, M., et al. (2010). Combining Brain–Computer Interfaces and Assistive Technologies: State-of-the-Art and Challenges. *Frontiers in Neuroscience, 4.* doi:10.3389/fnins.2010.00161

Miller, N. E. (1969). Learning of visceral and glandular responses. *Science, 163*(866), 434–445.

Mugler, E., Bensch, M., Halder, S., Rosenstiel, W., Bogdan, M., Birbaumer, N., and Kübler, A. (2008). Control of an internet browser using the P300 signal. *International Journal of Bioelectromagnetism, 10*(1), 56–63.

Mugler, E. M., Ruf, C. A., Halder, S., Bensch, M., and Kler, A. (2010). Design and implementation of a p300-based brain–computer interface for controlling an internet browser. *IEEE Transactions on Neural Systems and Rehabilitation Engineering, 18*(6), 599–609, doi:10.1109/TNSRE.2010.2068059

Münbinger, J. I., Halder, S., Kleih, S. C., Furdea, A., Raco, V., Hoesle, A., and Kubler, A. (2010). Brain painting: Evaluation of a new brain–computer interface application with ALS patients and healthy volunteers. *Frontiers in Neuroscience, 4,* 182. doi:10.3389/fnins.2010.00182

Nagai, Y., Goldstein, L. H., Fenwick, P. B., and Trimble, M. R. (2004). Clinical efficacy of galvanic skin response biofeedback training in reducing seizures in adult epilepsy: A preliminary randomized controlled study. *Epilepsy & Behavior, 5*(2), 216–223. doi:10.1016/j.yebeh.2003.12.003

Naito, M., Michioka, Y., Ozawa, K., Ito, Y., Kiguchi, M., and Kanazawa, T. (2007). A communication means for totally locked-in ALS patients based on changes in cerebral blood volume measured with near-infrared light. *IEICE Transactions on Information and Systems, 90*(7), 1028–1037.

Neumann, N., Kübler, A., Kaiser, J., Hinterberger, T., and Birbaumer, N. (2003). Conscious perception of brain states: Mental strategies for brain–computer communication. *Neuropsychologia, 41*(8), 1028–1036.

Nijboer, F., Birbaumer, N., and Kübler, A. (2010). The influence of psychological state and motivation on brain–computer interface performance in patients with amyotrophic lateral sclerosis—A longitudinal study. *Frontiers in Neuroscience, 4.* doi:10.3389/fnins.2010.00055

Nudo, R. J., Plautz, E. J., and Frost, S. B. (2001). Role of adaptive plasticity in recovery of function after damage to motor cortex. *Muscle & Nerve, 24*(8), 1000–1019.

Pasqualotto, E., Federici, S., and Olivetti Belardinelli, M. (2011a). Toward functioning and usable brain computer interfaces (BCIs): A literature review. *Disability & Rehabilitation: Assistive Technology* (Epub ahead of print). doi: 10.3109/17483107.2011.589486.

Pasqualotto, E., Federici, S., Simonetta, A., and Olivetti Belardinelli, M. (2011b). Usability of Brain–Computer Interfaces. In G. J. Gelderblom, M. Soede, L. Adriaens, and K. Miesenberger (Eds.), *Everyday Technology for Independence and Care: AAATE 2011*. (Vol. 29, pp. 481–8). Amsterdam, NL: IOS Press. doi:10.3233/978-1-60750-814-4-481

Pasqualotto, E., Simonetta, A., Federici, S., and Olivetti Belardinelli, M. (2009). Usability evaluation of BCIs. In P. L. Emiliani, L. Burzagli, A. Como, F. Gabbanini, and A. L. Salminen (Eds.), *Assistive Technology from Adapted Equipment to Inclusive Environments: AAATE 2009*. (Vol. 25, p. 882). Amsterdam, NL: IOS Press. doi:10.3233/978-1-60750-042-1-882

Pasqualotto, E., Simonetta, A., Gnisci, V., Federici, S., and Olivetti Belardinelli, M. (2011c). Toward a usability evaluation of BCIs. *International Journal of Bioelectromagnetism*, 13(3), 121–122. Retrieved from Ijbem.org website: HYPERLINK "http://ijbem.k.hosei.ac.jp/2006-/volume13/number3/2011_v13_no3_121-122.pdf" http://ijbem.k.hosei.ac.jp/2006-/volume13/number3/2011_v13_no3_121-122.pdf

Pfurtscheller, G., Allison, B. Z., Brunner, C., Bauernfeind, G., Solis-Escalante, T., Scherer, R., et al. (2010). The hybrid BCI. *Frontiers in Neuroscience*, 4(30). doi:10.3389/fnpro.2010.00003

Pfurtscheller, G., Müller, G. R., Pfurtscheller, J., Gerner, H. J., and Rupp, R. (2003a). 'Thought'-control of functional electrical stimulation to restore hand grasp in a patient with tetraplegia. *Neuroscience Letters*, 351(1), 33–36.

Pfurtscheller, G., Neuper, C., Guger, C., Harkam, W., Ramoser, H., Schlögl, A., et al. (2000). Current trends in Graz brain–computer interface (BCI) research. *IEEE Transactions on Rehabilitation Engineering*, 8(2), 216–219.

Pfurtscheller, G., Neuper, C., Müller, G. R., Obermaier, B., Krausz, G., Schlögl, A., et al. (2003b). Graz-BCI: State of the art and clinical applications. *IEEE Transactions on Neural Systems and Rehabilitation Engineering*, 11(2), 177–180. doi:10.1109/TNSRE.2003.814454

Phan, K. L., Fitzgerald, D. A., Gao, K., Moore, G. J., Tancer, M. E., and Posse, S. (2004). Real-Time fMRI of cortico-limbic brain activity during emotional processing. *Neuroreport*, 15(3), 527–532.

Plum, F., and Posner, J. B. (1966). *The diagnosis of stupor and coma*. Philadelphia: FA Davis.

Popescu, F., Fazli, S., Badower, Y., Blankertz, B., and Müller, K. R. (2007). Single trial classification of motor imagination using 6 dry EEG electrodes. *Plos One*, 2(7), e637. doi:10.1371/journal.pone.0000637

Rebsamen, B., Teo, C. L., Zeng, Q., Ang Jr, M. H., Burdet, E., Guan, C., et al. (2007). Controlling a wheelchair indoors using thought. *IEEE Intelligent Systems*, 18–24.

Robbins, R. A., Simmons, Z., Bremer, B. A., Walsh, S. M., and Fischer, S. (2001). Quality of life in ALS is maintained as physical function declines. *Neurology*, 56(4), 442–444.

Rockstroh, B., Elbert, T., Birbaumer, N., Wolf, P., Düchting-Röth, A., Reker, M., et al. (1993). Cortical self-regulation in patients with epilepsies. *Epilepsy Research*, 14(1), 63–72.

Rothwell, P. M., Coull, A. J., Giles, M. F., Howard, S. C., Silver, L. E., Bull, L. M., et al. (2004). Change in stroke incidence, mortality, case-fatality, severity, and risk factors in Oxfordshire, UK from 1981 to 2004 (Oxford Vascular Study). *Lancet*, 363(9425), 1925–1933. doi:10.1016/S0140-6736(04)16405-2

Ruiz, S., Lee, S., Soekadar, S.R., Caria, A., Veit, R., Kircher, T., Birbaumer, N., and Sitaram, R. (2011). Acquired self-control of insula cortex modulates emotion recognition and brain network connectivity in schizophrenia. *Human Brain Mapping*. (Epub ahead of print). doi:10.1002/hbm.21427

Sajda, P., Gerson, A., Müller, K. R., Blankertz, B., and Parra, L. (2003). A data analysis competition to evaluate machine learning algorithms for use in brain–computer interfaces. *IEEE Transactions on Neural Systems and Rehabilitation Engineering*, 11(2), 184–185. doi:10.1109/TNSRE.2003.814453

Schalk, G., McFarland, D. J., Hinterberger, T., Birbaumer, N., and Wolpaw, J. R. (2004). BCI2000: A general-purpose brain–computer interface (BCI) system. *IEEE Transactions on Biomedical Engineering*, 51(6), 1034–1043.

Scherer, M. J., Craddock, G., and Mackeogh, T. (2011). The relationship of personal factors and subjective well-being to the use of assistive technology devices. *Disability and Rehabilitation*, 33(10), 811–817. doi:10.3109/09638288.2010.511418

Scherer, M. J., Sax, C., Vanbiervliet, A., Cushman, L. A., and Scherer, J. V. (2005). Predictors of assistive technology use: The importance of personal and psychosocial factors. *Disability and Rehabilitation*, 27(21), 1321–1331. doi:10.1080/09638280500164800

Schlögl, A., Brunner, C., Scherer, R., and Glatz, A. (2007). *Biosig: An Open-Source Software Library for BCI Research*. Cambridge MA: MIT Press

Sellers, E. W., and Donchin, E. (2006). A p300-based brain–computer interface: Initial tests by ALS patients. *Clinical Neurophysiology*, 117(3), 538–548. doi:10.1016/j.clinph.2005.06.027

Simmons, Z., Bremer, B. A., Robbins, R. A., Walsh, S. M., and Fischer, S. (2000). Quality of life in ALS depends on factors other than strength and physical function. *Neurology*, 55(3), 388–392.

Sitaram, R., Zhang, H., Guan, C., Thulasidas, M., Hoshi, Y., Ishikawa, A., et al. (2007). Temporal classification of multichannel near-infrared spectroscopy signals of motor imagery for developing a brain–computer interface. *Neuroimage*, 34(4), 1416–1427. doi:10.1016/j.neuroimage.2006.11.005

Stephanidis, C., Salvendy, G., Akoumianakis, D., Bevan, N., Brewer, J., Emiliani, P. L., et al. (1998). Toward an information society for all: An international R&D agenda. *International Journal of Human-Computer Interaction*, 10(2), 107–134.

Strehl, U., Kotchoubey, B., Trevorrow, T., and Birbaumer, N. (2005). Predictors of seizure reduction after self-regulation of slow cortical potentials as a treatment of drug-resistant epilepsy. *Epilepsy & Behavior*, 6(2), 156–166. doi:10.1016/j.yebeh.2004.11.004

Strehl, U., Leins, U., Goth, G., Klinger, C., Hinterberger, T., and Birbaumer, N. (2006). Self-regulation of slow cortical potentials: A new treatment for children with attention-deficit/hyperactivity disorder. *Pediatrics*, 118(5), e1530–e1540. doi:10.1542/peds.2005–2478

Swartz, B. E., and Goldensohn, E. S. (1998). Timeline of the history of EEG and associated fields. *Electroencephalography and Clinical Neurophysiology*, 106(2), 173–176.

Vidal, J. J. (1973). Toward direct brain–computer communication. *Annual Review of Biophysics and Bioengineering*, 2(1), 157–180.

Vidal, J. J. (1977). Real-time detection of brain events in EEG. *Proceedings of the IEEE*, 65(5), 633

Vidal, J. J. (1999). Cyberspace bionics. *Human Factors in Information Technology*, 13, 203–218.

Weiskopf, N., Mathiak, K., Bock, S. W., Scharnowski, F., Veit, R., Grodd, W., et al. (2004a). Principles of a brain–computer interface (BCI) based on real-time functional magnetic resonance imaging (fMRI). *IEEE Transactions on Biomedical Engineering*, 51(6), 966–970. doi:10.1109/TBME.2004.827063

Weiskopf, N., Scharnowski, F., Veit, R., Goebel, R., Birbaumer, N., and Mathiak, K. (2004b). Self-Regulation of local brain activity using real-time functional magnetic resonance imaging (fmri). *Journal of Physiology, Paris*, 98(4–6), 357–373. doi:10.1016/j.jphysparis.2005.09.019

Weiskopf, N., Sitaram, R., Josephs, O., Veit, R., Scharnowski, F., Goebel, R., et al. (2007). Real-time functional magnetic resonance imaging: Methods and applications. *Magnetic Resonance Imaging*, 25(6), 989–1003. doi:10.1016/j.mri.2007.02.007

Weiskopf, N., Veit, R., Erb, M., Mathiak, K., Grodd, W., Goebel, R., and Birbaumer, N. (2003). Physiological self-regulation of regional brain activity using real-time functional magnetic resonance imaging (fMRI): Methodology and exemplary data. *Neuroimage*, 19(3), 577–586.

Wiedemann, H. R. (1994). Hans Berger. *European Journal of Pediatrics*, 153, 705

Wolpaw, J. R., Birbaumer, N., Heetderks, W. J., McFarland, D. J., Peckham, P. H., Schalk, G., et al. (2000). brain–computer interface technology: A review of the first international meeting. *IEEE Transactions on Rehabilitation Engineering*, 8(2), 164–173.

Wolpaw, J. R., Birbaumer, N., McFarland, D. J., Pfurtscheller, G., and Vaughan, T. M. (2002). brain–computer interfaces for communication and control. *Clinical Neurophysiology*, 113(6), 767–791.

Wolpaw, J. R., McFarland, D. J., Vaughan, T. M., and Schalk, G. (2003). The Wadsworth center brain–computer interface (BCI) research and development program. *IEEE Transactions on Neural Systems and Rehabilitation Engineering*, 11(2), 204–207. doi:10.1109/TNSRE.2003.814442

Wyndaele, M., and Wyndaele, J. J. (2006). Incidence, prevalence and epidemiology of spinal cord injury: What learns a worldwide literature survey? *Spinal Cord: The Official Journal of the International Medical Society of Paraplegia*, 44(9), 523–529. doi:10.1038/sj.sc.3101893

Zwi, M., Ramchandani, P., and Joughin, C. (2000). Evidence and belief in ADHD. *British Medical Journal*, 321(7267), 975–976.

18

New Rehabilitation Opportunities for Persons with Multiple Disabilities Through the Use of Microswitch Technology

G. E. Lancioni, N. N. Singh, M. F. O'Reilly, J. Sigafoos, D. Oliva, and G. Basili

CONTENTS

18.1 Introduction

Persons with profound and multiple disabilities, regardless of whether their disabilities are congenital or acquired, are often unable to interact with their immediate environment and control relevant stimuli because of their limited response skills (Lancioni et al. 2001a, 2001b, 2007b, 2007c; Mechling 2006). This lack of interaction (of response skills) has far-reaching social and practical implications. In fact, it emphasizes a condition of withdrawal and weakness, reduces the persons' opportunities of an active, constructive role within the environment, limits their overall perspectives of development or recovery, impoverishes their social appearance, and negatively affects their quality of life (Lancioni et al. 2001c, 2001d, 2008a, 2008b; Schalock et al. 2003; Lachapelle et al. 2005; Petry et al. 2009; McDougall et al. 2010).

Intervention procedures that are based on environmental enrichment and stimulation handled by staff and families are the most common forms of approach with these persons. These forms of approach are functional to improve the persons' input level and might also reduce problem behaviors that may be present in their repertoire (e.g., Ringdahl et al. 1997; Matson et al. 2006; Richman 2008). Despite these positive aspects, they also seem to have two correlated drawbacks. First, enrichment/stimulation conditions could easily make the individuals recipients of external input rather than active agents who pursue the input on their own initiative (i.e., purposefully). Second, those conditions would not support and motivate the development of any specific response schemes by the individuals. In fact, they would not need any such schemes to access environmental stimulation. This lack of opportunity/necessity may be seen as a critically negative perspective from a learning and education/rehabilitation standpoint (Glickman et al. 1996; Holburn et al. 2004; Lancioni et al. 2004c, 2008b, 2009b).

A possible way to help these individuals with profound and multiple disabilities deal with their situation is the use of microswitch technology or variations thereof such as voice output communication aids (VOCAs) (Leatherby et al. 1992; Sullivan and Lewis 1993; Sullivan et al. 1995; Lancioni et al. 2001a, 2008b; Mechling 2006). Microswitches are technical devices that are built to work as functional tools, that is, tools that allow persons with profound and multiple disabilities to acquire control of environmental events with minimal responses (i.e., responses that per se would not suffice to deal with those events) (Crawford and Schuster 1993; Lancioni et al. 2001b, 2002a; Mechling 2006). For example, a touch or pressure microswitch fixed to the armrest of a person's wheelchair and connected to a timer and a music device may enable the person to activate such a device and listen to music for brief periods of time (i.e., for periods such as those set in the timer) through small hand- or arm-movement responses. Similarly, an optic microswitch fixed to an eyeglasses' frame and connected to a timer and vibration devices may enable the person to activate brief periods of vibratory stimulation through prolonged eyelid closure. A touch-sensitive pad microswitch connected to the person's hand and linked to a timer and a series of visual stimuli may enable the person to turn on these stimuli for brief periods of time through minimal finger movements. None of the individuals involved in the examples described above would have been able to access the stimulation mentioned through a direct manipulation of the stimulus sources (i.e., music device, vibration tools, and visual displays or other forms of visual stimuli) (Lancioni et al. 2008b; Judge et al. 2010).

VOCAs (also known as speech-generating devices) are technical instruments that enable a person with multiple disabilities to produce synthesized or digitized verbal messages/requests through the performance of simple nonverbal responses (Schlosser and Sigafoos 2006; Lancioni et al. 2007a; Sigafoos et al. 2009; Valiquette et al. 2010). For example, the person may have a pressure device before his or her hand connected to an electronic control system equipped with a speech output instrument. Each time he or she applies some pressure on the device, this sends a signal to the electronic control system. This system in turn activates the speech output instrument, which emits a call to the person's caregiver to obtain attention and stimulation or to ask for his or her mediation in reaching specific environmental stimuli (Schlosser and Sigafoos 2006; Rispoli et al. 2010).

This chapter is divided into four sections. The first section focuses on studies using experimental microswitches developed to monitor small (nontypical) responses, such as eyelid and lip movements, and thus to suit persons with minimal motor behavior (Lancioni and Lems 2001; Lancioni et al. 2001c, 2009a, 2009b, 2010c). The second section analyzes studies that have combined two or more microswitches to allow the person direct access to different types of stimulation and choice opportunities (Sullivan et al. 1995; Lancioni et al. 2001, 2002a, 2006b, 2010a, 2010b). The third section reviews studies that have combined microswitches with VOCAs to allow the person direct access to stimulation as well as the possibility to call for social attention and interaction (Lancioni et al. 2008a, 2009f, 2010d). The fourth section discusses (1) the results obtained with the different forms of technology used and their applicability and possible impact in daily education/rehabilitation contexts, and (2) the possibility of using combinations of microswitches also for programs aimed at targeting increases of adaptive responding and reduction of problem behaviors or inadequate postures simultaneously. Table 18.1 lists relevant studies for each of the first three sections of the paper. Most of those studies are also summarized in the review sections that follow below.

TABLE 18.1

Studies Using Microswitch Technology for Persons with Multiple Disabilities

Studies	Participants	Age	Response Types
Experimental Microswitches for Small Responses			
Lancioni and Lems (2001)	2	4, 18	Vocalization
Lancioni et al. (2001c)	2	7, 10	Vocalization
Lancioni et al. (2004a)	1	18	Chin movements (as in chewing)
Lancioni et al. (2004b)	1	6	Chin movements (as in mouth opening)
Lancioni et al. (2004e)	1	17	Chin movements (as in chewing)
Lancioni et al. (2005a)	1	9	Repeated eye-blink pattern
Lancioni et al. (2006c)	2	7.5, 8	Chin movements
Lancioni et al. (2006f)	2	10, 12	Eyelid upward movement
Lancioni et al. (2007b)	2	6, 14	Forehead skin movements
Lancioni et al. (2007c)	2	5, 21	Hand-closure movements
Lancioni et al. (2009a)	1	68	Eyebrow lifting
Lancioni et al. (2009b)	1	26	Eyelid closures
Lancioni et al. (2010a)	1	25	Eyelid closures
Lancioni et al. (2010c)	1	41	Lip movements
Combinations of Microswitches			
Crawford and Schuster (1993)	3	4	2 responses per participant: Hand, wrist, or elbow movements
Sullivan et al. (1995)	1	3.5	2 responses: Head movements and hand movements
Lancioni et al. (2002a)	2	8, 12	3 responses per participant: Vocalization, head movements, and hand movements
Lancioni et al. (2002b)	2	8, 13	3 responses per participant: Vocalization, head movements, fist, elbow or hand movements and trunk move
Lancioni et al. (2004c)	2	7, 17	3 or 4 responses per participant: Vocalization, head movements, and one or two hand movements
Lancioni et al. (2004d)	2	19, 20	5 or 6 responses per participant: Word-like sounds
Lancioni et al. (2004f)	2	16, 20	3 or 9 responses per participant: Syllable-like or word-like sounds
Lancioni et al. (2006b)	3	7–16	2 responses per participant: Vocalization, chin and mouth movements, knee movements, and hand movements
Lancioni et al. (2009b)	1	45	2 responses: Head and foot movements mouth movements
Lancioni et al. (2010a)	1	21	2 responses: Eyelid and mouth movements
Lancioni et al. (2010b)	2	53, 56	2 responses per participant: Finger or hand movements, eyelid movements, and head movements
Combinations of Microswitches and VOCAs			
Lancioni et al. (2008a)	1	30	3 responses: Finger movements and different vocalizations
Lancioni et al. (2008c)	2	16, 18	3 responses per participant: Vocalization, head movements, and hand movements

(Continued)

TABLE 18.1 (CONTINUED)

Studies Using Microswitch Technology for Persons with Multiple Disabilities

Studies	Participants	Age	Response Types
Combinations of Microswitches and VOCAs (Continued)			
Lancioni et al. (2008d)	3	10–15	3 responses per participant: Trunk movements, head movements, leg/foot movements, and one or two hand movements
Lancioni et al. (2009b)	1	52	2 responses: Head movements and arm/hand movements
Lancioni et al. (2009c)	11	5–18	2 responses per participant: Head, foot, and hand movements and vocalization
Lancioni et al. (2009e)	2	35, 60	2 responses per participant: Hand and foot movements
Lancioni et al. (2009f)	1	32	3 responses: Eyelid movements and two hand movements
Lancioni et al. (2010d)	1	20	4 responses: Two hand movements and two head movements

18.2 Experimental Microswitches for Small (Nontypical) Responses

The most common examples of responses used in early microswitch programs have been head turning and hand pushing. The microswitches adopted for them generally consisted of commercially available pressure devices or similar kinds of instruments. These response-microswitch combinations, albeit apparently simple and immediate, may not suit a number of situations, namely those in which the person has only a minimal behavioral (motor) repertoire (Lancioni et al. 2005b, 2008b). In those situations, the professional is left with two options: (1) excluding the person from any microswitch programs, or (2) resorting to new microswitch devices that can detect small, nontypical responses, such as eyelid or chin movements, which may be much more feasible for the person (Lancioni et al. 2006f, 2009b). Table 18.1 provides a list of 14 studies, in each of which new/experimental microswitch technology was used for monitoring a single, nontypical response (Lancioni and Lems 2001; Lancioni et al. 2001c, 2004a, 2004b, 2004e, 2005a, 2006c, 2006f, 2007b, 2007c, 2009a, 2009b, 2010a, 2010c).

For example, Lancioni et al. (2001c) worked with two participants of seven and ten years of age. They had pervasive multiple disabilities with minimal motor repertoires, but they possessed spontaneous vocal responses, which were considered a relevant resource and targeted through a new (specifically built) microswitch. The new microswitch consisted of a battery-powered, sound-detecting device connected to a throat microphone (not affected by environmental noise), which was held at the participants' larynx, with a simple neckband. During the intervention phase, vocalization responses allowed the participants to access brief periods of preferred stimulation. Data showed that during that phase the participants' level of vocalization responses increased substantially and remained consistent. This increase was taken to suggest that the participants had learned to use these responses as means for stimulation access.

Lancioni et al. (2004b) conducted a program with a boy of six years of age, who usually sat in a reclined position with no obvious signs of movement of his head and limbs. The response that seemed most suitable for him to perform (and was already present in his repertoire) was chin movements, which resembled those occurring in a situation of mouth opening. The microswitch for this response included (1) a small box with a position sensor, which was attached to the side of a hat that the boy was to wear, and (2) a light band that passed under the boy's chin and connected the position sensor to the other side of the hat. Downward chin movements pulled the position sensor, thus activating the microswitch, which in turn caused the occurrence of preferred environmental stimuli. Data showed that the boy's chin-response frequency increased more than twofold during the intervention phases compared with the baseline periods.

Recently, a different microswitch was conceived to detect a response that can involve only movements of the lips or can also encompass chin and jaw movements and thus resemble the one mentioned above (Lancioni et al. 2010c). The microswitch was assessed with a 41-year-old woman who had suffered severe brain injury and coma after a car accident and had a diagnosis of a minimally conscious state with pervasive neuromotor disabilities. The microswitch included two optic sensors consisting of an infrared light-emitting diode and a mini infrared light-detection unit. The sensors were fixed to a metal support, which was attached to the woman's chin. When the woman had her mouth semi-open and the lips clearly apart (i.e., was in her most common position), the aforementioned sensors were directed at the upper lip and at the mouth cavity, respectively. The relative position, fixation point(s) of the sensors changed if the woman's lips moved closer together as well as if they moved further apart. These changes produced microswitch activations, which resulted in the occurrence of brief periods of preferred stimulation during the intervention phases. Data showed clear increases in the frequency of lip movements during those phases.

Lancioni et al. (2005a) reported an intervention with a boy of nine years of age, who presented with profound multiple disabilities and minimal motor behavior. The most reliable response for him seemed to be eye blinking. A specific response pattern (i.e., two blinks occurring within a 2-s interval) was targeted for the study because it was distinct from the common blinking behavior and occurred at a relatively low frequency. The microswitch for the response included (1) an optic sensor mounted on an eyeglasses' frame that the boy wore during the sessions, and (2) an electronic unit that emitted a signal when a response (two blinks within a 2-s interval) was detected. Response emission allowed access to brief periods of preferred stimulation during the intervention periods. Data showed that, during those periods, the child's response rates increased very markedly.

Lancioni et al. (2006f) set up a program with two children of 10 and 12 years of age and targeted upward eyelid movements as the response through which they could produce environmental changes (i.e., causing brief periods of preferred stimulation). The microswitch technology involved optic sensors mounted on eyeglasses comparable to those reported in the study by Lancioni et al. (2005a). However, the functioning of such technology was somewhat different so that it could detect the response targeted for the two participants. This consisted of raising one eyelid or both eyelids, as would occur when looking at something high up. In this study, the optic sensor was not to detect the eyelid closures (i.e., blinks) as in the study of Lancioni and colleagues (2005a), but rather the transition from the eyelid to the eye. Such a transition occurred each time the child performed a looking-up response. Both participants presented extensive response increases during the intervention periods (i.e., when the performance of the target response allowed them brief access to preferred stimuli).

The need of targeting double blinking or upward eyelid movements as specific responses may be fairly obvious in cases in which the conventional blinking response (i.e., single blinks) has a relatively high baseline frequency. However, when the baseline frequency of single blinks is low, this form of response might be targeted without foreseeable difficulties. In line with this view, Lancioni et al. (2009b) used a single-blink response with a man of 26 years of age who had suffered severe brain injury and coma after a road accident and had a diagnosis of a minimally conscious state with pervasive neuromotor disabilities. The microswitch was an adapted version of the optic sensor described above (Lancioni et al. 2005a, 2006f). The performance of single blink responses allowed the man to access brief periods of preferred stimulation during the intervention phases. The response frequencies during those phases increased rapidly and remained high.

Lancioni et al. (2007b) investigated the possibility of using small upward or downward movements of the forehead skin as the response through which participants of 6 and 14 years of age could control relevant stimulation. The microswitch consisted of an optic sensor (barcode reader) with an electronic regulation unit and a small tag with horizontal bars that was kept on the participants' forehead. The optic sensor was held in front of the tag. During the intervention, small movements of the tag (consequent to small upward or downward movements of the forehead skin) triggered the microswitch system and caused brief periods of preferred stimulation. Both participants had a clear response increase during the intervention phases of the study.

Lancioni et al. (2007c) reported the use of small hand-closure movements as the response with two participants of 5 and 21 years of age. The response consisted of the participants' fingers touching or pressing on a microswitch fixed to the palm of their hand. The microswitch involved a two-membrane thin device. The outer membrane (i.e., the one directly exposed to the participants' fingers) was a touch-sensitive sensor and was activated by contact with any of their fingers. The inner membrane was activated if the participants applied a pressure of approximately 20 g. Data showed that both participants successfully learned to use the microswitch as a way to access preferred stimulation during the intervention.

Lancioni et al. (2009a) investigated the use of eyebrow lifting as the target response with a 68-year-old man with a diagnosis of minimally conscious state and pervasive neuromotor disabilities after traumatic brain injury and coma. The microswitch adopted for this response was a modified version of the optic sensor used in the studies targeting eyelid closures and eyelid upward movements (see above). Eyebrow lifting was instrumental to allow the man brief access to preferred visual stimuli (i.e., video-clips with sport events and comic sketches) during the intervention periods of the study. Data showed that the response frequency increased largely during the intervention as compared with the baseline period.

Lancioni et al. (2010a) reported new research efforts aimed at building alternatives to the aforementioned experimental microswitches. These alternatives were to overcome a perceived limit of the aforementioned microswitches, specifically, their need to be held close to the part of the body producing the response (e.g., eyelids, lips, and forehead) through support frames (e.g., eyeglasses). Those support frames may be viewed as slightly invasive (not always pleasant) for the participant and not always practical or reliable for staff personnel responsible of their use within the programs. In fact, they may be difficult to place/maintain whenever the participant has dystonic movements or a head posture unsuitable to the stability of the frame. The alternatives investigated involved camera-based technology. This technology was used to monitor eyelid-closure responses by a man of 25 years of age. The man's left eyelid was provided with a green color spot greater than 1.5 cm^2. The spot would be minimally visible when the eye was open and maximally visible when the eye was closed. The variation of the spot dimension from minimal to maximal levels was recorded as the response. The participant increased the frequency of such response during the intervention phases of the study (i.e., when the response allowed access to preferred stimuli) as opposed to the baseline periods.

18.3 Combinations of Microswitches

The use of a single microswitch is normally directed at promoting a connection between a specific response and a set of stimuli. The stimuli are accessible to the person only in relation to his or her performance of the response during the intervention sessions. The possibility of establishing two or more responses with two or more microswitches would be highly relevant within any educational and occupational program. It would allow the participant to extend and vary his or her behavioral engagement, enrich and diversify his stimulation input, and eventually choose between the different stimuli available on the basis of preferences and other practical conditions. Table 18.1 provides a list of 11 studies assessing the combined use of two or more microswitches (Crawford and Schuster 1993; Sullivan et al. 1995; Lancioni et al. 2002a, 2002b, 2004c, 2004d, 2004f, 2006b, 2009b, 2010a, 2010b).

For example, Sullivan et al. (1995) worked with a girl who was 3.5 years of age at the start of the study. The two responses selected for the girl consisted of head backward movements and hand-pushing/stroking movements. These responses were used in combination with commercially available pressure microswitches. The microswitches were simultaneously available and the girl could activate either one of them depending on the response she performed. The responses allowed her to access different types of preferred stimuli. The results showed that she increased the frequency of both responses during the intervention conditions.

Lancioni et al. (2002a) reported a study in which two children of 8 and 12 years of age were involved. The three responses targeted for each participant concerned vocalization, hand movements (pushing/stroking), and head movements. Each response allowed access to a specific set of stimuli. The responses were introduced in sequence. Once the first two responses/microswitches had been introduced individually, the participants were provided with the opportunity to use them both and choose between them and the stimuli connected with them. Eventually, the third response/microswitch also was introduced and then combined with the other two. Once the intervention had covered all responses/microswitches, the participants could use any of them at any time. This response freedom ensured an extensive and differentiated engagement and an important opportunity to choose among three sets of preferred stimuli. Data indicated that both participants succeeded in acquiring the responses and had an increased and consistent use of all three of them.

Lancioni et al. (2004f) conducted a study with two participants of 16 and 20 years of age who possessed different vocal emissions. The goal of the study was to use the participants' emissions as different responses allowing them access to different stimulus sources. Three vocal emissions (one-syllable sounds) were selected for one of the participants and nine word-like emissions were selected for the second participant. To make the vocal emissions (responses) functional, computer systems were developed that worked as combinations of microswitches and could on the whole discriminate the emissions. The software program used for the discrimination of the emissions of the first participant was based on locally recurrent neural networks and time sequences of cepstral parameters. The software program used for the discrimination of the emissions of the second participant was based on a commercially available speech recognition program, which was combined with a specially developed control program. The participants increased the frequencies of their responses during the intervention (i.e., when positive environmental stimuli followed those utterances). The systems' percentages of correct response discrimination were approximately 70%.

Lancioni et al. (2006b) worked with three participants who were between 7 and 16 years of age and targeted two responses for each of them. The responses involved vocalization and repeated chin movements, light knee movement, minimal movement of a grid hanging close to the participant's face (while the participant was lying on her back), and mouth closing, and hand opening. The microswitches used for vocalization and chin movements matched those previously described for the same responses (Lancioni and Lems 2001; Lancioni et al. 2004a). The microswitches used for mouth closing and hand opening consisted of specially adapted versions of the aforementioned microswitch for chin movements. The microswitches used for knee and grid movements were combinations of tilt devices. The microswitches were introduced individually. After the introduction of the second microswitch, the participants were provided with the simultaneous availability of both microswitches. The participants could choose between the microswitches and related responses and, more importantly, between the sets of stimuli connected to the different microswitch/response combinations. Eventually, the study assessed whether the participants' preference for one response or the other was uniquely related to the stimuli following that response (i.e., the higher preference for those stimuli) or was also determined by a preference for the response as such. All three participants were very successful in acquiring the responses selected for them. They also showed clear differences in the frequencies of the responses. Those differences were apparently due to the stimuli available for the responses for two of the participants. The differences seemed to be due to a combined impact of the stimuli and of the response for the third participant.

Lancioni et al. (2009b) arranged a program for a post-coma man of 45 years of age, who presented with a minimally conscious state and extensive neuromotor disabilities. The responses targeted for him were head and foot movements. The microswitches used for these responses consisted of pressure devices at the wheelchair's headrest and a combination of tilt and pressure devices on the man's right foot. During intervention, head movements activating the headrest's sensors allowed access to video-clips; foot movements activating the combination of sensors on it allowed access to audio-recordings. The microswitches were introduced individually and then made available simultaneously. The man learned to use both responses (increasing their frequencies) and related microswitches during the initial intervention phases. He continued to have high responding levels during the final intervention phase (i.e., when both microswitches were available simultaneously within the sessions) with a possible preference trend for the foot-movement response.

Lancioni et al. (2010b) worked with two post-coma adults of 56 and 53 years of age who presented with a minimally conscious state and extensive neuromotor disabilities. The responses targeted for the first participant consisted of finger and head movements; the responses targeted for the second participant consisted of eyelid upward movements and hand stroking. The microswitches used for the finger movements and hand stroking involved touch-sensitive pads. The microswitch used for eyelid movements was an optic sensor (see Lancioni et al. 2006f). The microswitch used for head movements consisted of mini tilt devices. The microswitches were introduced individually. Once responding had consolidated on each of them, their use was alternated; that is, sessions with one microswitch/response were alternated with sessions with the other microswitch/response.

Results were largely encouraging. Each participant increased his responding with both microswitches through the intervention periods.

Lancioni et al. (2010a) worked with a man of 21 years of age whose physical condition had deteriorated markedly and the use of optic sensors fixed on support frames to monitor his responses (i.e., eyelid opening and mouth opening) had become difficult and not always reliable. The new camera-based microswitch technology (mentioned above) was used with him to monitor the aforementioned eyelid and mouth responses. During sessions in which mouth opening was targeted, the camera-based technology was used together with two small color spots on the participant's nose and lower lip, respectively. When the camera system recorded an increase in the distance between the two spots greater than a preset level, a mouth-opening response was recorded. During sessions in which eyelid opening was targeted, the camera-based technology was used together with a color spot on the left eyelid. When the dimensions of the spot were smaller than a preset level, the camera system recorded an eyelid-opening response. During sessions in which both responses were targeted, the camera-based technology was used in combination with the dots on the nose and lip as well as the spot on the eyelid. Each response (camera-technology activation) allowed access to brief stimulation events. The events differed for the two responses. Data showed a successful use of the technology with the frequency of both responses increasing widely during the intervention program.

18.4 Combinations of Microswitches and VOCAs

The successful use of single and multiple microswitches can be considered strong evidence in support of the effectiveness of these technological resources. Indeed, they may be instrumental to allow persons with severe/profound multiple disabilities opportunities of positive engagement, independent stimulation access, and choice. Microswitch-based programs may be seen as a critical component of any rehabilitation context for two main reasons. First, they can be complementary to the direct intervention of rehabilitation and care staff. In fact, these people cannot be expected to guarantee a consistent/continuous educational presence (Lancioni et al. 2008b). Second, they can be instrumental to help the participants develop forms of activity and independence through the acquisition of specific responses (Holburn et al. 2004; Lancioni et al. 2008b). The recognition of these extremely important functions may not totally eliminate a sense of caution about these programs. Such caution stems from the knowledge that they promote the person's access to environmental (nonhuman) stimuli but largely ignore any possible desires of the person for contact with the caregiver.

Caution would seem to be more realistically required when the implementation of these programs involves the use of relatively long sessions and/or a large number of sessions during the day. In those situations (and probably in less concerning ones as well), a reassuring approach might consist of supplementing conventional microswitch technology with a VOCA. The microswitch technology would ensure that the participant continues to independently access environmental stimuli. The VOCA would enable the participant to ask for caregiver contact whenever he or she desires to have such a contact. Table 18.1 provides a list of eight studies that have combined microswitch and VOCA devices to accommodate participants' desires and caregivers' duties. Specifically, those studies have (1) sought to provide the participants a wider range of occupational opportunities as well as contact with the caregivers, and (2) required the caregivers a level of commitment and responsibility presumably compatible with other daily duties (i.e., much more practicable than direct interaction with the participant or consistent availability within a program based exclusively on the use of VOCA devices) (Lancioni et al. 2008a, 2008c, 2008d, 2009b, 2009c, 2009e, 2009f, 2010d).

For example, Lancioni et al. (2008a) reported a program carried out with a 30-year-old man who was in a minimally conscious state and suffered extensive neuromotor disabilities after traumatic brain injury and coma. Initially, the man was provided with a microswitch, which allowed him to access brief periods of video-images. The microswitch consisted of touch sensors attached to the index finger of the right hand and activated by small movements/contacts of the thumb of the same hand. Then a VOCA device was introduced. The VOCA consisted of a sound-detecting sensor using a throat microphone and an airborne microphone. Activation of the sensor led to the occurrence of verbal messages (requests of interaction) directed to the man's mother or the man's sister depending on the length of the vocalization response. The mother and the sister could respond by presenting highly preferred items or low-impact items. Eventually, the microswitch and the VOCA were simultaneously available. The man learned to use the microswitch and the VOCA. Indeed, he used the VOCA to preferentially call the mother or the sister depending upon the stimuli that they offered. He also continued to use those instruments successfully during the last part of the study when they were simultaneously available.

Lancioni et al. (2008c) arranged a program, which included two microswitches and a VOCA for two participants of 16 and 18 years of age. The responses selected for the microswitches consisted of head and hand movements for both participants. The responses selected for the VOCA consisted of vocalization for one participant and a specific hand movement for the other participant. Initially, the intervention focused on each of the two microswitches individually. When responding had increased, they were made available simultaneously. Subsequently, the intervention focused on the VOCA. Once responding to it had increased, the VOCA and the two microswitches were made available simultaneously. The participants could choose among the three opportunities. Activation of the microswitches allowed the participants to access different sets of preferred stimuli (e.g., musical and visual items). Activation of the VOCA triggered a vocal output apparatus, which emitted a short phrase that requested for the attention of the caregiver. The caregiver responded to the requests in different ways (i.e., only verbally or verbally and physically). The verbal responses consisted of complimentary/support sentences and occurred for about two-thirds of the VOCA requests. The verbal and physical responses consisted of talking to and touching/caressing or kissing the participant briefly and occurred for about one-third of the VOCA requests. The use of the two types of responses was based on practical considerations. The verbal responses could also be easily administered during caregiver engagement in other duties. The outcome of the study was positive for both participants. They learned to use the microswitches and the VOCA. Nearly three-fourths of their total responses were directed to the microswitches and about one-fourth were related to the VOCA.

Lancioni et al. (2009b) implemented a program involving the use of a microswitch and a VOCA with a post-coma man of 52 years of age. The man had a diagnosis of minimally conscious state and extensive neuromotor disabilities. The responses required for activating the two devices were head movements and arm movements, respectively. Microswitch activations allowed the participant to have brief exposures to recordings of comic sketches. VOCA activations (triggering a verbal call for the caregiver) were followed by the caregiver approaching the man, talking to him, and engaging him briefly in activities such as watching pictures, magazines, or video-clips. The intervention initially focused on the use of the microswitch. Subsequently, the intervention emphasis was on the use of the VOCA. Eventually, the program alternated sessions with the microswitch and sessions with the VOCA. The outcome was satisfactory with the man acquiring and maintaining responding in relation to both the microswitch and the VOCA.

Lancioni et al. (2009c) conducted a study with 11 participants whose ages ranged between approximately 5 and 18 years. All participants were provided with one microswitch and one VOCA. Head, foot and hand movements, and vocalizations constituted the main types of responses for activating those devices. The intervention started always with the use of the microswitch. When responding to this had increased, the intervention focused on the VOCA. Finally, the microswitch and the VOCA were simultaneously available. The activation of the microswitch allowed the participants a brief access to preferred stimulation. This varied across participants and included, among other things, vibratory inputs, musical items, voices and noises, and lights. The activation of the VOCA caused the emission of a short phrase requesting the attention of the caregiver. The response of the caregiver could be verbal or verbal and physical (i.e., the same way as in the study reported above; Lancioni et al. 2008a). Data showed that all participants acquired successful microswitch and VOCA responding. The frequency of microswitch responding was always higher than the frequency of VOCA responding (i.e., as in the previous study). Such an outcome could reflect a lower impact of the VOCA consequences, which were probably softened by the decision to apply only verbal consequences to most participant requests. The positive implications of the findings are that VOCA requests (1) could be satisfactorily combined with microswitch use (i.e., independent management of environmental stimulation), and (2) could be maintained via a combination of feedbacks, most of which (i.e., the verbal responses) were extremely economical and practical to implement for the caregiver.

Lancioni et al. (2009e) carried out an intervention program with two post-coma individuals (a man and a woman) of 35 and 60 years of age who were diagnosed to be in a minimally conscious state and presented with extensive motor disabilities. Both participants were initially led to use a microswitch, which allowed them to access brief periods of preferred stimulation (e.g., music). The microswitches consisted of a touch-sensitive device fixed onto the leg of the man and a touch- and pressure-sensitive device fixed into the palm of the woman's hand. When they could use the microswitch, the VOCA was introduced. This consisted of (1) a wobble-like device attached to the stomach of the man that could be activated by a general hand movement, and (2) tilt devices attached to the foot of the woman that could be activated through slight foot movement. VOCA activation produced a call for caregiver attention. In response to the call, the caregiver talked to and engaged the participant in watching or listening to various stimuli. In the final phase of the program, the microswitch and the VOCA were simultaneously present for each participant. The participants learned to use both forms of technology, thus increasing their independent access to stimulation and their positive interaction with the caregiver.

Lancioni et al. (2010d) reported the case of a 20-year-old man who was taught to use the single versus the repeated execution of simple motor schemes as different responses. Initially, the intervention focused on establishing a single and a double finger movement as two separate microswitch responses. Those responses were recorded by a touch-sensitive microswitch and led to different types of video-clips. Then, the intervention focused on establishing a single and a double head movement as two different VOCA responses. Those responses were recorded through a pressure-sensitive device placed on the participant's headrest, which triggered vocal systems calling different caregivers. The caregivers interacted with the participant and presented him different stimuli. The intervention program continued with the simultaneous availability of the microswitch and VOCA systems. At that point, the participant could perform any of the responses acquired (choosing at any occasion among four different options). Data showed that he was successful in acquiring the microswitch and VOCA responses. The overall frequency of the microswitch responses was somewhat higher than that of the VOCA responses.

18.5 Discussion

18.5.1 Outcome of the Studies

The positive results generally reported by the studies using microswitches and related forms of technology such as VOCAs underline the importance of adopting these forms of assistive technology for persons with severe/profound multiple disabilities (Lancioni et al. 2009a, 2009b, 2009c; Sigafoos et al. 2009; Shih et al. 2010). Obtaining a successful outcome in intervention programs such as those examined in this overview is much more likely if a number of conditions are met. One of those conditions concerns the response requirement (demand), which should be within easy reach for the participant. More specifically, the likelihood of success is greater if the response difficulty is moderate (i.e., if the response is in the person's repertoire and requires a fairly low level of effort to be performed) (Lancioni et al. 2005b, 2008b, 2010d). A second condition concerns the stimulus events available for the participant's response(s). These events should have a reinforcing power (i.e., should be highly preferred/attractive) and their positive/attractive value for the participant should exceed the efforts required of him or her to perform the response(s) (Kazdin 2001). A third condition concerns the intervention length. This length needs to be tailored to the participant's learning characteristics and essentially should be significantly longer for the participants with a more severe (disadvantaged) condition (Kazdin 2001; Lancioni et al. 2001a, 2009a; Saunders et al. 2003; Catania 2007).

The positive outcomes, as documented above (i.e., in terms of participants' response frequencies; see review of the studies), are the most immediate and common form of evidence. Other apparently critical pieces of evidence, which were recorded only in some of the studies, could be (1) the indices of happiness or unhappiness of the participants, and (2) the opinion of staff personnel, family members, or other raters about the technology, its application impact and overall effects (Lancioni et al. 2006d, 2006e, 2007d, 2008b; Dillon and Carr 2007). For example, Lancioni et al. (2006d) assessed the mood of the three children involved in a microswitch-based study, in which each participant (child) had a microswitch to use for producing brief periods of preferred stimulation. The results showed that two of the participants had clear increases in indices of happiness during the intervention. The third participant had a decrease (a virtual elimination) of indices of unhappiness (i.e., frowning and crying) during the intervention. Similarly, Lancioni et al. (2007d) explored the mood of nine participants ranging in age from about 4 to about 19 years during the baseline and intervention with microswitch-based programs. The performance of microswitch-related responses during the intervention phases allowed the participants to access brief periods of preferred stimulation.

Data showed that all nine participants increased their microswitch responding during the intervention. Seven of them also showed increases in indices of happiness during those periods.

Measuring the opinion of staff, parents, or other plausible raters such as physiotherapists and psychology students through social validation procedures helps define (1) the level of acceptance/support that these people have of the programs evaluated in the study, and (2) their likely backing of the implementation of those programs within daily contexts. For example, Lancioni et al (2006a) conducted a study in which 140 teacher trainees and 84 parents were involved in rating microswitch-based programs versus interaction/stimulation conditions for participants with multiple disabilities. All teacher trainees and parents scored the two conditions on a seven-item questionnaire concerning the participants' enjoyment of the two conditions, the possible impact and practical benefits of those conditions, and the raters' personal view of those conditions in terms of likeableness. Data indicated that both teacher trainees and parents provided the microswitch programs with higher (more positive) scoring on all seven items. These scores seemed to constitute a very strong endorsement of the microswitch-based programs and a level of evidence totally in line with the positive outcomes of the programs in terms of participants' response frequencies.

18.5.2 Implications of the Studies and Practical Perspectives

The aforementioned overview and comments stress first of all the importance of identifying and targeting single, nontypical responses for conducting successful microswitch-based interventions with persons with minimal motor behavior. The studies adopting those responses have collected a new level of encouraging evidence as to the possibility of helping the aforementioned (most affected) persons (i.e., persons who could not possibly be involved in intervention programs relying on typical motor responses and traditional microswitches) (Lancioni et al. 2005b, 2008b). Enabling these persons to be active and responsible of their environmental stimulation through various periods of the day (i.e., various intervention sessions) could represent a very relevant achievement with multiple implications in terms of the individuals' social status and quality of life as well as from a technical standpoint (Lachapelle et al. 2005; Petry et al. 2005, 2009).

On an individual level, it might be argued that the person's ability to be constructively engaged and to independently determine his or her level of stimulation can increase his or her overall satisfaction, improve his or her general mood, and present a more advanced social image (Wehmeyer and Schwartz 1998; Szymanski 2000; Browder et al. 2001; Zekovic and Renwick 2003; Karvonen et al. 2004; Petry et al. 2005, 2009; Lancioni et al. 2006d, 2006e, 2007d). From a technical standpoint, one may underline and appreciate the relevance of having (1) isolated and successfully targeted a series of specific responses, and (2) built and assessed interfaces (microswitch devices) for those responses. Such interfaces proved viable to allow the participants to use those small responses to control relevant environmental events and maintain constructive engagement. Among the interfaces, the new camera-based technology may deserve special attention; it allows the possibility of monitoring small responses through the use of one or two color marks rather than through support frames in contact with the participant's face and head (Lancioni et al. 2010a).

The nontypical responses assessed in the studies reviewed above consisted of vocalization, chin and lip movements, eyelid and eyebrow movements, small hand-closure movements, and forehead skin movements. Although those responses represent a range of opportunities for multiple intervention programs, additional (new) responses as well as response variations should be investigated to provide alternatives to those mentioned above and thus allow a wider applicability of this approach (i.e., making it suitable also to individuals who require a response different from those mentioned above). For example, one could investigate the usability of prolonged eyelid closures for participants for whom this type of response may be much more plausible than double blinks or upward looking (see above). Prolonged closures could be detected through adapted versions of the optic-microswitch technology used for the other eyelid responses or through the new camera-based microswitch technology. Another new response that could be targeted concerns small hand-opening movements. This response could be particularly suitable for participants who tend to have their hands closed (i.e., persons who keep their fingers against the palm of their hand). The technical solutions to monitor this new response could include (1) a modified version of the microswitch now used for hand-closure responses (with the new microswitch version activated as the person decreases his or her pressure on it or ends his her contact with it, and (2) the aforementioned camera-based microswitch technology.

The possibility of using multiple responses through multiple microswitches can be seen as an important enrichment in the application of microswitch-based programs. In fact, multiple responses/microswitches allow a person to extend the forms and broaden the amount of his or her activity engagement and to widen the range of sensory input (preferred stimulation) obtainable. The availability of different types of stimuli (each related to one specific response) may also have beneficial effects in terms of response motivation while limiting the risks of stimulus satiation. In such a condition, the person would be allowed to operate choices (thus satisfying his or her possible stimulus preferences), to increase his or her level of enjoyment by exploiting the opportunities of stimulus variation, and to modulate his performance also in terms of response comfortableness (Stafford et al. 2002; Cannella et al. 2005). Choice, self-determination, stimulus variation, and response comfortableness are critical elements (variables) that could easily promote a sense of personal fulfillment, improve the person's mood, and ultimately enhance the person's quality of life (Green and Reid 1999; Algozzine et al. 2001; Kazdin 2001; Hoch et al. 2002; Ross and Oliver 2003; Lancioni et al. 2004c, 2006a; Dillon and Carr 2007).

A potential drawback of programs involving multiple responses with multiple microswitches is that they do not include any provisions for (1) checking whether the person has a desire to be in contact with the caregiver, and (2) satisfying such a possible desire. However, acknowledging this potential drawback does not mean that most of the programs with multiple microswitches/responses are affected by it. In fact, such a drawback may have an impact only in programs that include (1) participants who are accustomed to and obviously enjoy social contact, and (2) caregivers who are able to integrate the provision of verbal attention or verbal and physical attention to requests of contact within their daily work schedule. Whenever the aforementioned conditions (for participants and caregivers) exist, one could avoid the drawback by transforming programs with multiple microswitches into programs with combinations of microswitches and VOCAs (cf. Schlosser and Sigafoos 2006; Lancioni et al. 2008b; Sigafoos et al. 2009). The combination of a VOCA for requesting caregiver attention or mediation with regular microswitches that consent direct access to environmental stimuli may be considered a realistic and straightforward process. The studies reviewed earlier provide encouraging evidence with regard to this point (e.g., Lancioni et al. 2008b, 2009b, 2010c). An intervention program based on the use of microswitches and a VOCA can include fairly long and/or multiple sessions a day without any risk of isolating the participant and preventing him or her from human interactions.

18.5.3 Other Relevant Procedural Aspects for Daily Programs

In dealing with persons with severe/profound multiple disabilities, one can find that the lack of constructive engagement with the outside world is often combined with forms of problem behavior, such as eye poking and hand mouthing, or problem (inadequate) posture such as head tilting (Lancioni et al. 2009d). In an attempt to deal with these situations, one might resort to the use of microswitch clusters (i.e., a strategy not reviewed above). Such a strategy relies on the use of two or more microswitches to monitor simultaneously the positive/adaptive response that should be increased and the problem behavior/posture that should be reduced. The technology to realize viable cluster solutions may be considered reasonably accessible both in terms of complexity and costs (see Lancioni et al. 2008b, 2008e). Initially, the cluster program focuses on increasing the adaptive response that leads to preferred stimulation. Subsequently, the adaptive response allows access to preferred stimulation only if it occurs in the absence of the problem behavior/posture. Moreover, the stimulation following an adaptive response free from the problem behavior/posture would last the scheduled time only if the problem behavior/posture does not appear during that time period. One may argue that such a strategy represents a most constructive and positive approach to help persons with severe/profound multiple disabilities improve their performance and advance their development. In fact, the use of microswitch clusters allows the intervention conditions for increasing adaptive responding and for reducing problem behavior/posture to be integrated within the same program.

For example, Lancioni et al. (2007e) used microswitch clusters with two participants of 8 and 12 years of age to (1) increase adaptive responses, which consisted of forms of object manipulation, and (2) reduce problem behavior, which consisted of hand or object mouthing. The adaptive responses were monitored through a wobble-like microswitch or a vibration microswitch. The problem behavior was monitored through optic microswitches, which were arranged in different ways for the two participants so as to suit their behavioral expressions. Initially, the program ensured that the participants would obtain brief periods of preferred stimulation for each of their object manipulation responses irrespective of whether these responses occurred in the presence or in the absence of the problem behavior. Once the object manipulation responses had been strengthened, their emission would produce positive stimulation only if free from the problem behavior. Moreover, such stimulation would be interrupted prematurely if the problem behavior occurred during its presentation. Both participants were able to increase the frequency of their adaptive manipulation responses and to reduce their problem behavior to low levels.

Lancioni et al. (2008e) carried out a study that was aimed at extending the application and evaluation of microswitch clusters to promote adaptive responding and curb inappropriate (unhealthy) postures. The study involved three participants of about 8–17 years of age with multiple disabilities. The participants' adaptive responses concerned various foot and hand movements. The inappropriate posture was head forward tilting. Initially, the participants had access to a brief period of preferred stimulation after each adaptive response (regardless of their posture). Subsequently, only the adaptive responses that occurred in the absence of the inappropriate posture were followed by the stimulation scheduled for them. The stimulation lasted the full period if the participant remained free from the inappropriate posture through that time. Lack of posture control led to a premature interruption of the stimulation. Data showed that all three participants increased their overall frequencies of adaptive responses eventually performing most of those responses free from the inappropriate posture. Such a posture (i.e., head forward tilting) remained absent through most of the stimulation periods and through most of the session times. These positive findings were supported by an expert validation assessment of the program, which was conducted by physiotherapist trainees and professionals. Both groups indicated that such a program could represent a useful complement to formal motor rehabilitation procedures and thus become a regular part of the intervention package.

18.6 Conclusions

In conclusion, the studies analyzed within this chapter underline in an unequivocal manner the importance that forms of assistive technology, such as microswitches and VOCAs (and possibly microswitch clusters), can have within programs for persons with severe/profound multiple disabilities. Programs adopting microswitches can help these persons acquire constructive occupation and control access to stimulation independently. The benefits of such programs would grow considerably if combinations of microswitches (rather than single microswitches) are used. Programs adopting microswitches and VOCAs can help the persons on their occupation, access to stimulation, as well as on their social contact with relevant caregiving figures. Programs adopting microswitch clusters can improve the performance and advance the development of those persons by enhancing their adaptive responses and curbing their problem behavior/postures.

New research initiatives could be envisaged to improve the aforementioned forms of technology and their applications. For example, one might investigate new solutions to extend and upgrade the microswitches for monitoring minimal, nontypical responses. One such solution for these responses could be relying on the employment of camera-based technology. This technology would ensure high reliability and eliminate the need of using devices on the person's body (e.g., optic sensors fixed on eyeglasses; see Lancioni et al. 2010a; Leung and Chau 2010). One could also design various forms of microswitch-cluster programs to help reduce different posture problems and deterioration of persons with extensive motor disabilities (Begnoche and Pitetti 2007; Leyshon and Shaw 2008).

Summary of the Chapter

Forms of assistive technology such as microswitches and VOCAs may be essential resources to help persons with profound and multiple disabilities learn to control relevant stimuli of their environment and ask for social contact through simple (minimal) responses. This chapter is divided into four sections. The first section focuses on studies using experimental microswitches developed to monitor small (nontypical) responses, such as eyelid and lip movements, and thus to suit individuals with minimal motor behavior. The second section analyzes studies that have combined two or more microswitches to allow the person direct access to different types of stimulation and choice opportunities. The third section examines studies that have combined microswitches with VOCAs to allow the person direct access to stimulation as well as the possibility to call for social attention and interaction. The fourth section discusses (1) the results obtained with the different forms of technology used and their applicability and possible impact in daily education/rehabilitation contexts, and (2) the possibility of using combinations of microswitches also for programs aimed at simultaneously targeting increases of adaptive responding and reduction of problem behaviors or inadequate postures.

References

Algozzine, B., Browder, D., Karvonen, M., Test, D. W., and Wood, W. M. (2001). Effects of interventions to promote self-determination for individuals with disabilities. *Review of Educational Research, 71*, 219–277.

Begnoche, D., and Pitetti, K. H. (2007). Effects of traditional treatment and partial body weight treadmill training on the motor skills of children with spastic cerebral palsy: A pilot study. *Pediatric Physical Therapy, 19*, 11–19.

Browder, D. M., Wood, W. M., Test, D. W., Karvonen, M., and Algozzine, B. (2001). Reviewing resources on self-determination: A map for teachers. *Remedial and Special Education, 22*, 233–244.

Cannella, H. I., O'Reilly, M. F., and Lancioni, G. E. (2005). Choice and preference assessment research with people with severe to profound developmental disabilities: A review of the literature. *Research in Developmental Disabilities, 26*, 1–15.

Catania, A. C. (2007). *Learning* (4th Interim ed.). New York: Sloan Publishing.

Crawford, M. R., and Schuster, J. W. (1993). Using microswitches to teach toy use. *Journal of Developmental and Physical Disabilities, 5*, 349–368.

Dillon, C. M., and Carr, J. E. (2007). Assessing indices of happiness and unhappiness in individuals with developmental disabilities: A review. *Behavioral Interventions, 22*, 229–244.

Glickman, L., Deitz, J., Anson, D., and Stewart, K. (1996). The effect of switch control site on computer skills of infants and toddlers. *American Journal of Occupational Therapy, 50*, 545–553.

Green, C. W., and Reid, D. H. (1999). A behavioral approach to identifying sources of happiness and unhappiness among individuals with profound multiple disabilities. *Behavior Modification, 23*, 280–293.

Hoch, H., McComas, J. J., Johnson, L., Faranda, N., and Guenther, S. L. (2002). The effects of magnitude and quality of reinforcement on choice responding during play activities. *Journal of Applied Behavior Analysis, 35*, 171–181.

Holburn, S., Nguyen, D., and Vietze, P. M. (2004). Computer-assisted learning for adults with profound multiple disabilities. *Behavioral Interventions, 19*, 25–37.

Judge, S., Floyd, K., and Wood-Fields, C. (2010). Creating a technology-rich learning environment for infants and toddlers with disabilities. *Infants and Young Children, 23*, 84–92.

Karvonen, M., Test, D. W., Wood, W. M., Browder, D., and Algozzine, B. (2004). Putting self-determination into practice. *Exceptional Children, 71*, 23–41.

Kazdin, A. E. (2001). *Behavior Modification in Applied Settings* (6th ed.). New York: Wadsworth.

Lachapelle, Y., Wehmeyer, M. L., Haelewyck, M. C., Courbois, Y., Keith, K. D., Schalock, R., Verdugo, M. A., and Walsh, P. N. (2005). The relationship between quality of life and self-determination: An international study. *Journal of Intellectual Disability Research, 49*, 740–744.

Lancioni, G. E., Bellini, D., Oliva, D., Singh, N. N., O'Reilly, M. F., and Sigafoos, J. (2010a). Camera-based microswitch technology for eyelid and mouth responses of persons with profound multiple disabilities: Two case studies. *Research in Developmental Disabilities, 31*, 1509–1514.

Lancioni, G. E., and Lems, S. (2001). Using a microswitch for vocalization responses with persons with multiple disabilities. *Disability and Rehabilitation, 23*, 745–748.

Lancioni, G. E., Olivetti Belardinelli, M., Stasolla, F., Singh, N. N., O'Reilly, M. F., Sigafoos, J., and Angelillo, M. T. (2008a). Promoting engagement, requests and choice by a man with post-coma pervasive motor impairment and minimally conscious state through a technology-based program. *Journal of Developmental and Physical Disabilities, 20,* 379–388.

Lancioni, G. E., O'Reilly, M. F., and Basili, G. (2001a). An overview of technological resources used in rehabilitation research with people with severe/profound and multiple disabilities. *Disability and Rehabilitation, 23,* 501–508.

Lancioni, G. E., O'Reilly, M. F., and Basili, G. (2001b). Use of microswitches and speech output systems with people with severe/profound intellectual or multiple disabilities: A literature review. *Research in Developmental Disabilities, 22,* 21–40.

Lancioni, G. E., O'Reilly, M. F., Cuvo, A. J., Singh, N. N., Sigafoos, J., and Didden, R. (2007a). PECS and VOCA to enable students with developmental disabilities to make requests: An overview of the literature. *Research in Developmental Disabilities, 28,* 468–488.

Lancioni, G. E., O'Reilly, M. F., Oliva, D., and Coppa, M. M. (2001c). A microswitch for vocalization responses to foster environmental control in children with multiple disabilities. *Journal of Intellectual Disability Research, 45,* 271–275.

Lancioni, G. E., O'Reilly, M. F., Oliva, D., and Coppa, M. M. (2001d). Using multiple microswitches to promote different responses in children with multiple disabilities. *Research in Developmental Disabilities, 22,* 309–318.

Lancioni, G. E., O'Reilly, M. F., Oliva, D., Singh, N. N., and Coppa, M. M. (2002a). Multiple microswitches for multiple responses with children with profound disabilities. *Cognitive Behaviour Therapy, 31,* 81–87.

Lancioni, G. E., O'Reilly, M. F., Sigafoos, J., Singh, N. N., Oliva, D., and Basili, G. (2004a). Enabling a person with multiple disabilities and minimal motor behaviour to control environmental stimulation with chin movements. *Disability and Rehabilitation, 26,* 1291–1294.

Lancioni, G. E., O'Reilly, M. F., Singh, N. N., Buonocunto, F., Sacco, V., Colonna, F., Navarro, J., Lanzilotti, C., and Megna, G. (2010b). Post-coma persons with minimal consciousness and motor disabilities learn to use assistive communication technology to seek environmental stimulation. *Journal of Developmental and Physical Disabilities, 22,* 119–129.

Lancioni, G. E., O'Reilly, M. F., Singh, N. N., Buonocunto, F., Sacco, V., Colonna, F., Navarro, J., Lanzilotti, C., Olivetti Belardinelli, M., Bosco, A., Megna, G., and De Tommaso, M. (2009a). Evaluation of technology-assisted learning setups for undertaking assessment and providing intervention to persons with a diagnosis of vegetative state. *Developmental Neurorehabilitation, 12,* 411–420.

Lancioni, G. E., O'Reilly, M. F., Singh, N. N., Buonocunto, F., Sacco, V., Colonna, F., Navarro, J., Oliva, D., Megna, G., and Bosco, A. (2009b). Technology-based intervention options for post-coma persons with minimally conscious state and pervasive motor disabilities. *Developmental Neurorehabilitation, 12,* 24–31.

Lancioni, G. E., O'Reilly, M. F., Singh, N. N., Groeneweg, J., Bosco, A., Tota, A., Smaldone, A., Stasolla, F., Manfredi, F., Baccani, S., and Pidala, S. (2006a). A social validation assessment of microswitch-based programs for persons with multiple disabilities employing teacher trainees and parents as raters. *Journal of Developmental and Physical Disabilities, 18,* 383–391.

Lancioni, G. E., O'Reilly, M. F., Singh, N. N., Oliva, D., Baccani, S., Severini, L., and Groeneweg, J. (2006b). Micro-switch programmes for students with multiple disabilities and minimal motor behaviour: Assessing response acquisition and choice. *Pediatric Rehabilitation, 9,* 137–143.

Lancioni, G. E., O'Reilly, M. F., Singh, N. N., Oliva, D., Coppa, M. M., and Montironi, G. (2005a). A new microswitch to enable a boy with minimal motor behavior to control environmental stimulation with eye blinks. *Behavioral Interventions, 20,* 147–153.

Lancioni, G. E., O'Reilly, M. F., Singh, N. N., Oliva, D., Piazzolla, G., Pirani, P., and Groeneweg, J. (2002b). Evaluating the use of multiple microswitches and responses for children with multiple disabilities. *Journal of Intellectual Disability Research, 46,* 346–351.

Lancioni, G. E., O'Reilly, M. F., Singh, N. N., Sigafoos, J., Didden, R., Oliva, D., Campodonico, F., de Pace, C., Chiapparino, C., and Groeneweg, J. (2009c). Persons with multiple disabilities accessing stimulation and requesting social contact via microswitch and VOCA devices: New research evaluation and social validation. *Research in Developmental Disabilities, 30,* 1084–1094.

Lancioni, G. E., O'Reilly, M. F., Singh, N. N., Sigafoos, J., Didden, R., Oliva, D., and Montironi, G. (2007b). Persons with multiple disabilities and minimal motor behavior using small forehead movements and new microswitch technology to control environmental stimuli. *Perceptual and Motor Skills, 104,* 870–878.

Lancioni, G. E., O'Reilly, M. F., Singh, N. N., Sigafoos, J., Didden, R., Oliva, D., Montironi, G., and La Martire, M. L. (2007c). Small hand-closure movements used as a response through microswitch technology by persons with multiple disabilities and minimal motor behavior. *Perceptual and Motor Skills, 104,* 1027–1034.

Lancioni, G. E., O'Reilly, M. F., Singh, N. N., Sigafoos, J., Oliva, D., Antonucci, M., Tota, A., and Basili, G. (2008b). Microswitch-based programs for persons with multiple disabilities: An overview of some recent developments. *Perceptual and Motor Skills, 106,* 355–370.

Lancioni, G. E., O'Reilly, M. F., Singh, N. N., Sigafoos, J., Oliva, D., Baccani, S., Bosco, A., and Stasolla, F. (2004b). Technological aids to promote basic developmental achievements by children with multiple disabilities: Evaluation of two cases. *Cognitive Processing, 5,* 232–238.

Lancioni, G. E., O'Reilly, M. F., Singh, N. N., Sigafoos, J., Oliva, D., and Severini, L. (2008c). Enabling two persons with multiple disabilities to access environmental stimuli and ask for social contact through microswitches and a VOCA. *Research in Developmental Disabilities, 29,* 21–28.

Lancioni, G. E., O'Reilly, M. F., Singh, N. N., Sigafoos, J., Oliva, D., and Severini, L. (2008d). Three persons with multiple disabilities accessing environmental stimuli and asking for social contact through microswitch and VOCA technology. *Journal of Intellectual Disability Research, 52,* 327–336.

Lancioni, G. E., O'Reilly, M. F., Singh, N. N., Sigafoos, J., Tota, A., Antonucci, M., and Oliva, D. (2006c). Children with multiple disabilities and minimal motor behavior using chin movements to operate microswitches to obtain environmental stimulation. *Research in Developmental Disabilities, 27,* 290–298.

Lancioni, G. E., Saponaro, F., Singh, N. N., O'Reilly, M. F., Sigafoos, J., and Oliva, D. (2010c). A microswitch to enable a woman with acquired brain injury and profound multiple disabilities to access environmental stimulation with lip movements. *Perceptual and Motor Skills, 110,* 488–492.

Lancioni, G. E., Singh, N. N., O'Reilly, M. F., La Martire, M. L., Stasolla, F., Smaldone, A., and Oliva, D. (2006d). Microswitch-based programs as therapeutic recreation interventions for students with profound multiple disabilities. *American Journal of Recreation Therapy, 5,* 15–20.

Lancioni, G. E., Singh, N. N., O'Reilly, M. F., and Oliva, D. (2004c). A microswitch program including words and choice opportunities for students with multiple disabilities. *Perceptual and Motor Skills, 98,* 214–222.

Lancioni, G. E., Singh, N. N., O'Reilly, M. F., and Oliva, D. (2005b). Microswitch programs for persons with multiple disabilities: An overview of the responses adopted for microswitch activation. *Cognitive Processing, 6,* 177–188.

Lancioni, G. E., Singh, N. N., O'Reilly, M. F., Oliva, D., and Montironi, G. (2004d). A computer system serving as a microswitch for vocal utterances of persons with multiple disabilities: Two case evaluations. *Journal of Visual Impairment and Blindness, 98,* 116–120.

Lancioni, G. E., Singh, N. N., O'Reilly, M. F., Oliva, D., Montironi, G., and Chierchie, S. (2004e). Assessing a new response-microswitch combination with a boy with minimal motor behavior. *Perceptual and Motor Skills, 98,* 459–462.

Lancioni, G. E., Singh, N. N., O'Reilly, M. F., Oliva, D., Montironi, G., Piazza, F., Ciavattini, F., and Bettarelli, F. (2004f). Using computer systems as microswitches for vocal utterances of persons with multiple disabilities. *Research in Developmental Disabilities, 25,* 183–192.

Lancioni, G. E., Singh, N. N., O'Reilly, M. F., Oliva, D., Smaldone, A., Tota, A., Martielli, G., Stasolla, F., Pontiggia, G., and Groeneweg, J. (2006e). Assessing the effects of stimulation versus micro-switch-based programmes on indices of happiness of students with multiple disabilities. *Journal of Intellectual Disability Research, 50*, 739–747.

Lancioni, G. E., Singh, N. N., O'Reilly, M. F., and Sigafoos, J. (2009d). An overview of behavioral strategies for reducing hand-related stereotypes of persons with severe to profound intellectual and multiple disabilities. *Research in Developmental Disabilities, 30*, 20–43.

Lancioni, G. E., Singh, N. N., O'Reilly, M. F., Sigafoos, J., Buonocunto, F., Sacco, V., Colonna, F., Navarro, J., Megna, G., Chiapparino, C., and De Pace, C. (2009e). Two persons with severe post-coma motor impairment and minimally conscious state use assistive technology to access stimulus events and social contact. *Disability and Rehabilitation: Assistive Technology, 4*, 367–372.

Lancioni, G. E., Singh, N. N., O'Reilly, M. F., Sigafoos, J., Buonocunto, F., Sacco, V., Colonna, F., Navarro, J., Oliva, D., Signorino, M., and Megna, G. (2009f). Microswitch- and VOCA-assisted programs for two post-coma persons with minimally conscious state and pervasive motor disabilities. *Research in Developmental Disabilities, 30*, 1459–1467.

Lancioni, G. E., Singh, N. N., O'Reilly, M. F., Sigafoos, J., Didden, R., Oliva, D., Severini, L., Smaldone, A., Tota, A., and Lamartire, M. L. (2007d). Effects of microswitch-based programs on indices of happiness of students with multiple disabilities: A new research evaluation. *American Journal on Mental Retardation, 112*, 167–176.

Lancioni, G. E., Singh, N. N., O'Reilly, M. F., Sigafoos, J., Didden, R., Smaldone, A., and La Martire, M. L. (2010d). Helping a man with multiple disabilities to use single vs repeated performance of simple motor schemes as different responses. *Perceptual and Motor Skills, 110*, 105–113.

Lancioni, G. E., Singh, N. N., O'Reilly, M. F., Sigafoos, J., Oliva, D., Costantini, A., Gatto, S., Marinelli, V., and Putzolu, A. (2006f). An optic microswitch for an eyelid response to foster environmental control in children with minimal motor behaviour. *Pediatric Rehabilitation, 9*, 53–56.

Lancioni, G. E., Singh, N. N., O'Reilly, M. F., Sigafoos, J., Oliva, D., Gatti, M., Manfredi, F., Megna, G., La Martire, M. L., Tota, A., Smaldone, A., and Groeneweg, J. (2008e). A microswitch-cluster program to foster adaptive responses and head control in students with multiple disabilities: Replication and validation assessment. *Research in Developmental Disabilities, 29*, 373–384.

Lancioni, G. E., Singh, N. N., O'Reilly, M. F., Sigafoos, J., Oliva, D., Severini, L., Smaldone, A., and Tamma, M. (2007e). Microswitch technology to promote adaptive responses and reduce mouthing in two children with multiple disabilities. *Journal of Visual Impairment and Blindness, 101*, 628–636.

Leatherby, J. K., Gast, D. L., Wolery, M., and Collins, B. C. (1992). Assessment of reinforcer preference in multi-handicapped students. *Journal of Developmental and Physical Disabilities, 4*, 15–36.

Leung, B., and Chau, T. (2010). A multiple camera tongue switch for a child with severe spastic quadriplegic cerebral palsy. *Disability and Rehabilitation: Assistive Technology, 5*, 58–68.

Leyshon, R. T., and Shaw, L. E. (2008). Using the ICF as a conceptual framework to guide ergonomic intervention in occupational rehabilitation. *Work: Journal of Prevention, Assessment and Rehabilitation, 31*, 47–61.

Matson, J. L., Minshawi, N. F., Gonzalez, M. L., and Mayville, S. B. (2006). The relationship of comorbid problem behaviors to social skills in persons with profound mental retardation. *Behavior Modification, 30*, 496–506.

McDougall, J., Evans, J., and Baldwin, P. (2010). The importance of self-determination to perceived quality of life for youth and young adults with chronic conditions and disabilities. *Remedial and Special Education, 31*, 252–260.

Mechling, L. C. (2006). Comparison of the effects of three approaches on the frequency of stimulus activation, via a single switch, by students with profound intellectual disabilities. *The Journal of Special Education, 40*, 94–102.

Petry, K., Maes, B., and Vlaskamp, C. (2005). Domains of quality of life of people with profound multiple disabilities: The perspective of parents and direct support staff. *Journal of Applied Research in Intellectual Disabilities, 18*, 35–46.

Petry, K., Maes, B., and Vlaskamp, C. (2009). Measuring the quality of life of people with profound multiple disabilities using the QOL-PMD: First results. *Research in Developmental Disabilities, 30,* 1394–1405.

Richman, D. M. (2008). Early intervention and prevention of self-injurious behaviour exhibited by young children with developmental disabilities. *Journal of Intellectual Disability Research, 52,* 3–17

Ringdahl, J. E., Vollmer, T. R., Marcus, B. E., and Roane, H. S. (1997). An analogue evaluation of environmental enrichment: The role of stimulus preference. *Journal of Applied Behavior Analysis, 30,* 203–216.

Rispoli, M. J., Franco, J. H., van der Meer, L., Lang, R., and Camargo, S. P. H. (2010). The use of speech generating devices in communication interventions for individuals with developmental disabilities: A review of the literature. *Developmental Neurorehabilitation, 13,* 276–293.

Ross, E., and Oliver, C. (2003). The assessment of mood in adults who have severe or profound mental retardation. *Clinical Psychology Review, 23,* 225–245.

Saunders, M. D., Timler, G. R., Cullinan, T. B., Pilkey, S., Questad, K. A., and Saunders, R. R. (2003). Evidence of contingency awareness in people with profound multiple impairments: Response duration versus response rate indicators. *Research in Developmental Disabilities, 24,* 231–245.

Schalock, R., Brown, I., Brown, R., Cummins, R. A., Felce, D., Matikka, L., Keith, K. D., and Parmenter, T. (2003). Conceptualization, measurement, and application of quality of life for persons with intellectual disabilities: Reports of an international panel of experts. *Mental Retardation, 40,* 457–470.

Schlosser, R. W., and Sigafoos, J. (2006). Augmentative and alternative communication interventions for persons with developmental disabilities: Narrative review of comparative single-subject experimental studies. *Research in Developmental Disabilities, 27,* 1–29.

Shih, C.-H., Chang, M.-L., and Shih, C.-T. (2010). A new limb movement detector enabling people with multiple disabilities to control environmental stimulation through limb swing with a gyration air mouse. *Research in Developmental Disabilities, 31,* 875–880.

Sigafoos, J., Green, V. A., Payne, D., Son, S. H.,O'Reilly, M. F., and Lancioni, G. E. (2009). A comparison of picture exchange and speech-generating devices: Acquisition, preference, and effects on social interaction. *Augmentative and Alternative Communication, 25,* 99–109.

Stafford, A. M., Alberto, P. M., Fredrick, L. D., Heflin, L. J., and Heller, K. W. (2002). Preference variability and the instruction of choice making with students with severe intellectual disabilities. *Education and Training in Mental Retardation and Developmental Disabilities, 37,* 70–88.

Sullivan, M. W., Laverick, D. H., and Lewis, M. (1995). Fostering environmental control in a young child with Rett syndrome: A case study. *Journal of Autism and Developmental Disorders, 25,* 215–221.

Sullivan, M. W., and Lewis, M. (1993). Contingency, means-end skills and the use of technology in infant intervention. *Infants and Young Children, 5,* 58–77.

Szymanski, L. S. (2000). Happiness as a treatment goal. *American Journal on Mental Retardation, 105,* 352–362.

Valiquette, C., Sutton, A., and Ska, B. (2010). A graphic symbol tool for the evaluation of communication, satisfaction and priorities of individuals with intellectual disability who use a speech generating device. *Child Language Teaching and Therapy, 26,* 303–319.

Wehmeyer, M. L., and Schwartz, M. (1998). The relationship between self-determination, quality of life, and life satisfaction for adults with mental retardation. *Education and Training in Mental Retardation and Developmental Disabilities, 33,* 3–12.

Zekovic, B., and Renwick, R. (2003). Quality of life for children and adolescents with developmental disabilities: Review of conceptual and methodological issues relevant to public policy. *Disability and Society, 18,* 19–34.

19

Methods and Technologies for Leisure, Recreation, and an Accessible Sport

C. M. Capio, G. Mascolo, and C. H. P. Sit

CONTENTS

19.1 Introduction

19.1.1 Self-Efficacy Theory

A well-established area of sport psychology has built research on the role of self-efficacy in successful sports participation. Initially proposed by Bandura (1997), self-efficacy refers to the belief than an individual has in his or her the ability to execute a task to generate a specific outcome. This belief of having some amount of control over one's own functioning has been described to have a pervasive influence in an individual's task performance. Studies of the self-efficacy construct in sport have included physical proficiency and different aspects of game performance such as strategy selection, prediction of opponent's actions, and pressure management (Short and Ross-Stewart 2009).

Self-efficacy beliefs have been theorized to be products of an individual's cognitive processing of diverse sources of efficacy information (Feltz et al. 2008). The four principal sources of efficacy information as proposed by Bandura (1997) are (1) past performance accomplishments, (2) vicarious experiences, (3) verbal persuasion, and (4) psychological and emotional states. Among individuals with disabilities, efficacy information may be markedly different. In particular, the most influential of efficacy information sources has been identified to be past performance accomplishments, and their influence on self-efficacy beliefs has been confirmed through a meta-analysis of sport studies (Moritz et al. 2000). Self-efficacy is embedded in performance results (Bandura 1997), and as a person gains more experiences of a certain task, performance becomes a stronger predictor of self-efficacy (Short and Ross-Stewart 2009). This suggests that for individuals with disabilities, compromised performance outcomes may have a negative impact on their self-efficacy beliefs. However, an environment that promotes accessible sport for individuals with disabilities through the use of assistive technology and adapted programs may facilitate successful task performances that build over time. Although the self-efficacy beliefs of individuals with disabilities may continue to influence their performance outcomes, consistent experiences of accessible sport may contribute to enhancing their inclinations to participate in physical activities.

19.1.2 Facilitating Psychological Recovery through Sport

Participation in sport and physical activity has been suggested to be a factor that contributes toward psychological recovery for individuals who have acquired disabilities. Life changes can be overwhelming with an acquired disability because of heightened dependence on others and altered abilities to perform daily living activities. Persons in such a situation have been known to find new motivations in engaging in sport and physical activity, possibly because involvement in sport and exercise has been shown to facilitate a rediscovery of a sense of self-identity (Carless and Sparkes 2008) and boost self-esteem (Fox 2000; Richardson et al. 2005). With a host of other benefits (e.g., physiologic and social) associated with being physically active, the positive effects on the process of psychological recovery among individuals who experienced disabling injuries highlights the need for approaches to make sport and physical activity participation accessible.

Anecdotal stories have shown that individuals with disabilities struggle with finding the best techniques and technologies that would aid their successful performances in sport and physical activity. On some occasions, devices have been designed by the users themselves who best understood the needs and demands associated with their conditions. Nevertheless, paradigm shifts in the society have led to movements and institutionalized approaches at identifying methods and technologies that promote the participation of individuals with disabilities in sport and physical activity.

19.2 Adapted Physical Activity: When Physical Activity Is for Everyone

The direct and critical role of physical activity (PA) in the primary prevention of cardiovascular conditions, diabetes, obesity, and cancer has been established among adults (Dunn and Blair 2002). This has been confirmed in a recent review of the World Health Organization (WHO), and the positive effect of physical activity in musculoskeletal health and psychological well-being has been identified (Bull et al. 2004). Evidence has shown that PA participation may lead to improved physical fitness, muscular strength, and overall quality of life (Pedersen and Saltin 2006). Suffice it to say, substantial evidence indicates that physical inactivity is directly related to the global burden of disease, disability, and death.

In children, participation in PA is considered to have a positive impact on childhood health (Ekelund et al. 2004; Metcalf et al. 2004) and have beneficial effects on their future health status (Strong et al. 2005) by promoting lifetime PA participation (Huang et al. 2009). On the other hand, physical inactivity has been implicated in the increasing epidemic of overweight and obesity (Wang and Lobstein 2006; WHO 2010) and metabolic morbidities among children and adolescents (Strong et al. 2005). The multidimensional benefits of regular participation in PA by children and adolescents impacts the areas of health, socialization, discipline, and physical fitness (Sallis and Patrick 1994; Martens 1996). Evidence-based data indicate strong favorable effects on musculoskeletal and cardiovascular health (Strong et al. 2005). The benefits of PA among children are universal such that they encompass those with chronic diseases and disabilities as well (Murphy and Carbone 2008; Huang et al. 2009).

19.2.1 Adapted Physical Activity

Adapted physical activity (APA) programs deal with specific populations and have evolved from being integrated in rehabilitation interventions into services that support persons of all ages who need adaptation in PA participation in any kind of setting (Hutzler and Sherrill 2007). It has been considered as one of the most viable service delivery systems for persons with disabilities (Sherrill 2004), but the clientele may also include those who are obese, aged, or very young. Essentially, APA is directed toward making participation in physical activities possible for everyone. Although APA programs have been initially focused on facilitating better physical function, they have also been recognized as effective enablers of improved well being, enhanced self-worth, and a sense of empowerment (Pensgaard and Sorensen 2002; Winnick 2005). As a field of study and practice, APA has also evolved into a multi-, inter-, or cross-disciplinary movement, which reflects the varied stakeholders who are concerned with the goal of universal promotion of PA (Sherrill 2004).

Extensive research in PA has led to convincing evidence supporting the importance of being physically active in terms of health and well-being, and challenges have shifted toward the dissemination of evidence-based interventions (Rabin et al. 2006). However, the current status of research in APA is relatively less definitive and has been focused on establishing epidemiologic data (Sharav and Bowman 1992; Bandini et al. 2005; Foley et al. 2008) and clarifying measurement issues (Horvat et al. 1993; Fernhall and Unnithan 2002; Mackey et al. 2009; Capio et al. 2010). Factors related to APA participation by different groups have also been examined to gain an improved understanding and promote the removal of barriers to active involvement in PA (Law et al. 2006; Warms et al. 2007; Sit et al. 2009). Cross-sectional descriptive studies have suggested that APA programs lead to multidimensional benefits for individuals with disabilities (Bjornson et al. 2008; Groff et al. 2009). More recently, a growing number of intervention studies have also manifested indicators of positive effects of APA programs for specific participant groups (Driver and Ede 2009; Daniel et al. 2010).

19.2.2 Types of APA Programs

Physical activity has been defined as any body movement produced by the forces of skeletal muscles resulting in increased energy expenditure above the resting level (Bouchard and Shephard 1994). This definition is broad enough for types of PA to include active transport (e.g., walking and cycling), housework, recreational games and activities, dance, and deliberate sport or exercise (Cavill et al. 2006). As such, APA programs have been varied not only in terms of population groups, but in terms of types of PA as well. Although this appears to lead to inadequacy in terms of confirmatory and definitive evidence for interventions, this is also an indicator of the wide range of opportunities for concerned individuals to promote PA among persons with disabilities. Consequently, such variation of APA programs also leads to a greater potential to engage a range of sectors in the society.

For example, outdoor recreation has been shown to be beneficial for people with disabilities (Loy et al. 2003; McAvoy et al. 2006), and people are motivated to join because the activity results in social, psychological, and physiological benefits (Manfredo and Driver 1996). Adults with physical disabilities who have been engaged in outdoor recreational fishing in Germany reported through a questionnaire that participation in this activity led to benefits in terms of social interaction, self-improvement, experiencing nature and relaxation, and challenge-related aspects (Freudenberg and Arlinghaus 2010). The participant sample consisted mainly of people with mobility-related disabilities; thus, nearly half reported that engagement in outdoor recreational fishing required the use of special devices (e.g., wheelchairs) and structural modifications (e.g., ramps) on the fishing sites. Participants also used fishing techniques that had less demands on physical mobility.

Deliberate exercise consisting of aerobic and resistance training programs may also constitute an APA program. Implemented among adults with traumatic brain injury, such program was conducted 3 times per week over eight weeks (Driver and Ede 2009). Considering the participants' characteristics, individualized treatments were conducted and heart rates were kept within 50–70% of each individual's maximum heart rate. Results of this study indicated that the APA program led to a significant decrease of indices of the participants' tension, depression, anger, fatigue, and confusion. Improvements were also found in the participants' vigor and friendliness.

APA in the form of deliberate exercise may also consist of flexibility and strengthening exercises. Such program was implemented among elderly individuals aged 65 years or older (Benedetti et al. 2008). Postural deformities, flexed posture in particular, are common impairments associated with aging (Balzini et al. 2003). As such, the APA program consisted of exercises for the trunk that were based on a protocol that focused on proprioceptive input (Sinaki et al. 2005). The exercise protocol was adapted by limiting the number of exercises to suit the elderly participants. Each session lasted for 1 h and was conducted twice per week for a period of three months. Clinical and instrumental measurements indicated that the program resulted in significant improvements in postural alignment and decreased musculoskeletal impairment.

APA in the form of play (e.g., ball games, racket sports, video games) has been implemented in a hospital setting among children with cancer (Speyer et al. 2010). Participants joined individualized APA sessions for a minimum of 3 times per week during hospitalization. Parameters of each session were designed considering each individual child's choice and capacities, previous physical practices, and phase of the disease. Participation in APA was shown to lead to higher indices of health-related quality of life, specifically in terms of physical functioning, social-physical roles, self-esteem, and dimensions of mental health, behavior, and bodily pain.

Evidence-based recommendations on PA among children have suggested that an adequate amount of PA may be accumulated in school during physical education classes, along with recess time, intramural sports, and after-school programs (Strong et al. 2005). Consistent with this, one of the most prevalent forms of APA is school-based instructional adapted physical education, which has previously implied the use of classrooms and instructions that were dedicated to school-aged children with disabilities (Sherrill 2004). The recent years have seen a shift in the paradigm and attitudes of society toward disabilities (Kudlacek et al. 2010) such that a growing number of students with disabilities are being included into mainstream education (Kudlacek et al. 2002; Meegan and MacPhail 2006). Consequently, PA promotion through physical education classes is directly affected by the competencies of teachers to implement inclusive education. Studies have indicated that physical education teachers face challenges in including students with disabilities in general physical education, which could possibly result in significantly lower levels of participation in sports and PA participation among persons with disability (Kudlacek et al. 2010). This limitation is expected to be addressed by current strategies that aim to prepare teachers, coaches, and therapists who will work with persons with disabilities in educational settings.

Sports activities constitute a major form of PA, and among persons with disabilities, sports participation leads to physical benefits, enhanced psychological well-being, and improved social skills (Vanderstraeten and Oomen 2010). Biological factors associated with disabilities often lead to greater secondary health risks due to physical inactivity (Wrotniak et al. 2006) that may be combated by sports participation. Furthermore, sports have been seen to contribute to muscle strengthening, coordination, and balance (Giacobbi et al. 2008).

19.3 Sport and Disability

APA in the form of sports has shown remarkable growth, which is evident in the increasing number of people with disabilities who participate in sports (Nasuti and Temple 2010) and in the Olympic-level status of movements that have developed for individuals with intellectual and physical disabilities. The Special Olympics and the Paralympics have both become global stages that showcase and celebrate the abilities of athletes with different disabilities.

Among persons with intellectual disabilities, needs for organized PA have been addressed by Special Olympics programs through opportunities for sports competition (Farrell et al. 2004). Although the Special Olympics World Games is held every two years, sports training and competition opportunities at local community and school levels are encouraged and represent methods of engaging a greater number of eligible athletes (Special Olympics 2011a). A range of programs is also implemented to support the successful participation of individuals with intellectual disabilities in PA, such as the Healthy Athlete program, which includes fitness-training sessions (Special Olympics 2010). For the 2011 World Games, athletes competed in 21 Olympic-type team or individual sports (Special Olympics 2011b) that are summarized in Table 19.1. Adaptation is apparent in how athletes are classified in divisions with other athletes of similar abilities, which allows for fair competition and chances to win within each division. Although participation in Special Olympics programs has been associated with enhanced self-esteem, self-confidence, and positive self-perceptions among the athletes (Klein et al. 1993; Dykens and Cohen 1996), parents also reported perceptions of improved quality of life for their children and increased social support for families of individuals with disabilities (Klein et al. 1993; Murphy et al. 2007).

The Paralympic Games, which has been seen as the summit of disability sport (Gold and Gold 2007), has provided a stage for organized and competitive sports among athletes with physical disabilities. Twenty sports are included in Paralympics 2012 as listed in Table 19.1. The agenda of the Paralympic Games has been described as one that has evolved from therapeutic sports to elite-level competitions that carry intrinsic prestige.

TABLE 19.1

Olympic-Type Sports That Are Included in the Most Recent Special
Olympics and Paralympics

Special Olympics 2011	Paralympics 2012
• Aquatics (swimming)	• Paralympic archery
• Athletics (marathon/ half-marathon)	• Paralympic athletics
• Badminton	• Boccia
• Basketball	• Paralympic cycling—road
• Bocce	• Paralympic cycling—track
• Bowling	• Paralympic equestrian
• Cycling	• Football 5-a-side
• Equestrian	• Football 7-a-side
• Football (5-aside, 7-aside, 11-aside)	• Goalball
• Golf	• Paralympic judo
• Gymnastics	• Powerlifting
• Handball	• Paralympic rowing
• Judo	• Paralympic sailing
• Kayaking	• Paralympic shooting
• Powerlifting	• Paralympic swimming
• Roller skating	• Paralympic table tennis
• Sailing	• Volleyball—sitting
• Softball	• Wheelchair basketball
• Table tennis	• Wheelchair fencing
• Tennis	• Wheelchair rugby
• Volleyball	• Wheelchair tennis

This growth has led to some new challenges associated with a perceived overemphasis on measuring the excellence of performance in sports on the basis of the able-bodied model (McCann 1996). Considering such model, it implies that those who are more severely impaired are more likely to be eliminated from elite-level competition. Following the mainstream sports philosophy, qualifying standards are set to determine who may be qualified to join the competition. Probably related to this elite-level model as well as to the extent of physical disabilities, adaptation of sports in the Paralympics has generated greater utilization of assistive technology. Classification systems have also been subject to ongoing research directed at setting up fair competition amidst a wide range of physical abilities and limitations.

19.3.1 Historical Perspective

Sport for individuals with disabilities has been known to have its roots in Sir Ludwig Guttman's move to incorporate sports activities as an aid in the treatment and rehabilitation of patients with spinal cord injury (Guttman 1976). Sports, in the form of archery, snooker, and table tennis, were used to enhance the physiologic and anatomical aspects of musculoskeletal healing (Richter et al. 2005). The initial efforts of Guttman led to movement that created the first international games for persons with spinal cord injury. Initially known as the Stoke Mandeville Games Federation, the movement has evolved to an international level and has been renamed as the International Stoke Mandeville Wheelchair Sports Federation (ISMWSF) (IWASF 2011). The contributions of ISMWSF in the development of sports for individuals with disabilities have been recognized by the International Olympic Committee (IOC) through the Fearnley Cup award for outstanding achievement in the service of the Olympic ideal in 1956. From these early pioneering events, sport participation for individuals with disabilities has continually evolved and developed into its current state.

Sports participation for the disabled has changed from being a clinical rehabilitation tool to an increasingly competition-oriented activity that calls for specialized coaching and training (McCann 1996). Although it was introduced by Guttman in 1944 as a component of patient rehabilitation programs, sports came to be practiced by people with disability even after rehabilitation and eventually developed into their current organized and competitive nature (Vanderstraeten and Oomen 2010) that is characteristic of both the Special Olympics and the Paralympic Games.

19.3.2 Classification Systems within Paralympic Sports

Specific biological demands are associated with particular physical disabilities (Burkett 2010) and efforts to create fair competition have led to athlete classification systems in which athletes within a common range of performance potential were grouped together (McCann 1984). By minimizing the effect of impairment severity on the outcome of competition, participation in sport is promoted among persons with disabilities (Tweedy and Vanlandewijck 2010).

The original Paralympic classification system used a medical model and defined five classes of disability (Tweedy 2003). The classifications grouped athletes as those with (1) amputation, (2) cerebral palsy, (3) spinal cord injury, (4) visual impairment, or (5) any other condition that does not fit in any of the preceding four groups. As sports for the disabled ceased from being an extension of medical rehabilitation, the classification system also shifted into a functional model. Using a functional classification system, athletes' classes are determined not by the medical diagnosis but by the extent of impact of impairments on sports performance (Tweedy and Vanlandewijck 2010). Currently, functional classification systems are being used and are sport-specific because a single impairment may have different degrees of impact on each kind of sport. Although an athlete's classification is recognized to significantly affect the degree of success that he or she is likely to achieve, Paralympic classification systems are still based on judgments of recognized experts. However, research is needed to establish valid and reliable methods to assess and classify impairments (Beckman and Tweedy 2009). As such, current research activities of the Paralympic movement are driven toward the development of evidence-based classification systems.

Initial research output concerning sport classification systems illustrates the relationship of consequences of impairment with sport-specific performance determinants (Vanlandewijck et al. 2010). In a pilot study, the impact of trunk strength impairment on wheelchair acceleration was examined. Within the research process, the main determinants of wheelchair sports were defined, and acceleration of the wheelchair from standstill was found to be crucial. The impact of trunk muscle strength on the acceleration determinant was quantified. Furthermore, a standardized, valid, and reliable measure of the determinant was established. This study has illustrated the importance of understanding the impact of impairment on specific activities in establishing guidelines for evidence-based classification systems. In another preliminary study, five tests (standing broad jump, four bounds for distance, 10-m speed skip, running in place, and split jumps) were evaluated to determine which combination explained the greatest amount of variance in running performance (Beckman and Tweedy 2009). The tests were found reliable and a substantial amount of explained variance (as much as 75%) in running performance by a sample of persons with disability was found, implying the potential utility of these tests in developing classification systems among Paralympic athletes. Although it appears that the current status of disabled sports classification systems is in the early stages of development toward an evidence-based system, this evolution stands to push sports participation among persons with disability to greater heights.

19.3.3 Sports Participation among Persons With Disabilities

Sports among persons with disabilities affect not only the participating individual, but also society. Through sports, persons with disabilities are seen to accomplish things that persons without disabilities may have previously thought impossible (Parnes and Hashemi 2007), which breaks down assumptions and stereotypes of disability (Gold and Gold 2007). Sports participation has been shown to improve health among individuals with disabilities (Taylor et al. 2004). Moreover, sports performance allows them to learn skills for social interaction, develop particular amounts of independence, and become empowered to lead (Fukuchi 2007). In particular, children with disabilities who participate in sports are exposed to opportunities to form friendships, express creativity, and develop a self-identity that leads to enhanced psychological well-being (Dykens et al. 1998).

Although sports participation among persons with disabilities is becoming more prevalent these days, it is still less pervasive than the sports involvement of the general population (Vanderstraeten and Oomen 2010). Relatively less financial support and sponsorship, media attention, and spectator attendance tend to result in limited opportunities for people with disabilities to participate in sports (Schell et al. 1999; Thomas and Smith 2003). Nevertheless, the continued growth of adapted sports at the Olympic level appears to influence the design of barrier-free physical facilities and the overall accessibility of the built environment (Gold and Gold 2007).

Participating in sports carries with it risks of injuries that are experienced by able-bodied athletes and persons with disabilities alike (Vanderstraeten and Oomen 2010). Currently, research is still inadequate to adequately characterize injury patterns and risk factors for injury among athletes with disabilities (Vanlandewijck 2006). It has yet to be confirmed whether the risks of injuries are relatively greater and more complicated among persons with disabilities. This issue is further made complex by the use of adaptive equipment and particular concerns associated with athletes' impairments such as thermoregulation, spasticity, or heterotopic ossification (Vanderstraeten and Oomen 2010). Although further research is warranted to characterize sports injuries in disability sports, preparticipation evaluation procedures have been designed to identify potential contraindications and precautions related to an athlete's sports activities (Jacob and Hutzler 1998; Klenck and Gebke 2007).

The Sports Medical Assessment Protocol (SMAP) is a widely used preparticipation evaluation and includes an interview, cardiorespiratory assessment, and physical-functional tests (Jacob and Hutzler 1998). In addition to the identification of essential precautions, SMAP also aids the design of an athlete's training program. Another basis for preparticipation considerations is the "participation possibility chart" that was developed by the American Academy of Orthopedic Surgeons (Wind et al. 2004). This guide identifies sports options for individuals with particular physical disabilities. For instance, children with Down syndrome who have atlanto-axial instability are encouraged to take part in sports that do not have contact or collision (American Academy of Pediatrics 2001). Strategies to minimize the risks of injuries during sports activities are also implemented before participation. For instance, when athletes include children with spina bifida, the environment should be latex-free because there is a 25–65% prevalence of latex allergies in this diagnostic group of participants (Patel and Greydanus 2002).

19.4 Sport and Disability Techniques and Technologies for a "Sport for All"

Ongoing developments in the revision of the classification systems within Paralympic sports may be seen as a technique, at the institutional level, to facilitate sport for all. In other cases, sports participation is also enhanced through the creation of novel games for specific disability groups. For instance, Torball was developed in the 1970s as a ballgame for individuals with visual impairments (IBSA 2011). Similar to traditional ballgames that are played in courts with goals, this game was adapted by using a bell ball, naturally using the auditory system for feedback. Another specific Paralympic sport is Boccia, which is a target ball bowling sport that was developed initially for individuals with cerebral palsy (IBC 2007). It is currently being played by individuals in wheelchairs because of physical disabilities at international levels, with over 50 countries having local and/or national competitions (CPISRA 2009).

In addition to the techniques that develop opportunities for sports, assistive technology continues to evolve in addressing the needs of individuals with disabilities in conducting their activities of daily living and in sports performance (Burkett 2010). Mobility is a basic need for individuals with disabilities to take part in society, and it sets the stage for PA participation (Authier et al. 2007) that aids the prevention of long-term health problems, especially among those who are wheelchair-dependent (van Der Woude et al. 2006).

Although wheelchairs and prostheses have been fundamental in promoting independent performance of daily tasks (Haisma et al. 2006; Pasquina et al. 2006), the role of technology in sports performance is apparent in increasing sports opportunities for individuals who rely on power wheelchairs (Barfield et al. 2005). Greater gait efficiency and ambulation speed has also been facilitated by the development of energy-storing prosthetic feet (Brodtkorb et al. 2008), pushing the performance of Paralympic athletes to extents such that it has become controversial (Burkett 2010). Technology development, in facilitating sports for all, may also be described as dynamic because it responds to the demands of elite athletes who aim to go higher, faster, and longer (Vanlandewijck et al. 2001; Burkett et al. 2003).

19.4.1 Power Wheelchair Sports

The focus on wheelchair development may have been driven by the needs of individuals with mobility limitations, who are at risk of developing a sedentary lifestyle and limited opportunities for PA participation (Barfield et al. 2005). Inevitably, the enabling effect of wheelchairs has been extended by technology development toward competitive sports. Power wheelchair athletes include individuals with physical disabilities associated with various conditions such as cerebral palsy, muscular dystrophy, and spinal cord injury. Diverse characteristics of such disabling conditions have generated much interest in examining exercise responses and energy expenditure associated with wheelchair competition, and it has been established that factors associated with the ability of wheelchair athletes include cardiorespiratory fitness, anaerobic capacity, and upper limb coordination

(Coutts et al. 1983; Goosey et al. 2000). Pelvic and trunk strength have also been identified as relevant determinants of wheelchair sports performance (Vanlandewijck et al. 2010).

Remarkable developments in wheelchair technology have been observed in recent decades, but the central concept of a hand-propelled mechanism has remained (van Der Woude et al. 2006). Modifications of the conventional wheelchair design may largely be a response to requirements of sporting use, and many innovations have been found to originate from sports practice. For instance, wheelchair basketball and wheelchair tennis require rapid acceleration and quick changes in direction, which have been addressed by a fifth wheel at the back of the wheelchair, which prevents the wheelchair from flipping backward during play (Burkett 2010). On the other hand, fitting front and side bumper guards that have hooks used to trap opponent players have addressed the high-impact nature of wheelchair rugby. Modern wheelchairs have evolved toward achieving less weight, greater stability, and longer usability. In terms of specific technical modifications, much research attention has focused on modifying the design of tires and wheels and examining its effects on biomechanical functions and kinematic output.

In particular, the wheel camber is an important parameter in seeking the optimal design of a wheelchair (Faupin et al. 2004). Defined as the angle of the main wheel to the vertical (Higgs 1983), the camber directly influences other wheelchair parameters; for example, increased camber results in a slight reduction of seat height and an increased wheel-base (Faupin et al. 2004). Increased camber results in the mechanical gain of greater lateral stability (Trudel et al. 1997) and functional benefits of improved hand protection from contact/collision injuries (Veeger et al. 1989). Although earlier studies indicate beneficial effects of increased rear wheel camber, recent studies have reported findings that demonstrated negative effects on kinetic and kinematic aspects. Increased rolling resistance has been found proportional to increased rear wheel camber, which translates to decreased velocity of wheelchair propulsion and a congruent increase in required power output by the user (Faupin et al. 2004). Consistent with these findings, prolonged hand-wheel contact and pushing time have also been observed as an effect of greater rolling resistance (Veeger et al. 1989).

Power wheelchairs continue to evolve as a consequence of changing demands of sports participation for individuals with disabilities. Although the changes have been dramatic and studies have examined effects on the wheelchair itself and the users, it appears that the design of power wheelchairs will continue to change because the optimal standard remains dynamic.

19.4.2 Prosthetic Technology

Technology as an aid for mobility has also been evident in the form of prostheses, which have facilitated independent ambulation among individuals with lower limb amputations (Camporesi 2008). The unique requirements and demands of sports events (e.g., javelin throw and discus throw) have led to the development of sport-specific prostheses. For instance, the J-leg technology was the result of the need to support lower limb rotation in the discus throw, which is distinctly different from the demands associated with the javelin throw (Burkett et al. 2003). The J-leg prosthesis has a fixed knee unit that provides stability during rotation and consists of an energy-storing foot, which provides the desired ground push-off before the discus throw release.

The use of prosthetic technology is equally relevant and perhaps highly controversial among runners. Energy-storing prosthetic feet have been shown to result in significant increases in running speed among sprinters (Brown et al. 2009). The controversy surrounding its use in running revolves around the issue of performance enhancement afforded by prosthetic technology and the associated unfair advantage gained by users. Debates emerged before the 2008 Beijing Olympic and Paralympic Games, addressing the question of whether Oscar Pistorius, who was using an energy-storing prosthesis, should be allowed to compete in the Olympic Games along with able-bodied athletes (Edwards 2008; Lippi and Mattiuzzi 2008; Jones and Wilson 2009). Although Pistorius was subsequently allowed to compete in the Olympic Games, eventually, his performance did not meet the qualifying time.

Benefits of prosthetic technology in sports are also apparent in jumping events (e.g., long jump). In this field, athletes have utilized the developments in technology by adopting changes in jumping techniques, wherein the touch-down foot has shifted from the anatomic to the prosthetic limb (Nolan and Lees 2007). Prosthetic limbs have been found to be more effective than anatomical limbs in terms of absorption and release of ground reaction force. Consequently, a mechanical advantage is achieved by generating higher take-off velocities.

It appears that prosthetic technology and sport-specific techniques continue to advance toward greater sports performance. However, associated research gaps are still apparent in terms of the human-technology interface. In the case of wheelchairs, physiologic and biomechanical responses among users have been quantified. In contrast, prosthesis users' responses to the technology have yet to be adequately measured. In particular, the interface between the prosthesis and the individual is found at the stump-socket relationship. The stump-socket connection transmits the ground reaction forces to the amputee and produces the energy required to move the prosthetic limb (Burkett 2010). The environmental factors of air pressure, temperature, and humidity clearly may elicit changes in the volume of the stump, consequently affecting the biomechanical interface. Furthermore, although proprioceptive feedback appears to be fundamental in determining an athlete's performance, sensorimotor aspects of the stump-socket interface have yet to be quantified. It appears that further studies in these areas of concern are needed to determine the impact of prosthetic technology in facilitating sports participation for everyone and threshing out the issue of any unfair advantage that might be afforded by technology.

19.4.3 Technology for Developing Countries

Mobility devices, such as wheelchairs, are generally accessible and affordable in developed countries, but they are difficult to obtain in low-income developing countries because of economic constraints (Kelly and Lindley 1994; Authier et al. 2007). A substantial number of individuals with disabilities who are in need of wheelchairs are from these developing countries (Kim and Mulholland 1999; Wheelchair Foundation 2011), where users are often dependent on government or nongovernment organizations to purchase the equipment (Krizack 2007). Consequently, individuals with disabilities are prevented by immobility from taking part in education, employment, and recreation opportunities. This problem has been well recognized and various organizations have implemented programs to provide basic mobility solutions for developing countries (Authier et al. 2007). The largest-scale projects have been advocated by the International Paralympic Committee (IPC), highlighting the role of sports participation among individuals with disabilities in driving technology development for these low-income countries.

One such project aimed to design a sports wheelchair for use of individuals with disabilities in low-income countries (Authier et al. 2007). Based in India, the design used materials that were typically available in the country. This approach has been suggested as an essential strategy in wheelchair design in developing countries because it not only keeps the costs low, but it also ensures that the chair will be locally maintained (Pfaelzer and Krizack 2000). The corresponding local labor cost was also much lower relative to developed countries, and the combination with local materials resulted in a wheelchair design that cost less than 20% of similar equipment in the United States. It has been advocated that the cost of technology should not be a hindrance for individuals with disability to take part in sports and physical activity (Sport and Development 2011). Essentially, projects such as this one need to be pursued to enhance the participation of individuals with disabilities from less developed nations, leading toward the ideal of "sport for all."

19.5 Conclusions

Sport represents one form of physical activity, and among individuals with disabilities, this has been facilitated by adaptation strategies. Disability sport continues to grow in terms of both participation and competition. Such positive change appears to be dynamic, as methods, strategies, and technologies continue to evolve from research findings.

Summary of the Chapter

This chapter initiated the discussion on methods and technologies that facilitate accessible sport through self-efficacy theories that provide the motivation for enabling sports participation for all. The proposition that adapted physical activity (APA) programs sets up the stage for making PA participation possible for everyone was developed. Diverse forms of APA have been documented to have beneficial effects among individuals with disabilities, and sports activities appear to be an important form of PA. The wide extent of sports participation among individuals with disabilities is evident in the Special Olympics and Paralympics.

Such prestigious status of sports for individuals with disabilities has generated a corresponding body of research that has started to move towards evidence-based practice. The inherent competitive nature of sports has also been evident, consequently resulting in the use of technology to address evolving demands of athletes with disabilities. While it appears that PA is indeed for everyone, and is achieved through sports as supported by technology, further research is desired to enhance different parameters of the current status.

References

American Academy of Pediatrics. (2001). Health supervision for children with down syndrome. *Pediatrics, 107*(2), 442–449.

Authier, E. L., Pearlman, J., Allegretti, A. L., Rice, I., and Cooper, R. A. (2007). A sports wheelchair for low-income countries. *Disability Rehabilitation, 29*(11–12), 963–967.

Balzini, L., Vannucchi, L., Benvenuti, F., Benucci, M., Monni, M., Cappozzo, A., et al. (2003). Clinical characteristics of flexed posture in elderly women. *Journal of the American Geriatrics Society, 51*(10), 1419–1426.

Bandini, L. G., Curtin, C., Hamad, C., Tybor, D. J., and Must, A. (2005). Prevalence of overweight in children with developmental disorders in the continuous national health and nutrition examination survey (NHANES) 1999–2002. *Journal of Pediatrics, 146*(6), 738–743.

Bandura, A. (1997). *Self-Efficacy: The Exercise of Control.* New York: W.H. Freeman.

Barfield, J. P., Malone, L. A., Collins, J. M., and Ruble, S. B. (2005). Disability type influences heart rate response during power wheelchair sport. *Medicine and Science in Sports and Exercise, 37*(5), 718–723.

Beckman, E. M., and Tweedy, S. M. (2009). Towards evidence-based classification in Paralympic athletics: Evaluating the validity of activity limitation tests for use in classification of Paralympic running events. *British Journal of Sports Medicine, 43*(13), 1067–1072.

Benedetti, M. G., Berti, L., Presti, C., Frizziero, A., and Giannini, S. (2008). Effects of an adapted physical activity program in a group of elderly subjects with flexed posture: Clinical and instrumental assessment. *Journal of Neuroengineering and Rehabilitation, 5*, 32.

Bjornson, K. F., Belza, B., Kartin, D., Logsdon, R., McLaughlin, J., and Thompson, E. A. (2008). The relationship of physical activity to health status and quality of life in cerebral palsy. *Pediatric Physical Therapy, 20*(3), 247–253.

Bouchard, C., and Shephard, R. (1994). Physical activity, fitness and health: The model and key concepts. In C. Bouchard, R. Shephard and T. Stephens (Eds.), *Physical Activity, Fitness and Health. International Proceedings and Consensus Statement* (pp. 77–88). Champaigne, IL: Human Kinetics.

Brodtkorb, T. H., Henriksson, M., Johannesen-Munk, K., and Thidell, F. (2008). Cost-effectiveness of C-leg compared with non-microprocessor-controlled knees: A modeling approach. *Archives of Physical Medicine and Rehabilitation, 89*(1), 24–30.

Brown, M. B., Millard-Stafford, M. L., and Allison, A. R. (2009). Running-specific prostheses permit energy cost similar to nonamputees. *Medicine and Science in Sports and Exercise, 41*(5), 1080–1087.

Bull, F. C., Armstrong, T., Dixon, T., Ham, S., Neiman, A., and Pratt, M. (2004). Physical inactivity. In M. Ezzati, A. Lopez, A. Rodgers and C. J. L. Murray (Eds.), *Comparative Quantification of Health Risks: Global and Regional Burden of Disease Attributable to Selected Major Risk Factors* (Vol. 1, pp. 729–882). Geneva, Switzerland: WHO.

Burkett, B. (2010). Technology in Paralympic sport: Performance enhancement or essential for performance? *British Journal of Sports Medicine, 44*(3), 215–220.

Burkett, B., Smeathers, J., and Barker, T. (2003). Walking and running inter-limb asymmetry for Paralympic trans-femoral amputees, a biomechanical analysis. *Prosthetics and Orthotics International, 27*(1), 36–47.

Camporesi, S. (2008). Oscar Pistorius, enhancement and post-humans. *Journal of Medical Ethics, 34*(9), 639.

Capio, C. M., Sit, C. H., and Abernethy, B. (2010). Physical activity measurement using MTI (actigraph) among children with cerebral palsy. *Archives of Physical Medicine and Rehabilitation, 91*(8), 1283–1290.

Carless, D., and Sparkes, A. C. (2008). The physical activity experiences of men with serious mental illness: Three short stories. *Psychology of Sport and Exercise, 9*(2), 191–210.

Cavill, N., Kahlmeier, S., and Racioppi, F. (2006). Physical activity and health in Europe: Evidence for action. Geneva, Switzerland: WHO.

Coutts, K. D., Rhodes, E. C., and McKenzie, D. C. (1983). Maximal exercise responses of tetraplegics and paraplegics. *Journal of Applied Physiology, 55*(2), 479–482.

CPISRA. (2009). *About Boccia.* Retrieved from http://www.cpisra.org/index.php?id = 80

Daniel, F., Vale, R., Giani, T., Bacellar, S., and Dantas, E. (2010). Effects of a physical activity program on static balance and functional autonomy in elderly women. *Macedonian Journal of Medical Science, 3*(1), 21–26.

Driver, S., and Ede, A. (2009). Impact of physical activity on mood after TBI. *Brain Injury, 23*(3), 203–212.

Dunn, A., and Blair, S. (2002). Translating evidenced-based physical activity interventions into practice: The 2010 challenge. *American Journal of Preventive Medicine, 22*(4S), 8–9.

Dykens, E. M., and Cohen, D. J. (1996). Effects of Special Olympics International on social competence in persons with mental retardation. *Journal of the American Academy of Child and Adolescent Psychiatry, 35*(2), 223–229.

Dykens, E. M., Rosner, B. A., and Butterbaugh, G. (1998). Exercise and sports in children and adolescents with developmental disabilities—Positive physical and psychosocial effects. *Child and Adolescent Psychiatric Clinics of North America, 7*(4), 757–771, viii.

Edwards, S. D. (2008). Should Oscar Pistorius be excluded from the 2008 Olympic games? *Sport Ethics and Philosophy, 2*(2), 112–125.

Ekelund, U., Brage, S., and Wareham, N. J. (2004). Physical activity in young children. *Lancet, 363*(9415), 1163; author reply 1163–1164.

Farrell, R. J., Crocker, P. R. E., McDonough, M. H., and Sedgwick, W. A. (2004). The driving force: Motivation in special Olympians. *Adapted Physical Activity Quarterly, 21*(2), 153–166.

Faupin, A., Campillo, P., Weissland, T., Gorce, P., and Thevenon, A. (2004). The effects of rear-wheel camber on the mechanical parameters produced during the wheelchair sprinting of handibasketball athletes. *Journal of Rehabilitation Research and Development, 41*(3B), 421–428.

Feltz, D. L., Short, S., and Sullivan, P. J. (2008). *Self-Efficacy in Sport.* Champaign, IL: Human Kinetics.

Fernhall, B., and Unnithan, V. B. (2002). Physical activity, metabolic issues, and assessment. *Physical Medicine and Rehabilitation Clinics of North America, 13*(4), 925–947.

Foley, J. T., Bryan, R. R., and McCubbin, J. A. (2008). Daily physical activity levels of elementary school-aged children with and without mental retardation. *Journal of Developmental and Physical Disabilities, 20*(4), 365–378.

Fox, K. R. (2000). Self-esteem, self-perceptions and exercise. *International Journal of Sport Psychology, 31*(2), 228–240.

Freudenberg, P., and Arlinghaus, R. (2010). Benefits and constraints of outdoor recreation for people with physical disabilities: Inferences from recreational fishing. *Leisure Science, 32*(1), 55–71.

Fukuchi, K. (2007). *My Hope for an Inclusive Society.* Paper presented at the Sport in the United Nations Convention on the Rights of Persons with Disabilities.

Giacobbi, P. R., Stancil, M., Hardin, B., and Bryant, L. (2008). Physical activity and quality of life experienced by highly active individuals with physical disabilities. *Adapted Physical Activity Quarterly, 25*(3), 189–207.

Gold, J. R., and Gold, M. M. (2007). Access for all: The rise of the Paralympic Games. *Perspectives in Public Health, 127*(3), 133–141.

Goosey, V. L., Campbell, I. G., and Fowler, N. E. (2000). Effect of push frequency on the economy of wheelchair racers. *Medicine and Science in Sports and Exercise, 32*(1), 174–181.

Groff, D. G., Lundberg, N. R., and Zabriskie, R. B. (2009). Influence of adapted sport on quality of life: Perceptions of athletes with cerebral palsy. *Disability and Rehabilitation, 31*(4), 318–326.

Guttman, L. (1976). *Textbook of Sport for the Disabled.* Aylesbury, UK: HM & M Publishers Ltd.

Haisma, J. A., van der Woude, L. H., Stam, H. J., Bergen, M. P., Sluis, T. A., & Bussmann, J. B. (2006). Physical capacity in wheelchair-dependent persons with a spinal cord injury: A critical review of the literature. *Spinal Cord, 44*(11), 642–652.

Higgs, C. (1983). An analysis of racing wheelchairs used at the 1980 Olympic games for the disabled. *Research Quarterly for Exercise and Sport, 54*(3), 229–233.

Horvat, M., Croce, R., and Roswal, G. (1993). Magnitude and reliability of measurements of muscle strength across trials for individuals with mental retardation. *Perceptual and Motor Skills, 77*(2), 643–649.

Huang, J. S., Sallis, J., and Patrick, K. (2009). The role of primary care in promoting children's physical activity. *British Journal of Sports Medicine, 43*(1), 19–21.

Hutzler, Y., and Sherrill, C. (2007). Defining adapted physical activity: International perspectives. *Adaptive Physical Activity Quarterly, 24*(1), 1–20.

IBC. (2007). Boccia. Retrieved from http://www.bocciainternational.com/boccia.html

IBSA. (2011). Torball. Retrieved from http://www.ibsa.es/eng/deportes/torball/presentacion.htm

IWASF. (2011). International Stoke Mandeville Wheelchair Sports Federation (ISMWSF) History. Retrieved from http://www.iwasf.com/iwasf/index.cfm/about-iwas/history/ismwsf-history/

Jacob, T., and Hutzler, Y. (1998). Sports-medical assessment for athletes with a disability. *Disability and Rehabilitation, 20*(3), 116–119.

Jones, C., and Wilson, C. (2009). Defining advantage and athletic performance: The case of Oscar Pistorius. *European Journal of Sport Science, 9*(2), 125–131.

Kelly, N., and Lindley, B. (1994). Health volunteers overseas: Bringing rehabilitation to the world. *ARN News* 6–7.

Kim, J., and Mulholland, S. J. (1999). Seating/wheelchair technology in the developing world: Need for a closer look. *Technology & Disability, 11*, 21–27.

Klein, T., Gilman, E., and Zigler, E. (1993). Special Olympics—An evaluation by professionals and parents. *Mental Retardation, 31*(1), 15–23.

Klenck, C., and Gebke, K. (2007). Practical management: Common medical problems in disabled athletes. *Clinical Journal of Sports Medicine, 17*(1), 55–60.

Krizack, M. (2007, August 10). The importance of user choice for cost-effective wheelchair provision in low income countries. *Whirlwind Wheelchair International Newsletter.*

Kudlacek, M., Jesina, O., and Flannagan, P. (2010). European inclusive physical education training. *Advanced Rehabilitation, 3*, 14–17.

Kudlacek, M., Valkova, H., Sherrill, C., Myers, B., and French, R. (2002). An inclusion instrument based on planned behaviour: Theory for prospective Czech physical educators. *Adaptive Physical Activity Quarterly 19*, 280–299.

Law, M., King, G., King, S., Kertoy, M., Hurley, P., Rosenbaum, P., et al. (2006). Patterns of participation in recreational and leisure activities among children with complex physical disabilities. *Developmental Medicine and Child Neurology, 48*(5), 337–342.

Lippi, G., and Mattiuzzi, C. (2008). Pistorius ineligible for the Olympic Games: The right decision. *British Journal of Sports Medicine, 42*(3), 160–161.

Loy, D. P., Dattilo, J., and Kleiber, D. A. (2003). Exploring the influence of leisure on adjustment: Development of the leisure and spinal cord injury adjustment model. *Leisure Science, 25*(2–3), 231–255.

Mackey, A. H., Hewart, P., Walt, S. E., and Stott, N. S. (2009). The sensitivity and specificity of an activity monitor in detecting functional activities in young people with cerebral palsy. *Archives of Physical Medicine and Rehabilitation, 90*(8), 1396–1401.

Manfredo, M. J., and Driver, B. L. (1996). Measuring leisure motivation: A meta-analysis of the Recreation Experience Preference Scales. *Journal Leisure Research, 28*(3), 188.

Martens, R. (1996). Turning kids on to physical activity for a lifetime. *Quest, 48*, 303–310.

McAvoy, L., Holman, T., Goldenberg, M., and Klenosky, D. (2006). Wilderness and persons with disabilities. *International Journal of Wilderness, 12*, 23–31, 35.

McCann, C. (1984). Classification of the locomotor disabled for competitive sports: Theory and practice. *International Journal of Sports Medicine, 5*(Suppl), 167–170.

McCann, C. (1996). Sports for the disabled: The evolution from rehabilitation to competitive sport. *British Journal of Sports Medicine, 30*(4), 279–280.

Meegan, S., and MacPhail, A. (2006). Irish physical educators' attitude toward teaching students with special educational needs. *European Physical Education Review, 12*(1), 75–97.

Metcalf, B., Voss, L., Jeffery, A., Perkins, J., and Wilkin, T. (2004). Physical activity cost of the school run: Impact on schoolchildren of being driven to school (EarlyBird 22). *British Medical Journal, 329*(7470), 832–833.

Moritz, S. E., Feltz, D. L., Fahrbach, K. R., and Mack, D. E. (2000). The relation of self-efficacy measures to sport performance: A meta-analytic review. *Research Quarterly for Exercise and Sport, 71*(3), 280–294.

Murphy, N. A., and Carbone, P. S. (2008). Promoting the participation of children with disabilities in sports, recreation, and physical activities. *Pediatrics, 121*(5), 1057–1061.

Murphy, N. A., Christian, B., Caplin, D. A., and Young, P. C. (2007). The health of caregivers for children with disabilities: Caregiver perspectives. *Child Care Health Development, 33*(2), 180–187.

Nasuti, G., and Temple, V. A. (2010). The risks and benefits of snow sports for people with disabilities: A review of the literature. *International Journal of Rehabilitation Research, 33*(3), 193–198.

Nolan, L., and Lees, A. (2007). The influence of lower limb amputation level on the approach in the amputee long jump. *Journal of Sports Science, 25*(4), 393–401.

Parnes, P., and Hashemi, G. (2007). Sport as a means to foster inclusion, health and well-being of people with disabilities Report for the Sport for Development and Peace International Working Group (SDP IWG) Secretariat (pp. 124–157).

Pasquina, P. F., Bryant, P. R., Huang, M. E., Roberts, T. L., Nelson, V. S., and Flood, K. M. (2006). Advances in amputee care. *Archives of Physical Medicine and Rehabilitation, 87*(3 Suppl 1), S34–S43; quiz S44-S35

Patel, D. R., and Greydanus, D. E. (2002). The pediatric athlete with disabilities. *Pediatric Clinics of North America, 49*(4), 803–827.

Pedersen, B. K., and Saltin, B. (2006). Evidence for prescribing exercise as therapy in chronic disease. *Scandinavian Journal of Medicine and Science of Sports, 16*, 3–63.

Pensgaard, A. M., and Sorensen, M. (2002). Empowerment through the sport context: A model to guide research for individuals with disability. *Adaptive Physical Activity Quarterly, 19*(1), 48–67.

Pfaelzer, P., and Krizack, M. (2000, June 1). Wheelchair riders in control: WWI's model of technology transfer. *Whirlwind Wheelchair International Newsletter*.

Rabin, B. A., Brownson, R. C., Kerner, J. F., and Glasgow, R. E. (2006). Methodologic challenges in disseminating evidence-based interventions to promote physical activity. *American Journal of Preventive Medicine, 31*(4 Suppl), S24–S34.

Richardson, C. R., Faulkner, G., McDevitt, J., Skrinar, G. S., Hutchinson, D. S., and Piette, J. D. (2005). Integrating physical activity into mental health services for persons with serious mental illness. *Psychiatric Services, 56*(3), 324–331.

Richter, K. J., Sherrill, C., McCann, C., Mushett, C. A., and Kaschalk, S. M. (2005). Recreation and sport for people with disabilities. In J. A. DeLisa, B. M. Gans and N. E. Walsh (Eds.), *Physical Medicine and Rehabilitation: Principles and Practice*. Philadelphia: Lippincott Williams & Wilkins.

Sallis, J. F., and Patrick, K. (1994). Physical activity guidelines for adolescents: Consensus statement. *Pediatric Exercise Science, 60*, 302–314.

Schell, L. A., Schell, L. A. B., and Duncan, M. C. (1999). A content analysis of CBS's coverage of the 1996 Paralympic games. *Adaptive Physical Activity Quarterly, 16*(1), 27–47.

Sharav, T., and Bowman, T. (1992). Dietary practices, physical-activity, and body-mass index in a selected population of Down-syndrome children and their siblings. *Clinical Pediatrics, 31*(6), 341–344.

Sherrill, C. (2004). *Adapted Physical Activity, Recreation, and Sport: Cross-Disciplinary and Lifespan* (6th ed.). New York: McGraw-Hill.

Short, S., and Ross-Stewart, L. (2009). A review of self-efficacy based interventions. In S. D. Mellalieu and S. Hanton (Eds.), *Advances in Applied Sport Psychology: A Review*. London: Routledge.

Sinaki, M., Brey, R. H., Hughes, C. A., Larson, D. R., and Kaufman, K. R. (2005). Significant reduction in risk of falls and back pain in osteoporotic-kyphotic women through a Spinal Proprioceptive Extension Exercise Dynamic (SPEED) program. *Mayo Clinic Proceedings, 80*(7), 849–855.

Sit, C. H. P., Lau, C. H. L., and Vertinsky, P. (2009). Physical activity and self-perceptions among Hong Kong Chinese with an acquired physical disability. *Adaptive Physical Activity Quarterly, 26*(4), 321–335.

Special Olympics. (2010). Healthy Athletes. Retrieved from http://www.specialolympics.org/healthy_athletes.aspx

Special Olympics. (2011a). General Rules. Retrieved from http://www.specialolympics.org/general_rules.aspx

Special Olympics. (2011b). Sports Offered. Retrieved from http://www.athens2011.org/en/sports.asp

Speyer, E., Herbinet, A., Vuillemin, A., Briancon, S., and Chastagner, P. (2010). Effect of adapted physical activity sessions in the hospital on health-related quality of life for children with cancer: A cross-over randomized trial. *Pediatric Blood Cancer, 55*(6), 1160–1166.

Sport and Development. (2011). Sport and disability technical considerations: Equipment and technology Retrieved from http://www.sportanddev.org/en/learnmore/sport_and_disability2/technical_considerations___sport___disability/equipment_and_technology/

Strong, W. B., Malina, R. M., Blimkie, C. J., Daniels, S. R., Dishman, R. K., Gutin, B., et al. (2005). Evidence based physical activity for school-age youth. *Journal of Pediatrics, 146*(6), 732–737.

Taylor, N. F., Dodd, K. J., and Larkin, H. (2004). Adults with cerebral palsy benefit from participating in a strength training programme at a community gymnasium. *Disability & Rehabilitation, 26*(19), 1128–1134.

Thomas, N., and Smith, A. (2003). Preoccupied with able-bodiedness? An analysis of the British media coverage of the 2000 Paralympic Games. *Adaptive Physical Activity Quarterly, 20*(2), 166–181.

Trudel, G., Kirby, R. L., Ackroyd-Stolarz, S. A., and Kirkland, S. (1997). Effects of rear-wheel camber on wheelchair stability. *Archives of Physical Medicine and Rehabilitation, 78*(1), 78–81.

Tweedy, S. M. (2003). Biomechanical consequences of impairment: A taxonomically valid basis for classification in a unified disability athletics system. *Research Quarterly for Exercise and Sport, 74*(1), 9–16.

Tweedy, S. M., and Vanlandewijck, Y. C. (2010). International Paralympic Committee position stand—Background and scientific principles of classification in Paralympic sport. *British Journal of Sports Medicine, 45*(4), 259–269.

Vanderstraeten, G. G., and Oomen, A. G. M. (2010). Sports for disabled people: A general outlook. *International Journal of Rehabilitation Research, 33*(4), 283–284.

van der Woude, L. H. V., de Groot, S., and Janssen, T. W. (2006). Manual wheelchairs: Research and innovation in rehabilitation, sports, daily life and health. *Medical Engineering and Physics, 28*(9), 905–915.

Vanlandewijck, Y. (2006). Sport science in the Paralympic movement. *Journal of Rehabilitation Research and Development, 43*(7), xvii–xxiv.

Vanlandewijck, Y., Theisen, D., and Daly, D. (2001). Wheelchair propulsion biomechanics—Implications for wheelchair sports. *Sports Medicine, 31*(5), 339–367.

Vanlandewijck, Y., Verellen, J., and Tweedy, S. (2010). Towards evidence-based classification – the impact of impaired trunk strength on wheelchair propulsion. *Advances in Rehabilitation, 3*(1), 1–5.

Veeger, H. E. J., van der Woude, L. H. V., and Rozendal, R. H. (1989). Wheelchair propulsion technique at different speeds. *Scandinavian Journal of Rehabilitative Medicine, 21*(4), 197–203.

Wang, Y., and Lobstein, T. (2006). Worldwide trends in childhood overweight and obesity. *International Journal of Pediatric Obesity, 1*(1), 11–25.

Warms, C. A., Belza, B. L., and Whitney, J. D. (2007). Correlates of physical activity in adults with mobility limitations. *Family and Community Health, 30*(2 Suppl), S5–16.

Wheelchair Foundation. (2011). Retrieved from http://www.wheelchairfoundation.org/about/faq

Wind, W. M., Schwend, R. M., and Larson, J. (2004). Sports for the physically challenged child. *Journal of the American Academy of Orthopedic Surgeons, 12*(2), 126–137.

Winnick, J. P. (2005). An introduction to adapted physical education and sport. In J. P. Winnick (Ed.), *Adapted Physical Education and Sport* (4th ed., pp. 3–20). Champaigne, IL: Human Kinetics.

World Health Organization (WHO). (2010). *Global Recommendations on Physical Activity for Health.* Geneva, Switzerland: World Health Organization.

Wrotniak, B. H., Epstein, L. H., Dorn, J. M., Jones, K. E., and Kondilis, V. A. (2006). The relationship between motor proficiency and physical activity in children. *Pediatrics, 118*(6), e1758–1765.

Index